CARDIOLOGY
for the primary care
PHYSICIAN
Fourth edition

Editor

Joseph S. Alpert, MD
Professor and Chairman
Department of Medicine
University of Arizona
Health Sciences Center
Tucson, Arizona

with 77 contributors

Developed by Current Medicine LLC, Philadelphia

Current Medicine LLC
400 Market Street, Suite 700
Philadelphia, PA 19106

CURRENT MEDICINE LLC

400 Market Street, Suite 700 • Philadelphia, PA 19106

Director of Editorial, Design, Production . . . .*Wendy Vetter*

Senior Developmental Editor . . . .*Elizabeth Rexon*

Commissioning Supervisor Books . . . .*Annmarie D'Ortona*

Cover Design . . . .*Christine Keller-Quirk*

Design and Layout . . . .*Christine Keller-Quirk*

Illustrators . . . .*Wiesia Langenfeld and Maureen Looney*

Production Manager . . . .*Lori Holland*

Assistant Production Manager . . . .*Margaret La Mare*

Indexer . . . .*Holly Lukens*

Library of Congress Cataloging-in-Publication Data

Cardiology for the primary care physician / editor, Joseph S. Alpert, with 77
  contributors.--4th ed.
      p. ; cm.
  Includes bibliographical references and index.
  ISBN 1-57340-212-5
    1. Cardiology. 2. Primary care (Medicine) 3. Heart--Diseases. I. Alpert, Joseph S.
    [DNLM: 1. Heart Diseases--diagnosis. 2. Cardiology--methods. 3. Diagnosis,
  Differential. 4. Heart Diseases--therapy. 5. Primary Health Care. WG 210 C2677 2005]
  RC667.C3834 2005
  616.1'2--dc22

                                                                                    2004057127

ISBN 1-57340-212-5

Printed in Hong Kong by Paramount.

10 9 8 7 6 5 4 3 2 1

For more information please call 1 (800) 427-1796 or (215) 574-2266
www.current-science-group.com

PREFACE

With the aging of populations throughout the world, cardiovascular disease is becoming even more common than it was in the past. In primary care practices with many older patients, cardiovascular disease will be present in the majority of patients. *Cardiology for the Primary Care Physician* was designed and first published in 1996 specifically for the primary care practitioner who cares for this population of patients. The text has been revised and renewed three times since its initial publication.

This fourth edition of *Cardiology for the Primary Care Physician* has been extensively reworked and formatted from the third edition. Each of the chapter authors has revisited his or her chapter, adding up-to-date material and references and

deleting obsolete information. The text is full of the latest diagnostic and therapeutic concepts that should be useful to the clinically active primary care physician. *Cardiology for the Primary Care Physician* can be read cover-to-cover, or it can be employed as a reference aid when a particular problem is encountered. The numerous tables and figures should assist the busy practitioner in getting the needed information quickly and efficiently.

As with all scholarly activities, this text is the result of close collaboration between the authors, the editor, and the publisher. Many individuals have contributed to its creation. I would like to acknowledge in particular the outstanding efforts of Jane Barth, Barbara Raney, and Annmarie D'Ortona.

Joseph S. Alpert, MD

Tucson, Arizona

CONTRIBUTORS

Joseph S. Alpert, MD
Robert S. and Irene P. Flinn Professor
   of Medicine
Head, Department of Medicine
University of Arizona Health Sciences Center
Tucson, Arizona

Jack E. Ansell, MD
Professor and Vice Chair
Department of Medicine
Boston University Medical Center
Boston, Massachusetts

Mohammad Asif, MD, FACC
Clinical Assistant Professor
Department of Medicine
University of Medicine and Dentistry of
   New Jersey;
Attending Cardiologist
Newark Beth Israel Medical Center
Newark, New Jersey

Kathryn L. Bates, DO
Assistant Professor of Clinical Medicine
Department of Medicine
University of Arizona Health Sciences Center
Tucson, Arizona

Richard C. Becker, MD
Professor
Department of Medicine
Duke University Medical School;
Director, Duke Cardiovascular
   Thrombosis Center
Duke Clinical Research Institute
Durham, North Carolina

Bonnie J. Bidinger, MD
Assistant Professor of Medicine
Division of Rheumatology
Department of Internal Medicine
University of Massachusetts Medical School
University of Massachusetts Medical Center
Worcester, Massachusetts

Charles M. Blatt, MD
Assistant Clinical Professor of Medicine
Department of Medicine
Harvard Medical School
Associate Physician
Brigham & Women's Hospital
Boston, Massachusetts

Adam M. Brodsky, MD
Fellow in Cardiovascular Medicine
Department of Medicine
Division of Cardiology
Northwestern University Feinberg School
   of Medicine
Chicago, Illinois

Brad S. Burlew, MD
Professor of Medicine
University of Tennessee College of
   Medicine;
Chief, Department of Cardiology
Regional Medical Center
Memphis, Tennessee

Nagib T. Chalfoun, MD
Fellow
Department of Cardiology
Mount Sinai School of Medicine
New York, New York

Melvin D. Cheitlin, MD, MACC
Emeritus Professor of Medicine
Department of Medicine
University of California at San Francisco;
Former Chief of Cardiology
San Francisco General Hospital
San Francisco, California

John S. Child, MD
Professor
Department of Medicine
UCLA School of Medicine;
Streisand/AHA Chair in Cardiology
Ahmanson-UCLA Adult Congenital Heart
   Disease Center
Los Angeles, California

Julius J. Chosy, MD
Professor Emeritus
Department of Medicine
University of Wisconsin
Madison, Wisconsin

Peter F. Cohn, MD
Professor
Department of Medicine
State University Hospital at Stonybrook
Stonybrook, New York

Ranjan Dahiya, MD
Fellow
Department of Cardiology
University of Arizona Health Sciences Center
Tucson, Arizona

Deborah M. DeMarco, MD
Associate Professor
Department of Medicine/Rheumatology;
Associate Dean, GME
University of Massachusetts Medical School
Worcester, Massachusetts

Richard B. Devereux, MD
Professor
Department of Medicine
Director, Echocardiography Laboratory
The New York Hospital/Cornell
   Medical Center
New York, New York

Gordon A. Ewy, MD
Professor
Department of Medicine
University of Arizona School of Medicine;
Director, Sarver Heart Center
University of Arizona Health Sciences Center
Tucson, Arizona

Michael A. Fifer, MD
Associate Professor
Department of Medicine
Harvard Medical School;
Director, Coronary Care Unit
Massachusetts General Hospital
Boston, Massachusetts

Edward A. Fisher, MD
Associate Clinical Professor
Department of Medicine
Mount Sinai School of Medicine;
Associate Attending Physician
Mount Sinai Medical Center
New York, New York

Jonathan E. E. Fisher, MD
Clinical Instructor
Department of Cardiology
Mount Sinai School of Medicine
Staff Physician
Fisher Cardiology
New York, New York

Marc Fisher, MD
Professor
Department of Neurology
University of Massachusetts Memorial
   Healthcare
Worcester, Massachusetts

Gerald F. Fletcher, MD
Professor of Medicine
Department of Cardiovascular Medicine
Mayo Clinic College of Medicine;
Director, Preventive Cardiology
Mayo Clinic
Jacksonville, Florida

Barry A. Franklin, MD
Professor
Department of Physiology
Wayne State University
Detroit, Michigan;
Director, Cardiac Rehabilitation and
   Exercise Laboratories
William Beaumont Hospital
Royal Oak, Michigan

Martin E. Goldman, MD
Dr. Arthur and Hilda Master Professor
   of Medicine
Department of Cardiology
Mt. Sinai School of Medicine;
Director, Echocardiography Laboratory
Mt. Sinai Medical Center
New York, New York

Thomas B. Graboys, MD
Associate Clinical Professor of Medicine
Department of Medicine
Harvard Medical School;
Associate Physician
Brigham and Women's Hospital
Boston, Massachusetts

Hongsheng M. Guo, MD
Fellow in Cardiology
Department of Medicine
University of Iowa
Iowa City, Iowa

Rajiv Gupta, MD
Cardiology Fellow
Division of Cardiology
The University of Texas Medical Branch
   School of Medicine
Galveston, Texas

Robert C. Hendel, MD
Professor of Medicine
Department of Medicine;
Director, Coronary Care Unit
Rush University Medical Center
Chicago, Illinois

L. David Hillis, MD
Professor and Vice Chair
Department of Internal Medicine
University of Texas Southwestern
  Medical Center
Dallas, Texas

Norman K. Hollenberg, MD, PhD
Professor
Department of Medicine
Harvard Medical School;
Director of Physiologic Research
Brigham & Women's Hospital
Boston, Massachusetts

Thomas A. Holly, MD
Assistant Professor of Medicine
Division of Cardiology
Department of Medicine
Northwestern University Feinberg School
  of Medicine
Chicago, Illinois

Howard R. Horn, MD
The L.W. Diggs Alumni Professor of
  Medicine and Chair of Excellence in
  Medical Education
Associate Vice Chancellor for Health Affairs
University of Tennessee Health
  Sciences Center
Memphis, Tennessee

Russell D. Hull, MD, MBBS, MSc
Professor of Medicine
Department of Internal Medicine
University of Calgary School of Medicine;
Director, Thrombosis Research Unit
Foothills Medical Centre
Calgary, Alberta
Canada

Michael H. Humphreys, MD
Professor of Medicine
University of California San Francisco
Chief, Division of Nephrology
San Francisco General Hospital
San Francisco, California

Steven B. Johnson, MD
Professor of Surgery
Chief, Division of Surgical Critical Care
Department of Surgery
University of Maryland School of Medicine
Baltimore, Maryland

William B. Kannel, MD
Professor of Medicine and Public Health
Boston University School of Medicine
Medical Director, Emeritus
Framingham Heart Study
Boston, Massachusetts

Harry R. Kimball, MD, MACP
Adjunct Professor of Medicine
Department of Internal Medicine
University of Pennsylvania;
President Emeritus
American Board of Internal Medicine
Philadelphia, Pennsylvania

Deping Lee, MD
Assistant Professor
Department of Medicine/Research Medicine
University of Southern California
Los Angeles, California

Carl V. Leier, MD
Overstreet Professor of Medicine and
  Pharmacology
Departments of Cardiology and Internal
  Medicine
The Ohio State University College of
  Medicine
The Ohio State University Hospitals
Columbus, Ohio

A. James Liedtke, MD
Professor of Medicine
Department of Medicine
University of Wisconsin Medical School
Madison, Wisconsin

Joy L. Logan, MD
Associate Professor
Department of Medicine
University of Arizona Health Sciences Center
Tucson, Arizona

Robert G. Luke, MD, MACP, FRCP
Professor and Chairman
Department of Internal Medicine
University of Cincinnati Medical Center
Cincinnati, Ohio

Jorge E. Massare, MD
Senior Resident
Department of Internal Medicine
Wayne State University
Detroit Medical Center
Detroit, Michigan

Eric L. Michelson, MD
Adjunct Professor
Department of Medicine
Thomas Jefferson University
Philadelphia, Pennsylvania;
Senior Director, Clinical Development
AstraZeneca LP
Wilmington, Delaware

Maher Nahlawi, MD
Attending Cardiologist
Condell Medical Center
Libertyville, Illinois

Navin C. Nanda, MD
Professor of Medicine
Department of Medicine
University of Alabama, Birmingham;
Director, Heart Station/Echocardiography
  Laboratory
University of Alabama Hospital
Birmingham, Alabama

J.V. Nixon, MD, FACC, FAHA
Professor of Medicine
Division of Cardiology
Department of Internal Medicine;
Director, Echocardiography Laboratories
  and the Heart Station
Medical College of Virginia
Richmond, Virginia

John B. O'Connell, MD
Tranchida Professor and Chair
Department of Internal Medicine
Wayne State University School of Medicine;
Physician-in-Chief
Detroit Medical Center
Detroit, Michigan

Adafisayo M. Oduwole, MD
Assistant Professor of Clinical Medicine
Section of Cardiology
Department of Medicine
Morehouse School of Medicine
Atlanta, Georgia

Elizabeth O. Ofili, MD, MPH
Professor
Department of Medicine
Morehouse School of Medicine
Atlanta, Georgia

Jae K. Oh, MD
Professor and Consultant
Mayo Medical Center
Rochester, Minnesota

Brian Olshansky, MD
Professor of Medicine
Department of Internal Medicine
University of Iowa
Staff Physician
University of Iowa Hospitals and Clinics
Iowa City, Iowa

Peter Ott, MD
Assistant Professor
Department of Internal Medicine
University of Arizona Health Sciences Center
Sarver Heart Center
Tucson, Arizona

John A. Paraskos, MD
Professor of Medicine
Department of Medicine
University of Massachusetts Medical Center;
Director of Ambulatory Cardiology
University of Massachusetts Memorial
  Healthcare
Worcester, Massachusetts

J. Norman Patton, MD
Chair, Division of Cardiovascular Diseases
Department of Internal Medicine
Mayo Clinic
Jacksonville, Florida

Thomas G. Pickering, MD, DPhil
Professor of Medicine
Department of Medicine
Weilll Medical College of Cornell
  University
New York, New York

William R. Pitts, MD
Senior Fellow
Department of Cardiology
University of Texas Southwestern Medical
　Center
Dallas, Texas

Eric N. Prystowsky, MD
Consulting Professor of Medicine
Duke University Medical Center
Durham, North Carolina;
Director, Clinical Electrophysiology
　Laboratory
St. Vincent's Hospital
Indianapolis, Indiana

Muhammad Ramzan, MD
Assistant Professor
Department of Neurology
University of Massachusetts
Worcester, Massachusetts

Stuart Rich, MD
Professor of Medicine
Department of Medicine
Rush Medical College;
Director, Rush Heart Institute
Center for Pulmonary Heart Disease
Chicago, Illinois

Clifford J. Rosen, MD
Professor
Department of Nutrition
University of Maine
Orono, Maine;
Director, Maine Center for Osteoporosis
　Research and Education
St. Joseph Hospital
Bangor, Maine

Mark F. Sasse, MD
Cardiology Fellow
Section of Cardiology
Department of Medicine
Rush University Medical Center
Chicago, Illinois

John Speer Schroeder, MD
Professor of Medicine
Division of Cardiovascular Medicine
Stanford University School of Medicine
Stanford, California

**Ernst R. Schwarz, MD, PhD, FESC,
FACC**
Professor of Medicine
Division of Cardiology
The University of Texas Medical Branch
　School of Medicine
Galveston, Texas

Arnold L. Silva, MD, PhD
Assistant Professor
Department of Medicine
University of Arizona Health Sciences
　Center
Tucson, Arizona

Sidney C. Smith, Jr., MD
Professor
Department of Medicine/Cardiology;
Director, Center for Cardiovascular Science
　and Medicine
University of North Carolina
Chapel Hill, North Carolina

John A. Spittell, Jr., MD
Professor Emeritus
Department of Medicine
Mayo Medical School;
Consultant, Cardiovascular Diseases
Mayo Clinic
Rochester, Minnesota

Peter C. Spittell, MD
Assistant Professor of Medicine
Department of Medicine
Mayo Medical School;
Consultant, Cardiovascular Diseases
Mayo Clinic
Rochester, Minnesota

Kelly Anne Spratt, DO
Clinical Assistant Professor of Medicine
University of Pennsylvania
Presbyterian Medical Center
Philadelphia, Pennsylvania

Paul D. Stein, MD
Professor
Department of Internal Medicine
Wayne State University
Detroit, Michigan;
Director of Research
St. Joseph Mercy Oakland
Pontiac, Michigan

Neil J. Stone, MD
Professor of Clinical Medicine
Department of Cardiology
Northwestern University Feinberg School
　of Medicine
Chicago, Illinois

Maria Stys, MD
Fellow in Cardiology
State University Hospital at Stonybrook
Stonybrook, New York

Tomasz Stys, MD
Assistant Professor
Department of Medicine
State University Hospital at Stonybrook
Stonybrook, New York

Pantel S. Vokonas, MD
Professor of Medicine and Public Health
Boston University School of Medicine
Boston University Medical Center
Boston, Massachusetts

Park W. Willis, IV, MD
Professor of Medicine and Pediatrics
Associate Chief of Cardiology
Director, Adolescent and Adult Congenital
　Cardiac Clinic
Medical Director, Cardiac Graphics
　Laboratory
Director, Adult Training Program in
　Cardiovascular Medicine
University of North Carolina School of
　Medicine
Chapel Hill, North Carolina

Gregg M. Yamada, MD
Assistant Professor of Clinical Medicine
University of Hawaii;
Pacific Cardiology LLC
Private Practice
Honolulu, Hawaii

CONTENTS

Evaluating the Patient with Cardiovascular Disease

Joseph S. Alpert

Key Points

- The history is the most important diagnostic test for making the correct diagnosis.
- Effort syncope can occur in patients with valvular aortic stenosis or hypertrophic cardiomyopathy.
- Cough can be a symptom of pulmonary congestion or heart failure.
- 5 g/dL or more of unsaturated hemoglobin in the circulation allows the clinician to recognize cynanosis.
- The physician should know the potential economic or personal cost of a particular diagnostic test and the likelihood that the test will be definitive in making the correct diagnosis.

The evaluation of a cardiovascular patient involves a careful history, physical examination, and laboratory studies such as chest radiogram, electrocardiogram (ECG), and a number of standard blood tests (*eg*, a lipid profile). More specialized procedures, such as a Doppler echocardiographic study, enable the physician to make a precise cardiovascular diagnosis. Because specialized diagnostic tests are often expensive and can entail significant risk for the patient, they are usually reserved for individuals with clinically significant or symptomatic cardiovascular disease. Such tests are chosen with an eye to their cost–benefit ratio, including test-related morbidity.

THE CARDIOVASCULAR HISTORY

The history is the most important diagnostic tool for making the right diagnosis [1]. A correct diagnosis can be made in more than 50% of patients after a careful history is taken. With a detailed history, the physician seeks to understand the abnormal physiology that is producing the patient's symptoms. For example, when asking a patient about chest pain, the examiner should determine the specific quality, frequency, duration, and location of the pain, as well as precipitating factors related to it (*eg*, inspiration, recumbence, exertion, or emotional upset). A family history of heart disease, hypertension, diabetes mellitus, sudden death, rheumatic fever, congenital heart lesions, or lipid disorder often suggests hereditary predisposition to cardiovascular disease.

In addition, physicians should estimate the level of functional disability resulting from the patient's symptoms. Consider the difficulty that the patient experiences in carrying out the tasks of daily living. The level of disability is often expressed in terms of the traditional New York Heart Association Functional Classification, which includes four classes of functional ability and disability [2] (Table 1). Another system for classifying disability divides functional class into four levels that relate to specific activities and metabolic equivalents (METs)

[3] (Table 2). Moreover, very specific functional status can be obtained by measuring total body oxygen consumption (VO_2) at peak obtainable exercise levels [4].

SPECIFIC CARDIOVASCULAR SYMPTOMS

Dyspnea

Dyspnea is shortness of breath out of proportion to the level of exertion [5]. Common causes of dyspnea include left ventricular (LV) failure, mitral or aortic valve disease, and acute or chronic pulmonary disease, such as chronic obstructive pulmonary disease (COPD) or asthma. Other frequently observed causes of dyspnea include pulmonary embolism, interstitial lung disease, and anxiety. Patients with cardiac dyspnea often complain of associated orthopnea or paroxysmal nocturnal dyspnea. In some patients, it may be difficult to decide whether dyspnea is secondary to heart or to lung disease. Indeed, many patients may have coexisting heart and lung disease such as COPD and coronary artery disease (CAD). Information from the patient's history (eg, previous myocardial infarction [MI] or rheumatic fever), the physical examination, and laboratory results (eg, findings on the chest radiograph indicative of severe chronic lung disease) help to establish the cause of dyspnea [6].

Chest Discomfort

Coronary artery disease is a common cause of chest discomfort. Decisions about diagnostic testing and patient management depend on estimations of the likelihood that a patient's chest discomfort is caused by ischemic heart disease. The physician should decide whether the patient is having angina pectoris. Determining factors are specific characteristics of the chest pain: central location; radiation to arms, neck, or jaw; and a squeezing, pressing, or indigestion-like character. If the discomfort is predictably brought on by exertion, relieved by rest or nitroglycerin, and is severe enough to cause the patient to cease activity, the diagnosis is probably exertional angina. If the pain occurs spontaneously, is less predictably relieved by rest or nitroglycerin, and is milder, the patient may have atypical angina [7]. If the pain is not anginal in nature, the patient is said to have chest discomfort of noncardiac origin.

The discomfort of MI is usually similar to that associated with angina pectoris, although it is generally more severe and is often accompanied by dyspnea, nausea, or diaphoresis. Chest pain associated with pulmonary disorders such as pneumonia and pulmonary embolism is usually pleuritic in nature.

TABLE 1 THE NEW YORK HEART ASSOCIATION FUNCTIONAL CLASSIFICATION OF HEART DISEASE

Cardiac Status	Prognosis
Uncompromised	Good
Slightly compromised	Good with therapy
Moderately compromised	Fair with therapy
Severely compromised	Guarded with therapy

TABLE 2 A FUNCTIONAL CLASSIFICATION OF HEART DISEASE*

Class	Minutes on Treadmill[†]	Specific Activity	MET[‡]
I	> 6	Carrying 24-lb object up eight steps	10
		Walking 5 mi	9
		Carrying 80-lb object	8
		Shoveling snow, spading dirt	7
II	3–6	Walking 4 mi/h	5.0–6.0
		Raking, weeding the garden	5.0–6.0
		Sexual intercourse	5.0–5.5
		Carrying anything up eight steps	5.0–5.5
II	1–3	Stripping and making bed	4.0–5.0
		Pushing power lawn mower	4.0
		Showering without stopping	3.6–4.2
		Walking 2.5 mi	3.0–3.5
		Dressing without stopping	2.0–2.3
IV	< 1	None of the above	< 2

*Based on the patient's ability to meet metabolic demands of selected specific activities.
[†]Bruce protocol.
[‡]One MET represents the energy expended in burning 3.5 mL O_2/kg/min.
MET—metabolic equivalent.

Chest wall pain is often confused with angina pectoris. Differences in location, duration, and quality can usually differentiate chest wall pain from angina pectoris. Pain originating from the distal esophagus (esophageal reflux or spasm) can be similar to the discomfort of angina pectoris. However, eating rather than exertion is often the cause of distal esophageal pain. Anxiety, the hyperventilation syndrome, or both are often associated with chest pain that may also mimic angina pectoris, although the pain caused by anxiety or hyperventilation is usually sharp and fleeting or prolonged and highly localized.

Palpitations

Sensing an irregular heartbeat is termed *palpitation*. At times, the patient senses an irregularity in cardiac rhythm (*eg*, extrasystoles); at other times, he or she senses rapid, forceful cardiac activity (*eg*, sinus tachycardia). Patients frequently report that their heart is skipping, fluttering, pounding, or racing.

It is useful to have the patient describe the regularity or irregularity and the approximate rate of the palpitation. Associated light-headedness or syncope should be ascertained. Paroxysmal supraventricular dysrhythmias (*eg*, atrial fibrillation) are usually described as sudden in onset and termination. Sinus tachycardia is more gradual in onset and termination. Patients may not sense palpitations during ventricular tachycardia. Rather, they may experience dyspnea, syncope, or severe fatigue. Palpitations sensed during anxiety states relate to the patient's heightened awareness of cardiac activity. Normal sinus rhythm or sinus tachycardia is usually present. A routine ECG or additional testing (*ie*, electrocardiographic ambulatory monitoring or exercise testing) may be indicated [8].

Syncope

Syncope is usually the result of a cardiac or neurologic condition, including seizure disorders, vasodepressor syncope (the simple faint), and cardiac dysrhythmias such as ventricular tachycardia or complete heart block [9]. Historical points that favor a cardiac origin for syncope include sudden onset without warning, a sensation of rapid heart action before loss of consciousness, and lack of an aura or observed seizure activity, although seizures may occur during dysrhythmias as a result of decreased cerebral perfusion.

Effort syncope can occur in patients with valvular aortic stenosis or LV outflow obstruction (*ie*, hypertrophic cardiomyopathy with subaortic stenosis). Vasodepressor syncope usually occurs when the patient is physically or emotionally uncomfortable. Associated autonomic nervous symptoms such as sweating, nausea, and yawning are often present.

Cough

Cough is more often pulmonary than cardiac in origin (*eg*, asthma or pneumonia). However, cough may be a manifestation of pulmonary vascular congestion secondary to LV failure or mitral stenosis. In this setting, cough may be part of the symptom complex of paroxysmal nocturnal dyspnea. Cough secondary to pulmonary vascular congestion is often nonproductive. However, when pulmonary vascular congestion is severe and incipient pulmonary edema develops, small amounts of frothy white sputum may be produced. Occasionally, patients with cardiac disease experience hemoptysis during coughing. Hemoptysis, too, is often the result of pulmonary disease such as bronchiectasis or tumor. Cardiovascular causes for hemoptysis include pulmonary embolism, mitral stenosis, and, occasionally, LV failure. Approximately 10% of patients treated with angiotension-converting enzyme (ACE) inhibitors develop a recurrent, nonproductive cough that may prevent them from sleeping.

Peripheral Edema

Peripheral edema is often a late finding in patients with LV failure. In this setting, it is the result of concomitant right ventricular (RV) failure. However, the most common cause of peripheral edema is venous insufficiency. When peripheral edema is the result of RV failure, elevated jugular venous pressure is often present. Other cardiac causes of peripheral edema include constrictive pericarditis and primary RV failure secondary to pulmonary arterial hypertension. Noncardiovascular diseases that cause peripheral edema include chronic renal failure, nephrotic syndrome, profound hypoalbuminemia, and Cushing's disease.

Cyanosis and Clubbing

A level of 5 g/dL or more of unsaturated hemoglobin in the arterial circulation usually allows the examiner to diagnose cyanosis. Cyanosis is said to be peripheral when it is seen only in the extremities. Peripheral cyanosis is the result of decreased blood flow to the skin secondary to vasoconstriction. Common causes of peripheral cyanosis include shock and exposure to cold. Peripheral cyanosis is transient and not associated with clubbing of the fingernails.

Central cyanosis involves the entire body and is the result of abnormal saturation of venous blood during its pulmonary transit or from right-to-left cardiac or pulmonary shunts. Fingers and toes are often clubbed. Clubbing can be familial and not associated with decreased arterial oxygen saturation.

PHYSICAL EXAMINATION OF THE HEART

Physical examination of the heart provides important information about the cardiovascular system. Together with a thorough medical history, the physical examination provides the initial database and suggests further diagnostic tests and therapeutic maneuvers. A complete physical examination is indicated in cardiovascular patients in order to recognize systemic manifestations of cardiac disease or systemic illness that is affecting the cardiovascular system.

Jugular Venous Pulse

Two types of information are obtained from the jugular venous pulse (JVP): the quality of the waveform and the central venous pressure (CVP). JVP is best observed in the right internal jugular vein. With normal CVP, the JVP is assessed with the patient's trunk raised less than 30°. With elevated CVP, the patient's trunk must be raised higher, sometimes to as much as 90°. The JVP is accentuated by turning the patient's head away from the examiner and shining a flashlight obliquely across the skin overlying the vein.

Two waves per heartbeat are generally visible in the JVP: the A wave and the V wave. The A wave appears as a brief "flicker" and represents increased venous pressure resulting from right atrial contraction. The V wave is a longer surge that follows the A wave and represents increased venous pressure transmitted to the right atrium during RV contraction. The decrease in pressure after the A wave is called the X descent, and the decrease in pressure after the V wave is denoted as the Y descent. JVP waves can be timed by means of simultaneous palpation of the carotid artery. The A wave immediately precedes the carotid pulse, and the V wave follows the pulse. In many patients with normal central venous pressure, the A wave may be so diminutive that only a single wave, the V wave, is observed.

Occasionally, difficulty may be experienced in differentiating venous and arterial pulsations in the neck. Several observations and findings may be helpful: 1) the arterial pulse is more localized; whereas it forcefully strikes the examining fingers, palpation obliterates the venous pulse; 2) compression at the base of the neck does not alter the arterial pulse but it obliterates the venous pulse; 3) arterial pulses do not change with patient position, but venous pulses often disappear when the patient assumes an upright posture (either sitting upright or standing). The diagnosis of a variety of pathologic states is assisted by observation of abnormalities in the JVP (Table 3).

Central venous pressure is estimated by observing the vertical distance from the top of the V wave in the JVP to the top of the sternum. In an individual with normal CVP, the V wave rises 1 to 2 cm above the sternal angle. When the V wave rises more than halfway to the angle of the jaw in a patient who is not recumbent, elevated CVP is present. In patients with some pathologic conditions (eg, cardiac tamponade, constrictive pericarditis), CVP may be so high that A and V waves are above the angle of the jaw. In this setting, exaggerated X and Y descents may suggest the diagnosis. As a rule of thumb, for a patient sitting upright, a JVP visible at the sternal angle represents a CVP of approximately 10 mm Hg.

During inspiration, the height of the JVP typically declines as a result of increasingly negative intrathoracic pressure. In patients with certain pathologic conditions such as chronic constrictive pericarditis and occasionally tricuspid stenosis, congestive heart failure, RV dysfunction, or infarction, the JVP actually increases with inspiration. This important clinical finding is known as Kussmaul's sign.

Arterial Pressure Pulse

The central arterial pressure pulse (ie, aortic pressure) is characterized by a rapid increase to a rounded peak with a less rapid decline. The carotid arterial pulse retains a number of the qualities of the aortic pulse. Thus, information about the adequacy of ventricular contraction and possible obstruction in the LV outflow tract may be assessed by palpation of the carotid artery. By the time the pulse wave is transmitted to peripheral arteries (eg, the radial arterial pulse), much of this initial information is lost; however, pulsus alternans is best evaluated in the peripheral arteries.

A variety of pathologic conditions alter the characteristics of the carotid pulse. These conditions, and the corresponding modifications of the carotid pulse, are listed in Table 4. In patients with hypertension, simultaneous palpation of radial and femoral arterial pulses helps to rule out coarctation of the aorta.

TABLE 3 ABNORMAL JUGULAR VENOUS PULSATIONS	
Finding	**Comment or Significance**
Markedly raised central venous pressure, accentuated X and Y descents	? Cardiac tamponade
	? Constrictive pericarditis
	? Endocardial fibroelastosis
	? Severe right heart failure
Large A waves	? Pulmonary valvular stenosis
	? Hypertension
	? Various arrhythmias in which atria contract against closed AV valve (eg, junctional rhythm, AV dissociation)
Absent A wave	AF
Large V wave	TR

AF—atrial fibrillation; AV—atrioventricular; TR—tricuspid regurgitation.

Precordial Palpation

Information concerning the location and quality of the LV impulse is available through precordial palpation. In addition, the intensity of murmurs may be gauged by palpating associated thrills. Palpation is best accomplished using the fingertips, with the patient either supine or in the left lateral decubitus position. Simultaneous auscultation can aid in the timing of events. A list of abnormalities and their significance as detected by precordial palpation is found in Table 5.

Auscultation

The first heart sound (S1) occurs at the time of closure of the mitral and tricuspid valves. It is probably generated by the closure of the valves. S1 is frequently split (with mitral closure preceding tricuspid), but this may be hard to appreciate and is of little clinical relevance. More important is variation in intensity of the first heart sound. S1 varies with

the PR interval of the ECG. The shorter the PR interval, the louder the S1. The best example of S1 variation with PR interval occurs in a patient with complete heart block in which atrial and ventricular contractions are dissociated.

S1 may be loud and "snapping" in quality in mitral stenosis, indicating both that the valve is pliable and that it remains wide open at the beginning of isovolumic LV contraction. Conversely, a diminished or absent S1 in a patient with mitral stenosis suggests a rigidly calcified valve that cannot "snap" shut.

Other situations in which S1 may be diminished include mitral regurgitation, slow heart rates (long PR interval), poor sound conduction through the chest wall (thick chest wall musculature or large breasts), and a slow rise of LV pressure. A summary of clinical information derived from variations in S1 is found in Table 6.

In contrast to S1, in which splitting is less important than changes in intensity, S2 reveals variations in

---

TABLE 4 ABNORMALITIES IN THE CAROTID PULSE

Finding	Comment or Significance
Pulsus bisferiens (two systolic peaks)	AR and hypertrophic obstructive cardiomyopathy
Pulsus parvus (small, weak pulse)	Any condition causing diminished LV stroke volume or narrow pulse pressure (ie, hypovolemia, mitral or aortic valve stenosis, restrictive pericarditis, recent MI); may also be caused by atherosclerosis of the carotid artery or diseases of the aortic arch
Pulsus tardus (delayed systolic peak of pulse)	Aortic outflow obstruction (eg, AS)
Pulsus paradoxus (larger than normal decrease in systolic arterial pressure during inspiration)	Pericardial tamponade, airway obstruction, superior vena caval obstruction; also asthma or COPD
Pulsus alternans (consistent alternation in pulse pressure amplitude despite regular rhythm)	Severe LV decompensation for any reason; after paroxysmal tachycardia

AR—aortic regurgitation; AS—aortic stenosis; COPD—chronic obstructive pulmonary disease; LV—left ventricle; MI—myocardial infarction.

TABLE 5 ABNORMALITIES IN PRECORDIAL PALPATION

Finding	Comment or Significance
LV thrust	LV hypertrophy
Displacement of LV pulse downward and to the left	LV dilatation; LV failure; volume overload (AR or decompensated MR)
Presystolic impulse	Pressure overloaded states (hypertension, AS)
Double systolic impulse	Hypertrophic obstructive cardiomyopathy
Systolic bulge (dyskinetic impulse)	CAD, recent MI (most commonly felt above and medial to the point of maximal impulse)
Parasternal lift	MR (occurs after the LV apical impulse); RV dilatation (mitral stenosis, PE)
Thrills	AS, PS; VSD, severe MR

AR—aortic regurgitation; AS—aortic stenosis; CAD—coronary artery disease; LV—left ventricle; MI—myocardial infarction; MR—mitral regurgitation; MS—mitral stenosis; PE—pulmonary embolism; PS—pulmonary stenosis; RV—right ventricle; VSD—ventricular septal defect.

both splitting and intensity that provide important clinical information.

The second heart sound (S2) occurs at the time of closure of the aortic and pulmonic valves. In normal circumstances, aortic closure precedes pulmonic closure (A2 followed by P2). Under normal circumstances, the split in S2 is maximal at the end of inspiration and minimal at the end of expiration. This phenomenon reflects an underlying movement of P2 with respect to a relatively constant A2. During inspiration, RV filling increases and P2 is delayed, causing the widely split S2. During expiration, less RV filling occurs and P2 moves back toward A2, causing a diminished split in S2. This "normal" or "physiologic splitting" of S2 is invariably present in individuals younger than age 30 years, provided heart rates are not fast. It is best appreciated over the "pulmonic area" (upper left sternal border) and can be heard with either the stethoscope bell or the diaphragm.

A common abnormality of S2 is failure of splitting to close at the end of expiration. This "fixed splitting" occurs for one of two reasons: P2 is delayed or A2 is early. A split of S2 on expiration may also represent a normal variant. In the latter setting, however, some difference in the degree of splitting should occur between inspiration and expiration.

Fixed splitting of S2 caused by delayed P2 is found in four clinical settings: patients with 1) acute right heart pressure overload (eg, pulmonary embolism), 2) right bundle branch block, 3) atrial septal defect (ASD), and 4) pulmonic stenosis.

Paradoxical splitting of S2 is said to be present when S2 splits on expiration and closes on inspiration. Note that whereas fixed splitting is the result of delay in normal

TABLE 6 ABNORMALITIES OF S1

Finding	Comment or Significance
Loud S1	Short PR interval
Loud "snapping" S1	MS (pliable valve)
Variation in intensity of S1	Complete heart block
Diminished intensity of S1	MR, slow heart rate (long PR interval), poor conduction of sound through chest wall, slow rise of LV pressure, MS (rigidly calcific valve), severe or acute aortic regurgitation

LV—left ventricle; MR—mitral regurgitation; MS—mitral stenosis.

TABLE 7 ABNORMALITIES OF S2

Finding	Comment or Significance
Abnormalities in timing	
Fixed splitting	Acute right-heart overload (eg, PE)
	RBBB
	ASD (often widely split)
	PS
Paradoxical splitting	AS
	LBBB
Closely split with closure at midinspiration (variant of paradoxical splitting)	CAD
	Hypertension
Abnormalities in intensity	
Increased A2	Hypertension
	Aortic dilatation
Increased P2	Pulmonary hypertension
	Normal finding in thin-chested individual
Decreased A2	AS
Decreased P2	PS

AS—aortic stenosis; ASD—atrial septal defect; CAD—coronary artery disease; LBBB—left bundle branch block; PE—pulmonary embolism; PS—pulmonary stenosis; RBBB—right bundle branch block.

closure of the pulmonic valve, paradoxical splitting is caused by delayed closure of the aortic valve. Paradoxical splitting always occurs in the presence of cardiac disease. The most common states in which paradoxical splitting is encountered are aortic stenosis and left bundle branch block (LBBB). Paradoxical splitting takes place in about 25% of individuals with these conditions. Paradoxical splitting may also occur in patients with CAD, hypertension, or both. In these individuals, a closely split S2 may be observed to close to a single sound at midinspiration. A similar finding is often made in the early stages of aortic stenosis or in incomplete LBBB.

Alterations in the intensity of S2 can also yield important clinical information. A2 is frequently soft in patients with aortic stenosis. The presence of a normal A2 when aortic stenosis is clinically suspected raises the question of outflow obstruction at a site other than the valve. P2 may be augmented in intensity in patients with pulmonary hypertension and diminished in individuals with pulmonic stenosis. Finally, P2 may appear unusually loud in thin-chested individuals without cardiac disease. A summary of clinical information derived from alterations in S2 is found in Table 7.

The third heart sound (S3, or ventricular gallop) is low pitched and best heard at the apex with the stethoscope bell. The S3 is probably the result of rapid filling and stretching of an abnormal LV during early diastole. The cadence of the S3 has been likened to the "Y" in "Kentucky." An S3 may also be heard in patients with any condition producing rapid ventricular filling (mitral regurgitation and ASD). It is frequently an early sign of LV failure. Third heart sounds may also be present in those with ASD, mitral or aortic insufficiency, ventricular septal defect (VSD), and patent ductus arteriosus. An S3 can also be a normal variant in healthy young adults. A loud, early diastolic sound can also be heard in patients with constrictive pericarditis. This "pericardial knock" may be mistaken for an S3.

The fourth heart sound (S4, atrial gallop, presystolic gallop) is also the result of altered ventricular compliance. Its cadence has been likened to the soft "A" of "appendix." It is a low-pitched sound that is best heard with the stethoscope bell. It is loudest at the apex and may be accentuated by placing the patient in the left lateral decubitus position. The presence of an S4 implies effective atrial contraction; it is never heard in those with atrial fibrillation. An S4 may be heard in patients with any condition that causes reduced compliance of either ventricle: aortic stenosis, systemic or pulmonary hypertension, CAD, hypertrophic cardiomyopathy, acute mitral regurgitation, and MI.

Snaps, Clicks, and Other Adventitious Sounds

An opening snap of the mitral valve is frequently heard in patients with mitral stenosis. The opening snap arises from the stiff mitral valve's descent into the LV in early diastole. The opening snap is best heard in the fourth intercostal space halfway between the apex and the left sternal border.

The interval between S2 and the OS is related to the severity of mitral stenosis. The more severe the stenosis, the shorter the S2–OS interval.

Ejection clicks are high-pitched sounds occurring in early systole. They are associated with stenosis of either the aortic or the pulmonic valve, with hypertension, or with dilatation of either the aorta or the pulmonary artery or both. Aortic clicks are best heard at the apex, and pulmonic clicks are most audible at the left upper sternal border. Pulmonic clicks vary with respiration and are best heard during expiration. Aortic clicks do not vary with respiration.

Midsystolic clicks, often accompanied by a late systolic murmur, occur in patients with prolapse of the mitral valve. The clicks may result from sudden tensing of the chordae tendineae or snapping of the prolapsing leaflet. The clicks may be single or multiple and may occur at any time during systole, although they generally occur later in systole than ejection clicks.

Systolic Murmurs

Systolic murmurs are classified according to their time of occurrence, sound quality, and duration. The most fundamental distinction is between systolic ejection murmurs and pansystolic murmurs. Ejection murmurs ordinarily occur in midsystole; they begin shortly after S1 and are usually crescendo–decrescendo ("diamond-shaped"), ending before S2. Pansystolic murmurs begin with S1, extend throughout systole, and are characteristically uniform in intensity. Systolic ejection murmurs have been likened to the chug of a stream engine laboring up a hill, and pansystolic murmurs have been likened to the high-pitched wail of the engine's whistle (Table 8).

Systolic Ejection Murmurs

Systolic ejection murmurs (SEMs) begin after the semilunar (aortic and pulmonic) valves open at the end of isovolumic systole. Their intensity parallels the amount of blood being ejected through the stenosis, peaking in midsystole. SEMs arise in the following settings: 1) aortic or pulmonic stenosis, 2) dilatation of the aorta or pulmonary artery distal to the valve, 3) increased rate of ventricular ejection (heart block, fever, anemia, exercise, and thyrotoxicosis), and 4) healthy individuals.

Pansystolic murmurs occur when blood flows through a VSD or retrograde through the mitral or tricuspid valve. The constant intensity and long duration of these murmurs reflect the large pressure difference across the orifice where the sound originates. The murmur continues as long as pressure in the chamber of origin exceeds that in the recipient chamber.

Early systolic murmurs are of short duration beginning with or shortly after S1 and ending by midsystole. They have been reported in 1) patients with mitral stenosis probably secondary to coexistent mitral regurgitation, 2) patients with small VSDs, and 3) individuals without cardiac disease.

Late systolic murmurs are also of short duration, beginning in midsystole and extending to or through S2. They may be heard in those with mitral valve prolapse (frequently accompanied by midsystolic clicks) or coarctation of the aorta.

Systolic murmurs arising from the right side of the heart generally increase with inspiration, and those originating from the left side decrease or do not change. Many systolic murmurs are totally innocent (as in pregnant woman, growing children, and individuals with abnormal chest configurations).

Diastolic Murmurs

Diastolic murmurs are classified according to their position in diastole as early, mid, or late. An alternative classification emphasizes the cause: regurgitant murmurs from semilunar valve insufficiency versus ventricular filling murmurs. Whereas regurgitant murmurs are generally early, diastolic ventricular filling murmurs occur in mid and late diastole (Table 9). Early diastolic murmurs begin immediately after S2. The most common causes are aortic

or pulmonic valve regurgitation. The murmur is usually high pitched and blowing in quality with a decrescendo configuration. The intensity of the murmur reflects the size of the valvular leak, the acoustic properties of the chest, and the pressure difference across the valve. The distinction between pulmonic and aortic regurgitation may be extremely hard to make and may require echocardiography for definitive determination.

Mid and Late Diastolic Murmurs

Mid and late diastolic murmurs are produced by forward flow of blood through the atrioventricular (mitral and tricuspid) valves. They arise from either augmented blood flow or a stenosed valve. As a rule, the murmur is low pitched and rumbling in quality. It does not begin until the valve from which it originates opens (sometimes with an audible snap) and ventricular pressure has decreased below atrial pressure in early diastole. Conditions in which mid or late diastolic murmurs may arise include mitral or tricuspid

TABLE 8 SYSTOLIC MURMURS

Early Systolic	Ejection (Midsystolic)	Pansystolic	Late Systolic
1. VSD (small)	Dilatation of vessel	1. VSD	1. MVP
	1. Pulmonary artery dilatation	2. MR	2. Coarctation of the aorta
	2. Aortic dilatation	3. TR	
	Stenosis of valve		
	1. PS		
	2. AS		
	Increased flow across valve		
	1. Heart block		
	2. Fever		
	3. Anemia		
	4. Exercise		
	5. Thyrotoxicosis		
	6. Normal		

AS—aortic stenosis; MR—mitral regurgitation; MVP—mitral valve prolapse; PS—pulmonic stenosis; TR—tricuspid regurgitation; VSD—ventricular septal defect.

TABLE 9 DIASTOLIC MURMURS

Early Diastolic	Mid and Late Diastolic
1. PR	1. MS
2. AR	2. TS
	3. Atrial myxoma
	4. MR
	5. Large left-to-right shunt

AR—aortic regurgitation; MR—mitral regurgitation MS—mitral stenosis; PR—pulmonic regurgitation; TS—tricuspid stenosis.

stenosis, left atrial myxoma, mitral regurgitation (increased flow), and large left-to-right shunts (increased flow).

Continuous Murmurs

Murmurs are considered continuous when they are audible throughout all phases of the cardiac cycle. They generally arise when a continuous pressure differential allows blood to flow constantly from a high to a low pressure zone, as may occur in patients with a variety of congenital defects, most commonly patent ductus arteriosus, anomalous origin of the left coronary artery, and coronary arteriovenous fistula. Other conditions that may cause continuous murmurs include ruptured aneurysm of a sinus of Valsalva, proximal coronary artery stenosis, and pulmonary artery branch stenosis.

An analogous phenomenon is a venous hum. This continuous, low-pitched murmur results from an increased velocity of venous blood flow. It is an innocent finding, usually heard in the lower anterior portion of the neck. Venous hum is accentuated by deep inspiration in most patients and may be obliterated by the Valsalva maneuver or by pressure on the internal jugular vein.

Physiologic and Pharmacologic Manipulation of Heart Sounds and Murmurs

Various physiologic and pharmacological maneuvers are available to accentuate heart sounds and murmurs [10]. A partial listing of these maneuvers, together with their physiologic consequences, is found in Table 10. Maneuvers that are useful in the analysis of specific murmurs and heart sounds are listed in Table 11. Physiologic and pharmacologic manipulations may help untangle difficult problems in differential diagnosis when normal auscultatory findings are ambiguous. Unfortunately, the use of these maneuvers has declined because of the more widespread use of Doppler echocardiography.

CLINICAL JUDGMENT

The combination of knowledge, experience, and common sense enables physicians to recognize many common illnesses. Of course, experienced physicians are aware of the uncertainty involved in making a diagnosis. There is a small but definite probability that a patient does not have a common illness but rather a serious and complex disease.

Decisions made in an environment fraught with uncertainty should never be considered as objective and incontrovertible facts. Rather, such decisions should be viewed as probability statements (ie, the favored horse will probably win the race). New information or further examination of existing data may lead to an alteration in the probability statement.

Another aspect of clinical judgment relates to the manner in which the physician approaches the patient. Biased, intellectually arrogant, or unfeeling attitudes on the part of the physician represent an error in clinical judgment because such attitudes interfere with data

TABLE 10 MANIPULATION OF HEART SOUNDS AND MURMURS		
Maneuver	**Physiologic Consequence**	**Comment**
Physiologic maneuvers		
Respiration	Inspiration: right heart filling increased, left heart filling decreased	Right heart murmurs increased; left heart murmurs decreased or unchanged
Rapid changes in position (*eg*, elevation of legs, standing, squatting)	Changes in RV filling (RV filling increased by lying, leg elevation, or squatting; venous return decreased by standing)	Gallop sounds, murmurs of pulmonic and aortic stenosis, all increased by lying, leg elevation, or squatting; IHSS murmur increased by standing
Valsalva maneuver	Initially causes sharp increase in BP (phase I), then impairs venous return and BP decreases (phase II)	During phase II, murmurs of PS, AS, and MR diminish but murmurs of IHSS increase
Pharmacologic maneuvers		
Phenylephrine	Increased systemic arterial pressure	Murmur of AR and MR increased
Isoproterenol	Increased myocardial contraction	Murmur of IHSS increased
Amyl nitrite	Potent vasodilator; decreased systolic pressure; reflex increase in heart rate	Murmurs of AR and MR decreased; all ejection murmurs increased; VSD murmur decreased

AR—aortic regurgitation; AS—aortic stenosis; BP—blood pressure; IHSS—idiopathic hypertrophic subaortic stenosis; MR—mitral regurgitation; PS—pulmonic stenosis; RV—right ventricle; VSD—ventricular septal defect.

collection and appropriate therapy [11]. Clinical judgment usually requires medical knowledge, some experience, common sense, and an awareness of one's own biases. It may also require moral reasoning.

Despite the fact that most physicians would like to believe that they are dispassionate and objective with respect to their clinical judgment, it must be acknowledged that we are all prone to subjective forces. Value judgments, prejudices, likes, and dislikes all influence clinical judgment at some level. The most one can hope for is to be aware of subjective influences and to attempt to recognize when they are influencing the decision-making process.

Cost Benefit and the Differential Diagnosis

Another factor that should be considered in the evaluation of the patient is the ratio of cost to benefit. Cost in this context refers both to economic cost and to pain and suffering. Both entities extract something from the patient—money or physical or psychological distress. Physicians need to know the potential economic or personal cost of a particular diagnostic test and the likelihood that the test will be definitive in making the diagnosis or changing the treatment. Ideally, an inexpensive and painless test is best; however, the test chosen depends on the risk–benefit ratio as well as on cost and discomfort.

Physicians should consider whether the results of a specific test will alter the patient's therapy or comfort. A test that is not associated with a reasonable likelihood of altering either therapy or patient comfort should not be performed. It should be stressed that patient comfort has both physical and psychological or emotional components. Therefore, a test that does not alter therapy but that confirms a rather benign diagnostic entity and thereby eliminates a frightening one is certainly worth performing.

Another rule of clinical judgment is that it is foolish and wasteful to order two tests that produce the same information [12]. If the physician has obtained an echocardiogram

Condition	Maneuver
TABLE 11 MANEUVERS FOR ANALYSIS OF HEART SOUNDS AND MURMURS	
AS	Valvular: midsystolic murmur louder with sudden squatting, leg raising, or amyl nitrite; fades during Valsalva maneuver
	Hypertropic subvalvular: systolic murmur louder with sitting or squatting, during Valsalva maneuver, or with amyl nitrite; softens with sudden squatting or leg elevation
AR	Blowing diastolic murmur increases with sudden squatting, fades with amyl nitrite
	Austin Flint murmur fades with amyl nitrite
MS	Diastolic murmur made louder with tachycardia, exercise, left lateral position, coughing, or amyl nitrite
MR	Rheumatic systolic murmur louder with sudden squatting, softer with amyl nitrite
	Mid to late systolic MVP: late systolic murmur becomes mid or holosystolic with upright position, with amyl nitrite, and during Valsalva maneuver; midsystolic click occurs earlier with these maneuvers; murmur fades with lying flat
PS	Midsystolic murmur increases with amyl nitrite, except with marked RV hypertrophy; also may increase with first few beats after Valsalva release
PR	Congenital: early or middiastolic murmur (harsh, low-pitched) increases on inspiration and with amyl nitrite
	Pulmonary hypertensive: high-frequency early diastolic blowing murmur not influenced by respiration; inconstant response to amyl nitrite
TS	Middiastolic and presystolic murmurs increase during inspiration and with amyl nitrite
TR	Systolic murmur increases during inspiration and with amyl nitrite
VSD	Small defect without pulmonary hypertension: murmur fades with amyl nitrite
	Large defect with hyperkinetic pulmonary hypertension: murmur louder with amyl nitrite
	Large defect with severe pulmonary vascular disease: little change with above agents
Gallop rhythm	Ventricular filling sounds: ventricular gallop and atrial gallop are accentuated by lying flat with passive leg raising; decreased by sitting or standing; right-sided gallop sounds usually increased during inspiration, left-sided during expiration
	Summation gallop may separate into ventricular gallop (S3) and atrial gallop (S4) sounds when heart rate slowed by carotid sinus massage

AR—aortic regurgitation; AS—aortic stenosis; MR—mitral regurgitation; MS—mitral stenosis; MVP—mitral valve prolapse; PR—pulmonic regurgitation; PS—pulmonic stenosis; RV—right ventricle; TR—tricuspid regurgitation; TS—tricuspid stenosis; VSD—ventricular septal defect.

to evaluate ventricular function, a radionuclide ventriculo-gram is not needed because the latter test yields informa-tion similar to that derived from the echocardiogram. The two tests are (in this instance but not always) redundant. The rational work-up is like a carefully reasoned argument in a debate: it proceeds logically from one point to the next without redundancy or confusion.

REFERENCES

1. Sandler G: The importance of the history in the medical clinic and the cost of unnecessary tests. *Am Heart J* 1980, 100:928–931.

2. Criteria Committee of the New York Heart Association: Major changes made by the Criteria Committee of the New York heart Association. *Circulation* 1974, 49:390.

3. Goldman L, Hashimoto B, Cooks EF, *et al.*: Comparative repro-ducibility and validity of systems for assessing cardiovascular functional class: advantages of a new specific activity scale. *Circu-lation* 1981, 64:1227–1234.

4. Wasserman K, Hansen JE, Sue DY, *et al.*: *Principles of Exercise Testing and Interpretation*. Philadelphia: Lea & Febiger; 1987.

5. Manning HL, Schwartzstein RM: Pathophysiology of dyspnea. *N Engl J Med* 1995, 333:1547–1553.

6. Mulrow CD, Lucey CR, Farnett LE: Discriminating causes of dyspnea through clinical examination. *J Gen Intern Med* 1993, 8:383–392.

7. Campeau L: Grading of angina pectoris [letter]. *Circulation* 1976, 54:522.

8. Sox HC Jr: Exercise testing in suspected coronary artery disease. *Dis Mon* 1985, 31:1–93.

9. Silver KH, Alpert JS: Syncope. *J Intensive Care Med* 1992, 7:138.

10. Dohan MC, Criscitiello MG: Physiological and pharmacological manipulations of heart sounds and murmurs. *Mod Concepts Cardiovasc Dis* 1970, 39:121.

11. Sheehan TJ, Husted S, Candee D, *et al.*: Moral judgment as a predictor of clinical performance. *Eval Health Prof* 1980, 3:393.

12. Lee TH, Goldman L: Serum enzyme assays in the diagnosis of acute myocardial infarction. *In Common Diagnostic Tests: Use and Interpretation*, edn 2. Edited by Sox HC. Philadelphia: American College of Physicians; 1990.

Referrals

Julius J. Chosy
Harry R. Kimball

Key Points

- Effective referral and consultation are important for optimum health care delivery, control of costs, and quality of care.
- Accurate communication is essential; referring physicians should state clearly what it is they want to know and what they want the consultant to do.
- Consultants must define the task, address the referring physician's concerns, and know what responsibility for care is to be assumed.
- Consultants should use problem lists, make recommendations that are succinct, to the point, and specific, and then follow up if possible.
- Consultants should transmit what is important to both the patient and the referring physician.
- Should disagreements about medical management occur between physicians, a second opinion should be obtained.

Effective consultation and referral among physicians and other medical providers facilitates the delivery of high-quality health care to patients and improves the outcomes of care [1,2••]. By matching patient needs with appropriate choice of consultants, primary physicians can protect patients from the adverse effects of unnecessary care and ensure that costly medical services are used judiciously [3,4]. These outcomes are especially important at a time of explosive growth in biomedical knowledge and technology, public concern about patient safety, and limited health care budgets. In response to rising costs, managed care has come to dominate health care in the United States and has profoundly influenced physician practice [5•]. We now have capitation, gatekeeping, preauthorization of referrals, provider panel limitations, restricted formularies, physician profiling, practice guidelines, case management, disease management, and shifting of patients from one managed care organization to another [5•]. Physicians have thought themselves demeaned by the gatekeeper role, with less freedom of choice in consultants, and diminished personal relationships with other physicians, resulting in less communication and information exchange and ability to influence the referral process [6].

In turn, the dissatisfaction with managed care, in particular with gatekeeping, by patients, physicians, employers, and governments [5•,7•], and the limited evidence of significant reductions in subspecialty use by gatekeeping or capitated primary physician payments [8,9], has changed managed care. Many managed care organizations have eliminated financial disincentives to primary care physicians for use of specialty or hospital care, relaxed the requirements for access to specialty services, or have abandoned gatekeeping altogether [5•,9,10].

Physicians in training are exposed to a variety of consultation services, but few training programs offer formal instruction about how optimal outcomes of referral and consultation can be achieved [11]. In this chapter the principles, process, and pitfalls of patient referral and consultation are discussed.

REFERRAL

Referrals may involve requests for a wide range of services, from a limited consultation (for example, to a nutrition service for diet assessment) to a complete transfer of patient care responsibility. The outcome of these arrangements among the primary physician, the patient, and the consultant is generally improved care for the patient; however, poor communication between the participants can lead to misunderstanding, disruptions in continuity, duplication of care, delayed or missed diagnoses, or even lapses in care [3,4,12•].

Consultation and referral patterns, their variability, and the clinical decision processes that govern them are not well understood. Patient characteristics, physician specialty, length of training experience, reimbursement issues, and type of health coverage (fee-for-service, health maintenance organization, preferred provider organization, and so forth) appear to be important [3,13,14•,15,16,17•]. Two studies suggest that the greater a practitioner's diagnostic certainty or knowledge in a specialty area, the higher the referral rate to that specialty [18,19].

The reasons for referral and consultation are varied and complex (Table 1) [20,21,22•,23]. They mainly involve seeking advice or help in diagnosis or patient management, performing a procedure, reassurance, pleasing someone, patient education, and divestiture of responsibility for care.

A special category of consultation is informal, or "curbside," consultation (eg, in person, by phone, or email). Its advantages are efficiency, low cost, and in some managed care settings, avoidance of financial loss. Some disadvantages are the risks of incomplete or inaccurate communication, possible loss of compensation, and legal liability. Whether such informal consult is used appropriately, or negatively impacts health care quality, is unknown [24•].

The literature includes many articles about when to refer patients with a particular problem or disease. The chief plea of consultants is that patients be referred "soon enough." "Soon enough" depends on the problem in question, the condition of the patient, and the skills of the primary physician and consultant. Certainly, when a physician is feeling a certain level of discomfort, it is time to refer. When the patient's condition is getting worse or at a plateau and further improvement might be possible, it is time to refer. A physician should not wait until the patient has become resentful or is compelled to ask for a referral. Patients are increasingly aware of possible treatment options because such information is easily available through the Internet and other media. Physicians should not be afraid to seek a second opinion: to do so will either validate their care and thereby their reputation, or it will lead to patients' getting the care they need, or both.

A somewhat sensitive reason for referral is the wish to be free of a particularly troublesome, litigious, or hypochondriacal patient. It is an appropriate reason to refer when the physician can no longer provide the attentive listening and objective responses good medical care requires. In fairness to both the patient and the consultant, the reason should be made clear to the consultant.

What should be done when a patient asks for a referral that is not indicated or a second opinion that is believed unnecessary? Unless a plan satisfactory to the patient can be devised, it is probably best to arrange it. Similarly, should a patient ask to see a specific consultant believed to be inappropriate or poorly matched to the patient's needs, it is prudent to be upfront with the patient and suggest alternatives.

Steps in Referral

The process of referral and consultation involves five essential steps (Table 2) [3,21,25•,26]. Problems may occur at any point, usually because of failures in communication or discordant expectations [3,12•,20,21,22•,25•,26–29]. The most important step is formulating the question being asked. The consultant can't provide what is wanted if physi-

TABLE 1   REASONS FOR REFERRAL
Diagnosis or confirmation of diagnosis
Recommendations for therapy or management
Implementation of therapy or management
Performance of a specialty procedure
Routine specialty examination
Prior care by subspecialty consultant
Reassurance for patient, relative, or physician
Request by patient
Education of patient or physician
Medical-legal reasons
Transfer of patient care

TABLE 2   THE FIVE STEPS OF REFERRAL AND CONSULTATION
1. Referring physician and patient recognize need for consultation
2. Referring physician communicates reason for consultation and clinical information about patient to consultant
3. Consultant evaluates patient's condition
4. Consultant clearly communicates findings and recommendations to referring physician in a timely manner
5. Patient, referring physician, and consultant decide about continuing care

cians themselves don't know or have not asked for it clearly. The physician must ask, "What is it I want to know, and what is it I want the consultant to do?"

For example, in requesting a neurology consultation, rather than saying, "Diabetic patient with progressive lower extremity weakness," say, "Insulin-dependent diabetic with steroid-dependent chronic obstructive pulmonary disease and three-month history of progressive lower extremity weakness. Considering diabetic plexopathy versus steroid myopathy. Would appreciate your opinion and suggestions for evaluating and managing this problem."

In requesting a rehabilitation medicine consultation, it is less helpful to say, "Admitted for pneumonia, needs rehab" than to say "76-yo patient admitted for treatment of pneumonia who is now deconditioned because of extended bedrest. Wishes to be discharged home. Lives alone. Please evaluate for self care and mobility and intervene as necessary."

When choosing a consultant, the primary physician's responsibility is to ensure the best possible outcome for the patient. In these days of managed care there may be limitations on referral choices. In a system with referral limitations, the physician remains obliged to provide the right consultation options for the patient, even if it means recommending a consultant outside of the patient's health plan.

Physicians choose consultants based on reputation, the recommendations of colleagues, and their own personal experience. Consultants are sought who will give a skilled and thoughtful response, whose personality fits the patient well, and who will keep the referring physician informed.

The mode of contact with the consultant varies with circumstances and personal style. Commonly, contact is by telephone, which has the advantage of speed and the opportunity to clarify questions and expectations. In other instances formal letters or consultation forms are used. Some physicians use verbal instructions to their patients to convey the purpose of a consultation, but this carries a great risk for miscommunication.

It is important to provide the consultant with all relevant clinical information (Table 3), including results of diagnostic tests and procedures to avoid unnecessary duplication [25•,30]. It is helpful for the consultant to know of any previous therapy that has failed so that the same therapy is not recommended again. Consultants must know what responsibility for care they are to assume. It is courting disaster, for example, for the consulting physician to write aminoglycoside orders while thinking, incorrectly, that the primary physician will monitor blood levels and renal function. The consultant needs to know if a request is an emergency, urgent, or routine, as emergency consults must be seen immediately and urgent ones urgently. It is helpful for the consultant to know what the referring physician has told the patient about the referral so that the patient's expectations can be anticipated. Similarly, it is helpful for the consultant to know about any preferences or special attitudes of the patient, such as inordinate fear, fixed opinions of tests or treatments, or unreasonable expectations of outcome.

CONSULTATION

Now we turn to the consultant's role and the rules of effective consultation (Table 4) [12•,19–21,27–30,31••]. The consultant's first task is to understand what the referring physician wants. That is not always evident in the written consultation request or referral letter. A phone call to the referring physician may be needed to ascertain what the questions are and what specifically the consultant is being asked to do and when.

Next, consultants should carefully review the problem by interviewing and examining the patient, reviewing old records, or tracking down missing information when necessary. Because of their expertise and special perspective, consultants may recognize the significance of information overlooked or misinterpreted by others. They can also give the patient another chance to provide key information. The problem of one patient referred to find the cause of chronic postcholecystectomy right upper quadrant pain was illuminated when the consultant, after listening to the patient, confirmed the presence of a tender mass just where the patient said it was; at laparotomy, a stitch abscess was removed. Similarly, a telephone call to another hospital's

TABLE 3 INFORMATION CONSULTANTS NEED FROM REFERRING PHYSICIAN
Specific reason for consultation
Current medical problems
Current medications
Diagnostic test and procedure results
Previous therapeutic failures
Specific responsibility for care consultant is to assume
How soon consultant needs to see patient
What patient has been told about referral
Any special patient attitude about the problem

TABLE 4 RULES FOR EFFECTIVE CONSULTATION
Define what referring physician wants
Establish urgency
Look for yourself
Address referring physician's concerns
Make specific and succinct recommendations
Limit number of recommendations to fewer than six, if possible
Include problem list
Call referring physician
Make follow-up visit

record room may confirm whether a lung nodule was present 2 years ago.

The consultant's recommendations should be succinct and directed to the questions posed by the referring physician. Compliance with recommendations increase when recommendations are fewer than six [28,29], identified as crucial [29], and focused on issues central to current patient care [27–29]; when drug dosages and regimens are specific [27,31••]; and when follow-up visits are made [27–29]. Use problem lists in consultation notes or letters. A group of British general practitioners overwhelmingly preferred a letter with a problem list over one containing the same information in the conventional narrative format [32]. Unless it is certain that the referring physician will see the consultant's note in suitable time, the referring physician should be telephoned. There is no substitute for direct contact to discuss recommendations and plans [27].

Secondary referrals or major interventions should not be undertaken that have not been mutually agreed upon beforehand [25•]. It is extremely disconcerting for a referring physician to learn that a patient referred for evaluation of an abnormal mammogram has had a radical mastectomy.

Finally, it is important to communicate with the patient as well as the referring physician [7•]. Many consultants report their conclusions and recommendations verbally to the patient. Others believe the results of the consultation should be conveyed to the patient by the referring physician, who knows the patient better, particularly if there is bad news. What and how much patients should be told varies according to the circumstances, but discretion and sensitivity are important. If in doubt, consultants should contact the referring physician before talking with the patient.

AWKWARD ISSUES

In the process of referral and consultation several awkward issues can be counted upon to arise. One is the problem of the referring physician or the consultant concluding that poor medical care has been given by the other. In this situation, as always, the patient's best interests come first, and an appropriate care plan should be recommended to the patient as gently and tactfully as possible without denigrating the character or clinical skills of the physician in question [31••]. What is to be done if a medical error or a situation that looks like an error is discovered? First, more investigation is warranted to be certain an error has, indeed, occurred. A conversation with the physician in question can establish whether the patient and/or the medical information accurately represents what happened. If an error is confirmed, the patient has a right to disclosure and there is a duty to disclose. If the error had significant consequences for the patient, some method for disclosure is imperative [7•]. Again, it is preferable that the error is acknowledged by the physician in question and the disclosure be by that physician alone or with the other.

Another problem is that of disagreement between a referring and a consulting physician over an important matter of management. Resolution of the conflict will most often be achieved by discussion between the two physicians [27,31••,33•]. But what if it cannot? The consulting physician should document any recommendations in the chart and has the right to discuss the recommendations with the patient, preferably with the permission of or in the presence of the referring physician. A second opinion should be sought [33•].

Last is the situation in which the patient wants the consultant to become the primary physician or to completely take over care when such was not intended by the referring physician. A sure way for a consulting physician's practice to suffer is to develop a reputation for "stealing" patients [25•,27]. The referral-consultant relationship should be explained to the patient, who should be urged to discuss concerns with the referring physician. Should the patient be unwilling to do so, however, it is not unethical to accept the patient in this circumstance.

It would be proper for the consultant to inform the referring physician of the patient's wishes and the reasons for them, along with a description of the consultant's attempts to return the patient to the referring physician.

To be a good consultant, make communication a priority, establish what the consultant's task is, be specific and to the point, follow up, and transmit what is important to the patient and to the referring physician.

GETTING PAID

Health care in the United States is also in trouble because of the constantly changing managed care organizations, insurers, and Medicare rules regarding reimbursement. Physicians asked what they found most helpful in getting their claims paid usually said, "Have a good coder." But even a good coder can't get optimum results if the right things haven't been done. Here are some suggestions that may help. First, when billing a consult versus a simple visit, be certain to meet the necessary three criteria to meet consult billing level. These criteria are 1) the service is provided by a physician whose opinion or advice regarding evaluation and/or management of a specific problem is requested by another physician or appropriate source. 2) A physician consultant may initiate diagnostic and/or therapeutic services. 3) The request for a consultation from the attending physician or other appropriate source and the need for consultation is documented in the patient's medical record. The consultant's opinion and any services that are ordered or performed must also be documented in the patient's medical record and communicated to the requesting physician or other appropriate source [34•]. This last reference contains many tips for what language to use and not use, what steps to take to back up consultation codes, when consults may be claimed, and so forth.

Second, read the articles "When to Bill for a Consultation" [35•] for tips to help you understand Medicare's rules for reimbursement, and "Best Practices in Claims Processing" [36•] for strategies to help you minimize claims delays and denials.

KEY REFERENCES

Recently published papers of outstanding interest, as identified in *References and Recommended Reading*, have been annotated.

•• Harrold L, Field T, Gurwitz J: Knowledge, patterns of care, and outcomes of care for generalists and specialists. *J Gen Intern Med* 1999, 14:499–511.

This review article evaluates the differences between generalist and specialist physicians in these three domains.

•• Pearson S: Principles of generalists-specialists relationships. *J Gen Intern Med* 1999, 14(suppl 1):513–520.

Discussion of the guiding principles of generalist-specialist relationships, the joint and separate duties in consultation and referral, and the duties of health plans in supporting these relationships.

REFERENCES AND RECOMMENDED READING

Recently published papers of particular interest have been highlighted as:
• Of interest
•• Of outstanding interest

1. Ahmed A, Allman RM, Kiefe CI, *et al.*: Association of consultation between generalists and cardiologists with quality and outcomes of heart failure care. *Am Heart J* 145:1086–1093.

2.•• Harrold L, Field T, Gurwitz J: Knowledge, patterns of care, and outcomes of care for generalists and specialists. *J Gen Intern Med* 1999, 14:499–511.

3. Franks P, Clancy C, Nutting P: Gatekeeping revisited-protecting patients from overtreatment. *N Engl J Med* 1992, 327:424–429.

4. Bodenheimer T, Lo B, Caslino L: Primary care physicians should be coordinators, not gatekeepers. *JAMA* 1999, 281:2045–2049.

5.• Dudley R, Luft H: Managed care in transition. *N Engl J Med* 2001, 344:1087–1092.

6. Anthony D: Changing the nature of physician referral relationships in the US: the impact of managed care. *Social Sci Med* 2003, 56:2033–2044.

7.• Jacobson J: Keeping the patient in the loop: ethical issues in outpatient referral and consultation. *J Clin Ethics* 2002, 13:301–309.

8. Forrest C, Nutting P, Werner J, *et al.*: Managed health plan effects on the specialty referral process: results from the Ambulatory Sentinel Practice Network Referral study. *Med Care* 2003, 41:242–253.

9. Ferris T, Chang Y, Blumenthal D, Pearson S: Leaving gatekeeping behind - effects of opening access to specialists for adults in a health maintenance organization. *N Engl J Med* 2001, 345:1312–1317.

10. Lawrence D: Gatekeeping reconsidered. *N Engl J Med* 2001, 345:1342–1343.

11. Lewis JB, Morrison RE, Arnold A: Using a general internal medicine consult service to teach residents and care for patients. *Am J Med Sci* 2003, 326:73–78.

12.• Epstein R: Communication between primary care physicians and consultants. *Arch Fam Med* 1995, 4:403–409.

13. Salem-Schatz S, Moore G, Rucker M, Pearson S: The case for case-mix adjustment in practice profiling. *JAMA* 1994, 272:871–874.

14.• Franks P, Williams G, Zwanziger J, *et al.*: Why do physicians vary so widely in their referral rates? *J Gen Intern Med* 2000, 15:163–168.

15. Braun BL, Fowles JD, Forrest CB, *et al.*: Which enrollees bypass their gatekeepers in a point-of-service plan? *Med Care* 2003, 41:836–841.

16. Trude S, Stoddard JJ: Referral gridlock–primary care physicians and mental health services. *J Gen Intern Med* 2003, 18:442–449.

17.• Haas JS, Phillips KA, Baker LC, *et al.*: In the prevalence of gatekeeping in a community associated with individual trust in medical care? *Med Care* 2003, 41:660–668.

18. Reynolds G, Chitnis J, Roland M: General practitioner outpatient referrals: do good doctors refer more patients to hospital? *BMJ* 1991, 302:1250–1252.

19. Calman N, Hyman R, Licht W: Variability in consultation rates and practitioner level of diagnostic certainty. *J Fam Pract* 1992, 35:31–38.

20. Lee T, Pappius E, Goldman L: Impact of inter-physician communication on the effectiveness of medical consultations. *Am J Med* 1983, 74:106–112.

21. McPhee S, Lo B, Saika G, Meltzer R: How good is communication between primary care physicians and subspecialty consultants(?) *Arch Intern Med* 1984, 144:1265–1268.

22.• Bourquet C, Gilchrist V, McCord G: The consultation and referral process: a report from NEON. *J Fam Pract* 1998, 46:47–53.

23. Donohue M, Kravitz K, Wheeler D, *et al.*: Reasons for outpatient referrals from generalists to specialists. *J Gen Intern Med* 1999, 14:281–286.

24.• Golub R: Curbside consultations and the viaduct effect. *JAMA* 1998, 280:229–286.

25.• Williams PT, Peet G: Differences in the value of clinical information: referring physicians versus consulting specialists. *J Am Board Fam Pract* 1994, 7:292–302.

26. Stoller JK, Striet R: Inpatient consultation–results of a physician survey and a proposed improvement. *J Healthcare Qual* 2003, 25:27–35.

27. Goldman L, Lee T, Rudd P: Ten commandments for effective consultations. *Arch Intern Med* 1983, 143:1753–1755.

28. Sears C, Charlson M: The effectiveness of a consultation: compliance with initial recommendations. *Am J Med* 1983, 74:870–876.

29. Pupa L, Coventry J, Hanley J, Carpenter J: Factors affecting compliance for general medicine consultations to non-internists. *Am J Med* 1986, 81:508–514.

30. Newton J, Eccles M, Hutchinson A: Communication between general practicioners and consultants: what should their letters contain? *BMJ* 1992, 304:821–824.

31.•• Pearson S: Principles of generalists-specialists relationships. *J Gen Intern Med* 1999, 14(suppl 1):513–520.

32. Lloyd B, Barnett P: Use of problem lists in letters between hospital doctors and general practitioners. *BMJ* 1993, 306:247.

33.• Stinson M: Conflicts in consultation. *J S C Med Assoc* 1996, Jan:14–17.

34.• *Coding Answer Book* Rockville, MD: Decision Health; 2003:Vol A-L:12801–12826.

35.• Moore K: When to bill for a consultation. *Fam Pract Management* 1999, 6:11.

36.• Backer L: Best practices in claims processing. *Fam Pract Management* 2003, 10:19–24.

Preoperative Consultation

Adam M. Brodsky
Maher Nahlawi
Thomas A. Holly

Key Points
- Clinical history, including functional capacity, is an important component of the evaluation.
- Noninvasive and invasive testing where appropriate can help to risk-stratify patients and guide possible therapy to reduce the perioperative risk.
- Preoperative consultation should also give an assessment of long-term prognosis, because this may affect decisions regarding type of surgery and possible preoperative interventions.

More than 25 million patients undergo noncardiac surgery in the United States each year. One million of these patients have known coronary artery disease (CAD), another 2 to 3 million have multiple risk factors for CAD, and another 6 million are at risk because they are older than 65 years [1,2]. Surgery imposes many stresses on the cardiovascular system (Table 1) and can tip the myocardial supply/demand balance over the line that separates tolerable function from ischemia and/or infarction. Thus, it is not surprising that the occurrence of perioperative cardiac events is the leading cause of death after noncardiac surgery [1].

Risk stratification is therefore an important part of the preoperative evaluation of patients. It requires knowledge of the planned operation and anesthesia and the stresses they impose on the cardiovascular system, the general medical condition of the patient, and the specific degree of CAD, myocardial dysfunction, and risk of ischemia that the individual brings to the procedure. Evaluation requires a thorough history and physical examination, and when appropriate, further noninvasive or invasive testing and medical stabilization. Such an evaluation also provides an assessment of long-term prognosis.

TYPE OF SURGERY

To stratify patients appropriately by risk, one must consider the risk of the specific surgical procedure (Table 2). Aortic and other major vascular, peripheral vascular procedures, prolonged surgical procedures associated with large fluid shifts or blood loss, and emergency operations are considered to carry a high risk for cardiac complications. Vascular surgery carries many potential stresses including blood loss, intraoperative hypotension, and large fluid shifts. Orthopedic, intraperitoneal, intrathoracic, head and neck, carotid endarterectomy, and prostate surgery are considered intermediate risk for perioperative cardiac complications. Orthopedic surgery often involves prolonged operative time with considerable blood loss and large fluid shifts and is often performed on elderly patients. Conversely, endoscopic, ophthalmologic, superficial, and breast surgical procedures generally are believed to carry low risks [2].

ANESTHESIA

Consideration of the risk of surgery necessitates some comment on the choice of anesthesia. There is little evidence that spinal or epidural anesthetic techniques are safer for cardiac patients [3–6]. Both spinal and epidural anesthesia can cause hypotension secondary to sympathetic blockade; furthermore, these techniques are not as easily reversible as is general anesthesia. In general, the choice of anesthesia has not been found to influence perioperative outcomes. However, Goldman *et al.* [7] did find that patients with a history of congestive heart failure (CHF) or severe left ventricular dysfunction were less likely to develop postoperative CHF when spinal or epidural anesthesia was used.

CLINICAL ASSESSMENT

The initial history, physical examination, and electrocardiogram (ECG) are essential components of the clinical assessment of patients undergoing major noncardiac surgery. The physician should focus on the identification of potentially serious cardiac disorders, including CAD (*eg*, prior myocardial infarction [MI], angina pectoris), congestive heart failure, symptomatic arrhythmias, or major valvular disease. In addition, disease severity, stability, and prior treatment are important components of the initial clinical assessment (Table 3). Other factors that help determine cardiac risk include age, comorbid conditions (*eg*, diabetes, renal dysfunction, pulmonary disease), and type of surgery. Functional capacity has also been shown to be a reliable predictor of perioperative and long-term events even after adjustment for other baseline clinical risk factors. Daily activity levels of less than four metabolic equivalents (METs) are generally associated with a higher risk of cardiac events (Table 4) [2].

The American College of Cardiology (ACC) and the American Heart Association (AHA) have produced joint guidelines for perioperative cardiac evaluation for noncardiac surgery, developed by the ACC/AHA Task Force on Practice Guidelines [2]. A stepwise Bayesian strategy that relies on assessment of clinical markers, prior coronary evaluation and treatment, functional capacity, and surgery-specific risk was developed. The preoperative

TABLE 1 SURGICAL STRESSES

Preoperative

Anxiety—increases blood pressure, heart rate, catecholamine levels

Sedation—may impair ventilation

Intraoperative

Anesthesia—can cause myocardial depression

Impaired ventilation—decreases oxygenation and causes acid-base disturbances

Blood pressure fluctuations—may cause myocardial ischemia due to decreased coronary blood flow (hypotension) or increased myocardial oxygen demand (hypertension)

Blood loss—decreases myocardial oxygen delivery

Compromised function of vital organs, especially secondary to hypotension

Acid-base disturbances

Reactions to drugs, blood products

Volume overload—increases preload; decreases oxygenation secondary to pulmonary congestion

Hypovolemia—decreases cardiac output; decreases flow to myocardium and other vital organs

Hyper- or hypothermia, shivering—increases myocardial oxygen demand

Postoperative

Hypovolemia related to blood loss, vomiting, diaphoresis, poor intake, excessive diuresis

Anemia secondary to blood loss—decreases myocardial oxygen delivery

Volume overload from excessive transfusion, fluid infusions

Sepsis—markedly increases myocardial oxygen demands

Venous or arterial thrombosis related to postoperative clotting factor changes and immobility

Endocarditis—can directly affect cardiac valvular function, as well as increasing metabolic demands

Reactions to drugs, blood products

Anxiety

Adapted from Ockene and Holly [34].

evaluation process is presented as a flow chart, which constitutes a framework for determining which patients are candidates for further cardiac testing. The algorithm is summarized in Table 5. The urgency of noncardiac surgery, previous coronary revascularization, previous coronary evaluation, type of surgery, functional capacity, and the clinical predictors of cardiac risk are all essential information for the decision to proceed with surgery or with further cardiac testing.

A number of studies have examined the relationship between CAD, especially antecedent MI, and the risk of surgery. Steen *et al.* [5] reviewed the records of 73,321 patients who underwent anesthesia and noncardiac surgery at the Mayo Clinic; 587 of these patients had suffered previous MIs. Thirty-six (6.1%) had a reinfarction, and 25 of the 36 (69%) died. The relationship of morbidity and mortality to the length of time between infarction and surgery in this study is shown in Table 6. It is likely that the explanation for the higher morbidity and mortality in these patients is related to residual ischemia, as well as left ventricular dysfunction. If at all possible, major surgery should be delayed for 6 months after an MI, although risk stratification with noninvasive testing may permit the identification of a low-risk subset that may safely undergo surgery earlier.

Patients with peripheral arterial disease (PAD) present a particularly interesting problem. These patients have a high incidence of associated CAD, but because their ability to exercise may be limited by claudication, they may have little or no angina. Routine coronary arteriography in patients with PAD has shown that the incidence of significant (but

TABLE 3 CLINICAL PREDICTORS OF INCREASED PERIOPERATIVE CARDIOVASCULAR RISK

Major
  Unstable coronary syndromes
    Recent MI (<1 month) with evidence of important ischemic risk by clinical symptoms or noninvasive study
    Unstable or severe angina (Canadian Cardiovascular Society class III or IV)
  Decompensated CHF
  Significant arrhythmias
    High-grade AV block
    Symptomatic ventricular arrhythmias
    Supraventricular arrhythmias with uncontrolled ventricular rate
  Severe valvular disease
Intermediate
  Mild angina pectoris (Canadian Cardiovascular Society class I or II)
  Prior MI by history or pathologic Q waves
  Compensated or prior HF
  Diabetes mellitus
Minor
  Advanced age
  Abnormal ECG (LVH, LBBB, ST-T abnormalities)
  Rhythm other than sinus (*eg*, AF)
  Low functional capacity (*eg*, unable to climb one flight of stairs with a bag of groceries)
  History of stroke
  Uncontrolled systemic hypertension

AF—atrial fibrillation; AV—atrioventricular; CHF—congestive heart failure; ECG—electrocardiogram; HF—heart failure; LBBB—left bundle branch block; LVH—left ventricular hypertrophy; MI—myocardial infarction.

TABLE 2 CARDIAC EVENT RISK* STRATIFICATION FOR NONCARDIAC SURGICAL PROCEDURES

High (reported cardiac risk is often > 5%)
  Emergent major operations, particularly in the elderly
  Aortic and major vascular surgeries
  Peripheral vascular surgery
  Anticipated prolonged surgical procedures associated with large fluid shifts or blood loss
Intermediate (reported cardiac risk is generally <5%)
  Carotid endarterectomy
  Head and neck surgeries
  Intraperitoneal and intrathoracic surgeries
  Orthopedic surgery
  Prostate surgery
Low (reported cardiac risk is generally <1%)
  Endoscopic procedures
  Superficial procedures
  Cataract surgery
  Breast surgery

*Combined incidence of cardiac death and nonfatal myocardial infarction.

TABLE 4 METABOLIC EQUIVALENTS

METs	Activities
1	Activities of daily living (*eg*, eating, dressing, using the toilet)
1–3	Walking around the house, walking one block on level ground
4	Light housework (*eg*, washing dishes, dusting, cleaning); climbing one flight of stairs; jogging a short distance
5–10	Heavy housework (*eg*, scrubbing floors, moving furniture, lifting boxes); golf; bowling; dancing; doubles tennis
> 10	Singles tennis, swimming, skiing, basketball, football

Adapted from Eagle *et al.* [2].
METs—metabolic equivalents.

often asymptomatic) CAD may be more than 30%. In a study of 1000 cases from the Cleveland Clinic, Hertzer *et al.* [8] found that 34% of patients undergoing peripheral vascular surgery and clinically suspected of having CAD as well as 14% of those without clinical evidence for CAD had "severe, correctable" CAD documented by catheterization. Additionally, these patients carry a similar 10-year risk of cardiovascular death or myocardial infarction as do patients with established coronary artery disease [9].

NONINVASIVE TESTING

The value of exercise testing and, in particular, the determination of functional capacity in preoperative evaluation has been known for some time. In 1981, Cutler *et al.* [10] showed that ECG stress testing was especially valuable in the preoperative assessment of patients with PAD. Patients who achieved more than 75% of maximum predicted heart rate (MPHR) and had no ischemic ECG changes (35 of

	Functional capacity	High-risk surgery	Intermediate-risk surgery	Low-risk surgery
Major clinical predictors	N/A	Consider delaying or canceling surgery with medical management vs coronary angiography with treatment dictated by results		
Intermediate clinical predictors	Poor	Stress test	Stress test	Mild or no increased risk (go to OR)
	Moderate or greater	Stress test	Mild or no increased risk (go to OR)	Mild or no increased risk (go to OR)
Minor clinical predictors	Poor	Stress test	Mild or no increased risk (go to OR)	Mild or no increased risk (go to OR)
	Moderate or greater	Mild or no increased risk (go to OR)	Mild or no increased risk (go to OR)	Mild or no increased risk (go to OR)

TABLE 5 STEPWISE APPROACH TO PREOPERATIVE CARDIAC ASSESSMENT BASED ON THE PATIENT CHARACTERISTICS AND THE SURGICAL RISK

If the need for noncardiac surgery is an emergency, proceed to the OR regardless of the patient cardiac risk. Postoperative risk stratification and risk factor management should be implemented.

If the patient has undergone coronary revascularization within the previous 5 years without recurrent symptoms, proceed with surgery. No further testing is required.

If the patient has undergone recent coronary evaluation (*ie*, within the past 2 years) and the results were favorable with no change in symptoms, proceed with surgery.

"Poor" functional capacity: <4 METs. "Moderate or greater" functional capacity: able to perform >4 METs of activity.

"Stress test" refers to exercise or pharmacologic stress, depending on the patient. Nuclear or echocardiographic imaging may be useful in certain situations (*eg*, pharmacologic stress, baseline ECG abnormalities).

If the noninvasive stress test reveals high-risk findings, coronary angiography and possibly coronary revascularization should be considered.

ECG—electrocardiogram; METs—metabolic equivalents; OR—operating room.

TABLE 6 MYOCARDIAL REINFARCTION AND MORTALITY*

Time of surgery after infarct, *mo*	Patients, *n*	Postoperative reinfarctions, *n (%)*	Deaths, *n (%)*
0–3	15	4 (27)	4 (100)
4–6	17	2 (11)	1 (50)
7–12	31	2 (6)	2 (100)
13–18	30	1 (3)	0 (0)
19–24	17	1 (6)	1 (100)
>25	383	15 (4)	8 (53)
Unknown	93	11 (12)	9 (82)
Total	587	36 (6.1)	25 (69)

*Relation to interval from previous myocardial infarction.

105 patients) had no postoperative cardiac complications. In contrast, in the highest-risk group (26 patients with an ischemic ECG response at <75% of maximum predicted heart rate), there were 10 postoperative cardiac complications (38%), including seven MIs (27%), five of which were fatal. Others [11–14] have shown that failure to achieve 85% MPHR, 5 METs, or a heart rate of 100 are predictors of a poor outcome. ECG evidence of ischemia is less predictive than poor functional capacity, but when added to it, indicates even greater risk.

Dipyridamole-thallium testing has become an established noninvasive alternative to conventional stress testing for patients at high risk for CAD who cannot exercise because of PAD or orthopedic problems. Several studies have demonstrated the use of dipyridamole-thallium imaging in the preoperative assessment of cardiac risk. Reversible perfusion defects, indicating ischemia, are a significant predictor of perioperative cardiac events.

Although its sensitivity for detecting patients at increased risk is excellent, dipyridamole-thallium imaging for preoperative screening carries a relatively low specificity for clinical events. To improve the specificity and positive predictive value, some investigators have tried combining clinical markers with noninvasive testing, and others have demonstrated that quantifying the amount of myocardium at risk can better define patients at risk for perioperative cardiac events.

Eagle et al. [15] performed preoperative dipyridamole-thallium testing and clinical evaluation in 254 patients before major vascular procedures. Surgery was subsequently performed in 200. Of these 200 patients, 30 (15%) had early postoperative ischemic events; there were six deaths (3%) and nine nonfatal MIs (4.5%). Thallium redistribution was highly predictive of subsequent events, as were five clinical variables (ie, Q waves on ECG, history of ventricular ectopic activity, diabetes, age >70 years, angina). Use of both the clinical and thallium data yielded significantly higher specificity with no loss of sensitivity. The authors noted that for nearly half of the patients, very low or very

high operative risk could be predicted on the basis of clinical variables alone, making dipyridamole-thallium imaging unnecessary (Fig. 1).

A number of other studies have shown that there is a strong correlation between the extent of reversible thallium defects and the risk of cardiac death or MI. Brown and Rowen [16] developed a method to stratify perioperative risk based on the number of segments with transient thallium defects and a history of diabetes mellitus. The impact of combining these methods with clinical indices such as those described by Eagle et al. [15] has not been tested to date.

Dobutamine stress echocardiography (DSE) has been used to identify patients at risk for cardiac complications of surgery. Several studies have described the usefulness of DSE in diagnosing CAD. In the largest series, Poldermans et al. [17] demonstrated the ability of DSE to identify patients at high and low risk for vascular surgery. In their study, 24% of patients with new or worsened regional wall motion abnormalities suffered a perioperative MI or cardiac death compared with none of those who had a negative DSE result. All 27 patients with perioperative cardiac events (unstable angina, n=10; nonfatal MI, n=12; cardiac death, n=5) had positive test results (Fig. 2).

As with dipyridamole-thallium scintigraphy, it appears that DSE may not enhance the risk assessment in clinically low-risk patients. In contrast, however, DSE is useful in both intermediate- and high-clinical-risk patients because the absence of a new segmental wall motion abnormality with stress may be able to identify a very low-risk group regardless of the clinical risk stratification. On the other hand, the presence of a new wall motion abnormality identifies patients at high risk for perioperative cardiac events.

Ambulatory ECG monitoring also has been shown to identify ischemia in symptomatic patients with normal 12-lead ECGs and negative exercise tolerance test results [18] and in patients with silent ischemia [19]. Raby et al. [20] prospectively studied 176 patients undergoing elective vascular surgery. A total of 32 patients had ST segment

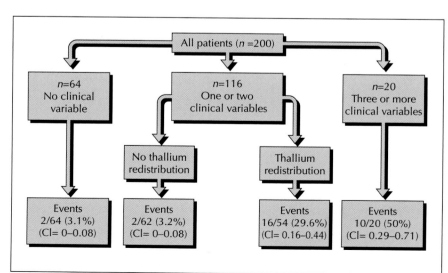

FIGURE 1 Algorithm for using clinical variables and results of dipyridamole-thallium imaging to stratify cardiac risk as applied to this group of 200 patients. Event refers to postoperative cardiac ischemic events including unstable angina, ischemic pulmonary edema, myocardial infarction, or cardiac death. Clinical variables are presence of Q wave on electrocardiogram, age > 70 years, history of angina, history of ventricular ectopic activity requiring treatment, and diabetes mellitus requiring treatment. CI—confidence interval. (Adapted from Eagle et al. [15].)

depression on preoperative ambulatory ECG monitoring. Of these, 12 patients had postoperative ischemic events (MI, unstable angina, or ischemic pulmonary edema) compared with only one of 144 patients who did not have preoperative ischemia on ambulatory monitoring. The sensitivity of ST depression on ambulatory monitoring was 92%, specificity was 88%, positive predictive value was 38%, and negative predictive value was 99%. The use of this test is limited, however, by a relatively low sensitivity and thus by the inability to reliably define a low-risk group, and because this test cannot be performed in patients with baseline ECG abnormalities. The current evidence does not support the use of ambulatory ECG as the only diagnostic test.

INVASIVE TESTING

In general, indications for preoperative coronary angiography are similar to those identified for the nonoperative setting. For certain patients at high risk or who are unable to undergo stress testing, it may be appropriate to proceed with coronary angiography rather than perform a noninvasive test. Patients with high-risk results during noninvasive testing, unstable angina pectoris, or nondiagnostic or equivocal noninvasive test in a high-risk patient undergoing a high-risk noncardiac surgery are appropriate indications for coronary angiography [21].

In summary, clinical information combined with appropriate noninvasive testing can select a subset of patients who are at high risk for a perioperative cardiac event. These patients, if appropriate, should undergo invasive testing with a view towards possible revascularization before their noncardiac surgery.

LONG-TERM PROGNOSIS

Although the immediate purpose of preoperative examination is to assess the patient's perioperative risk, determination of long-term prognosis is an important part of the eval-

uation because long-term prognosis affects the risk/benefit ratio of the contemplated procedure. This topic has been most extensively studied in vascular surgery patients. Hendel *et al.* [22,23] demonstrated the value of thallium scanning for this purpose. Although reversible defects are associated with perioperative cardiac events, fixed defects are associated with late events (Fig. 3). A poor long-term outlook may lead to the conclusion that the planned surgery is inappropriate, and such knowledge may help the patient and physician make decisions regarding the necessity of high-risk surgery or the benefit of major preoperative interventions (*ie*, percutaneous transluminal coronary angioplasty [PTCA] or coronary artery bypass surgery [CABG]).

MANAGEMENT

Appropriate management of patients perioperatively may include preoperative coronary revascularization as well as pharmacologic therapy. Equally important is appropriate postoperative management, as most perioperative cardiac events occur in the postoperative setting. This may be due to increased circulating catecholamines, and thus adequate pain control should be assured.

The appropriate role of CABG and PTCA in the preoperative management of the patient with coronary aretery disease undergoing noncardiac surgery is still debated, although there are many who feel that under appropriate circumstances mechanical revascularization prevents ischemic morbidity and mortality during subsequent noncardiac surgery.

Foster *et al.* [24] examined this issue in an analysis of data from the Coronary Artery Surgery Study (CASS). Patients without significant CAD had an operative mortality of 0.5%, similar to that of patients with significant CAD who had CABG performed before noncardiac surgery (0.9%). For patients with significant CAD undergoing noncardiac surgery without prior CABG, the operative mortality was 2.4%, significantly higher than in the other

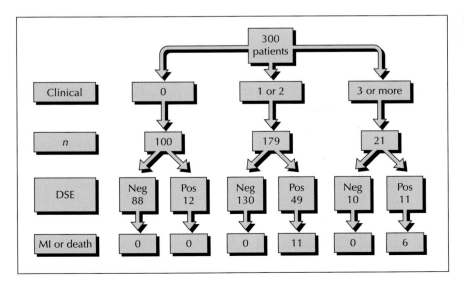

FIGURE 2 The interaction of clinical variables and dobutamine stress echocardiography (DSE) results with regard to perioperative outcomes. Clinical variables are age older than 70 years, angina, diabetes requiring treatment, Q waves on electrocardiogram (ECG), and a history of ventricular ectopy. MI—myocardial infarction; Neg—normal DSE; Pos—new wall motion abnormalities during DSE. (*Adapted from* Poldermans *et al.* [17].)

two groups. The incidence of perioperative MI and arrhythmia was similar in the three groups. Of note, the perioperative mortality associated with CABG itself was 1.4%.

A few studies have examined the use of PTCA before noncardiac surgery. Huber *et al.* [25] looked at the incidence of perioperative MI and death in a group of 50 high-risk patients undergoing 54 operations a median of 9 days after angioplasty. The overall frequency of perioperative MI was 5.6%, and the mortality was 1.9%. Although there was no control group, they concluded that patients who have had successful PTCA for severe CAD have a low risk of major cardiac complications associated with noncardiac surgery.

Another study from the Mayo Clinic [26] compared the cardiac morbidity, mortality, and survival of patients who underwent PTCA (*n*=14) or CABG (*n*=86) before abdominal aortic aneurysm repair. The rate of perioperative MI was 0% for the PTCA group and 5.8% for the CABG group, and no hospital deaths occurred in either group. However, the 3-year survival was not statistically different between the groups.

Kaluza *et al.* [27] retrospectively studied 40 consecutive patients from one institution who had undergone coronary stenting less than 6 weeks prior to elective or semielective noncardiac surgery. They found a high rate of catastrophic complications, such as major bleeding, ST segment elevation MI, or death (9/40 patients, including eight deaths). Acute stent thrombosis was felt to be the cause of all of the MIs in the cohort. Most patients had aspirin and/or ticlopidine held perioperatively. Notably, all deaths and MIs occurred in patients who had surgery less than 14 days after coronary stenting [27]. Wilson *et al.* [28] retrospectively looked at 207 patients at the Mayo clinic who had noncardiac surgery within 2 months of stent placement and found eight major adverse events, including six deaths, all of which occurred in patients who had surgery within 6 weeks of stent placement.

In summary, these studies are all limited in that they are not randomized, prospective trials, and many are statistically underpowered. The available data suggest that while antecedent balloon angioplasty may be safely performed, coronary stenting prior to elective noncardiac surgery carries a high risk of major complications, expecially if the surgery is performed within 2 to 6 weeks of stenting. This is an area that deserves further study. Of particular interest is the fact that newer stents, such as drug-eluting stents, have not been studied. These stents are generally felt to require a longer duration of antiplatelet therapy due to the possibility of drug-induced delayed endothelialization and the attendant risk of stent thrombosis. In general, elective noncardiac surgery should be delayed for at least 2 and preferably 6 weeks after percutaneous coronary revascularization. Although balloon angioplasty may seem like a safe alternative to coronary stenting in this setting, it must be appreciated that stenting may be unavoidable in some cases (due to suboptimal angiographic results or complications such as dissection), even if the original intent was to perform only ballon angioplasty. Nonetheless, mechanical intervention may be indicated in selected high-risk patients who are scheduled to undergo a major noncardiac operation, bearing in mind the morbidity and mortality of the myocardial revascularization procedure itself.

The management of drug therapy perioperatively deserves special comment. Many surgical patients are taking antihypertensives, beta-blocking agents for ischemia, or digoxin. Almost all cardiac medications should be continued up to the time of surgery and resumed as soon as possible after surgery. Beta-blockers or nitrates may be given intravenously or topically (nitroglycerine paste) during periods when the patient is unable to take oral medications.

The prophylactic use of certain beta-blockers may actually decrease the occurrence of perioperative ischemia [29–31]. Mangano *et al.* [32] performed a randomized, double-blind, placebo-controlled trial to compare the effect of atenolol on survival and cardiovascular morbidity in 200 patients with or at risk for CAD who were undergoing

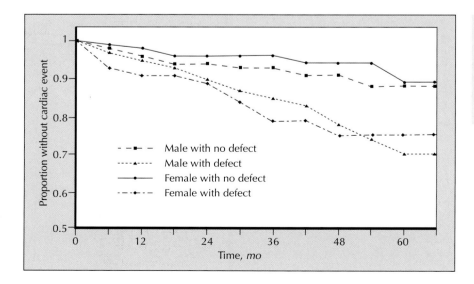

FIGURE 3 Myocardial infarction–free survival in men and women based on the presence or absence of a myocardial perfusion defect. A normal scan was associated with improved event-free survival in both men and women. (*Adapted from* Hendel *et al.* [23].)

noncardiac surgery. There was 78% reduction in overall mortality in the atenolol-treated patients at 1-year follow-up. Cardiac events were reduced by 67% within 1 year. These results were sustained at 2 years.

In another multicenter study, patients with at least one cardiac risk factor and a positive dobutamine stress echocardiogram for ischemia undergoing major vascular surgery were randomized to bisoprolol versus placebo. Bisoprolol reduced cardiac events in this high-risk group from 29% to 3% at 1 month [33]. The findings of these studies demonstrate the efficacy and safety of beta-blockers in patients with CAD who are undergoing major noncardiac surgery. Perioperative beta-blockade should be considered for such patients, and if the patient is taking a beta-blocker, it should be maintained perioperatively. It should be noted that atenolol and bisoprolol are the only beta-blockers that have been studied perioperatively in randomized trials. Furthermore, generalizability of these studies is unknown, as they were performed in a very select, high-risk group of patients. Nevertheless, it seems reasonable that beta-blockers be used in patients found to be at increased risk for perioperative coronary events.

Alpha-agonists have also been studied recently for use in perioperative cardiovascular risk reduction. Studies using both clonidine (an oral alpha-agonist) and mivazerol (an intravenous alpha-agonist) have been reported, which suggest that these agents may be useful in preventing perioperative cardiac events. These agents deserve further study before a firm recommendation can be made; however, they may be considered as an alternative to beta-blockers in selected patients [2].

History, physical examination, and ECG are all that are necessary for adequate preoperative risk assessment in the large majority of patients. Using some form of risk assessment criteria such as those in the ACC/AHA guidelines is helpful and may select out patients in whom further functional or anatomic information is needed. Exercise testing, dipyridamole-thallium imaging, echocardiography, dobutamine stress echocardiography, and cardiac catheterization provide additional information that can further define both the short-term perioperative risk as well as the long-term risk of future cardiovascular events. This information may then be used in the decision of whether or not to proceed with the planned surgery, as well as how best to treat the patient perioperatively and in the future.

REFERENCES

1. Mangano DT: Perioperative cardiac morbidity. *Anesthesiology* 1990, 72:153–184.

2. Eagle KA, Berger PB, Calkins H, *et al.*: ACC/AHA guideline update for perioperative cardiovascular evaluation for noncardiac surgery: a report of the American College of Cardiology/American Heart Association Task Force on Practice Guidelines (Committee to Update the 1996 Guidelines on Perioperative Cardiovascular Evaluation for Noncardiac Surgery). *J Am Coll Cardiol* 2002. 39:542–553.

3. Bode RH Jr, Lewis KP, Zarich SW, *et al.*: Cardiac outcome after peripheral vascular surgery: comparison of general and regional anesthesia. *Anesthesiology* 1996, 84:3–13.

4. O'Hara DA, Duff A, Berlin JA, *et al.*: The effect of anesthetic technique on postoperative outcomes in hip fracture repair. *Anesthesiology* 2000, 92:947–957.

5. Steen PA, Tinker JH, Tarhan S: Myocardial reinfarction after anesthesia and surgery. *JAMA* 1978, 239:2566–2570.

6. Goldman L, Caldera DL, Nussbaum SR, *et al.*: Multifactorial index of cardiac risk in noncardiac surgical procedures. *N Engl J Med* 1977, 297:845–850.

7. Goldman L, Caldera DL, Southwick FS, *et al.*: Cardiac risk factors and complications in non-cardiac surgery. *Medicine* 1978, 57:357–370.

8. Hertzer NR, Beven EG, Young JR, *et al.*: Coronary artery disease in peripheral vascular patients. *Ann Surg* 1984, 199:223–233.

9. Grundy SM, Becker D, Clark LT, *et al.*: Third Report of the National Cholesterol Education Program Expert Panel on Detection, Evaluation, and Treatment of High Blood Cholesterol in Adults (Adult Treatment Panel III). Bethesda: National Heart, Lung, and Blood Institute, National Institutes of Health. NIH Publication No. 02-5215; September, 2002.

10. Cutler BS, Wheeler HB, Paraskos JA, *et al.*: Applicability and interpretation of electrocardiographic stress testing in patients with peripheral vascular disease. *Am J Surg* 1981, 141:501–506.

11. Carliner NH, Fisher ML, Plotnick GD, *et al.*: Routine preoperative exercise testing in patients undergoing major noncardiac surgery. *Am J Cardiol* 1985, 56:51–58.

12. McPhail N, Calvin JE, Shariatmader A, *et al.*: The use of preoperative exercise testing to predict cardiac complications after arterial reconstruction. *J Vasc Surg* 1988, 7:60–68.

13. Gerson MC, Hurst JM, Hertzberg VS, *et al.*: Cardiac prognosis in noncardiac geriatric surgery. *Ann Intern Med* 1985, 103:832–837.

14. Kopecky SL, Gibbons RJ, Hollier LH: Preoperative supine exercise radionuclide angiogram predicts perioperative cardiovascular events in vascular surgery. *J Am Coll Cardiol* 1986, 7:226A.

15. Eagle KA, Coley CM, Newell JB: Combining clinical and thallium data optimizes preoperative assessment of cardiac risk before major vascular surgery. *Ann Intern Med* 1989, 110:859–866.

16. Brown KA, Rowen M: Extent of jeopardized viable myocardium determined by myocardial perfusion imaging predicts perioperative cardiac events in patients undergoing noncardiac surgery. *J Am Coll Cardiol* 1993, 21:325–330.

17. Poldermans D, Arnese M, Fioretti PM, *et al.*: Improved cardiac risk stratification in major vascular surgery with dobutamine-atropine stress echocardiography. *J Am Coll Cardiol* 1995, 26:648–653.

18. Stern S, Tzivoni D: Early detection of silent ischemic heart disease by 24-hour electrocardiographic monitoring of active subjects. *Br Heart J* 1974, 36:481–486.

19. Cohn PF: Silent myocardial ischemia: Classification, prevalence, and prognosis. *Am J Med* 1985, 79(suppl 3A):2–6.

20. Raby KE, Goldman L, Creager MA, *et al.*: Correlation between preoperative ischemia and major cardiac events after peripheral vascular surgery. *N Engl J Med* 1989, 321:1296–1300.

21. Scanlon PJ, Faxon DP, Audet A, *et al.*: Guidelines for coronary angiography: a report of the American College of Cardiology/American Heart association Task Force on Practice (Committee on Coronary Angiography) *J Am Coll Cardiol* 1999, 33:1756–1816.

22. Hendel RC, Whitfield SS, Villegas BJ, *et al.*: Prediction of late cardiac events by dipyridamole thallium imaging in patients undergoing elective vascular surgery. *Am J Cardiol* 1992, 70:1243–1249.

23. Hendel RC, Chen MH, L'Italien GJ, *et al.*: Sex differences in perioperative and long-term cardiac event-free survival in vascular surgery patients. *Circulation* 1995, 91:1044–1051.

24. Foster ED, Davis KB, Carpenter JA, *et al.*: Risk of noncardiac operation in patients with defined coronary disease: The coronary artery surgery study (CASS) registry experience. *Ann Thorac Surg* 1986, 41:42–50.

25. Huber KC, Evans MA, Bresnahan JF, *et al.*: Outcome of noncardiac operations in patients with severe coronary artery disease successfully treated preoperatively with coronary angioplasty. *Mayo Clin Proc* 1992, 67:15–21.

26. Elmore JR, Hallett JW, Gibbons RJ, *et al.*: Myocardial revascularization before abdominal aortic aneurysmorrhaphy: effect of coronary angioplasty. *Mayo Clin Proc* 1993, 68:637–641.

27. Kaluza GL, Joseph J, Lee JR, *et al.*: Catastrophic outcomes of noncardiac surgery soon after coronary stenting. *J Am Coll Cardiol* 2000, 35:1288–1294.

28. Wilson SH, Fasseas P, Orford JL, *et al.*: Clinical outcome of patients undergoing noncardiac surgery in the two months following coronary stenting. *J Am Coll Cardiol* 2003, 42:234–240.

29. Stone JG, Foex P, Sear JW, *et al.*: Myocardial ischemia in untreated hypertensive patients: effect of a single small oral dose of a beta-adrenergic blocking agent. *Anesthesiology* 1988, 68:495–500.

30. Pasternack PF, Grossi EA, Baumann FG, *et al.*: Beta blockade to decrease silent myocardial ischemia during peripheral vascular surgery. *Am J Surg* 1989, 158:113–116.

31. Pasternack PF, Imparato AM, Baumann FG, *et al.*: The hemodynamics of beta-blockade in patients undergoing abdominal aortic aneurysm repair. *Circulation* 1987, 76(suppl 3):1–7.

32. Mangano DT, Layug EL, Wallace A, *et al.*: Effect of atenolol on mortality and cardiovascular morbidity after noncardiac surgery. *N Engl J Med* 1996, 335:1713–1720.

33. Poldermans D, Boersma E, Bax JJ, *et al.*: The effect of bisoprolol on perioperative mortality and myocardial infarction in high-risk patients undergoing vascular surgery. *N Engl J Med* 1999, 341:1789–1794.

34. Ockene IS, Holly TA: Noncardiac surgery in the cardiac patient. In *Intensive Care Medicine*, edn 3. Edited by Rippe J, *et al.* Boston: Little, Brown; 1996.

Using and Interpreting Noninvasive Cardiac Tests

Robert C. Hendel
Mark F. Sasse

4

Key Points

- The clinician must use his or her clinical judgment in deciding how to use and interpret diagnostic tests, because no test is 100% accurate.

- Electrocardiograms can help to diagnose myocardial ischemia and arrhythmias, and suggest other conditions such as drug overdoses and electrolyte disturbances.

- Exercise or pharmacologic stress testing is used to diagnose coronary artery disease, offer prognostic information, and assess the need for or adequacy of revascularization.

- Echocardiography is used to assess systolic and diastolic function, evaluate valve function and pathology, and assess pericardial and myocardial pathology alone and in conjunction with exercise and pharmacologic stress testing.

- Nuclear cardiology is used to diagnose coronary artery disease, offer prognostic information after myocardial infarction and before noncardiac surgery, and in patients with known or suspected coronary disease.

- Technetium-99m–based radionuclides allow the physician to obtain information regarding ventricular function and myocardial perfusion from the same test.

- Cardiac magnetic resonance imaging, electron beam computed tomography, and multislice computed tomography are new imaging modalities that can be used in assessing coronary anatomy, cardiac structure, and myocardial function.

- Newer uses of noninvasive tests include imaging in the emergency department in patients with nondiagnostic electrocardiograms, and early imaging after myocardial infarction to assess the degree of myocardium damage and myocardial salvage.

- Serum proteins (C-reactive protein, myeloperoxidase, and brain natriuretic factor) offer new ways to diagnose cardiovascular disease and assess prognosis of patients at cardiac risk.

Noninvasive cardiac testing is playing an increasingly prominent role in the diagnosis, assessing prognosis, and treatment of patients with known or suspected heart disease. This trend is likely to continue given the current economic climate and the high expense and potential risk associated with invasive procedures. Technological advances in nuclear cardiology, radiology, echocardiography, laboratory chemistry, and electrocardiography now allow for enhanced diagnostic capabilities. Ample research also supports the prognostic value of these methods. New myocardial perfusion agents and improved instrumentation in nuclear cardiology have significantly improved the diagnostic accuracy for detection of coronary artery disease (CAD). Echocardiography has undergone rapid development; transesophageal probes are now able to detect thrombi or tumors as small as 1 mm. In addition, stress echocardiography is being used with increasing frequency and in a variety of patient populations. Magnetic resonance imaging (MRI), electron beam computed tomography (EBCT), and multislice spiral computed tomography (MSCT) have added new ways to image the heart and coronary arteries. Proteomics is an evolving field that will identify more patients at risk for cardiovascular disease.

This chapter reviews the different noninvasive cardiac modalities currently available and their applications as related to evaluation of coronary artery disease, valvular abnormalities, pericardial disorders, and arrhythmia evaluations.

TABLE 1 ELECTROCARDIOGRAPHIC LOCATION OF MYOCARDIAL INFARCTION

Inferior	II, III, aVF
Lateral	I, aVL, V_4–V_6
Septal	V_1–V_2
Anterior	V_2–V_4
Inferoposterior	II, III, aVF, V_1–V_2 ST depression
True posterior	Tall R wave in V_1

ELECTROCARDIOGRAPHY

The electrocardiogram (ECG) is the most commonly used diagnostic test in cardiology, providing a definitive diagnosis or helpful clues for many disorders. The ECG is predominantly used to diagnose myocardial ischemia or infarction, conduction disturbances, and arrhythmias, but also reveals clues to electrolyte imbalances, medication-induced abnormalities, and metabolic derangements.

Ischemia/Infarction

There are many possible electrocardiographic manifestations of myocardial ischemia including ST segment elevation, horizontal or downsloping ST segment depressions, symmetric T-wave inversion, normalization of a previously abnormal T wave (also called "pseudonormalization"), or QT prolongation. The location of myocardial injury may be ascertained by the ECG, as shown in Table 1. While a single ECG may provide a diagnosis, often a series of ECGs showing evolving changes or patterns is crucial. The

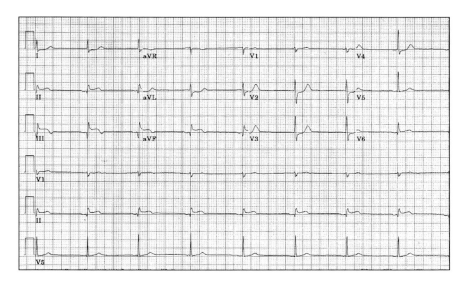

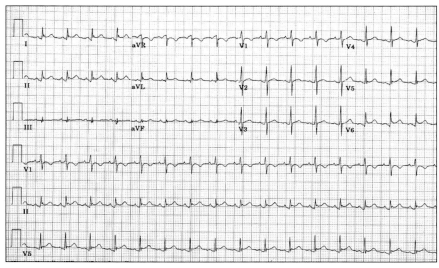

FIGURE 1 Evolutionary electrocardiographic changes associated with an acute myocardial infarction. Notice the ST segment elevations and small Q waves in the inferior leads, and the reciprocal ST segment depressions in the lateral leads. The ST depressions in leads V_1 and V_2 indicate posterior involvement as well. A cardiac catheterization revealed an occluded proximal right coronary artery. Temporal factors for these patterns are highly variable and may be influenced by acute interventions, such as thrombolytic therapy or angioplasty. See text for further details.

FIGURE 2 Electrocardiogram recording. The patient had a history of breast cancer and developed shortness of breath and severe, sharp chest pain worsened by motion and a supine position. Concave ST segment elevation is noted in virtually all leads, with prominent PR depression. The patient was diagnosed with pericarditis, and a moderate-sized pericardial effusion was noted on echocardiography.

classic sequence of ECG changes in the setting of an acute myocardial infarction (MI) begins with tall and peaked T waves (hyperacute) followed by convex ST segment elevations with ≥ 1 mm ST elevation in two or more contiguous leads (Fig. 1). The next step is the inversion of the T waves and the formation of Q waves. Other causes of ST segment elevations that may be confused with an acute MI are pericarditis (Fig. 2), electrolyte abnormalities, and a normal juvenile (variant) pattern. The presence of reciprocal changes with ST segment depression in leads other than those with ST segment elevation is a helpful clue for the diagnosis of acute infarction. Resting ST segment depression portends a poorer prognosis after MI than its absence [1,2]. Right ventricular involvement may be accurately diagnosed by the presence of ST elevation in the fourth right precordial lead [3].

Arrhythmias

In addition to diagnosing myocardial ischemia, the ECG may document and diagnose arrhythmias. Supraventricular tachyarrhythmias (SVT), which are usually narrow QRS complex rhythms, include atrial fibrillation, atrial flutter, atrial tachycardia, atrioventricular nodal reentrant tachycardia (AVNRT), and atrial reentrant tachycardia (also referred to as a bypass tract tachycardia, preexcitation, Wolff-Parkinson-White syndrome). AVNRT is the most common SVT and is characterized by an abrupt onset and abrupt termination. ECG manifestations feature an absence of a P wave or an inverted P wave just after the QRS. Preexcitation syndrome is characterized by delta waves on the ECG and a short P-R cycle. Adenosine may be used with the ECG to differentiate among several arrhythmias. If the SVT terminates abruptly, the rhythm was likely AVNRT. The transient atrioventricular (AV) block induced by adenosine also may uncover the "F" waves produced in atrial flutter. When a history of preexcitation is present, adenosine must be used with caution, because it may induce ventricular fibrillation.

When a wide QRS complex is present, it is often difficult to differentiate between ventricular tachycardia and SVT with aberrant conduction. However, criteria have been defined to improve the accuracy of the ECG diagnosis for wide complex tachycardias (Table 2) [4].

Chamber Enlargement/Left Ventricular Hypertrophy

Although there are established criteria for diagnosing chamber enlargement, the anatomic correlation tends to be poor. While characterization of ECG abnormalities associated with enlargement or hypertropy of the cardiac chambers is beyond the scope of this text, left ventricular hypertrophy (LVH) is a common and often-discussed entity [5]. Numerous diagnostic criteria have been proposed for the diagnosis of LVH (Table 3). The sensitivity of most criteria is in the range of 30% to 50%. In addition to prominent QRS voltage, the ST-segment and T-wave abnormalities seen reflect a shift of subendocardial to subepicardial repo-

larization. ECG evidence of LVH in hypertensive patients is associated with a threefold increase in overt CAD and an increased risk of death [6].

Bundle Branch Block

A bundle branch block is characterized by a prolonged (> 0.12 sec) QRS complex (Tables 4 and 5). A right bundle branch block (RBBB) is more common than left bundle branch block (LBBB) and is usually clinically unimportant. However, RBBB may be an early warning sign for the onset of symptomatic CAD and congestive heart failure [7]. The most common cause of a LBBB is CAD. In contrast to RBBB, a LBBB may confound the determination of myocardial infarction. In fact, a new LBBB when associated with classic symptomatology should be taken as evidence of an acute MI. Although difficult, it may be possible to diagnose myocardial ischemia with a LBBB:

TABLE 2 CRITERIA FOR VENTRICULAR TACHYCARDIA

Classic criteria suggesting ventricular tachycardia
QRS duration > 0.14 sec
Superior QRS axis
Fusion beats
Atrioventricular dissociation

Brugada criteria for diagnosis of ventricular tachycardia
1. Absence of an RS complex in all precordial leads
   If present, VT
   If absent, continue algorithm
2. R-to-S interval >100 ms (0.1 sec) in one precordial lead
   If present, VT
   If absent, continue algorithm
3. AV dissociation
   If present, VT
   If absent, continue algorithm
4. Morphology criteria (see below) for VT present in V_1, V_2, and V_6
If present, VT
If absent, then SVT with aberrant conduction

Morphology criteria
LBB type
R>0.3 sec in lead V_1 or V_2
Onset of R to nadir of
S>0.7 sec in V_1
No S wave in V_6
RBB type
R/S ratio in V_6<1
RSR, QR, or monophasic R in V_1

AV—atrioventricular; LBB—left bundle branch; RBB—right bundle branch; SVT—supraventricular tachycardia; VT—ventricular tachycardia.

TABLE 3 CRITERIA FOR LEFT VENTRICULAR HYPERTROPHY

Estes criteria*

1. Amplitude		3 points
Largest R or S in limb leads >20 mm		
S wave in V_1 or $V_2 \geq 30$ or R wave in V_5 or $V_6 \geq 30$ mm		
2. ST-T wave shifts (LV strain pattern) in the opposite direction of mean QRS		
Without digoxin		3 points
With digoxin		1 point
3. Left atrial involvement		3 points
4. Left axis deviation > 30°		2 points
5. QRS duration ≥ 0.09		1 point
6. Intrinsicoid deflection in leads V_5 or $V_6 \geq 0.05$		1 point

Cornell voltage criteria

S wave in V_3 plus R wave in aVL ≥ 28 in men, ≥ 20 in women

Sokolow and Lyons criteria

S wave in V_1 plus R wave in V_5 or $V_6 \geq 35$ mm

LVH in the presence of a LBBB

S wave in V_2 plus R in $V_6 \geq 45$ mm

Left atrial enlargement

QRS duration > 0.16 s

*Point scoring system: 5 points = LVH, 4 points probable LVH. LBBB—left bundle branch block; LVH—left ventricular hypertrophy.

TABLE 4 ELECTROCARDIOGRAPHIC DIAGNOSIS OF A LEFT BUNDLE BRANCH BLOCK

Diagnostic findings	**Clues to diagnosis**
QRS duration > 0.12 ms	Poor R-wave progression
Broad R wave in leads I, V_5, and V_6	Broad S wave in the right precordial leads
Absence of Q waves in same leads	Left axis deviation
Delay in intrinsicoid deflection in V_5 and V_6	QS pattern in the inferior leads
ST and T waves in the opposite direction of *major* QRS deflection	

TABLE 5 ELECTROCARDIOGRAPHIC DIAGNOSIS OF A RIGHT BUNDLE BRANCH BLOCK

QRS > 0.12 s

RSR in the right precordial leads

Delay in intrinsicoid deflection in leads I, V_5, and V_6

Broad or slurred S wave in leads I, aVL, V_5, or V_6

T-wave inversion in right precordial leads only

T-wave changes in the opposite direction of the terminal deflection of the QRS

Upward terminal deflection in aVR and downward in aVL

inferior ST elevation may represent an acute infarction, and T-wave deflections in the same direction as the primary QRS forces represent primary T-wave changes and are consistent with ischemia. It may be possible to diagnose an acute MI, even when LBBB [8•].

EXERCISE STRESS TESTING

Exercise stress testing is often indicated to establish the diagnosis of CAD using graded exercise treadmill or bicycle ergometry with a variety of exercise protocols (Table 6). For example, the Bruce protocol employs 3-minute stages with

TABLE 6 EXERCISE STRESS TESTING
Indications
Screening for coronary artery disease
Post-MI risk stratification
Provocation of arrhythmia
Evaluation of revascularization
Evaluation of medical therapy
Evaluation of functional capacity
Preoperative risk stratification
Contraindications
Unstable angina
Acute MI (within 2 days)
Congestive heart failure
Uncontrolled ventricular arrhythmia
Known left main coronary stenosis
Severe aortic stenosis (symptomatic)
Acute myocarditis
Acute aortic dissection
MI—myocardial infarction.

gradual increases in speed and grade. Patients who have recently had an MI or patients that may have difficulty keeping up can exercise with a modified Bruce protocol, which has no incline for the first two stages of exercise.

A positive ECG test is usually defined as ≥ 1 mm of horizontal or downsloping ST segment depression 0.08 seconds after the J point of the QRS (Fig. 3). Upsloping ST segment depression of ≥ 1.5 mm in magnitude 0.08 seconds after the QRS also indicates a positive test. The sensitivity and specificity of the test is approximately 75%. In addition to the ECG response, much clinical information is obtained from an exercise test, including the assessment of functional capacity, blood pressure changes, and the production of symptoms. Severe or multivessel CAD may be suggested by a marked reduction in exercise capacity (less than 6 minutes of exercise), a decrease in blood pressure during exercise, or severe and prolonged symptoms or ECG changes.

As with any test, the pretest probability strongly influences the outcome as well as what to do with the information. Patients with a high pretest likelihood of coronary disease and a negative test may still have CAD. Patients with an intermediate likelihood of CAD are the best candidates for exercise stress testing. Women and patients who are receiving digoxin, who have LVH, or who have resting ECG abnormalities have a higher incidence of false-positive ECG stress tests and may require adjunctive noninvasive imaging for the accurate assessment of CAD. Additional applications of exercise testing beyond the detection of coronary disease include risk stratification after MI, evaluation of arrhythmias, assessment of therapy, and determination of long-term prognosis. For example, patients who exercise to the end of stage III of a Bruce protocol have an excellent 5-year survival, irrespective of the degree of CAD. A comprehensive review of the indications, performance, and interpretation of exercise testing is presented in a recent series of practice guidelines [9].

New methods have sought to improve the diagnostic

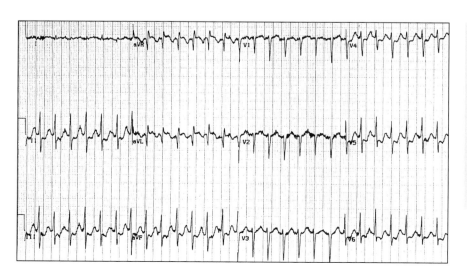

FIGURE 3 Electrocardiographic tracing at peak exercise (5 minutes) demonstrating 2 to 3 mm of downsloping ST segment depression in the inferolateral leads. The patient developed chest pain after 3 minutes of exercise and stopped soon thereafter. The patient is a 50-year-old male smoker who denied any history of angina. These changes persisted long into recovery, and at cardiac catheterization, the patient was found to have severe three-vessel coronary disease.

and, especially, the prognostic value of exercise stress testing. The use of three right precordial leads substantially improves the sensitivity of stress testing, from 52% to 89% in patients with single vessel CAD [10]. Additionally, the use of a treadmill exercise score (Duke treadmill score), incorporating exercise duration, symptoms, and ST segment changes [11•] with the speed of decrease in the postexercise heart rate is a good predictor of mortality [12].

NUCLEAR CARDIOLOGY

Myocardial perfusion imaging is used in conjunction with exercise electrocardiography or pharmacologic stress testing and can be performed using planar or single photon emission computed tomography (SPECT) imaging. Planar images are acquired in three primary views, while SPECT imaging collects a series of planar projections acquired as a camera rotates in an arc around the patient. SPECT images are then reconstructed three dimensionally and are typically displayed in three orientations: 1) short axis, 2) horizontal long axis, and 3) vertical long axis. SPECT allows for better localization of perfusion abnormalities and enhanced diagnostic sensitivity (approximately 85%).

There are two classes of agents used for perfusion imaging. Thallium-201 has been used for more than 30 years for perfusion imaging. More recently, technetium-99m (Tc-99m) compounds have been used such as Tc-99m sestamibi (Cardiolite; Bristol-Meyers-Squibb Medical Imaging, N. Billerica, MA), and Tc-99m tetrofosmin (Myoview; Amersham Healthcare, Arlington Heights, IL). Within the

normal physiologic range, myocardial uptake of tracer is proportional to coronary blood flow. Therefore, regional differences in myocardial blood flow caused by CAD will manifest regional differences in tracer uptake, resulting in defects on the initial scan. A second set of images obtained at rest after a second injection of a Tc-99m tracer will provide the comparison necessary to determine if the perfusion defect is permanent, such as after MI, or if it is reversible and consistent with ischemia (Fig. 4). Usually only one injection of thallium is used, but relative changes of tracer distribution occur with time. Ischemic myocardium is characterized by a slower washout of thallium, so that a second set of images acquired at a later time may show normalization or redistribution. Some myocardium may improve further if a third image is acquired as much as 24 hours later or if a second injection of thallium is administered immediately after the second image (viable myocardium). Several laboratories now perform dual isotope imaging with rest thallium/stress sestamibi in an attempt to decrease the amount of time required for each study and maximize the detection of myocardial viability, while optimizing image quality [13].

Although the Tc-99m-based agents are better suited for gamma camera imaging because of their physical properties, the extensive literature supports the diagnostic and prognostic value of thallium [14,15]. The Tc-99m agents now appear to have similar utility, and these tracers provide images of superior quality, and importantly, permit the assessment of ventricular function in addition to myocardial perfusion. Using techniques such as gated SPECT imaging

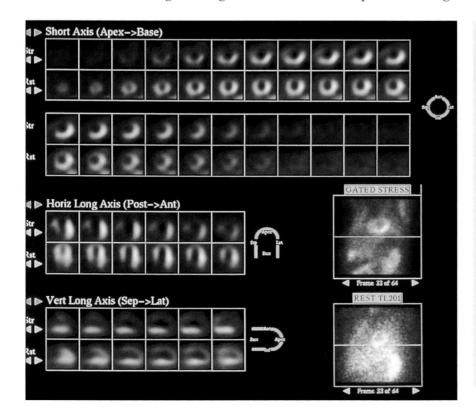

FIGURE 4 Gated single photon emission computed tomography (SPECT) dual isotope myocardial perfusion images. The patient is a 31-year-old male with a past medical history of Hodgkin's disease status post-mantle radiation, tobacco use, and hypercholesterolemia who presented with chest pain and dyspnea on exertion. The perfusion images reveal a severe partially reversible defect in the anterior wall and severe, totally reversible defects in the septal, apical, and antero-lateral walls of the left ventricle, indicating extensive ischemia and involvement of the left anterior descending (LAD) artery and possibly the left circumflex coronary artery. There was enlargement of the left ventricular cavity with stress (transient ischemic dilatation) consistent with multivessel coronary disease. The ejection fraction was 27%. The patient at cardiac catheterization had a 95% stenosis of the proximal LAD and a 95% proximal stenosis of a large ramus branch (supplying the anterolateral wall of the left ventricle).

[16], viable myocardium is found to thicken and brighten, and the global left ventricular ejection fraction may be quantitated with accuracy. This method has been shown to improve the recognition of artifacts, significantly increasing specificity [17]. Although assessment of wall motion can help improve the recognition of artifacts in myocardial perfusion imaging, photon attenuation by soft tissues overlying the heart still hampers accurate interpretation of the images. Several multicenter trials of attenuation correction programs have demonstrated improvement in specificity (or normalcy) without significant reductions in sensitivity [18,19]. Recent position papers now recommend the addition of attenuation correction technology to current gated SPECT imaging systems [20].

Beyond the identification of CAD, the great value of myocardial perfusion imaging is the ability of the technology to localize stenoses and to assess the extent and severity of perfusion abnormalities. These attributes allow the reliable prediction of outcomes of patients with known or suspected CAD. Myocardial perfusion imaging is used routinely in preoperative risk assessment, risk stratification after an MI, determination of therapeutic efficacy, evaluation of the functional significance of angiographically determined stenoses, and the assessment of myocardial viability. When assessing patients with suspected CAD, a normal perfusion study is associated with a very low risk (< 1%) for sustaining a cardiac event within the next year, with a greater than 10-fold increase in the risk of subsequent MI or death if an abnormal perfusion study finding is present [21]. These prognostic benefits are clearly supplemental to clinical and stress test data in low and intermediate risk populations and have independent value years after the test [22•,23]. The functional data derived from gated dual isotope studies has also added supplemental prognostic information to the perfusion study alone. The determination of transient cavity dilatation or an increased lung uptake of thallium following the stress portion of the study (lung:heart ratio of greater than 0.5) have been shown to be markers of multivessel disease and ventricular dysfunction, and therefore a worse prognosis. Even in patients with normal or mildly abnormal perfusion studies, transient cavity dilatation was an independent risk for death, myocardial infarction, or revascularization [24]. The ejection fraction and end systolic volume determined from gated SPECT imaging have demonstrated incremental prognostic value over perfusion imaging alone [25].

A number of recent trials [26•] have demonstrated that not only is myocardial perfusion imaging a valuable diagnostic and prognostic technique but that it also provides these data in a highly cost-effective manner, enabling an improved use of resources, such as angiography and revascularization.

Left ventricular dysfunction may improve after revascularization in patients who demonstrate myocardial viability. Although there is no true gold standard for the noninvasive identification of viability, positron emission

tomography (PET) is currently the most effective modality used. Thallium imaging, however, may be an inexpensive and simple alternative to PET and has been correlated with postoperative outcome and PET imaging [27]. There are two protocols for detecting viability: 1) a small dose of thallium is injected immediately after the second set of images is acquired of a regular stress test and a third image is acquired; and 2) thallium is injected at rest and then two sets of images are taken. Quantitation of sestamibi activity also may allow for the accurate detection of viable myocardium.

In patients who are unable, are unwilling, or should not undergo exercise, pharmacologic stress testing is a valuable alternative (Table 7). Two categories of pharmacologic stress agents are available: 1) vasodilators, including dipyridamole and adenosine, and 2) catecholamines, including dobutamine and arbutamine. The intravenous vasodilators cause regional disparities in blood flow when a coronary stenosis is present, causing a perfusion defect. These actions may be reversed by aminophylline; consequently caffeine and theophylline should be withheld before testing. Because of the direct bronchoconstriction produced by adenosine and dipyridamole, patients with severe lung disease or active wheezing should not undergo pharmacologic stress testing with the vasodilators. Vasodilator stress testing is recommended for patients with LBBB, because exercise testing may produce false-positive perfusion defects, wall-motion abnormalities, or ECG changes. Unlike adenosine and dypridamole, dobutamine and arbutamine cause an increase in myocardial oxygen consumption and produce ischemia and subsequent perfusion abnormalities and regional wall-motion disturbances. Rest-redistribution thallium imaging may assist in the identification of patients who may receive maximum benefit from revascularization. The catecholamines are most useful in conjunction with perfusion imaging in patients unable to receive dipyridamole or adenosine.

PET is a relatively new technique that can be used in the detection of CAD, the estimation of its severity, and for the assessment of myocardial viability in patients with left ventricular dysfunction. PET is considered the gold standard in the noninvasive assessment of viability, as this method can directly measure and quantitate markers of

TABLE 7 INDICATIONS FOR PHARMACOLOGIC STRESS TEST
Inability to exercise
Vascular, neurologic, or orthopedic patients
Limited exercise capacity
High risk from exercise
Aortic aneurysm, aortic stenosis, severe hypertension
Left bundle branch block

myocardial metabolism, such as fatty acid or glucose utilization. The most commonly used agent for detection of viability is fluorodeoxyglucose (FDG). FDG is a marker of regional exogenous glucose uptake. Areas that have reduced perfusion but normal or increased glucose uptake indicate viable tissue. Because of the limited availability of cyclotrons for production of tracers and the cost of PET equipment, it is unlikely that PET scanning will become a widespread and standard technique for the evaluation of CAD. However, it is now feasible to image FDG with a modified SPECT camera, making metabolic imaging more available for clinical use [28].

Radionuclide Angiography

Radionuclide angiography is used for the quantitative determination of left ventricular function, providing highly accurate and reproducible assessment of ventricular volumes and left ventricular ejection fraction. Although this technique has been largely replaced by echocardiography for the routine measurement of ventricular function, radionuclide angiography is still used to evaluate patients prior to, or those patients currently undergoing cardiotoxic chemotherapy. One technique is first-pass angiography, which involves analysis of counts during the first 15 to 20 seconds after an intravenous injection of a tracer. More frequently, gated equilibrium radionuclide angiography is performed where the R wave of the ECG is used as a "gate" for serial static images in relation to the cardiac cycle. Several hundred beats are collected and summed to allow for adequate counts. Both first-pass and equilibrium studies may be performed at rest or in conjunction with exercise, obtaining measurements of left ventricular ejection fraction at each stage of exercise. Abnormal exercise ejection fraction response or absolute value less than 50% have been shown to be powerful prognostic indicators [29,30].

Besides being able to measure left ventricular function, radionuclide angiography can evaluate left ventricular volumes, right ventricular function and volume, regurgitant fraction in patients with valvular incompetence, and left ventricular diastolic function. Because many patients who present with heart failure may in fact have diastolic dysfunction, it is often important to distinguish systolic from diastolic dysfunction, since the treatment of each process is dramatically different.

ECHOCARDIOGRAPHY
M-Mode, Two-Dimensional, Doppler, and Contrast Echocardiography

Echocardiography uses high-frequency ultrasonic waves for the real-time imaging of cardiac structures and blood cells as they transit the heart. A transducer applied to the chest wall emits and receives acoustic data, which then may be displayed in a variety of formats. M-mode echocardiography has largely been replaced by two-dimensional information, but may still be useful in measuring dimensions and wall thickness of cardiac chambers. Two-dimensional echocardiography provides an accurate representation of cardiac structures and reveals the anatomic relationships of various structures. Wall motion can be visualized and classified as normal, hypokinetic, akinetic, or dyskinetic. Although true quantitation is not yet a reality, this semiquantitative analysis, in conjunction with a segmental model, provides useful diagnostic and prognostic information. Doppler echocardiography provides physiologic information regarding valvular function and the patterns of blood flow through the heart. The signal is reflected off the moving erythrocytes and produces a slight shift in frequency, permitting determination of the direction and velocity of flow. There are three forms of Doppler imaging: 1) pulse wave, 2) continuous wave, and 3) color flow. Color-flow Doppler imaging permits visualization of this information superimposed on the two-dimensional echocardiogram. Doppler imaging is frequently used to detect valve regurgitation and quantitate the degree of valvular and subvalvular stenosis. The echocardiographically derived valve areas in the setting of mitral or aortic stenosis correlate well with data obtained from cardiac catheterization. Additionally, Doppler flows can be used to assess diastolic left ventricular function and estimate right ventricular and pulmonary artery pressures.

Echocardiography has a variety of applications including the evaluation of global and regional left ventricular function, determination of left ventricular mass and volume, detection of thrombi or tumors in cardiac chambers, assessment for the presence and degree of pericardial effusion, and the initial evaluation of valve pathology (stenosis, prolapse, flail, and incompetence). Echocardiography is useful for the evaluation of complications after acute MI, such as mitral regurgitation, papillary muscle dysfunction, rupture of the ventricular septum or papillary muscle (Fig. 5), or apical thrombus. Echocardiography is often used in critical care settings because of its portability. In a recent paper, the acute assessment of right ventricular function by transthoracic echo in patients with submassive pulmonary embolism helped guide therapy with thrombolytic therapy, which improved 30-day event-free survival [31].

Despite constant improvements of echocardiography equipment, suboptimal evaluations are still quite prevalent secondary to body habitus and underlying lung disease. The introduction of ultrasound contrast agents has substantially improved the quality of cardiac imaging studies. The majority of the contrast agents are air and fluorocarbon microbubbles encapsulated by a lipid or albumin shell. The microbubbles reflect ultrasonic waves allowing for enhanced imaging of the left ventricular cavity, endocardial border, and myocardial blood flow [32]. The primary indication for ultrasound contrast is for left ventricular opacification to determine ejection fraction. The accuracy of contrast enhanced left ventricular ejection fraction quantification has been validated in comparison to ejection fraction determined by MRI [33]. Since the microbubbles are smaller than red blood cells, the capillary and venule beds of the myocardium, and the ultrasonic waves, perfusion imaging of the myocardium is possible. Although it has been studied extensively, it is still not widely available. When compared with SPECT imaging, myocardial perfusion results are variable, which has limited its routine clinical use [34,35].

Transesophageal Echocardiography

Transesophageal echocardiography (TEE) is performed in the same manner as an upper endoscopic procedure. Because of the invasive nature of the procedure, certain precautions are necessary during the test. For example, oxygen saturation and blood pressure monitoring should be performed during and after the test, especially if the patient has received sedation. The risk of bacterial endocarditis is low, and in general, antibiotic prophylaxis is not indicated. However, patients with prosthetic valves or those in high-risk groups should receive antibiotics before and after the procedure. The only real contraindication to TEE is

esophageal pathology, although patients who have difficulty swallowing represent a challenging group. All probes are now equipped with biplane technology; anatomic relationships and pathology can be seen in multiple views and with less uncertainty. The newer TEE probes allow investigation in multiple planes, further enhancing diagnostic abilities. Doppler imaging also can be performed with the TEE probes (Fig. 6).

The indications for TEE are expanding rapidly (Table 8) [36]. Because of the anatomic relationship of the heart and the esophagus, many structures can be visualized in great detail. The most common use of TEE is to evaluate the heart as a source of embolism or to rule out endocarditis. The left atrium is the most posterior structure, and therefore is uniquely suited to examination by TEE. Most thrombi are located within the left atrial appendage, which is rarely seen on standard transthoracic echocardiography. A TEE-guided approach toward early cardioversion in patients with atrial fibrillation has been used successfully and is cost effective [37•]. TEE is ideal for examination of the intra-atrial septum for atrial septal defects, a patent foramen ovale, and intra-atrial septal aneurysms. TEE also

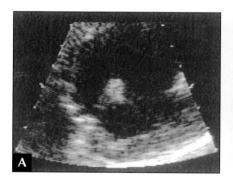 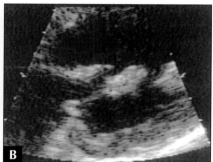

FIGURE 5 **A**, Systolic and **B**, diastolic images from a two-dimensional echocardiogram. Subcostal view demonstrates a ruptured papillary muscle from a patient who suffered a myocardial infarction 2 days before the echocardiogram was obtained.

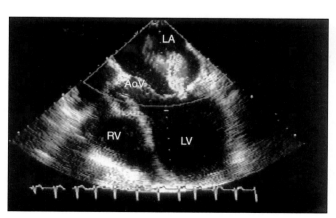

FIGURE 6 Color flow Doppler image from a transesophageal echocardiogram. The image reveals a normal left ventricle, a large left atrium, and a single broad turbulent jet of mitral regurgitation extending far back into the left atrium during systole. (*See* Color Plate.)

TABLE 8 INDICATIONS FOR TRANSESOPHAGEAL ECHOCARDIOGRAPHY
Potential source of embolism
Evaluate left atrium and left atrial appendage
Rule out left ventricle thrombus
Assess aorta for atheroma
Rule out atrial septal defect or patent foramen ovale
Complications of infective endocarditis
Evaluate LV and LV outflow tract
Rule out atrial septal defect or ventricular septal defect
Evaluate prosthetic valve function
Intraoperative monitoring
Evaluating congenital heart disease
Evaluating aorta for possible dissection, atheroma, or aneurysm
LV—left ventricle.

is useful in the setting of suspected infective endocarditis, because it may reveal vegetations as small as 1 to 2 mm. This method may also detect complications of endocarditis, such as ring abscesses, valve dehiscence, or leaflet perforation. Intraoperatively, TEE may be employed as a means of assessing for myocardial ischemia during surgery, as well as assisting in the determination of whether a valve needs replacement or repair during coronary bypass surgery.

Stress Echocardiography

Stress echocardiography is a recently developed modality permitting the assessment of coronary artery disease by means of regional wall-motion analysis [38]. Despite its potential advantages regarding cost and time efficiency, stress echocardiography has significant limitations: up to 30% of patients do not have adequate acoustic windows, and image interpretation is highly observer dependent.

Exercise echocardiography in comparison with exercise SPECT had a similar sensitivity (85% vs 87%) but a slightly greater specificity (77% vs 64%, respectively) [39•]. Unfortunately, limited outcome data are available regarding exercise echocardiography because of the recent origin of the method. In addition to exercise, pharmacologic stress echocardiography also may be performed, primarily using a dobutamine infusion. This catecholamine is delivered in increasing doses to allow for identification of new wall-motion abnormalities. Dobutamine stress echocardiograms have been used for a variety of scenarios including risk stratification before surgery, ischemia evaluation, and in patients who have recently undergone angioplasty [40•]. A variety of publications have supported the use of stress echocardiography for the prediction of cardiac death and nonfatal MI [41•]. Additionally, in patients with left ventricular dysfunction, low-dose dobutamine echocardiography can detect myocardial viability by demonstration of improved contractility. Its ability to detect viability is comparable to thallium studies and has been confirmed by outcomes and postoperative evaluation of left ventricular function [42•].

Contrast-enhanced stress echocardiography can help with the interpretation of suboptimal studies, especially during the stress portion of the study. The addition of myocardial perfusion data, as mentioned above, is still not standard in most echocardiography laboratories [32].

Electrophysiology

The field of cardiac electrophysiology has grown dramatically in the past 10 years. In addition to invasive electrophysiologic studies, several noninvasive techniques are currently available. Twenty-four–hour ambulatory or Holter monitoring is used for the evaluation of patients with bradycardia or tachycardia, detecting prolonged pauses or episodes of tachycardia. The presence of significant ventricular ectopy increases a patient's risk of sudden death [43•]. An alternative method for patients with less frequent symptoms or arrhythmia is the use of an event monitor, a recorder that the patient wears and can activate whenever he or she experiences symptoms. These data can then be transmitted telephonically and interpreted by a physician.

Tilt-table testing is used to evaluate the patient whose history suggests vasodepressor syncope (simple faint). The bed is gradually tilted to an angle of approximately 70° while the patient's heart rate and blood pressure are monitored. If this does not provoke symptoms, then isoproterenol is infused and the bed is again tilted until the test is over or the patient develops symptoms. Currently, most patients are treated with β-adrenergic blockers and then are retested to ascertain efficacy of drug therapy. If unsuccessful, other drugs can be assessed.

The role of signal average electrocardiograms (SAECG) in the prediction of sudden death is unclear. In post-MI patients with a narrow QRS complex on their ECG, the SAECG appears valuable in identifying a high-risk group. Although this technique may also be useful in patients with hypertrophic cardiomyopathy or nonischemic dilated cardiomyopathy, the predictive value of SAECG is not as powerful [44]. The presence of late potentials in the terminal portion of the QRS conveys an increased risk of sudden death. Other measure of increased risk is loss of heart rate variability (HRV) and T-wave alternans (alternating amplitudes from beat to beat). HRV is determined by having the patient lie flat with a standard ECG recording the heart rate. HRV is usually performed just before electrophysiology studies and has yet to demonstrate enough independent prognostic value to be of clinical use. T-wave alternans is measured during either bicycle or treadmill exercise. In multiple studies it has been shown to be an independent risk factor for ventricular arrythmias in high-risk patient populations [45–47].

Magnetic Resonance Imaging

During the late 1990s the literature confirming the usefulness of cardiac MRI has become more robust. Despite its explosive growth, it is still chiefly employed in evaluating cardiac tumors and masses, pericardial disease, congenital anomalies, and in the assessment of possible aortic dissection [48]. Since cardiac MRI does not require iodinated contrast, the indications are constantly evolving for cardiac imaging. Gadolinium-enhanced MRI has been successfully used to identify viable myocardium prior to revascularization (Fig. 7) [49]. Cardiac MRI identified 78% of the dysfunctional regions as viable, which is comparable to PET, the current gold standard for identifying viable myocardium [50]. Cardiac MRI also identifies subendocardial MIs with greater sensitivity than SPECT [51]. Routine use of this technology for angiography remains restricted secondary to technical limitations. In a recent study of 109 patients, 22% percent of the right coronary arteries and 32% of the middle segments of the circumflex coronary artery were not interpretable [52]. Recent publications have also demonstrated the likely clinical use of stress MRI for the detection of coronary disease [53].

COMPUTED TOMOGRAPHY

As with cardiac MRI, recent technologic advances in computed tomography (CT) have permitted its use as a diagnostic tool for imaging the heart and coronary arteries (Fig. 8). Initially CT has been used primarily in the diagnosis of aortic dissection, but with the advent of controlling for cardiac motion with gated studies and the introduction of reconstruction techniques, CT can now be used as a reliable diagnostic tool for the heart. The two modes of CT that are now in use for cardiac imaging are EBCT and MSCT [54].

EBCT was the first modality to be used for cardiac imaging. Its ability to image the heart and coronary arteries with good spatial resolution was due to very rapid scanning times. Conventional CT uses a standard rotating x-ray tube, which does not allow for rapid enough image acquisition. The electron gun and the stationary tungsten target generate x-rays in such a way that allows serial images to be

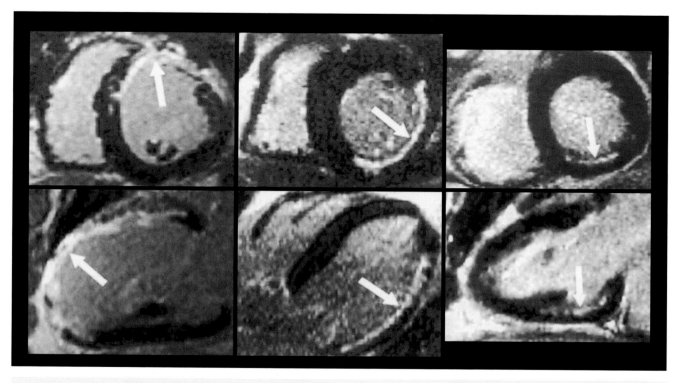

FIGURE 7 Typical contrast-enhanced images obtained by magnetic resonance imaging in a short-axis view (*upper panels*) and a long-axis view (*lower panels*) in three patients. Hyperenhancement is present (*arrows*) in various coronary-perfusion territories—the left anterior descending coronary artery, the left circumflex artery, and the right coronary artery—with a range of transmural involvement. (*From* Kim *et al.* [49]; with permission.)

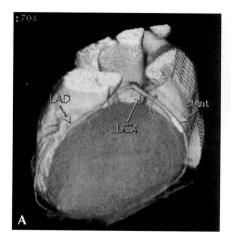

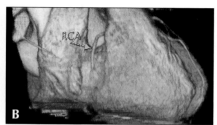

FIGURE 8 Contrast-enhanced computed tomography (CT) images of the heart and coronary arteries. **A,** Three-dimensional reconstruction CT images demonstrating the patent left anterior descending and left circumflex coronary artery. Note the stent in the mid-segment of the left circumflex artery. (*See* Color Plate.) **B,** Three-dimensional reconstruction CT images demonstrating the right coronary artery. (*See* Color Plate.)

obtained in 100 ms [55]. This rapid acquisition protocol allows quantification of coronary calcification, a marker of atherosclerosis, without the use of intravenous contrast. Therefore, this method has been suggested as a screening tool for the presence of CAD. Recent prospective studies of EBCT have shown that coronary calcification provides independent prognostic information when added to traditional risk factors [56,57] (Fig. 9). However, two meta-analyses have shown poor specificity (70%–75%) for detecting obstructive CAD, limiting its use as a general screening tool [55,58]. Although there is no defined group at this time that may benefit from quantification of coronary calcification, the best use of this technology may be in patients where the decision to embark on long-term interventions such as aspirin, statins, and antihypertensives can be made on the basis of a positive scan. Although not standard at this time, the addition of contrast to EBCT can identify high-grade coronary artery stenoses [59].

Retrospectively gated MSCT has become an alternative modality for assessing coronary calcification and coronary artery stenoses. The present generation of spiral CT systems have 16 detectors, and the acquisition speed has significantly decreased allowing similar spatial resolution to the EBCT [54]. The major advantage is that MSCT is more prevalent and less costly to maintain. MSCT has been used to detect coronary calcium, but when compared with EBCT it did not prove to be a feasible alternative [60]. Given its limitations for calcium quantification MSCT will be used primarily for coronary angiography. Although a recent study demonstrates an 80% positive predictive value and a 97% negative predictive value for stenoses ≥ 50%, the technology has limitations secondary to the inability to adequately image all segments of the coronary tree [61].

PROTEOMICS

Proteomics is the rapidly evolving field that uses levels of serum proteins to diagnose and predict outcomes of disease in individual patients. The three tests that are gaining wider clinical use are C-reactive protein (CRP), B-type or brain natriuretic factor (BNP), and myeloperoxidase. CRP, an acute phase reactant, has demonstrated in two prospective trials (Women's Health Study and the Physician's Health Study) that those participants with the highest baseline plasma concentration have a two to three times higher risk of having a cardiovascular event compared with those with the lowest levels [62,63]. Since statins can lower the CRP, and potentially reduce the incidence of acute coronary events, obtaining baseline levels in high-risk patients may help guide therapy [64]. BNP is a protein that is localized to the ventricular myocardium. Levels have been successfully used to distinguish between congestive heart failure and noncardiac dyspnea in the emergency department. When using a cutoff of 100 pg/mL the test had a sensitivity of 90% and a specificity of 76% for differentiating between conges-

tive heart failure and noncardiac dyspnea [65]. BNP has also demonstrated the ability to predict outcomes following an acute coronary syndrome. Patients with levels greater than 80 pg/mL are more likely to die, have a recurrent myocardial infarction, or progress to heart failure than those with levels of 80 pg/mL or less [66]. Myeloperoxidase, an inflammatory marker that is found in leukocyte enzymes and in coronary plaques, has demonstrated the ability to predict major adverse cardiac events 84.5% of the time when added to the troponin T assay [67].

CLINICAL APPLICATIONS
Diagnosis of Coronary Artery Disease

The technological advancements in cardiac testing have permitted the practitioner to detect CAD at different stages of its presentation. In the past, symptomatic patients were those mainly subjected to cardiac imaging studies to detect subclinical disease. Now with proteomics and adjunct imaging studies such as EBCT, asymptomatic patients can be risk stratified for cardiovascular disease.

The approach to the asymptomatic patient begins with assessing the clinical risk factors before proceeding with noninvasive testing. The Framingham risk score comprising age, total cholesterol, smoking status, and systolic blood pressure creates a score with estimates of 10-year risk of CAD events [68]. CRP and coronary calcification determined by EBCT have incremental independent prognostic information when added to the Framingham risk score [56,62]. If patients have significant cardiac risk, exercise or pharmacologic stress testing with adjunct imaging can be employed to diagnose obstructive coronary disease (ie, stenosis ≥ 50%). The asymptomatic diabetic patient should be considered differently, since

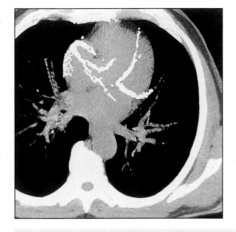

FIGURE 9 An electron beam computed tomography image of extensive calcification (*white area*) of the left anterior descending coronary artery and the left circumflex coronary artery. The coronary artery calcium score is greater than 400. Values greater than 100 are considered markedly abnormal.

diabetics without prior MI have the same risk of MI as patients who have had previous MI [69]. Although not recommended at this time by the American College of Cardiology/American Heart Association, a recent study demonstrated that extent of perfusion abnormalities by SPECT independently predicted cardiac events in diabetic patients [9,70].

The approach to the symptomatic patient is better defined. Clinical assessment of the patient's pretest probability can be determined by the clinical prediction rule developed by Diamond and Forrester based on the type of chest pain, age, and relief with nitroglycerin or rest [71]. Assuming the patient has an intermediate probability, exercise or pharmacologic testing can be ordered depending on the patient's ability. Low-risk people should not require testing, and high-risk patients should go straight to cardiac catheterization since a negative study does not totally rule out the presence of disease in this population.

Diagnosis of Acute Myocardial Infarction

ST segment elevation is the hallmark of acute infarction, permitting triage and rapid intervention with thrombolytic therapy or angioplasty. However, the initial electrocardiogram is diagnostic of an acute MI in only 50% to 60% of patients, with serial ECGs identifying an additional 10%. Right ventricular involvement is an important clinical entity and may be detected using right-sided ECG leads and confirmed by the presence of ≥ 1 mm ST elevation in V_{3R} or V_{4R} in the setting of an inferior infarction [3].

The gold standard for the diagnosis of an acute MI in the past has been the measurement of serum creatine kinase (CK)–MB isoenzymes. The typical pattern consists of an increase in CK-MB within 4 to 8 hours of an acute MI and peak activity at 12 to 24 hours. Despite its routine use, the sensitivity and specificity vary depending on test timing. Therefore, additional serologic tests have become available for the early detection of acute injury such as CK-MB isoforms (limited to research protocols), troponin-T, troponin-I, and serum myoglobin. Troponin-T and -I are cardiac specific. They tend to rise at 8 to 12 hours after the onset of symptoms. One advantage is that these tests can remain elevated for 10 to 14 days following an event [72]. Myoglobin found in cardiac and skeletal muscle may be

detected as early as 2 hours after the onset of symptoms [72]. A recent meta-analysis of serial biomarker determinations summarizes the sensitivity and specificity of the various tests (Table 9) [73].

Since biomarker determinations have variable test characteristics, adjunct imaging studies may be performed to visualize a wall-motion abnormality with echocardiography or a scintigraphic perfusion defect after administration of sestamibi, both of which confirm an acute ischemic syndrome in the absence of prior infarction [74]. A recent multicentered trial confirms the routine use of myocardial perfusion imaging in the emergency room setting. In patients with suspected acute coronary syndromes and nondiagnostic electrocardiograms, acute resting myocardial perfusion imaging improves clinical decision making helping to reduce the number of unnecessary hospitalizations without sacrificing quality of care [75].

Risk Stratification After Myocardial Infarction

Prognosis after MI is predominantly dependent on three factors: 1) left ventricular ejection fraction; 2) the presence of residual ischemia; and 3) the presence of ventricular arrhythmias. The left ventricular ejection fraction is inversely proportional to long-term survival and may be assessed by radionuclide ventriculography, contrast ventriculography, or echocardiography. An ejection fraction of less than 40% is associated with increased risk; however, this value is not an absolute cutoff, but a continuum. Recurrent symptoms or objective evidence of myocardial ischemia as demonstrated on a stress test (exercise or pharmacologic, with or without imaging) in patients with significant ventricular ectopy, complex ectopy, or recurrent ventricular tachycardia on Holter monitoring also have a poor prognosis. Ironically, suppression of ventricular ectopy by antiarrythmic medications may increase the risk of death. A signal-average ECG that detects late potentials in the terminal portion of the QRS is useful for predicting the risk of sudden death after MI. Programmed electrical stimulation (EP study) has been used for risk stratification, but the value of a negative study is unclear.

Diagnosis of Pericardial Diseases

The ECG remains the most important test for the diagnosis of pericarditis, which is confirmed by the presence of diffuse concave ST segment elevation in multiple leads and PR segment depression. There are no reciprocal changes in other leads, as would be expected in acute MI. Pericarditis should not be mistaken for an acute MI, because the risk of a hemopericardium is high if the patient were to receive thrombolytic therapy or heparin. Pericardial thickening also may be evaluated by CT or MRI.

Echocardiography is extremely sensitive for diagnosing pericardial effusions. Certain echocardiographic criteria suggest the diagnosis of tamponade, including right atrial or ventricular diastolic collapse, and augmented respiratory variation of diastolic flow through the mitral valve.

TABLE 9 SERUM BIOMARKERS FOR ACUTE MYOCARDIAL INFARCTION

Biomarker	Rise time, h	Sensitivity, %	Specificity, %
CK-MB	4–8	79	96
Myoglobin	2–4	89	87
Troponin I	8–12	90–100	83–96
Troponin T	8–12	93	85

Assessment of Valvular Heart Disease

Echocardiography is ideally suited for assessment of valvular regurgitation and stenosis, demonstrating the morphology and anatomic relationships of the valves and related structures. Additionally, Doppler echocardiography provides a physiologic assessment of the severity of turbulent blood flow. In valvular stenosis, transvalvular gradients may be determined and valve areas calculated, with a high correlation with data obtained during cardiac catheterization. The degree of valvular incompetence also may be assessed, since Doppler flows demonstrate the extent of regurgitant flow. Radionuclide angiography allows serial assessment of ventricular function and has been used in conjunction with exercise testing for aortic insufficiency to assist in decisions regarding the timing of valve replacement surgery. Radionuclide angiography also is useful for quantitation of the regurgitant fraction and ventricular volume. Intraoperative TEE can be used to determine the need for valve replacement while the patient is undergoing another procedure, such as coronary artery bypass graft surgery. After implantation of a prosthetic valve, echocardiography may be used to assess function, although the acoustic window may mandate a transesophageal approach. Transthoracic echocardiography and TEE are often used to search for sources of emboli or the presence of vegetations in suspected endocarditis.

Preoperative Risk Stratification

The assessment of cardiac risk factors in patients undergoing noncardiac surgery is an important duty for most primary care physicians. The majority of indices for risk assessment have been devised for the general surgical population. However, these clinical parameters may be insufficient in many other patient cohorts, and additional information may be necessary [76]. Exercise stress testing remains useful for preoperative assessment, but many patients cannot undergo rigorous exercise. Pharmacologic testing, with dipyridamole, adenosine, or dobutamine, in conjunction with perfusion imaging has excellent prognostic value. Similarly, dobutamine stress echocardiography may effectively stratify patients based on operative risk. The recently revised guidelines on preoperative assessment are a good resource for the approach to risk stratification [77].

REFERENCES AND RECOMMENDED READING

Recently published papers of particular interest have been highlighted as:

- • Of interest
- •• Of outstanding interest

1. Cohen M, Hawkins L, Greenberg S, Fuster V: Usefulness of ST-segment changes in ≥ leads on the emergency room electrocardiogram in either unstable angina pectoris or non Q wave myocardial infarction in predicting outcome. *Am J Cardiol* 1991, 67:1368–1373.

2. Krone R, Greenberg H, Dwyer E, *et al.*: Long-term prognostic significance of ST segment depression during acute myocardial infarction. *J Am Coll Cardiol* 1993, 22:361–367.

3. Zehender M, Kasper W, Kauder E, *et al.*: Right ventricular infarction as an independent predictor of prognosis after acute inferior myocardial infarction. *N Engl J Med* 1993, 328:981–988.

4. Brugada P, Brugada J, Mont L, *et al.*: A new approach to the differential diagnosis of a regular tachycardia with a wide QRS complex. *Circulation* 1991, 83:1649–1659.

5. Casale P, Devereux R, Kligfeld P: Electrocardiographic detection of left ventricular hypertrophy: development and prospective validation of improved criteria. *J Am Coll Cardiol* 1985, 6:572–580.

6. Ghali J, Liao Y, Simmons B, *et al.*: The prognostic role of left ventricular hypertrophy in patients with and without coronary artery disease. *Ann Intern Med* 1992, 117:831–836.

7. Schneider JF, Thomas HE, Kreger BE, *et al.* New acquired right bundle branch block: The Framingham Study. *Ann Intern Med* 1980, 92:37–44.

8.• Sgarbossa EB, Pinski SL, Barbagelata A, *et al.*: Electrocardiographic diagnosis of evolving acute myocardial infarction in the presence of left bundle-branch block. *N Engl J Med* 1996, 334:581–587.

9. Gibbons RJ, Balady GJ, Bricker JT, *et al.*: ACC/AHA guideline update for exercise testing: a report of the American College of Cardiology/American Heart Association Task Force on Practice Guidelines (Committee on Exercise Testing). 2002. American College of Cardiology. http://www.acc.org/clinical/guidelines/exercise/dirIndex.htm.

10. Michaelides A, Psomadaki ZD, Dilaveris PE, *et al.*: Improved detection of coronary artery disease by exercise electrocardiography with the use of right precordial leads. *N Engl J Med* 1999, 340:340–345.

11.• Shaw LJ, Peterson ED, Shaw LK, et al.: Use of a prognostic treadmill score in identifying diagnostic coronary disease subgroups. *Circulation* 1998, 98:1622–1630.

12. Cole CR, Blackstone EH, Pashkow EJ, *et al.*: Heart-rate recovery immediately after exercise as a predictor of mortality. *N Engl J Med* 1999, 341:1351–1357.

13. Berman D, Kiat H, Friedman J, *et al.*: Separate rest thallium-201/stress technetium-99m sestamibi dual isotope myocardial perfusion single photon emission computed tomography: a clinical validation study. *J Am Coll Cardiol* 1993, 22:1455–1464.

14. Iskandrian A, Chae S, Heo J, *et al.*: Independent and incremental prognostic value of exercise single-photon emission computed tomographic (SPECT) thallium imaging in patients with coronary artery disease. *J Am Coll Cardiol* 1993, 22:665–670.

15. Machecourt J, Longere P, Fagret D, *et al.*: Prognostic value of thallium-201 single photon emission computed tomographic myocardial perfusion imaging according to extent of myocardial defect. *J Am Coll Cardiol* 1994, 23:1096–1106.

16. Chua T, Kiat H, German OG, *et al.*: Gated technetium-99m sestamibi for simultaneous assessment of stress myocardial perfusion, postexercise regional ventricular function and myocardial viability. *J Am Coll Cardiol* 1994, 23:1107–1114.

17. Taillefer R, DePuey EG, Udelson JE, *et al.*: Comparative diagnostic accuracy of TI-201 and Tc-99m sestamibi SPECT imaging (perfusion and ECG gated SPECT) in detecting coronary artery disease in women. *J Am Coll Cardiol* 1997, 29:69–77.

18. Hendel, RC, Berman DS, Cullom S, *et al.*: Multicenter trial to evaluate the efficacy of correction for photon attenuation and scatter in SPECT myocardial perfusion imaging. *Circulation* 1999, 99:2742–2749.

19. Links JM, Becker LC, Rigo, *et al.*: Combined corrections for attenuation, depth-dependent blur, and motion in cardiac SPECT: a multicenter trial. *J Nucl Cardiol* 2000, 7: 414–425.

20. Hendel RC, Corbett JR, Culllom J, *et al.*: The value and practice of attenuation correction for myocardial perfusion SPECT imaging: a joint position statement from the American Society of Nuclear Cardiology and the Society of Nuclear Medicine. *J Nucl Cardiol* 2002, 9:135–143.

21. Iskader S, Iskandrian AE: Risk assessment using single-photon emission computed tomographic technetium-99m sestamibi imaging. *J Am Coll Cardiol* 1998, 32:57–62.

22.• Hachamovich R, Berman DS, Kiat H, *et al.*: Exercise myocardial perfusion SPECT in patients without known coronary artery disease. *Circulation* 1996, 93:905–914.

23. Vanzetto G, Ormezzano O, Fagret D, *et al.*: Long term additive prognostic value of thallium-201 myocardial perfusion imaging over clinical and exercise stress test in low to intermediate risk patients: study in 1137 patients with 6-year follow-up. *Circulation* 1999, 100:1521–1527.

24. Aiden, A, Bax JJ, Hayes, SW, *et al.*: Transient ischemic dilatation ratio of the left ventricle is a significant predictor of future cardiac events in patients with otherwise normal myocardial perfusion SPECT. *J Am Coll Cardiol* 2003, 42:1818–1825.

25. Sharir, T, Germano G, Kavangh PB, *et al.*: Incremental prognostic value of post-stress left ventricular ejection fraction and volume by gated myocardial perfusion single photon emission computed tomography. *Circulation* 1999, 100:1035–1042.

26.• Shaw LJ, Hachamovitch R, Berman DS, *et al.*: The economic consequences of available diagnostic and prognostic strategies for the evaluation of stable angina patients: an observational assessment of the value of pre-catheterization ischemia. *J Am Coll Cardiol* 1999, 33:661–669.

27. Dilsizian V, Bonow R: Current diagnostic techniques of assessing myocardial viability in patients with hibernating or stunned myocardium. *Circulation* 1993, 87:1–20.

28. Delbeke D, Videlefsky S, Patton JA, *et al.*: Rest myocardial perfusion metabolism imaging using simultaneous dual-isotope acquisition SPECT with technetium-99m-MIBI/fluorine-18FDG. *J Nucl Med* 1995, 36:2110–2119.

29. Lee K, Pryor D, Peiper K, *et al.*: Prognostic value of radionuclide angiography in medically treated patients with coronary artery disease: a comparison with clinical and catheterization variables. *Circulation* 1990, 82:1705–1717.

30. Bonow R: Radionuclide angiography for risk stratification of patients with coronary artery disease. *Am J Cardiol* 1993, 72:735–739.

31. Konstantinides S, Geibel A, Heusel F, Kasper W: Heparin plus alteplase compared with heparin alone in patients with submassive pulmonary embolism. *N Eng J Med* 2002, 347:1143–1150.

32. American Society of Echocardiography: Contrast echocardiography: current and future applications. *J Am Soc Echocardiogr* 2000, 13:331–342.

33. Hundley WG, Kizilbash AM, Afridi I, *et al.*: Administration of intravenous perfluorocarbon contrast agent improves echocardiographic determination of left ventricular volumes and ejection fraction: comparison with cine magnetic resonance imaging. *J Am Coll Cardiol* 1998, 32:1426–1432.

34. Heinle SK, Noblin J, Goree-Best P, *et al.*: Assessment of myocardial perfusion by harmonic power Doppler imaging at rest and during adenosine stress: comparison with 99mTc-sestamibi SPECT imaging. *Circulation* 2000, 102: 55–60.

35. Marwick TH, Brunken R, Meland N, *et al.*: Accuracy and feasibility of contrast echocardiography for detection of perfusion defects in routine practice. *J Am Coll Cardiol* 1998, 32:1260–1269.

36. Peterson GE, Brickner ME, Reimold SC: Transesophageal echocardiography: clinical indications and applications. *Circulation* 2003, 107:2398–2402.

37.• Silverman DJ, Manning WF: Role of echocardiography in patients undergoing elective cardioversion of atrial fibrillation. *Circulation* 1998, 98:479–486.

38. Ryan T, Armstrong W, O'Donnell J, Feigenbaum H: Risk stratification after acute myocardial infarction by means of exercise two-dimensional echocardiography. *Am Heart J* 1987, 114:1305–1316.

39.• Fleischmann KE, Hunink MG, Kuntz KM, Douglas PS: Exercise echocardiography or exercise SPECT imaging? : A meta-analysis of diagnostic test performance. *JAMA* 1998, 280: 913–920.

40.• Marcovitz P, Shayna V, Horn R, *et al.*: Value of dobutamine stress echocardiography in determining the prognosis of patients with known or suspected coronary artery disease. *Am J Cardiol* 1996, 78:404.

41.• Poldermans D, Fioretti PM, Boersma E, *et al.*: Long-term prognostic value of dobutamine-atropine stress echocardiography in 1737 patients with known or suspected coronary artery disease. *Circulation* 1999, 99:757–762.

42.• Vanoverschelde JJ, D'Hondt AM, Marwick T, *et al.*: Head-to-head comparison of exercise-redistribution-reinjection thallium single photon emission computed tomography and low dose dobutamine echocardiography for prediction of reversibility of chronic left ventricular ischemic dysfunction. *J Am Coll Cardiol* 1996, 28:432–442.

43.• Bikkina M, Larson M, Levy D: Prognostic implications of asymptomatic ventricular arrhythmias: the Framingham Heart Study. *Ann Intern Med* 1992, 117:990–996.

44. Podrid PJ, Bumio F, Fogel R, *et al.*: Evaluating patients with ventricular arrhythmia: role of the signal averaged electrocardiogram, exercise test, ambulatory electrocardiogram, and electrophysiologic studies. *Cardiol Clin* 1992, 10:371–395.

45. Rosenbaum DS, Jackson LE, Smith JM, *et al.*: Electrical alternans and vulnerability to ventricular arrhythmias. *N Engl J Med* 1994, 330:235–241.

46. Rosenbaum DS, Albrecht P, Cohen RJ: Predicting sudden cardiac death from T-wave alternans of the surface electrocardiogram: promise and pitfalls. *J Cardiovasc Electrophysiol* 1996, 7:1095–1111.

47. Hohnloser SH, Klingenheben T, Li Y-G, *et al.*: T-wave alternans as a predictor of recurrent ventricular tachyarrhythmias in ICD recipients: prospective comparison with conventional risk markers. *J Cardiovasc Electrophysiol* 1998, 9:1258–1268.

48. Castillo E, Bluemke DA: Cardiac MR Imaging. *Radiol Clin North Am* 2003, 41:17–28.

49. Kim RJ, Wu, E, Rafael A, *et al.*: The use of contrast enhanced magnetic resonance imaging to identify reversible myocardial dysfunction. *N Engl J Med* 2000, 343:1445–1453.

50. Tamiki N, Kawamoto M, Tadamura E, *et al.*: Predication of reversible ischemia after revascularization: perfusion and metabolic studies with positron emission tomography. *Circulation* 1995, 91:1675–705.

51. Wagner A, Mahrholdt H, Holly TA, *et al.*: Contrast enhanced MRI and routine single photon emission computed tomography (SPECT) perfusion imaging for the detection of subendocardial myocardial infarcts: an Imaging study. *Lancet* 2003, 361:374–379.

52. Kim WY, Danias PG, Stuber M, *et al.*: Coronary magnetic resonance angiography for the detection of coronary stenoses. *N Engl J Med* 2001, 345:1863–1869.

53. Nagel E, Lehmkuhl HB, Bocksch W, *et al.*: Noninvasive diagnosis of ischemia-induced wall motion abnormalities with the use of high-dose dobutamine stress MRI. *Circulation* 1999, 99:763–770.

54. Schoepf UJ, Becker CR, Hofmann LK, Yucel, EK: Multidetector-row CT of the heart. *Radiol Clin North Am* 2003, 41:491–505

55. O'Rourke, R, Brundage BH, Froelicher, V, *et al.*: American College of Cardiology/American Heart Association expert consensus document on electron-beam computed tomography for the diagnosis and prognosis of coronary heart disease. *Circulation* 2000, 102:126–140.

56. Shaw LJ, Raggi, P, Schisterman, E, *et al.*: Prognostic value of cardiac risk factors and coronary artery calcium screening for all-cause mortality. *Radiology* 2003, 228:826–833.

57. Kondos GT, Hoff, JA, Sevrukov A, *et al.*: Electron-beam tomography coronary artery calcium and cardiac events. *Circulation* 2003, 107: 2571–2576.

58. Nallamothu BK, Saint, S, Bielak LF, *et al.*: Electron-beam computed tomography in the diagnosis of coronary artery disease: A meta-analysis. *Arch Intern Med* 2001, 161:833–838.

59. Achenbach S, Moshage W, Ropers D, *et al.*: Value of electron-beam computed tomography for the noninvasive detection of high-grade coronary-artery stenoses and occlusions. *N Engl J Med* 1998, 339: 1964–1971.

60. Goldin JG, Yoon HC, Greaser LE, *et al.*: Spiral versus electron-beam CT for coronary artery calcium scoring. *Radiology* 2001, 221:213–221.

61. Nieman K, Cademartiri F, Lemos PA, *et al.*: Reliable noninvasive coronary angiography with fast submillimeter multislice spiral computed tomography. *Circulation* 2002, 106:2051–2054.

62. Ridker PM, Nader R, Rose L, *et al.*: Comparison of C - reactive protein and low-density lipoprotein cholesterol levels in the prediction of first cardiovascular events. *N Engl J Med* 2002, 347:1557–1565.

63. Ridker PM, Cushman M, Stampfer MJ, *et al.*: Inflammation, aspirin and the risk of cardiovascular disease in apparently healthy men. *N Engl J Med* 1997, 336:973–979.

64. Ridker PM, Rifai N, Clearfield M, *et al.*: Measurement of C-reactive protein for the targeting of statin therapy in the primary prevention of acute coronary events. *N Engl J Med* 2001, 344:1959–1965.

65. Maisel AS, Krishnaswamy P, Nowak RM, *et al.*: Rapid measurement of B-type natriuretic peptide in the emergency diagnosis of heart failure. *N Engl J Med* 2002, 347:161–167.

66. De Lemos JA, Morrow DA, Bentley JH, *et al.*: The prognostic value of B-type natriuretic peptide in patients with acute coronary syndromes. *N Engl J Med* 2001, 345:1014–1021.

67. Brennan ML, Penn MS, Van Lente F, *et al.*: Prognostic value of myeloperoxidase in patients with chest pain. *N Engl J Med* 2003, 349: 1595–1604.

68. Executive summary of the third report of the National Cholesterol Education Program (NCEP) expert panel on the detection, evaluation, and treatment of high blood cholesterol in adults (adult treatment panel III). *JAMA* 2001, 285:2486–2497.

69. Haffner SM, Seppo L, Tapani, R, *et al.*: Mortality from coronary heart disease in subjects with type 2 diabetes and in nondiabetic subjects with and without prior myocardial infarction. *N Engl J Med* 1998, 339:229–234.

70. Giri, S, Shaw LJ, Murthy DR, *et al.*: Impact of diabetes on the risk stratification using stress single-photon emission computed tomography myocardial perfusion imaging in patients with symptoms suggestive of coronary artery disease. *Circulation* 2002, 105:32–40.

71. Diamond GA, Forrester JS: Analysis of probability as an aid in the clinical diagnosis of coronary artery disease. *N Engl J Med* 1979, 300:1350–1358.

72. Braunwald E, Antman EM, Beasley JW, *et al.*: ACC/AHA 2002 guidelines update for the management of patients with unstable angina and non-ST segment elevation myocardial infarction: a report of the American College of Cardiology/American Heart Association Task Force on Practice Guidelines (Committee on the Management of Patients With Unstable Angina). 2002. http://www.acc.org/clinical/guidelines/unstable/unstable.pdf.

73. Balk EM, Ioannidis JP, Salem D, *et al.*: Accuracy of biomarkers to diagnose acute cardiac ischemia in the emergency department: a meta-analysis. *Ann Emerg Med* 2001, 37:478–493.

74. Tatum J, Jesse R, Kontos M, *et al.*: Comprehensive strategy for the evaluation and triage of the chest pain patient. *Ann Emerg Med* 1997, 29:116–125.

75. Udelson JE, Beshansky JR, Ballin DS, *et al.*: Myocardial perfusion imaging for evaluation and triage of patients with suspected acute cardiac ischemia. *JAMA* 2002, 288:2693–2700.

76. Eagle K, Coley C, Newell J, *et al.*: Combining clinical and thallium data optimizes preoperative assessment of cardiac risk before major vascular surgery. *Ann Intern Med* 1989, 110:859–866.

77. Eagle KA, Berger PB, Calkins H, *et al.*: ACC/AHA guideline update for perioperative cardiovascular evaluation for noncardiac surgery: a report of the American College of Cardiology/American Heart Association Task Force on Practice Guidelines (Committee to Update the 1996 Guidelines on Perioperative Cardiovascular Evaluation for Noncardiac Surgery). 2002. American College of Cardiology. http://www.acc.org/clinical/guidelines/perio/dirIndex.htm.

SELECT BIBLIOGRAPHY

ACC/AHA/ASNC: Guidelines for clinical use of cardiac radionuclide imaging: a report on of the American College of Cardiology/American Heart Association Task Force on Practice Guidelines (ACC/AHA/ASNC Committeee to Revise the 1995 Guidelines for the Clinical Use of Radionuclide Imaging). 2003. American College of Cardiology http://www.acc.org/clinical/guidelines/radio/rni_fulltext.pdf.

Foster E: Transesophageal echocardiography. *Cardiol Clin North Am* 2000, 1:867–910.

Gerber TC, Kuzo RS, Karstaedt N, *et al.*: Current results and new developments of coronary angiography with use of contrast enhanced computed tomography of the heart. *Mayo Clin Proc* 2002, 77:55–71.

Heller GV, Hendel RC. Nuclear Cardiology: Clinical Applications. New York: McGraw-Hill; 2004

Pellikka PA, Roger VL, Oh JK, *et al.*: Stress echocardiography. Part II. Dobutamine stress echocardiography: techniques, implementation, clinical applications, and correlations. *Mayo Clin Proc* 1995, 70:16–27.

Roger VL, Pellikka PA, Oh JK, *et al.*: Stress echocardiography. Part I. Exercise echocardiography: techniques, implementation, clinical applications, and correlations. *Mayo Clin Proc* 1995, 70:5–15.

Zimetbaum PJ, Josephson ME: Use of electrocardiogram in acute myocardial infarction. *N Engl J Med* 2003, 348:933–940.

Evaluation of the Patient with Nontraumatic Chest Pain

John A. Paraskos

5

Key Points

- Many of the economic and medical resources used in evaluating patients with chest pain are unnecessary.

- A carefully obtained history is crucial to assessing the likelihood of coronary disease before any testing is obtained (*ie*, the pretest likelihood for coronary disease).

- The pretest likelihood is assessed from the patient's age, gender, character of the pain or discomfort, and associated risk factors.

- Both the choice and interpretation of noninvasive tests to establish the diagnosis depend on the pretest likelihood and the perceived urgency or instability of the clinical presentation.

- The choice and timing of coronary arteriography depend on the urgency of the clinical presentation and the inability of noninvasive tests to establish the diagnosis reliably.

Considering the potentially lethal consequences of error, evaluating a patient with nontraumatic chest pain is one of the most common as well as one of the most challenging problems in clinical medicine. A recent study [1••] found that 2.1% of 889 patients who presented to an emergency room with an acute myocardial infarction (MI) were mistakenly sent home. This relatively low percentage is countered by the fact that acute MI or unstable angina is confirmed in less than one third of patients admitted with suspected acute coronary syndromes. It is no surprise, therefore, that the identification of patients whose chest pain results from myocardial ischemia consumes a tremendous amount of economic and medical resources. Many of the resources expended in cardiac evaluation, however, are unnecessary or misused. The most important evaluative tools are also the least expensive: a careful and focused medical history augmented by physical examination and simple laboratory procedures.

Angina pectoris is a diagnosis of medical history. An effective clinician can often make the proper assessment with a careful history and a thorough knowledge of the likelihood of coronary artery disease (CAD) in a given population. Whenever a patient presents with chest pain, the clinician is faced with the task of assessing the likelihood 1) that the individual has coronary disease, 2) that the pain as described is cardiac in origin, or 3) that the patient may have another serious condition that presents with similar symptoms. This task is complicated by the multiplicity of problems that can cause chest pain (Table 1). After a careful initial evaluation, many patients must be treated as if they have myocardial ischemia until the diagnostic dilemma is resolved by further observation, diagnostic studies, or response to therapy. Subsequent investigations in patients in whom coronary disease has been excluded have demonstrated that esophageal spasm and gastroesophageal reflux disease are the most commonly associated abnormalities [2,3•]. Empiric therapy with antisecretory agents rather than costly investigation has been shown to be the most cost-effective strategy for such patients [4•].

EMERGENCY EVALUATION

Patients with recent or ongoing chest pain must be subjected to rapid evaluation and triage. This includes a focused but incisive history and physical examination. While this is being performed, administration of supplemental oxygen, placement of a stable intravenous line, and the initiation of electrocardiographic (ECG) monitoring should be carried out promptly for anyone in whom a cardiac cause is at all likely. A full ECG and sending off of blood for the measurement of cardiac markers are also performed rapidly. The ordering of chest radiographs, echocardiograms, computed tomography scans, and so on depends on the clinical scenario and the stability of the patient. Rapid diagnosis of MI and exclusion of aortic dissection are most important when considering among the options of antithrombotic therapy, thrombolytic therapy, catheter intervention with rapid revascularization, and prompt surgical intervention.

If the patient's chest pain has subsided and vital signs are stable, the clinician needs to assess the possibility of a life-threatening coronary syndrome. The more unstable the pattern of chest pain, the more urgently the initial work-up should include prompt and definitive evaluation. For such patients, hospitalization, anticoagulation, and early coronary arteriography are often warranted.

TABLE 1 CAUSES OF CHEST PAIN

Cardiovascular
Coronary artery disease
    Obstructive, spastic, nonathero-
        sclerotic, and congenital
    Cocaine abuse
Severe aortic stenosis or aortic
    insufficiency
Hypertrophic cardiomyopathy
Aortic dissection
Pericarditis
Myocarditis
Dressler's syndrome
Pulmonary embolism
Pulmonary hypertension
Thoracic aneurysm
Hepatic engorgement
Mitral valve prolapse

Pulmonary
Pneumonitis
Pleurisy
Pulmonary infarction or hemorrhage
Pulmonary embolism or *in situ*
    thrombosis
Tracheitis and tracheobronchitis
Spontaneous pneumothorax
Intrathoracic tumor

Gastrointestinal
Hiatal hernia with reflux esophagitis
Esophageal spasm
Esophageal perforation
Esophagitis
Irritable esophagus
Mallory-Weiss syndrome
Peptic ulcer disease
Gastritis
Cholecystitis and biliary colic
Pancreatitis
Gas entrapment syndromes
    Gastric distention
    Hepatic or splenic flexure distention

Musculoskeletal
Costochondritis (Tietze's syndrome)
Costochondral or xiphisternal
    arthralgia
Sternoclavicular arthralgia
Manubriosternal arthralgia
Costovertebral arthritis
Epidemic myalgia
Fibromyalgia
Myositis
Thoracic outlet syndromes
Sternal or rib fractures
Slipping rib syndrome
Precordial catch syndrome (muscle
    spasm)
Muscle strain
Ostealgia from neoplasm,
    inflammation, or infarction
Sternal marrow pain (acute leukemia)
Trauma

Neurologic
Radicular syndrome
Thoracic disk disease
Brachial plexus syndrome
Intercostal neuritis
Reflex autonomic dysfunction
    (shoulder-hand syndrome)
Neurofibromatosis
Herpes zoster involving thoracic
    dermatome with postherpetic pain

Functional or psychiatric
Anxiety with periapical hyperesthesia
Hyperventilation with increased muscle
    tension
Panic attacks
Cardiac neurosis
Psychogenic regional pain syndrome
Malingering
Depression

Miscellaneous
Diaphragmatic spasm or flutter
Superficial thrombophlebitis (Mondor's
    syndrome)
Mediastinitis
Mediastinal emphysema
Mediastinal tumors

CHARACTERISTICS OF CHEST PAIN CAUSED BY MYOCARDIAL ISCHEMIA

Angina pectoris is usually substernal and transient. It may be stable or unstable.

Stable Angina Pectoris

Stable angina pectoris is often brought on by exercise and relieved by rest or nitrates. It may be provoked by a large meal and be mistaken for indigestion. If the coronary disease is stable, the pain episodes are usually short-lived and provoked by exertion or meals. A stable pattern, by definition, has been unchanged in frequency, duration, and severity for at least several months.

Unstable Angina Pectoris

Unstable angina is characterized by a less predictable course with a higher likelihood of going on to an acute MI or sudden death. The instability is usually the result of a complication in the coronary artery (eg, plaque rupture, coronary thrombosis, or spasm). Features that mark instability include new-onset angina; accelerating angina (occurring more frequently or at lower workloads); rest angina; angina that wakes the patient from sleep; prolonged anginal episodes; anginal episodes not responsive to nitrates; and angina associated with severe nausea, weakness, dyspnea, sweating, palpitation, syncope, or pulmonary edema.

Acute Myocardial Infarction

Acute MI is characterized by pain similar to that of angina pectoris. However, it is usually much more severe and longer lasting (1 hour or more). The pain of MI usually includes a number of features of instability and is more often accompanied by nausea and sweating. Patients suspected of having an acute MI or unstable angina are admitted for intensive care monitoring because short-term survival is enhanced by early intervention.

When evaluating chest pain, the clinician must determine if the patient's pain is 1) typical for myocardial ischemic pain; 2) atypical for but possibly caused by ischemic pain; 3) unlikely to be ischemic in origin; or 4) likely to be of a serious nature.

Even typical angina pectoris does not always indicate serious coronary disease; rather, it may be associated with less threatening causes (eg, mitral valve prolapse [MVP], nonthreatening stable coronary disease). Alternatively, chest pain may be caused by other life-threatening conditions that require immediate attention (eg, aortic dissection, critical aortic stenosis, accelerating hypertension, pulmonary thromboembolism, pulmonary hypertension). After addressing these questions, the clinician can judge whether hospitalization is warranted, whether intensive care unit monitoring is wise, and which emergency procedures are required. Many episodes of myocardial ischemia and even MI are asymptomatic. Alternatively, myocardial ischemia may be painless but provoke other symptoms such as profound weakness, severe diaphoresis, nausea, or malaise. These symptoms are considered anginal equivalents and often alert the clinician to the correct diagnosis.

LOCATION AND RADIATION

Pain caused by myocardial ischemia is typically located in the lower substernal area with radiation to either or both arms (more often the left than the right, especially in the ulnar distribution). Another typical site of radiation is to the anterior aspect of the neck or lower jaw. Ischemic pain rarely extends beyond the area from the lower jaw to the epigastrium (C3-T6); the extreme possible limits are from the occiput to the epigastrium (C2-T8) (Fig. 1). In patients with atypical presentations, myocardial ischemic pain may be localized in the jaw, teeth, mid or upper back, shoulder, elbow, or wrist, mimicking a dental or orthopedic problem. However, ischemic pain is not so sharply localized that its area can be covered by a fingertip. Sharply localized inframammary pain is particularly unlikely to be ischemic in origin. Chest pain that radiates from the sternum to the back or vice versa may indicate aortic dissection.

CHARACTER

Ischemic pain is usually described as heavy or constricting (ranging from crushing to mild pressure). It may also be described as expansible or burning, but rarely as sharp or stabbing. The pain is "deep" and "visceral" and is commonly associated with sweating, dyspnea, nausea, and occasionally hiccuping. Although the patient may find it difficult to take a deep breath when the pain is severe, the pain is not pleuritic.

DURATION

A single episode of transient myocardial ischemia (angina pectoris) usually lasts 2 to 30 minutes, with extremes of 30 seconds to more than 1 hour. Lightening-like stabs are clearly nonischemic. Episodes of discomfort lasting more than 30 minutes should raise the suspicion of MI or unstable angina. Therefore, if a patient has suffered for months from multiple episodes of pain lasting hours at a time and fails to demonstrate ECG evidence for recent or remote MI, the pain is unlikely to be ischemic in origin.

TIME-INTENSITY CURVE

Typically, angina pectoris builds in intensity for several minutes, remains at a peak for up to 20 to 30 minutes, and then wanes and disappears over several additional minutes. The pain of acute MI also waxes over the course of minutes but remains much longer. Chest pain that abruptly reaches maximum intensity should raise the suspicion of aortic dissection.

INCITING FACTORS

Inciting factors of the pain are often important clues to the correct diagnosis. Physical effort is the usual inciting factor for a transient episode of myocardial ischemia caused by fixed coronary obstructive disease. Exertion is more likely to cause angina early in the morning and with use of the arms or isometric activity. For many patients, working with the arms above shoulder level is more likely to provoke angina than other activities. Emotional stress, exposure to cold, walking up a grade or against the wind, and exertion after a large meal are other common initiating or contributing factors. Ischemic pain that develops at rest or wakes the patient from sleep is more suggestive of MI, unstable angina, or (occasionally) coronary spasm (ie, variant angina).

Chest pain worsened by respiration is not ischemic. Such pain, brought on by a deep breath or cough, is usually sharp and caused either by pleural or pericardial inflammation or a chest wall condition such as a fractured rib, costochondritis, or intercostal neuritis. Ischemic pain is not aggravated by a single motion of an arm, neck, or torso, and such a pattern strongly suggests a musculoskeletal cause. Pain that can be reproduced or worsened by local palpation is also not ischemic; however, during an acute MI, some patients may have mild local precordial tenderness of obscure cause.

PATTERNS OF RELIEF

Patterns of relief are also valuable in assessing the cause of chest pain. Prompt relief within 2 to 10 minutes of rest is most characteristic of effort-induced angina pectoris. A more gradual disappearance over several hours, or even days, is more typical of musculoskeletal pain. Occasionally, effort-induced ischemic pain disappears while the physical activity continues; this is known as "walk-through" or "second wind" angina. Relief within several minutes of the administration of sublingual nitrates is characteristic of patients with angina pectoris; however, the pain of spastic gastrointestinal (GI) disorders may also respond dramatically to nitrates. Prompt relief with induced bradycardia (as with Valsalva's maneuver or carotid sinus pressure) is also described in patients with angina. The pain of an acute MI is unlikely to be totally relieved by nitrates and usually requires narcotics. Relief of pain with food or antacids suggests esophagitis or peptic disease. Partial relief by sitting forward is more typical of pericarditis or pancreatitis. Occasionally, pericarditis develops as a complication of MI, and these patients can have pericardial chest pain with both pleuritic and positional components.

NONISCHEMIC CHEST PAIN

Nonischemic chest pain syndromes include sharply localized pain, especially costochondral or inframammary; pain radiating outside the limits of C2 to T8; momentary catches or stabs of pain; pain incited by motion, respiratory effort, or local pressure; and recurrent, long-lasting, unabating pain (many hours to days) in the absence of ECG evidence of ischemia or infarction. A single convincing nonischemic feature should cancel several ischemic-like features if it is clearly part of the same chest pain symptom complex.

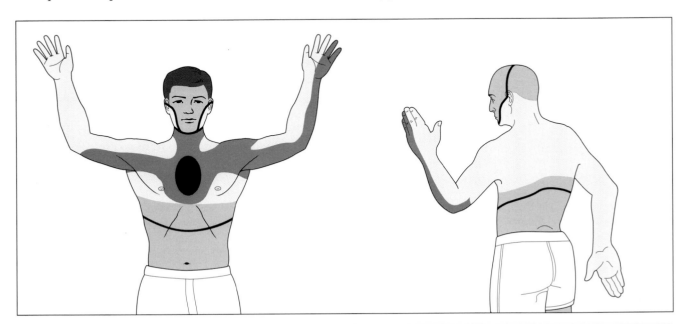

FIGURE 1 Location and radiation of ischemic pain. The *black area* represents the most frequent location of ischemic pain. *Dark shading* represents the most common sites of radiation, and *pink shading* includes all but the rarest areas of sites of radiation (C3–T6). The *heavy lines* encompass the rarest sites of radiation (C2–T8).

ATYPICAL CHEST PAIN

"Atypical angina pectoris" is a phrase often used to refer to pain caused by myocardial ischemia with clinical features not typical of ischemic chest pain (Table 2). Characteristics of a chest pain syndrome sometimes cannot be clearly classified as either nonischemic or typical for ischemia. The more atypical the patient's pain, the less likely it is to be ischemic in origin. Whether these patients are treated as having coronary disease depends on the clinician's judgment. If the pain is somewhat atypical yet has enough features to keep the clinician unsure, it is best to treat the patient as if coronary disease is the cause until further tests have lowered the likelihood considerably.

The likelihood of significant coronary disease has been estimated at a pooled mean prevalence of 89% for all patients with chest pain typical for angina, 50% for those with chest pain atypical for angina, and 16% for all other subjects [5•]. The prevalence was heavily influenced by age and gender (Fig. 2). The estimate of the prevalence of significant coronary disease has important implications for the interpretation of noninvasive tests for patients with myocardial ischemia [6••] (Figs. 3 and 4).

PHYSICAL EXAMINATION

The physical examination may be unremarkable during an episode of life-threatening myocardial ischemia or an evolving MI. Circulatory instability and shock, marked respiratory distress, cyanosis, or life-threatening arrhythmias must initiate urgent intervention and rapid transfer to

TABLE 2   CLINICAL CLASSIFICATION OF CHEST PAIN

Typical angina pectoris
    Substernal chest discomfort with a characteristic quality
        and duration that is…
    Provoked by exertion or emotional stress and…
    Relieved by rest or nitroglycerin
Atypical angina
    Meets two of the above characteristics
Noncardiac chest pain
    Meets only one or none of the typical angina
        characteristics
 	
Adapted from Diamond [26].

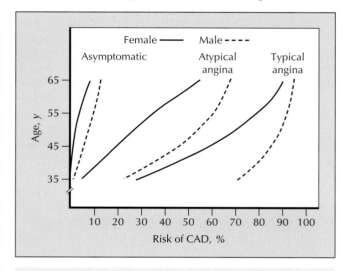

FIGURE 2 Influence of age, gender, and symptoms on risk of coronary artery disease (CAD). (*Adapted from* Epstein [6••].)

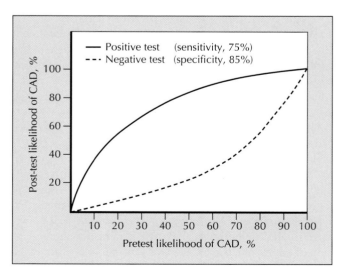

FIGURE 3 Influence of pretest likelihood of coronary artery disease (CAD) on the post-test likelihood of CAD for a test with 75% sensitivity and 85% specificity. (*Adapted from* Epstein [6••].)

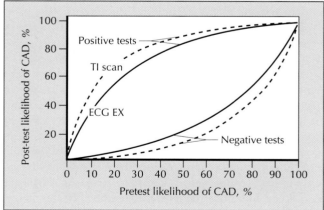

FIGURE 4 Influence of pretest likelihood of coronary artery disease (CAD) on the post-test likelihood of CAD for electrocardiographic exercise testing (ECG EX) and thallium perfusion scintigraphy (Tl scan). (*Adapted from* Epstein [6••].)

the most suitable area of the hospital for intensive care. For these patients, a focused physical examination can be performed as other necessary interventions are being carried out. The physical examination often provides further useful clues to the diagnosis. For those with nonischemic causes of chest pain, the physical examination may help lead to the correct diagnosis. Cases of chest wall tenderness, musculoskeletal disease, breast disease, thoracic outlet syndromes, or neurologic syndromes may be disclosed by abnormal physical findings. Disorders of the GI tract often fail to provide characteristic findings; however, upper quadrant or epigastric tenderness or marked tympany suggests bowel distention or inflammation.

Cardiovascular examination may first call attention to a noncoronary cause for myocardial ischemia. The diagnosis of aortic dissection may be suggested by absent pulses or the inequality of blood pressure (BP) of the arms or legs. Suspicion of aortic dissection is heightened if aortic regurgitation or an enlarging pleural effusion exist. A late-peaking aortic systolic murmur associated with a diminished intensity of the second heart sound and a delayed carotid upstroke may provide the first clue to the presence of critical aortic stenosis. Hypertrophic cardiomyopathy also may be associated with angina pectoris in the absence of coronary obstructive disease and is likely to be manifested by a brisk carotid upstroke and a harsh systolic murmur at the left sternal edge that typically increases with Valsalva's maneuver. A patient with MVP may be recognized by the characteristic non-ejection click with or without a mid to late systolic murmur at the apex. Pericardial or pleural friction rubs may unmask serosal inflammation, but friction rubs may also be caused by transmural MI or proximal aortic dissection with bleeding into the pericardial sac. It should also be remembered that valvular lesions or hypertrophic cardiomyopathy may coexist with significant and symptomatic coronary disease.

Although it is common for patients with CAD to present without abnormal physical findings, it often gives evidence of ventricular dysfunction. The findings may present transiently during ischemic episodes or they may be more prolonged because of "stunned" myocardium or MI. Fourth heart sounds are ubiquitous in patients with significant symptomatic coronary disease, and they are apt to become more prominent during ischemic episodes. Third heart sounds, paradoxically split second heart sounds, holosystolic murmurs, pulsus alternans, a decrease in systemic BP, pulmonary congestion, pallor, as well as cold and clammy skin are often encountered in patients during severe myocardial ischemia. Transient increases in BP may also occur. Evidence for severe hypercholesterolemia (eg, xanthelasmata, tuberous xanthomata) certainly raises the suspicion of associated atherosclerotic disease but does not confirm that the patient's pain is ischemic in origin. Femoral or carotid bruits or diminished peripheral pulses indicate the presence of atherosclerosis and, therefore, a higher likelihood of CAD.

Although tachycardia and tachypnea are nonspecific findings, they may be signs of left ventricular failure. Tachycardia itself may provoke myocardial ischemia. Bradycardias often develop during the early stages of an inferior or posterior wall infarction.

During the acute ischemic episode, rapid and severe pulmonary congestion (flash pulmonary edema) often with incipient or frank shock, suggests a previously compromised left ventricle or severe ischemia involving a large portion of the left ventricle, as may occur in patients with left main or proximal left anterior descending occlusion or proximal occlusion of a dominant right coronary artery. A rare physical finding of severe stenosis of the left main or left anterior descending coronary artery is an early to mid-diastolic high-pitched murmur; this is best heard along the left sternal border. It is produced by turbulent flow in the severely stenotic coronary artery and is essentially a coronary bruit. The murmur is diastolic in timing because flow in the left coronary system occurs predominantly in diastole. Because of its location and timing, the murmur is usually confused with that of aortic regurgitation.

ELECTROCARDIOGRAPHIC, RADIOLOGIC, AND ECHOCARDIOGRAPHIC STUDIES

Electrocardiography

Electrocardiography performed at rest and in the absence of stress or ongoing chest pain, is an insensitive test for the presence of CAD. Most patients with CAD have normal resting ECGs. The presence of abnormal Q waves may indicate previous MI, but their absence is not helpful in excluding significant CAD. Arrhythmias and conduction abnormalities are nondiagnostic findings.

Aside from the history and physical examination, the ECG is the most valuable tool for initial patient assessment during chest pain. Evidence for ischemia may be in the form of horizontal or downsloping ST-segment depression of at least 1 mm (Fig. 5), with or without abnormally inverted or peaked (hyperkalemic appearing) T waves (Fig. 6). More subtle findings include nonspecific T-wave flattening or inversion and inverted U waves (Fig. 7). These latter findings are nonspecific and are only mildly supportive of the diagnosis of myocardial ischemia.

Myocardial injury or infarction usually causes ST-segment elevation and eventual development of abnormal Q waves. Reciprocal changes in the early to mid-precordial leads (V-1 through V-4) suggests true posterior wall infarction. In all the multivariate analytic systems for the evaluation of chest pain, the ECG plays a pivotal role. Although a normal ECG taken during an episode of chest pain is evidence against ischemic disease, it does not by any means exclude it. Indeed, during the early stages of a MI, the ECG may be appear normal. If the history and patient setting are suggestive, the diagnosis must be entertained despite a normally appearing ECG. A left bundle branch block makes the diagnosis of an acute MI or new ischemia difficult. However, its presence in a patient presenting with possible ischemia must be taken as presumptive evidence for ischemic heart disease, unless shown to be old or until proved otherwise.

Electrocardiography may be helpful in supporting a diagnosis of acute pericarditis with diffuse ST elevations and possible PR segment depression (ST depression and PR segment elevation in aVR). Occasionally, the ECG demonstrates acute right ventricular strain, which suggests massive pulmonary embolism. In acute right ventricular strain, the QRS vector is often altered so that an S wave appears in lead I while a significant Q wave with T-wave inversion develops in lead III (S1, Q3, T3 pattern of McGinn and White). T-wave inversion in leads II and aVF may also be present so that an inferior wall MI is simulated. Inverted T waves in the right precordial leads (V3 and V4) may occur, but ST segment deviations are absent or of small amplitude. ECG also may be valuable in the patient with chest pain by uncovering arrhythmias, conduction abnormalities, or hypertrophy patterns.

Chest Radiography

Chest radiographs are likely to be unremarkable during an acute ischemic episode or in an uncomplicated MI. Pulmonary vascular congestion, however, may occur in either. The heart shadow is usually normal. A large heart

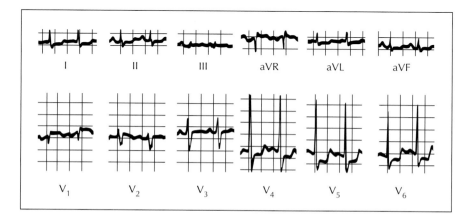

FIGURE 5 Exercise electrocardiogram demonstrating 2 to 3 mm of horizontal to downsloping ST segment depression in V_4 through V_6. (*Adapted from* Shamroth [25]; with permission.)

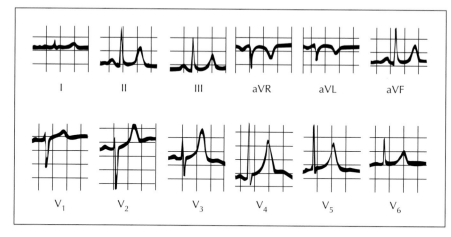

FIGURE 6 Electrocardiogram taken during ischemic chest pain demonstrates peaked T waves in II, III, aVF, and V_2 through V_6. (*Adapted from* Shamroth [25]; with permission.)

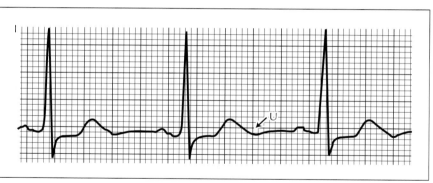

FIGURE 7 Electrocardiogram taken during ischemic chest pain demonstrates less than 1 mm horizontal ST depression associated with inverted U waves. (*Adapted from* Shamroth [25]; with permission.)

shadow during an ischemic episode or in the early stages of an infarct suggest antecedent myocardial damage, valvular disease, or pericardial effusion. Pulmonary infiltrates, pneumothorax, rib fractures, and metastatic lesions are other sources of chest pain that may be discovered by the chest film. Although a widened mediastinum on the posteroanterior view is usually seen in patients with aortic dissection, it is nonspecific and often seen in elderly patients. However, a normal mediastinal width makes aortic dissection less likely. If the patient is stable enough to be transported to the radiology department, a spiral CT scan can be used to look for aortic dissection.

Echocardiography

Echocardiography may be helpful in delineating the cause of cardiac chest pain. A transthoracic echocardiogram may reveal wall motion abnormalities during an episode of ischemic heart pain and in the early stages of MI, even when the ECG is still normal. Unsuspected valvular disease, pericardial effusion, widened aortic root, and, occasionally, dissection of the ascending aorta may be demonstrated. A transesophageal echocardiogram is useful and accurate in the early diagnosis of aortic dissection [7]. If the patient is stable enough to be transported to the radiology department, a spiral CT scan can also be used to look for aortic dissection.

Laboratory Studies

Arterial blood gases and pulse oximetry are usually at normal levels in patients with acute ischemic heart disease, unless significant left ventricular congestion or antecedent lung disease coexist. Hypoxia with associated hypocapnia is a nonspecific finding common to pulmonary congestion, pulmonary embolism, and other acute respiratory problems.

A complete blood count may be valuable in the differential diagnosis of chest pain. Severe anemia is occasionally first manifested by angina. Acute MI and pulmonary embolism both may be associated with a modest granulocytosis; however, a markedly elevated leukocyte count (>15,000/mL) with a shift to the left should raise the suspicion of an infectious origin.

Evaluation of cardiac enzymes during the initial patient assessment may be helpful as well, but routine measurements of creatine kinase MB (CK-MB) fraction and troponin levels are often normal in the early stages of an infarction. Myoglobin levels may be elevated within 3 hours of presentation, when the initial CK-MB level is negative. Myoglobin levels, however, are elevated with any muscle injury and are therefore highly nonspecific. Musculoskeletal causes of chest pain (eg, skeletal muscle injury, myositis, thoracic outlet syndrome) can be expected to raise both myoglobin and the total CK level. Measurement of CK-MB and troponin I or T followed by early exercise testing if it remains normal is a cost-effective strategy for patients with a low to moderate probability of an MI. In patients with a higher risk level, troponin levels are cost effective if the CK-MB level is normal and early exercise testing is not an option.

NONINVASIVE EVALUATION

For stable patients with clearly noncardiac chest pain or a very low probability of coronary disease, any further work-up can proceed on an outpatient basis, and empiric therapy is often in order. If the patient's history of chest pain represents a stable pattern of angina pectoris, the work-up can again proceed on an outpatient basis with use of noninvasive procedures. For patients with an intermediate likelihood of coronary disease and whose chest pain syndrome may represent an unstable pattern of angina, continued careful observation in an emergency room, chest pain unit, or in-patient facility is warranted until the possibility of cardiac etiology is either confirmed or excluded. The observation must include continuous monitoring of ECGs, frequent vital signs, determination of cardiac markers for myocardial injury and ST segment monitoring (with frequent 12- or 15-lead ECGs). Noninvasive procedures involve monitoring the ECG under either physiologic or pharmacologic stress. Simultaneous use of myocardial imaging techniques greatly improves the sensitivity, specificity, and predictive value of the tests. Stress testing within 6 to 12 hours after presentation to the hospital can be performed safely in stable patients (ie, those without failure, significant arrhythmias, or ischemic ECG changes at rest who are no longer in pain and whose cardiac enzymes have failed to demonstrate myocardial injury) [8]. Selection of the most appropriate test depends on the patient's exercise capacity, ability to tolerate pharmacologic intervention, and, especially, the pretest likelihood of significant obstructive coronary disease.

The choice of a suitable noninvasive test for a patient with ischemic disease is decided by the predictive accuracy of the test for that patient. The predictive accuracy of the test is determined by the patient's pretest likelihood for coronary disease, which is determined by the patient's gender, age, chest pain characteristics, family history, and other risk factors [6••]. Angina pectoris is rare before age 35 years, especially in women; however, its likelihood increases with each decade of life. Between ages 35 and 65 years, men have a higher likelihood of CAD; after age 65 years, it is distributed relatively equally among men and women. The presence and number of risk factors also increase the likelihood of disease. Combining these factors, the clinician can arrive at a level of suspicion (ie, low, intermediate, or high) for CAD. Various tests for ischemia provide a degree of positive or negative confirmation of that pretest likelihood (eg, the posttest likelihood deviates to a greater degree from the pretest likelihood).

Exercise Treadmill Test

The exercise treadmill test (ETT), or simple exercise ECG with treadmill (or bicycle ergometry), has the lowest predictive accuracy [6••] and the least ability to quantitate the severity of ischemia. ETT is more likely to be valuable in those with a normal resting ECG because resting ST-T abnormalities or left bundle branch block interferes with interpretation of the test. ETT is best reserved for those with a somewhat moderate or intermediate pretest likelihood of disease in whom the probability of a false-negative result is also low. A positive test carries a chance of being falsely positive and may require further testing with myocardial imaging.

If a patient develops angina such as chest pain associated with horizontal or developing ST-segment depression of more than 1 mm, the likelihood of CAD is high. If the test result is positive with marked ST depression at a low level of exercise, widespread ischemia is suggested. Other features of widespread ischemia are ischemic changes associated with a decrease in BP while exercise continues and prolonged post-exercise ischemic changes. For such patients, cardiac catheterization is usually the next step.

A person with high pretest likelihood of CAD still has a moderate possibility of having the disease, even in the absence of ischemic changes on the ETT. If it is necessary to establish the diagnosis of CAD, this person will require more sensitive tests with myocardial imaging or even coronary arteriography.

The ETT may also provide prognostic information in patients with suspected CAD. The Duke Prognostic Treadmill Score is an attempt to stratify patients into high, intermediate, and low prognostic risk groups based on their performance on treadmill exercise. The prognostic component is intended to assess the likelihood of the subjects succumbing from cardiac disease over the ensuing several years [9,10] (Table 3). The usefulness of the Dukes Score remains unclear. Several other more complex scoring systems have also been devised that claim to better stratify patients into low, intermediate, and high risk [11,12]. However, they are more difficult to derive and are not commonly used in exercise testing. In evaluating a patient with acute or recent onset of chest pain, the presence of any ischemic ECG response must be interpreted in light of the patient's medical history. If an acute infarct

has been excluded and the chest pain syndrome is consistent with unstable angina, any ischemic ECG change on an ETT warrants further investigation, no matter what the Duke Score. On the other hand, if a patient seems otherwise stable, an intermediate or high-risk score may also warrant further investigation [13].

Stress Imaging Studies

Imaging myocardial perfusion or performance during stress provides a higher positive and negative predictive value than exercise ECG alone [14–16]. This is particularly true for patients who have ECG abnormalities at rest or who are taking digoxin or diuretics. For those who are unable to exercise, the use of pharmacologic stress with imaging is indicated. Stress nuclear perfusion studies have a higher technical success than stress echocardiography and a higher sensitivity, especially when multiple wall motion abnormalities are present. On the other hand, stress echocardiography has a greater specificity and a greater ability to evaluate cardiac anatomy and function. Which test to use depends largely on local expertise and availability.

Exercise Perfusion Scintigraphy

Exercise perfusion scintigraphy with thallium or sestamibi carries a better predictive accuracy than simple ETT. In thallium scintigraphy, the radionuclide is injected into a peripheral vein the minute before termination of exercise. Myocardial imaging begins within minutes. The initial "stress" images are compared with those taken 4 hours later, when redistribution allows ischemic areas to take up the radionuclide. This imaging method allows a quantitative analysis of perfusion defects [17]. A negative test result, even in a patient with a high pretest likelihood of disease, decreases the possibility of myocardial ischemia considerably; other causes of chest pain should be strongly considered. Occasionally, however, the pretest likelihood is so compelling that other imaging techniques (eg, stress echocardiography, coronary arteriography) are needed to exclude a false-negative nuclear test.

Dipyridamole Perfusion Scintigraphy

Dipyridamole perfusion scintigraphy is often useful in patients who are unable to exercise adequately on a treadmill [18]. Dipyridamole causes maximum dilatation of the coronary arteries. In the presence of significant CAD, coronary flow reserve is limited and disparities occur in the distribution of the thallium. Predictive accuracy is equivalent to an exercise scintigram. Patients with severe obstructive lung disease or asthma often cannot tolerate dipyridamole; in such patients, stress may be accomplished with dobutamine or adenosine.

Stress Echocardiography

Stress echocardiography is performed with treadmill exercise or bicycle ergometry. Pharmacologic stress is usually performed with dobutamine, but dipyridamole or adeno-

---

TABLE 3 DIAGNOSTIC TREADMILL SCORE

From the total duration of treadmill exercise in minutes:
    Subtract 5 × maximal ST segment deviation in
        millimeters, whether during or after exercise
    From this, subtract 4 × treadmill angina index (0 for
        no angina; 1 for nonlimiting angina; 2 for exercise-
        limiting angina)
    Possible score from −25 (highest risk) to +15 (lowest risk)
      low risk +5 to +15 (2/3 of patients fell in this group and
        had 0.25% annual mortality rate)
      high risk −10 to −25 (4% of patients fell in this group
        and had a 5% annual mortality rate)
 	
(Data from Mark *et al.* [10].)

sine have also been used [19,20]. Studies suggest excellent predictive accuracy for the majority of patients in whom adequate echocardiographic imaging is possible. For patients with difficult imaging, contrast agents are used to improve the assessment of myocardial wall motion.

Other Noninvasive Techniques

Other noninvasive techniques, including positron emission tomography [21] and 24-hour ambulatory ECG (Holter monitoring) [22], are occasionally useful in the evaluation of patients with ischemic chest pain. A high coronary calcium score on CT scan will increase the pretest likelihood for disease in the intermediate risk group independently from age, gender, and other risk factors [23]. Holter monitoring is not appropriate for patients under observation and is too insensitive to be used routinely as an outpatient test for ischemia; however, it may be particularly valuable for patients who experience pain only at rest or who are strongly suspected of having episodes of silent ischemia.

When the likelihood of a cardiac condition is excluded or considered unlikely, further work-up of recurrent chest pain of obscure origin depends on the special characteristics of the patient and the pain. Esophageal manometry with or without provocation, ambulatory 24-hour esophageal monitoring of pH, and psychologic testing may be warranted for selected patients who continue to be uncomfortable and in whom simple measures to treat esophageal disease fail [24]. However, empiric therapy with antisecretory agents may be more cost effective for the majority of such patients whose symptoms point to an esophageal origin [4•].

Coronary Arteriography

The most reliable test for the diagnosis and quantification of CAD is cardiac catheterization with selective coronary arteriography. Indications for coronary arteriography include chest pain suspicious for CAD undiagnosed by thorough noninvasive evaluation, chest pain thought to result from coronary disease but unresponsive to medical therapy, unstable angina, and postinfarction angina. The more unstable the angina, the more reasonable it is to submit the patient to coronary arteriography early, even as one of the first diagnostic tests.

Coronary arteriography in at least two orthogonal views allows an excellent assessment of the extent of CAD as well as the potential for instability in the form of high-grade proximal stenoses, intraluminal thrombus, and ruptured or complicated plaques. Along with the patient's clinical course, this information is used to select medical therapy, catheter intervention (*eg*, angioplasty and stenting), or coronary artery bypass surgery in the management of the patient.

Conclusions

When a patient's chest pain has characteristics suspicious for myocardial ischemia and the patient's age, gender, and other risk factors make coronary disease possible, the clinician should exclude myocardial ischemia as a cause. If the characteristics suggest an unstable pattern of myocardial ischemia, the clinician should exclude acute or recent MI and assess the advisability of urgent antithrombotic therapy or the need for invasive diagnostic procedures. The patient's history, supported by simple physical examination and laboratory evaluation, is central to the process. The need for further consultation and more elaborate diagnostic procedures is determined by this initial evaluation. The more carefully the history is taken, the less likely it is that expensive procedures are ordered unnecessarily.

After the history, physical examination, and ECG, the choice of tests for diagnostic evaluation include ETT, ETT with imaging, and coronary arteriography. Imaging techniques with radionuclide or echocardiography greatly improve diagnostic accuracy. Although expensive, their use could limit the number of coronary arteriograms otherwise required.

References and Recommended Reading

Published papers of particular interest have been highlighted as:
• Of interest
•• Of outstanding interest

1.•• Pope JH, Aufderheide TP, Ruthazer R, *et al.*: Missed diagnoses of acute cardiac ischemia in the emergency department. *N Engl J Med* 2000, 342:1163–1170.

2. Schofield PM, Whorwell PJ, Brooks NH, *et al.*: Oesophageal function in patients with angina pectoris: a comparison of patients with normal coronary angiograms and patients with coronary artery disease. *Digestion* 1989, 42:70–78.

3.• Goyal RK: Changing focus on unexplained esophageal chest pain. *Ann Intern Med* 1996, 124:1008–1011.

4.• Borzecki AM, Pedrosa MC, Prashker MJ: Should noncardiac chest pain be treated empirically? A cost-effectiveness analysis. *Arch Intern Med* 2000, 160:844–852.

5.• Diamond GA, Forrester JS: Analysis of probability as an aid in the clinical diagnosis of coronary artery disease. *N Engl J Med* 1979, 300:1350–1358.

6.•• Epstein SE: Implications of probability analysis on the strategy used for noninvasive detection of coronary artery disease: role of single or combined use of exercise electrocardiographic testing, radionuclide cineangiography and myocardial perfiision imaging. *Am J Cardiol* 1980, 46:491–499.

7. Hashimoto S, Kumada T, Osakada G, *et al.*: Assessment of transesophageal Doppler echography in dissecting aortic aneurysm. *J Am Coll Cardiol* 1989, 14:1253–1262.

8. Gaspoz JM, Lee TH, Cook EF, *et al.*: Outcome of patients who were admitted to a new short-stay unit to "rule-out" myocardial infarction. *Am J Cardiol* 1991, 68:145–149.

9. Shaw LJ, Peterson ED, Shaw LK, *et al.*: Use of prognostic tread-mill score in identifying disgnostic coronary disease subgroups. *Circulation* 1998, 98:1622–1630.

10. Mark DB, Shaw L, Harrell FE Jr., *et al.*: Prognostic value of a treadmill exercise score in outpatients with suspected coronary artery disease. *N Engl J Med* 1991, 325:849–853.

11. Gibbons RJ, Balady GJ, Bricker TJ, *et al.*: ACC/AHA 2002 guideline update for exercise testing: summary article. A report of the American College of Cardiology/American Heart Association Task Force on Practice Guidelines (Committee to Update the 1997 Exercise Testing Guidelines). *J Am Coll Cardiol* 2002, 40:1531–1540.

12. Fearon WF, Gauri AJ, Myers J, *et al.*: A comparison of treadmill scores to diagnose coronary artery disease. *Clin Cardiol* 2002, 25:117–122.

13. Shaw LJ, Hachamovitch R, Iskandrian AE: *J Nucl Cardiol* 1997, 4:74–78.2

14. Beller GA, Zaret BL: Contributions of nuclear cardiology to diagnosis and prognosis of patients with coronary artery disease. *Circulation* 2000, 101:1465–1478.

15. Zaret BL, Wackers FJ: Nuclear cardiology (1). *N Engl J Med* 1993, 329:775–783.

16. Zaret BJ, Wackers FJ: Nuclear cardiology (2). *N Engl J Med* 1993, 329:855–863.

17. Mahmarian JJ, Boyce TM, Goldberg RK, *et al.*: Quantitative exercise thallium-201 single photon emission computed tomography for the enhanced diagnosis of ischemic heart disease. *J Am Coll Cardiol* 1990, 15:318–329.

18. Beller GA: Pharmacologic stress imaging. *JAMA* 1991, 265:633–638.

19. Mazeika PK, Nadazdin A, Oakley CM: Dobutamine stress echocardiography for detection and assessment of coronary artery disease. *J Am Coll Cardiol* 1992, 19:1203–1211.

20. Kontos MC, Hinchman D, Cunningham M, *et al.*: Comparison of contrast echocardiography with single-photon emission computed tomographic myocardial perfusion imaging in the evaluation of patients with possible acute coronary syndromes in the emergency department. *Am J Cardiol* 2003, 91:1099–1102.

21. Demer L, Gould K, Goldstein R, *et al.*: Assessment of coronary artery disease severity by positron emission tomography. comparison with quantitative arteriography in 193 patients. *Circulation* 1989, 79:825–835.

22. Deanfield JE, Rubierc, P, Oakley K, *et al.*: Analysis of ST segment changes in normal subjects: implications for ambulatory monitoring in angina pectoris. *Am J Cardiol* 1984, 54:1321–1325.

23. Greenland P, LaBree L, Azen SP, *et al.*: Coronary artery calcium score combined with Framingham score for risk prediction in asymptomatic individuals. *JAMA* 2004, 291:210–215.

24. Richter J: Overview of diagnostic testing for chest pain of unknown origin. *Am J Med* 1992, 92(suppI 5A):41–45.

25. Shamroth L, ed: *The Electrocardiology of the Coronary Diseases*, edn 1. Philadelphia: JB Lippincott; 1975.

26. Diamond GA: A clinically relevant classification of chest discomfort. *J Am Coll Cardiol* 1983, 1:574–575.

SELECT BIBLIOGRAPHY

Lee TH, Goldman L: evaluation of the patient with acute chest pain. *N Engl J Med* 2000, 342:1187–1195.

Constant J: The clinical diagnosis of non-anginal chest pain: the differentiation of angina from non-anginal chest pain by history. *Clin Cardiol* 1983, 6:11–16.

Rude RE, Pool WK, Muller JE, *et al*: Electrocardiographic and clinical criteria for recognition of acute myocardial infarction based on analysis of 3697 patients. *Am J Cardiol* 1983, 52:936–942.

Evaluation of the Patient with Heart Failure

Carl V. Leier

6

> ### *Key Points*
> - Heart failure is a clinical presentation of an underlying cardiovascular disorder or disease.
> - An effort should be made to diagnose the cause of heart failure, specifically to determine whether the heart failure is caused by a remedially reversible disorder or disease.
> - Neither cardiomegaly nor a depressed ejection fraction alone is indicative of inoperable underlying heart disease.
> - The medical history, a good cardiovascular examination, electrocardiogram, chest roentgenogram, and two-dimensional Doppler echocardiogram are essential components of the initial evaluation of the heart failure patient.
> - Unclear etiology, possible underlying reparable heart disease, symptomatic dysrhythmias and conduction disturbances, New York Heart Association (NYHA) functional class III and IV classification, unstable course, and the need for specialized cardiovascular testing should prompt cardiology consultation or referral to a heart failure–transplantation center.

Heart failure is one of the few cardiovascular conditions that are becoming more prevalent in our society. More than 70% of patients with heart failure are currently evaluated and managed by primary care physicians. This chapter provides recommendations for the evaluation and follow-up of patients with heart failure; these recommendations are in general agreement with published guidelines [1••,2•]. In this setting, optimal patient care and cost-effective management are inseparable because proper evaluation and therapy for heart failure keep patients alive, functional, employed, out of hospitals, and off transplant waiting lists.

INITIAL EVALUATION

The patient with ventricular dysfunction can present in several ways. Evaluation and therapy for each patient must be modified according to clinical presentation, acuity, and severity of heart failure; reversibility of the underlying disease process; and concomitant disease states. Nevertheless, general recommendations can be made to guide the optimal evaluation of the heart failure patient.

Medical History and Physical Findings
Important aspects of medical history

As in most conditions, the acuity and severity of symptoms determine the level of urgency in the evaluation and therapy for the patient with heart failure. A patient presenting with a 3-day history of orthopnea and 12 hours of resting dyspnea deserves more vigorous work-up and treatment than the patient with a 6-month history of steadily increasing pedal edema and easy fatigability, although both patients may ultimately undergo similar testing and often are placed on comparable long-term treatment.

Heart failure alone should never be considered a primary diagnosis. Heart failure is a symptom complex or syndrome; thus, it is always caused by some underlying cardiovascular disorder (*ie*, the primary diagnosis). On establishing the presence of heart failure by medical history and physical examination, the physician focuses on potential underlying causes, particularly reversible causes or those treatable with specific interventions (*eg*, coronary angioplasty-stent, valvular repair or replacement). In general, intermittent symptoms of recent onset are more likely to be caused by reversible lesions (*eg*, occlusive coronary artery disease, ischemic papillary muscle dysfunction with episodic mitral regurgitation) than are long-standing symptoms. Although surgically treatable, chronic valvular stenosis or insufficiency often presents with long-standing symptoms. A history of major coronary risk factors (*eg*, smoking, diabetes mellitus, family history), concomitant angina pectoris, and intermittent or nocturnal symptoms should suggest occlusive atherosclerotic coronary artery disease and resultant disorders (*eg*, intermittent myocardial ischemia, diastolic or systolic dysfunction, papillary muscle dysfunction with mitral regurgitation). "Flash" pulmonary edema is usually caused by occlusive coronary artery disease, uncontrolled severe hypertension (often secondary to renal artery stenosis), periodic noncompliance to diet and drug therapy, or a combination of these factors.

Although a recent viral illness should raise the consideration of viral myocarditis in a patient with new onset heart failure, the symptoms of a viral event are often indistinguishable from those experienced during an episode of congestive heart failure. Serologic testing for virus and endomyocardial biopsy for signs of inflammation are usually unrevealing in this setting. Our ability to diagnose postviral cardiomyopathy should improve as better diagnostic techniques are developed for viral infections and retroviral DNA/RNA alterations.

As many as 30% to 40% of patients with idiopathic dilated cardiomyopathy have a family history of cardiomegaly, heart failure, or sudden death [3], suggesting that some patients with dilated cardiomyopathy develop their illness by genetic transmission. However, until these defects are more precisely defined and biotechnologically correctable, the clinical approach to these patients is still the same as that to other patients with dilated cardiomyopathy.

Increasing age, obesity, diabetes mellitus, and a history of systemic hypertension should suggest that diastolic dysfunction may play a major pathophysiologic role, often the primary role, in the patient's heart failure. Many of these patients will have normal left ventricular systolic function (ejection fraction >45%) at rest.

Advancing age, increased severity of heart failure symptoms, a poor or refractory response to optimal medical management, and a history of syncope or cardiac arrest are some of the major historical points that portend a less favorable prognosis [1••,2•,3–6].

Key physical findings

The initial physical examination is generally directed at evaluating the extent and severity of heart failure and looking for clues for an underlying cause.

Indicators of extent and severity of heart failure

The severity and general character of a patient's heart failure are cumulatively assessed on physical examination by the presence and degree of a general appearance of well-being, anxiety or distress, pallor, cyanosis, tachypnea, Cheyne-Stokes respiratory pattern, tachycardia, narrow pulse pressure, pulsus alternans, pulsus paradoxus, systemic hypotension, hypokinetic and laterally displaced apical impulse, ventricular gallop sounds, mitral and tricuspid regurgitant murmurs, pulmonary rales, pleural effusion, elevated jugular venous pressure, hepatojugular reflux, hepatomegaly with or without tenderness and ascites, and pedal edema. It is important to record the initial (*ie*, baseline) positive and pertinent negative findings because they, along with body weight and symptoms, are the principal means of guiding therapy.

Clues for underlying cause of heart failure

Most patients with chronic congestive cardiac failure have evidence of both right and left heart failure. Patients with decompensated nonischemic dilated cardiomyopathy and patients with predominant right heart dysfunction (*eg*, cor pulmonale, right ventricular dysplasia) usually present with prominent signs of right heart failure, including jugular venous distention, hepatomegaly with or without ascites, or peripheral edema. If the patient presents with predominant signs and symptoms of left heart failure, the primary considerations for differential diagnosis are systemic hypertension, occlusive coronary artery disease, and an aortic or mitral valvular disorder.

Evidence of systemic atherosclerotic vascular disease implicates occlusive coronary artery disease as the cause of the patient's heart failure.

Systemic hypotension unrelated to drug therapy in the patient with adequate or high ventricular filling pressures suggests considerable cardiac dysfunction and an unfavorable prognosis; vasodilator and converting enzyme inhibitor therapy are often difficult to administer in such a patient. Elevated blood pressure may be a consequence of the neurohormonal reaction to cardiac failure (particularly during acute cardiac failure); however, long-standing or severe uncontrolled systemic hypertension is often a major contributor or the predominant cause of cardiac decompensation. The patient with hypertensive heart failure usually responds favorably to proper antihypertensive, afterload-reducing therapy.

Several systemic illnesses are associated with cardiac disease and failure; a few include various neuromuscular disorders (eg, muscular dystrophy, myotonia dystrophica, Friedreich's ataxia), thyroid disease, and amyloidosis. The presence of a hyperdynamic precordium and circulation (tachycardia and bounding, full pulses) raises the possibility of high-output heart failure and the various causes, including anemia, hyperthyroidism, and arteriovenous malformations; most of these conditions are treatable.

Blood/Serum Studies

Most patients with heart failure should have a baseline complete blood count, thyroid function studies, and measurement of serum electrolytes, urea nitrogen, creatinine, and magnesium. Hyponatremia, azotemia, and anemia of chronic disease are often indicative of a severe, advanced stage of heart failure. Brain natriuretic peptide (BNP) is produced and released by the ventricles during periods of high wall stress, as occurs with most forms of heart failure [7]. The laboratory determination of this substance in a blood sample (specifically plasma) can be helpful in distinguishing cardiac failure from other causes of dyspnea, exertional fatigue, and related symptoms. BNP levels generally fall during effective management of the heart failure. BNP may have prognostic value, correlating indirectly with long-term outcome.

Other laboratory tests that can be informative in certain situations include cardiac enzymes, sedimentation rate, C-reactive protein, serum iron studies, and occasionally viral serology tests when myocarditis is suspected; coagulation studies (ie, prothrombin time, activated partial thromboplastin time, and platelet count) if anticoagulation therapy is anticipated; hepatic enzymes to assess the patient with severe heart failure and liver congestion; and arterial blood gas and pH in severe heart failure complicated by respiratory distress or problematic low cardiac output.

Chest Roentgenography

In addition to excluding unrelated but complicating conditions (eg, lung neoplasia) in a generally middle-aged to older population, the chest roentgenogram gives the physician a reasonable assessment of heart size, cardiac chamber enlargement, pulmonary congestion, and pleural effusion, and it can render clues regarding cause (Fig. 1). Along with the physical examination, the chest roentgenogram is a reasonable (and least expensive) method of following heart size and pulmonary congestion during long-term management.

Electrocardiogram, Specialized Electrocardiographic Studies, and Electrophysiologic Testing

The electrocardiogram (ECG) establishes the cardiac rhythm at the time of the test and provides clues regarding hypertrophy and conduction disturbances (Fig. 2). Infarct patterns suggest occlusive coronary artery disease as the cause or contributing condition, although nonischemic cardiomyopathies are the most common disorders causing "pseudoin-

farct" patterns. Some studies have found atrial fibrillation and left ventricular conduction defects to be some of the predictors of a poor outcome in heart failure [4–6].

The electrocardiographic finding of ventricular conduction block (left bundle branch block, intraventricular conduction block, and perhaps right bundle branch block) with a QRS duration of over 120 msec in a patient with an ejection fraction under 35% and residing at functional capacity III-IV is very important in identifying the patient who may benefit from cardiac resynchronization therapy (an intervention provided by biventricular pacing).

In the case of acute heart failure, an early ECG is invaluable in determining whether a patient might benefit from immediate thrombolytic therapy or urgent cardiac catheterization with coronary intervention.

Signal-averaged electrocardiography (SAE) appears to have little predictive power in nonischemic cardiomyopathy [4,6,8,9]. The prognostic value in ischemic cardiomyopathy is probably better, but the information is of limited practical value because therapeutic interventions have not yet been shown to significantly alter the clinical course of the heart failure patient with an abnormal SAE. The analysis of heart rate variability can provide a laboratory correlate of severity of heart failure and perhaps prognosis [6,10]. This methodology is currently limited in its clinical application by general non-availability, non-reimbursement, and multiple variables. The approach to disordered heart rate variability in this setting is still optimization of congestive heart failure (CHF) therapy.

Holter ECG recordings are not recommended as a routine component of the initial evaluation of the heart failure patient, but are quite informative in directing antiarrhythmic therapy, pacemaker interventions, or defibrillator placement in patients experiencing dysrhythmia-induced symptoms [4,6,11–14]. ECG event recorders with memory are useful in assessing patients with infrequent, dysrhythmia-induced symptoms.

The role of invasive electrophysiologic testing is currently somewhat limited in the setting of CHF. It is occasionally combined with upright tilt testing for the patient with unexplained near-syncope or syncope and non-diagnostic Holter or event ECG recordings, although the approach to suspected dysrhythmia-induced syncope in heart failure is moving toward cardioverter-defibrillator insertion [13]. The results of the Multicenter Unsustained Tachycardia Trial (MUSTT) [14] suggest that patients with an ejection fraction of less than 40% after myocardial infarction should undergo Holter monitoring followed by EPS testing in those of nonsustained ventricular tachycardia. The patients with sustained (>30 seconds) ventricular tachycardia on Holter monitoring or extrastimuli-induced ventricular tachycardia appear to attain a significant survival benefit from placement of a cardioverter-debrillator unit. Results of the MADIT II trial raise consideration for inserting defibrillators to improve survival in all postinfarct patients with an ejection fraction less than 30% [15].

Echocardiography

Echocardiography is a pivotal diagnostic study in the initial evaluation of the heart failure patient. In addition to providing information on the size and function of the four heart chambers, echocardiography is the test of choice to determine whether mitral or tricuspid regurgitation (both can be inaudible on examination) and ventricular diastolic dysfunction play a role in the patient's presentation (Fig. 3). Echocardiography, particularly transesophageal, can be helpful in detecting cardiac sources of systemic and pulmonic embolization, not an uncommon complication of cardiac failure.

Exercise Testing

For patients who can adequately relate their symptoms to the physician, exercise testing is not an essential component of the initial evaluation. However, exercise testing can be helpful in corroborating a patient's symptoms, following the patient's therapy, assessing a patient's candidacy for employment or cardiac transplantation, and prescribing an exercise conditioning program [16–18]. Expiratory gas analysis is also not essential, but this technique provides a more precise evaluation of exercise capacity and effort [17,18]. Although influenced by age, physi-

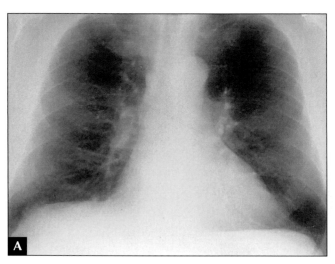
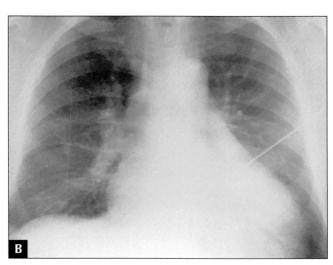
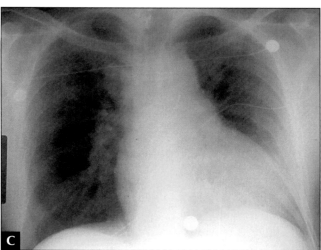
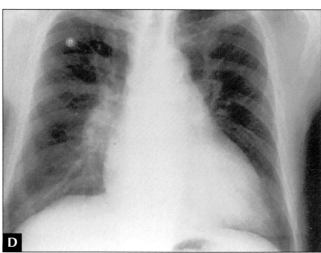

FIGURE 1 **A**, Relatively unremarkable chest roentgenogram of a 52-year-old tire dealer who presented to an emergency room 3 weeks earlier with acute "flash" pulmonary edema. At cardiac catheterization-angiography, high-grade obstructive lesions were noted along the proximal segments of the right coronary artery and left anterior descending coronary artery. **B**, Chest roentgenogram shows marked cardiomegaly, pulmonary venous engorgement, and pleural effusion of the base and minor fissure of the right chest; this 66-year-old salesman presented with decompensation of chronic heart failure secondary to nonischemic dilated cardiomyopathy. **C**, Moderate pulmonary edema on chest roentgenogram of a 49-year-old factory administrator who presented with a 9-month history of dyspnea on exertion, 4 hours of increasing dyspnea at rest, and chest "tightness." He had undergone coronary artery bypass surgery 8 years before this hospital admission. Electrocardiogram and cardiac enzyme analyses indicated an acute anterior myocardial infarction in addition to a prior inferior wall infarction. **D**, Chest roentgenogram of a 78-year-old retired restaurant owner afflicted with 9 to 10 months of increasing dyspnea on exertion, orthopnea, and pedal edema. Mild left ventricular systolic dysfunction (EF 45%), marked biventricular diastolic dysfunction, and normal epicardial coronary arteries were noted at cardiac catheterization.

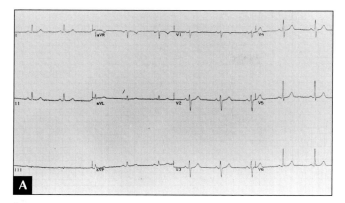

A

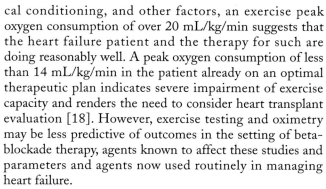

cal conditioning, and other factors, an exercise peak oxygen consumption of over 20 mL/kg/min suggests that the heart failure patient and the therapy for such are doing reasonably well. A peak oxygen consumption of less than 14 mL/kg/min in the patient already on an optimal therapeutic plan indicates severe impairment of exercise capacity and renders the need to consider heart transplant evaluation [18]. However, exercise testing and oximetry may be less predictive of outcomes in the setting of beta-blockade therapy, agents known to affect these studies and parameters and agents now used routinely in managing heart failure.

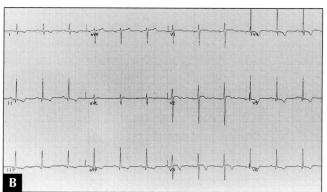

B

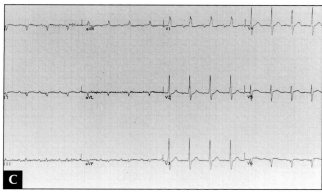

C

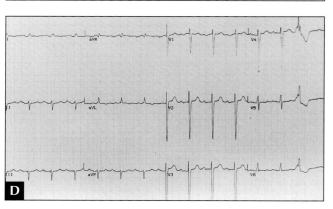

D

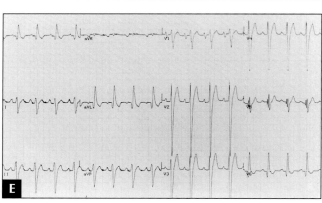

E

FIGURE 2 A, Normal electrocardiogram of a 68-year-old retired university professor who first presented with the sole complaint of 3 months of increasing dyspnea on exertion. Proximal high-grade obstructive coronary artery disease was noted at cardiac catheterization (*see* Fig. 4A). B, The electrocardiogram of a 52-year-old farmer with a 5-year history of increasing dyspnea on exertion, easy fatigability, and two episodes of severe decompensation (pulmonary edema). The left ventricular hypertrophy pattern noted on the electrocardiogram is a consequence of a 25- to 30-year history of inadequately controlled essential hypertension. C, Electrocardiogram of a 58-year-old laborer with a 3-week history of increasing weakness and pedal edema. Four weeks before admission, he experienced episodic severe chest pain and intermittent nausea and vomiting. The electrocardiogram shows an extensive posterolateral myocardial infarction, marked right axis deviation, and left posterior fascicular block. Physical examination, echocardiography, and cardiac catheterization further demonstrated moderate mitral regurgitation, elevated left and right ventricular end-diastolic and pulmonary artery pressures, depressed cardiac output, moderately increased left

ventricular diastolic volume, and reduced ejection fraction (24%) secondary to a ventricular remodeling and large akinetic zone involving the inferior, posterior, and lateral regions of the left ventricle. Complete occlusions of the proximal right coronary artery and left circumflex coronary artery were seen on coronary angiography. D, This electrocardiogram, showing biventricular enlargement, left axis deviation, a premature ventricular beat, abnormal P waves, and prolonged PR interval, was taken of a 42-year-old housewife with a 3-year history of progressively symptomatic dilated cardiomyopathy. She was referred for further treatment and transplantation evaluation. E, Myocardial dystrophy is the likely explanation for the electrocardiographic changes observed in this 20-year-old patient with Duchenne muscular dystrophy. Sinus tachycardia, abnormal P waves, left axis deviation, intraventricular conduction delay, lateral wall "pseudoinfarct" pattern, and biventricular enlargement are represented on the recording. In addition to musculoskeletal limitations, he had been afflicted with advancing symptoms and signs of heart failure for 3 to 4 years before this admission. He was dyspneic at rest and had orthopnea, hepatomegaly, and pedal edema on admission.

Cardiac Catheterization-Angiography

Most patients with heart failure deserve strong consideration for a diagnostic cardiac catheterization-angiography before their condition is declared irreparable. It is often impossible to distinguish nonischemic from ischemic forms of cardiac failure, and unless a reversible cause for heart failure is found, congestive heart failure has a grim long-term prognosis. An ejection fraction of 0.25 or less is no longer considered a contraindication to a revascularization procedure because revascularization can be effective in improving such a patient's ventricular dysfunction and heart failure if reversible myocardial ischemia, rather than infarction, is causing the ventricular dysfunction (Fig. 4) [19,20].

Patients with another end-stage illness limiting their overall clinical course and survival (*eg*, metastatic malignant neoplasia) and elderly patients who are not likely to survive a major surgical procedure may not benefit greatly from cardiac catheterization-angiography.

Patients who present with acute heart failure are more likely to have a remedially reparable cardiac lesion compared with patients with more chronic forms of heart failure. For patients presenting with acute pulmonary edema or cardiogenic shock, precise diagnostic definition of the cardiac lesions and urgent, specific intervention (*eg*, angioplasty-stent or valvular repair or replacement) offer the optimal and, often, the only means of improving an otherwise dismal clinical course and reduced survival [21,22].

Myocardial Biopsy

Without specific, proven-effective therapy as an end point for obtaining a specific diagnosis, there are no absolute indications for performing an endomyocardial biopsy in heart failure. On the other hand, transvenous endomyocardial biopsy is the best way of diagnosing or confirming several pathogenic cardiac conditions, including myocarditis, Löffler's eosinophilic endocarditis, amyloidosis, and other inflammatory and infiltrative disorders. Corticosteroid or any immunosuppressive therapy is not empirically indicated (*ie*, without an endomyocardial biopsy) for a patient who presents with dilated cardiomyopathy and suspected myocarditis. Most of these patients do not have histologic myocarditis, and the risk–benefit ratio of empiric corticosteroid or any other immunosuppressive therapy in cardiomyopathic heart failure likely exceeds that of an endomyocardial biopsy and directed therapy. Endomyocardial biopsy is a principal means of following cardiac rejection after transplantation.

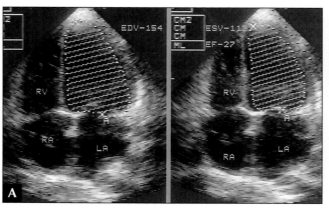

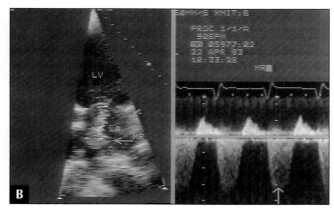

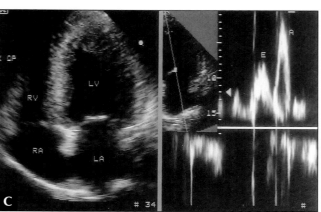

FIGURE 3 **A,** Two-dimensional echocardiographic apical four-chamber views in a 36-year-old patient who presented with congestive heart failure secondary to nonischemic dilated cardiomyopathy, demonstrating marked left ventricular (LV) enlargement and depressed systolic function with modest volume change from diastole (*left*) to systole (*right*). End-diastolic volume equals 154 mL; end-systolic volume, 111 mL; and ejection fraction (EF), 27%. **B,** Color Doppler (*left*) and continuous wave Doppler (*right*) images from a patient with dilated cardiomyopathy and considerable mitral regurgitation (*arrows*), which was barely audible on auscultation. (*See* Color Plate). **C,** Two-dimensional apical four-chamber view of a 53-year-old patient with long-standing systemic hypertension and heart failure demonstrating (*left*) marked concentric left ventricular hypertrophy (wall thickness, 1.5 cm; LV mass index, 154 g/m²). Systolic function was normal (EF, 65%), but pulsed Doppler of mitral inflow (*right*) demonstrates markedly diminished early filling velocities (E) and enhanced atrial contribution to filling (A) consistent with impaired diastolic relaxation. (*See* Color Plate.)

Pharmacohemodynamic Evaluation

Patients with refractory heart should benefit from intense pharmacohemodynamic study before being placed on a cardiac transplant waiting list or being declared to have terminal congestive heart failure [23,24]. Such patients should be referred to a comprehensive heart failure center to take advantage of expertise in the use of standard heart failure medication, pharmacohemodynamic evaluation of standard and experimental agents, therapeutic application of experimental compounds, and assessment and treatment of transplant candidates.

Other Testing Modalities

Myocardial imaging

Resting or stress radionuclide perfusion studies, magnetic resonance viability testing, and positron emission tomogra-phy (PET) can help in determining myocardial viability in patients who present with occlusive coronary artery disease complicated by heart failure [20,25]. A patient with operable occlusive coronary artery disease and a substantial amount of viable, threatened myocardium should be considered for a revascularization procedure.

Pulmonary function studies

Dyspnea and related symptoms of many patients are secondary to combined cardiac and pulmonic disease. After a patient's heart failure is optimally treated, pulmonary function studies are indicated in patients with any clinical evidence (eg, history of smoking, findings on physical examination) of lung disease. For patients with reduced expiratory flow rates, bronchodilators should be tested to determine the reversibility of impaired flow rates and whether certain

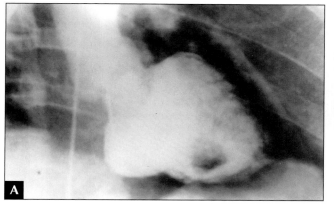

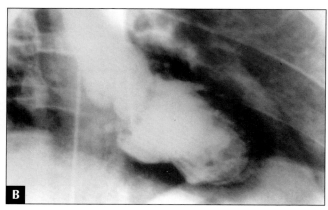

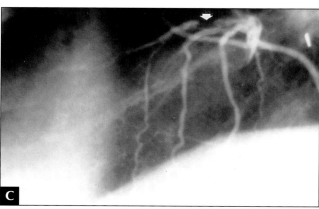

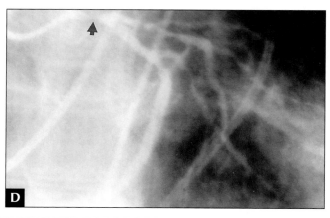

FIGURE 4 A through C, Angiographic frames of the patient presented in Figure 2A. Coronary artery bypass surgery was successful in bringing this patient from relative physical inactivity before surgery to a daily 2-mile run or 2000-yard swim within 9 months of his surgery. A, Contrast injection of left ventricle in diastole. Some chamber enlargement is present. B, Considerable anterior and apical hypokinesis are demonstrated in this end-systolic frame. The hypokinetic regions demonstrated thallium redistribution, indicating viable myocardium. The preoperative ejection fraction of 0.28 rose to 0.48 6 months after surgery. C, Left lateral view of a left coronary artery injection demonstrating an occlusive lesion of the proximal left anterior descending coronary artery (arrow).

Scattered plaques were noted along the proximal right coronary artery. The patient did not recall ever experiencing angina pectoris. D, Left coronary injection of a 76-year-old man who went to his local emergency room on two occasions with severe dyspnea, weakness, roentgenographic pulmonary edema, and transient electrocardiographic anterior ischemic changes. A high-grade obstructive lesion is present in the left main coronary artery (arrow) with additional obstructive disease in the proximal left anterior descending artery. A nondominant right coronary artery was completely occluded. He remains symptom-free with increased physical activity 18 months after coronary bypass surgery.

patients need bronchodilators as part of their overall therapeutic plan. Pulmonary function studies can be helpful in evaluating the safe application of beta-blockade theapy in the heart failure patient with chronic lung disease or airways disorders.

Sleep studies

Sleep disorders occur in over 60% of patients with heart failure. These conditions adversely affect cardiac function and hemodynamics (particularly right heart) and generally exacerbate the symptoms of the heart failure patient. Specifically directed interventions (eg, nocturnal oxygen, continuous positive airway pressure [CPAP], biphasic positive airway pressure [BiPAP]) can improve the clinical and cardiac status of the heart failure patient afflicted with a sleep disorder. Thus, sleep studies are indicated in the heart failure patient at particular risk (eg, concomitant obesity, oropharyngeal crowding) and in those relating symptoms of a sleep disorder (eg, restless sleep, snoring, daytime tiredness or somnolence).

FOLLOW-UP EVALUATION

The outpatient care of the patient with heart failure is facilitated by patient (and spouse) participation in the day-to-day management of the condition by adhering to dietary instructions, recording daily weights at home, promptly reporting new or worsening symptoms to the physician's office, continually learning about the condition and treatment, and, if feasible, joining a support group of heart failure patients.

General Clinical Evaluation

An immense amount of information can be quickly attained by observing the patient and spouse (or close family member or friend) during the initial greeting. A favorable or steady course and an unfavorable course (eg, worsening or new symptoms) can be sensed by the physician, then verified by further questioning and cardiovascular examination. The clinical impression extracted from this initial brief contact generally guides the direction, activities, and intensity of the outpatient visit.

The standard clinical question, "How are you doing?" is a reasonable way to start a focused recent medical history. Further questioning is then directed at the patient's (or spouse's) response, the course of prior symptoms, activity and sleep patterns, outpatient body weight recordings, dietary issues, and medications.

The focused follow-up cardiovascular examination in heart failure includes assessment of body weight, supine and upright heart rate and blood pressure, estimation of jugular venous pressure, palpation of carotid pulses and precordium, auscultation for the presence and intensity of gallop sounds and murmurs (particularly mitral and tricuspid regurgitation), palpation and measurement of the liver (vertical span along the right clavicular line), and

palpation of the legs and ankles for edema and tenderness. General appearance and the respiratory rate and pattern are gleaned from the patient during the examination. A lung examination for rales and pleural effusion follows a history of dyspnea at rest, increasing dyspnea, tachypnea, weight gain, and the finding of rales or effusion during a prior examination.

At this point, the clinician has most of the information needed to adjust the patient's activities, diet, and medication, order additional laboratory studies, and determine the timing of the subsequent visit. If the patient has recently experienced an unfavorable course, the decision is made to alter outpatient management or to admit the patient to the hospital.

Follow-up Laboratory Testing

A standard schedule of outpatient laboratory testing cannot satisfy the clinical needs of all patients with ventricular dysfunction and heart failure. Follow-up laboratory testing is best individualized to avoid inappropriate risk, expense, and use of laboratory time and resources for a low yield of useful information and clinical benefit. Common sense is the guiding principle. However, routine tests are necessary for patients receiving certain medications (eg, anticoagulation therapy) or for patients with more symptomatic or advanced stages of heart failure.

Chronic stable mild heart failure (NYHA functional class I or II)

Patients in the NYHA class I or II category require fewer outpatient visits and less laboratory testing. After a stable course is achieved, an occasional (eg, every 6 to 12 months) serum potassium and urea nitrogen (or creatinine) determination is usually the maximal laboratory requirement. An echocardiogram to determine chamber size and function is reasonable at greater than 18- to 24-month intervals.

Chronic moderate to severe heart failure (NYHA functional class III or IV)

Patients with NYHA functional class III or IV heart failure require more frequent follow-up visits than patients with milder heart failure. As the severity of heart failure increases, symptoms and complications escalate in frequency and intensity, the overall clinical condition becomes more unstable, and the medication requirements, adjustments, and side effects increase. Functional class III or IV patients are generally seen in the outpatient setting at 2-week to 3-month intervals. To avert hospitalization during a relatively unstable period, more frequent visits (as many as 1 to 2 per week) and laboratory testing may be required. Unless the patient enters an unstable decompensated phase, outpatient management may include an annual echocardiogram to assess cardiac chamber size and function and the degree of mitral and tricuspid regurgitation.

With effective history taking, intermittent exercise testing is not essential for the optimal treatment of most patients with chronic heart failure. An exercise study can be useful in assessing a patient with symptoms disparate from clinical or other laboratory findings and evaluating whether a patient should continue or seek employment, apply for employment disability, or undergo evaluation for cardiac transplantation.

Certain patients require other testing modalities to address specific complaints and problems. For example, Holter or event ECG recordings should be considered in the heart failure patient with palpitations and related symptoms, and ECG should be considered in a patient with a recent change in cardiac rhythm, a recent episode of prolonged angina, or suspected ventricular conduction defect (*eg*, left bundle branch block). Repeat cardiac catheterization and coronary angiography should be considered in a heart failure patient whose remote catheterization showed nonocclusive coronary lesions but now presents with angina, angina-equivalent symptoms, or unexpected decompensation.

Decompensation

The patient whose symptoms are escaping a previously effective therapeutic plan deserves special, more intense consideration and, often, referral to a cardiologist or heart failure center.

After review of the patient's symptoms, inquiries should be made into changes in personal and home situations. Family or marital difficulties, financial problems, dietary alterations or indiscretions, and intentional or inadvertent changes in medications or dosing schedule often provide clues for the mechanisms of the clinical deterioration. A focused cardiovascular examination is then performed to establish physical evidence of clinical deterioration (*eg*, body weight, level of jugular venous distention, liver size, rales, pedal edema) and to reveal complications of heart failure (*eg*, new onset atrial fibrillation, recent development of mitral regurgitation) that may explain or significantly contribute to the deteriorating course. Decompensation is not uncommonly precipitated by noncardiovascular conditions (*eg*, respiratory infection or recent addition of a nonsteroidal antiinflammatory drug).

If the explanation for the unfavorable course is not apparent from history and physical examination and to further assess the extent of decompression, laboratory testing is indicated and generally includes assessment of serum electrolytes, urea nitrogen, creatinine, complete blood count and, occasionally, hepatic enzymes; chest roentgenogram to evaluate heart size and degree of pulmonary congestion; and two-dimensional Doppler echocardiography to assess changes in chamber size and function and the presence and degree of mitral and tricuspid regurgitation.

If the patient's deteriorating clinical condition is threatening or does not respond in a reasonable time (1 to 3 days) to a rational change in therapy, the patient should be hospitalized for monitored observation, intravenous therapy directed at improving symptoms and the patient's cardiovascular status (*eg*, intravenously administered diuretics, vasodilators, nesiritide, dobutamine, or milrinone), additional diagnostic studies, and consideration for pharmacohemodynamic evaluation [23,24].

EVALUATING THE CARDIAC TRANSPLANTATION CANDIDATE

The complete evaluation of the heart failure patient for cardiac transplantation is best done via referral to a heart failure or transplantation specialist. Nevertheless, the referring physician can greatly assist in the preliminary assessment of the transplantation candidate. Basically, the typical candidate approved as a transplant recipient is a person younger than 65 years of age with symptomatic advanced heart failure refractory to optimal therapy. The patient is in otherwise good health without a chronic infection, infectious source, major chronic disease, or terminal illness. Compliance to physician and nurse instructions, stable psychological make-up, and an intact familial and social support structure are other important favorable features of an acceptable transplant-recipient candidate.

REFERENCES AND RECOMENDED READING

Recently published papers of particular interest have been highlighted as:
• Of interest
•• Of outstanding interest

1.•• ACC/AHA guidelines for the evaluation and management of chronic heart failure in the adult: executive summary. *J Am Coll Cardiol* 2001, 38:2101–2113.

2.• ACTION-HF Committee: Consensus recommendations for the management of chronic heart failure. *Am J Cardiol* 1999, 83(suppl 2A):1–37.

3. Unverferth DV, Wooley CF: Familial dilated cardiomyopathy. In *Dilated Cardiomyopathy*. Edited by Unverferth DV. Mt. Kisco, NY: Futura Publishing Co.; 1985:159–165.

4. Leier CV: The cardiomyopathies: mortality, sudden death, and ventricular arrhythmias. In *Cardiovascular Clinics: Contemporary Management of Ventricular Arrhythmias*. Edited by Greenspon AJ, Waxman HL. Philadelphia: FA Davis Co.; 1992:275–306.

5. Unverferth DV, Magorien RD, Moeschberger ML, *et al.*: Factors influencing the one-year mortality of dilated cardiomyopathy. *Am J Cardiol* 1984, 54:147–152.

6. Leier CV, Alvarez RJ, Binkley PB: The problem of ventricular dysrrhythmias and sudden death in cardiac failure: impact of current therapy. *Cardiology* 2000, 93:56–69.

7. Dao Q, Krishnaswamy P, Kazanegra R, *et al.*: Utility of B-type natriuretic peptide (BNP) in the diagnosis of CHF in an urgent care setting. *J Am Coll Cardiol* 2001, 37:379–385.

8. Gonska B, Bethge K, Figulla H, *et al.*: Occurrence and clinical significance of endocardial late potentials and fractionations in idiopathic dilated cardiomyopathy. *Br Heart J* 1988, 59:39–46.

9. Turitto G, Ahuja RK, Caref EB, El-Sherif N: Risk stratification for arrhythmic events in patients with nonischemic dilated cardiomyopathy and nonsustained ventricular tachycardia: role of programmed ventricular stimulation and the signal-averaged electrocardiogram. *J Am Coll Cardiol* 1994, 24:1523–1528.

10. Brouwer J, Van Veldhuisen DJ, Man in't Veld AJ, *et al.* for the Dutch Ibopamine multicenter trial group: Prognostic value of heart rate variability during long-term follow-up in patients with mild to moderate heart failure. *J Am Coll Cardiol* 1996, 28:1183–1189.

11. Holmes J, Kubo SH, Cody RJ, *et al.*: Arrhythmias in ischemic and nonischemic dilated cardiomyopathy: prediction of mortality by ambulatory electrocardiography. *Am J Cardiol* 1985, 55:146–151.

12. Hofmann T, Meinertz T, Kasper W, *et al.*: Mode of death in idiopathic dilated cardiomyopathy: a multivariate analysis of prognostic determinants. *Am Heart J* 1988, 116:1455–1463.

13. Stevenson WG, Stevenson LW, Middlekauff HR, *et al.*: Improving survival for patients with advanced heart failure: a study of 737 consecutive patients. *J Am Coll Cardiol* 1996, 26:1417–1423.

14. Buxton AE, Lee KL, Fisher JD, *et al.* for the Multicenter Unsustained Tachycardia Trial investigators: A randomized study of the prevention of sudden death in patients with coronary artery disease. *N Engl J Med* 1999, 341:1882–1890.

15. Moss AJ, Zareba W, Hall WJ, *et al.*: Prophylactic implantation of a defibrillator in patients with myocardial infarction and reduced ejection fraction. *N Engl J Med* 2002, 346:877–883.

16. Leier CV, Huss P, Magorien RD, *et al.*: Improved exercise capacity and differing arterial and venous tolerance during chronic isosorbide dinitrate therapy for congestive heart failure. *Circulation* 1983, 67:817–822.

17. Weber KT, Kinasewitz GT, Janicki JS, *et al.*: Oxygen utilization and ventilation during exercise in patients with chronic cardiac failure. *Circulation* 1982, 65:1218–1223.

18. Mancini DM, Eisen H, Kussmaul W, *et al.*: Value of peak exercise oxygen consumption for optimal timing of cardiac transplantation in ambulatory patients with heart failure. *Circulation* 1991, 83:778–786.

19. Holmes DR Jr, Detre KM, Williams DO, *et al.*: Long-term outcome of patients with depressed left ventricular function undergoing PTCA. *Circulation* 1993, 87:21–29.

20. Di Carli MF, Asgarzadie F, Schelbert HR, *et al.*: Quantitative relation between myocardial viability and improvement in heart failure symptoms after revascularization in patients with ischemic cardiomyopathy. *Circulation* 1995, 92:3436–3444.

21. Sanborn TA, Sleeper LA, Webb JG, *et al.*: Correlates of one-year survival in patients with cardiogenic shock complicating acute myocardial infarction. *J Am Coll Cardiol* 2003, 42:1373–1379.

22. Holmes DR Jr, Bates EF, Kleiman NS, *et al.* for the GUSTO-I Investigators: Contemporary reperfusion therapy for cardiogenic shock: the GUSTO-I trial experience. *J Am Coll Cardiol* 1995, 26:668–674.

23. Stevenson LW, Dracup KA, Tillisch JH: Efficacy of medical therapy tailored for severe congestive heart failure in patients transferred for urgent cardiac transplantation. *Am J Cardiol* 1989, 63:461–464.

24. Haas GJ, Leier CV: Invasive cardiovascular testing in chronic congestive heart failure. *Crit Care Med* 1990, 18:51–54.

25. Mody FV, Brunken RC, Stevenson LW, *et al.*: Differentiating cardiomyopathy of coronary artery disease from nonischemic dilated cardiomyopathy utilizing positron emission tomography. *J Am Coll Cardiol* 1991, 17:373–383.

SELECT BIBLIOGRAPHY

ACC/AHA guidelines for the evaluation and management of chronic heart failure in the adult: executive summary. *J Am Coll Cardiol* 1995, 26:1376–1398.

ACTION-HF Committee: Consensus recommendations for the management of chronic heart failure. *Am J Cardiol* 2001, 38:2101–2113.

Cowie MR, Mendez GF: BNP and congestive heart failure. *Prog Cardiovasc Dis* 2002, 44:293–321.

Heart Failure Society of America (HFSA) practice guidelines. HFSA guidelines for management of patients with heart failure caused by left ventricular systolic dysfunction–pharmacological approaches. *J Card Fail* 1999, 5:357–82.

Leier CV: Nuggets, pearls, and clinical vignettes of master heart failure clinicians. *Congest Heart Fail* 2001, 7:244–249, 7:297–308; 2002, 8:49–53, 8:98–124.

Poole-Wilson PA, Colucci WS, Massie BM, *et al.*: *Heart Failure: Scientific Principles and Practice.* New York: Churchill Livingstone, Inc; 1997.

Evaluation of the Patient with Hypotension and Shock

Richard C. Becker

7

> ### *Key Points*
> - Shock is a syndrome characterized by systemic hypotension, tissue hypoperfusion, and release of vasoactive inflammatory mediators.
> - Profound vasodilation, arteriovenus shunting, and increased capillary membrane permeability are features that typify septic, neurogenic, and anaphylactic shock, but may also be observed in cardiogenic shock.
> - Cardiogenic shock is predominantly caused by a critical reduction in cardiac output (relative to existing metabolic demands).
> - In shock states, prompt stabilization, diagnosis, and definitive treatment are prerequisites for patient survival.

Hypotension is defined as a reduction in systemic blood pressure to below a mean arterial pressure of 70 mm Hg. It is important to recognize, however, that individuals with preexisting hypertension can, in fact, be hypotensive at a higher mean arterial pressure (*ie*, in a relative state of hypotension).

Shock is a recognizable collection of symptoms, signs, and laboratory abnormalities (*ie*, syndrome) that is characterized by hypotension and tissue hypoperfusion. Tissue hypoperfusion is pathognomonic of shock states and is associated with widespread cellular and major organ dysfunction. Although this process is initially *reversible*, persistent hypoperfusion leads to *irreversible* cellular injury, microvascular thrombosis, multiorgan failure, and ultimately death.

DETERMINATES OF A NORMAL SYSTEMIC BLOOD PRESSURE

Systemic blood pressure is determined by the volume of blood ejected from the heart into the systemic circulation (cardiac output) and by the peripheral vascular resistance. Therefore, disturbances in blood pressure are caused by either a reduced cardiac output (the hallmark of cardiogenic shock) or a reduced peripheral vascular resistance (the hallmark of septic, neurogenic, and anaphylactic shock). It is important to recognize that any and all shock states may include both reduced inotropic and systemic vascular reserve.

Peripheral Vascular Resistance

Peripheral vascular resistance varies inversely with the fourth power of the arteriolar radius (resistance vessels). Therefore, vascular resistance is determined by vascular tone, which is directly influenced by:

1. Metabolic and mechanical autoregulatory mechanisms,
2. Neurogenic constrictor influences operating through norepinephrine,
3. Neurogenic vasodilator influences operating through acetylcholine and histamine, and
4. Circulating and locally released vasoactive substances, including catecholamines, angiotensin II, bradykinin, prostaglandins, and endothelin.

The autonomic nervous system plays a crucial role in the maintenance of systemic blood pressure because it directly influences both cardiac output and peripheral vascular resistance.

Blood Volume

An adequate intravascular volume is required to maintain cardiac output and systemic blood pressure. This is accomplished primarily through the renin-angiotensin-aldosterone system; other contributors include arginine vasopressin and brain-type natriuretic polypeptide.

TABLE 1 DETERMINANTS OF CARDIAC PERFORMANCE
Preload (ventricular filling)
Venous return
Total blood volume
Intrathoracic pressure
Intrapericardial pressure
Atrial contraction
Atrioventricular synchony
Afterload (ventricular wall stress; impedance)
Contractility (inotropic activity of myocardium)
Sympathetic nervous system
Circulating catecholamines
Local environment (anoxia, ischemia, acidemia)
Contractile mass
Inotropic response to stimulation
Heart rate

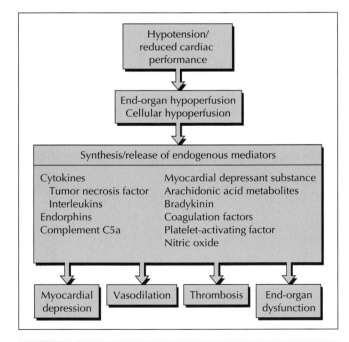

FIGURE 1 The shock state is initiated when tissue hypoperfusion stimulates the release of endogenous mediators, which in turn are responsible for myocardial depression, vasodilation, thrombosis, and end-organ dysfunction.

Cardiac Performance

The three primary determinants of cardiac performance are preload, afterload, and contractility. As cardiac output is the product of heart rate and stroke volume, the former is considered to be a fourth determinant of cardiac performance (Table 1).

SHOCK STATE: PHYSIOLOGY AND FUNDAMENTAL MECHANISMS

When systemic hypotension is prolonged and severe, a series of compensating mechanisms are initiated in an attempt to restore blood volume, increase peripheral vascular resistance, improve cardiac performance, and maintain vital organ perfusion. Marked stimulation of the autonomic and renin-angiotensin-aldosterone systems occurs in patients with cardiogenic shock. If adequate end-organ perfusion is not restored, endogenous mediators (contraregulatory mechanisms) are released from monocytes, macrophages, and neutrophils. As in septic shock, these mediators may contribute directly to the perpetuation of the shock state and be responsible for end-organ dysfunction (Fig. 1).

CLINICAL SIGNS AND SYMPTOMS

Hypotension and hypoperfusion are the two cardinal manifestations of shock states in general and of cardiogenic shock in particular. Hypotension is defined as a systolic blood pressure of less than 70 mm Hg. Because some patients experience end-organ (tissue) hypoperfusion at a higher blood pressure, a working definition of mean arterial pressure of 30 mm Hg or more below the baseline blood pressure may be preferred.

The presence of hypoperfusion can be determined indirectly from several key clinical observations: 1) altered mental status (agitation, restlessness, obtundation); 2) pale or mottled, cool, clammy skin; and 3) reduced urine output (<30 mL/h). Most patients with cardiogenic shock are tachycardic (> 100 bpm). The peripheral pulses are typically weak and thready, and tachypnea (> 20 respirations/min) is also common.

The common laboratory abnormalities include:
- Hypoxia, hypocarbia, metabolic acidosis
- Elevated serum lactate level

TABLE 2 RECOMMENDATIONS FOR STABILIZING CRITICALLY ILL PATIENTS
Assure adequate oxygenation (low threshold for tracheal intubation)
Obtain intravenous access (central access preferred)
Restore arterial pressure (mean, > 70 mm Hg)
Volume replacement
Vasopressor agents (dopamine, norepinephrine)
Correct acid–base abnormalities
Correct rhythm disturbances and conduction abnormalities

- Leukocytosis (mild to moderate), thrombocytopenia (disseminated intravascular coagulation)

CARDIOGENIC SHOCK AFTER MYOCARDIAL INFARCTION

The key to early diagnosis and treatment of patients with cardiogenic shock rests in the ability to identify patients at risk. In the GUSTO (Global Utilization of Streptokinase and TPA for Occluded coronary arteries)-1 trial, four major factors were associated with the development of shock: age (>70 years), systolic blood pressure (<100 mm Hg), heart rate (>100 bpm), and Killip classification (class II or III). Together these four variables accounted for more than 85% of the predictive information [1•].

The SHould we emergently revascularize Occluded Coronaries in cardiogenic shocK (SHOCK)-1 trial registry and randomized trial included 1190 and 232 patients, respectively. Predominant left ventricular failure (78.5%) was most common, with isolated right ventricular failure (28%), severe mitral insufficiency (6.5%), ventricular septal rupture (3.9%), and pericardial tamponade (1.4%) responsible less often for cardiogenic shock [2••]. Of these causes, ventricular septal rupture was associated with the highest mortality (87.3%).

The time course for cardiogenic shock onset follows a dichotomous pattern. In the SHOCK trial registry, overt shock developed a median of 6.2 h after myocardial infarction (MI) onset and occurred earliest among patients with left main coronary artery disease (1.7 h). Shock within 24 h of initial symptoms (74.1% of overall cohort) was associated with ST segment elevation and multiple infarct locations. In contrast, late shock (> 24 h) was associated with recurrent myocardial ischemia [3].

TABLE 3 COMMON CAUSES OF CARDIOGENIC SHOCK

Acute myocardial infarction
Ventricular septal rupture
Acute mitral insufficiency
Right ventricular infarction
Myocarditis
Dilated cardiomyopathy
Advanced valvular heart disease
    Aortic stenosis
    Aortic insufficiency
    Mitral stenosis
    Mitral insufficiency
Tachy- and bradyarrhythmias
Cardiac tamponade
Pulmonary embolism
Hypertrophic cardiomyopathy
End-stage hypertensive heart disease

The incidence of ST segment elevation MI has not changed substantially over the past decade; however, the relative proportion of infarctions without ST segment elevation continues to rise, particularly among patients older than 65 years. The GUSTO-IIb trial [4•] included 12,084 patients who did not present to the hospital with features of cardiogenic shock. Overall, 4.2% of patients with ST segment elevation developed shock compared with 2.5% of those without ST segment elevation (odds ratio 0.58). In the latter group, which included a greater proportion of patients with diabetes mellitus, advanced age, and multivessel coronary artery disease, shock developed much later in the hospital course (76.2 h vs 9.6 h in patients with ST segment elevation) and was more likely to result in death (73% vs 63%).

INITIAL STABILIZATION

Care of critically ill patients is unique in many ways. Unlike other clinical situations that permit a series of diagnostic tests to be performed before instituting treatment, cardiogenic shock is imminently life-threatening; therefore, prompt stabilization is required before a thorough diagnostic evaluation can be performed (Table 2).

DIFFERENTIAL DIAGNOSIS

A number of common diseases of the heart can cause hypotension and cardiogenic shock (Table 3). The most common is reduced myocardial performance caused by severe coronary artery disease, one or more prior MIs, or acute MI.

The incidence of cardiogenic shock complicating MI ranges from 5% to 15%. The degree of left ventricular compromise correlates with the overall extent of ventricular damage. The Starling mechanism of functional compensation fails when the surface area of necrosis exceeds 30%; however, substantial variability has been observed, suggesting that other mechanisms contribute substantially [5••,6]. Smaller infarctions may cause complications associated with shock, including ventricular septal rupture, free-wall rupture, and papillary muscle rupture.

A consistent pathologic observation among patients with fatal cardiogenic shock is progressive myocardial necrosis (Fig. 2). Persistent occlusion of the infarct-related

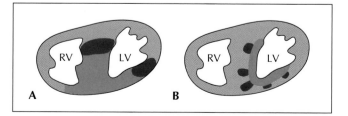

FIGURE 2 Patients with myocardial infarction complicated by cardiogenic shock demonstrate marginal extension at autopsy that can be either subepicardial (**A**) or lateral (**B**) in location. LV—left ventricle; RV—right ventricle.

TABLE 4 DIAGNOSTIC BENCHMARKS IN CARDIOGENIC SHOCK

	General physical appearance	Signs or history	Jugular venous pressure	Heart sounds	Lung examination	Chest radiograph	Electrocardiography	Other diagnostic tests
Myocardial infarction	Apprehensive Cool, moist skin Agitation	Symptom onset at rest Chest pain Dyspnea Hypotension Tachycardia	↑, ↔	S_3, S_4 gallops ± Holosystolic murmur (papillary muscle dysfunction)	Rales in > 50% of both lung fields	Pulmonary edema	ST-segment elevation ± Q waves Widespread ST-segment depression	Elevated creatine kinase Abnormal MB fraction (may not be elevated early) Focal wall motion abnormality on echocardiogram
Ventricular septal rupture	Anxious Diaphoretic	Recent MI (3–5 d)* Sudden change in clinical status Chest pain Dyspnea Tachycardia	↑	S_3, S_4 gallops Localized holosystolic murmur (new) Palpable systolic thrill (lower left sternal border)	Rales in > 50% of lung fields	Pulmonary edema	Persistent ST-segment elevation Pseudonormalization of T waves	L→R shunt on echocardiogram O_2 saturation "step-up"
Mitral insufficiency (acute)	Anxious Diaphoretic	Sudden dyspnea Recent inferior/ inferoposterior MI or History of mitral valve prolapse or History of blunt/ penetrating trauma	↑, ↔	S_1 decreased S_3 gallop Holosystolic murmur obscuring S_2 (A_2 component)	Rales in > 50% of lung fields	Pulmonary edema	Recent MI Nonspecific ST-T wave abnormality	Mitral insufficiency ± flail mitral leaflet on echocardiogram
Right ventricular infarction	Apprehensive Diaphoretic	Chest pain Nausea	↑↑	S_3, S_4 gallops (right sided)	Clear or basilar rales	Clear	Inferior injury pattern with posterior extension ≥0.5 mm ST elevation in V_3R, V_4R Bradyarrhythmias Conduction abnormalities (2°, 3° heart block)	Inferoposterior hypokinesis and right ventricular hypokinesis on echocardiogram
Myocarditis	Apprehensive Cool, moist skin	Viral prodrome Progressive shortness of breath Low-grade temperature Narrow pulse pressure	↑	S_3, S_4 gallops	Rales in > 50% of lung fields	Pulmonary edema Heart size normal or enlarged	Sinus tachycardia Nonspecific ST/T changes Pseudoinfarction pattern Bundle-branch block	Chamber dilation Hypokinesis on echocardiogram
Dilated cardiomyopathy	Diaphoretic Cool Peripheral mottling	History of chronic heart failure Narrow pulse pressure Chronic venous stasis pigmentation–ulceration	↑↑	S_3, S_4 gallops Holosystolic murmur (mitral, tricuspid regurgitation)	Rales in > 50% of lung fields	Pulmonary edema Cardiomegaly	Sinus tachycardia/ tachyarrhythmias (atrial/ventricular) Low voltage Bundle-branch block Diffuse ST/T-wave changes	Four-chamber dilation on echocardiogram

*May occur earlier (24–48 hours) following thrombolytic therapy.

(Continued on next page)

TABLE 4 DIAGNOSTIC BENCHMARKS IN CARDIOGENIC SHOCK (CONTINUED)

	General physical appearance	Signs or history	Jugular venous pressure	Heart sounds	Lung examination	Chest radiograph	Electrocardiography	Other diagnostic tests
Hypertrophic cardiomyopathy	Anxious Diaphoretic	History of chest pain, dyspnea, syncope Family history of sudden death Apical "triple" beat Rapid carotid upstroke	↑, ↔ (prominent A wave)	Prominent S_4 gallop Holosystolic blowing murmur at apex Holosystolic harsh murmur left sternal border (↑ Valsalva)	Rales in > 50% of lung fields	Pulmonary edema	Left ventricular hypertrophy Q waves inferolateral leads	Septal hypertrophy on echocardiogram Outflow tract obstruction on Doppler studies
Aortic stenosis	Pale Diaphoretic	Carotid shudder, delayed upstroke	↑	S_1 soft; single S_2 (P_2) S_3, S_4 gallops Harsh, late–peaking systolic murmur (radiation to carotid arteries)	Rales in > 50% of lung fields	Pulmonary edema	Left ventricular hypertrophy	Aortic valve thickening Reduced leaflet motion Pressure gradient across aortic valve
Aortic insufficiency	Diaphoretic	History of hypertension, endocarditis, or trauma Chest ± back pain Dyspnea Asymmetric blood pressure/pulses Paralysis/sensory deficits	↑, ↔	S_1 soft or absent S_2 (P_2) prominent S_3, S_4 gallops Early, low-pitch diastolic murmur	Rales in > 50% of lung fields	Pulmonary edema "Calcium" sign with aortic dissection	Nonspecific ST/T–wave changes	Aortic dissection Aortic insufficiency Transesophageal echocardiogram
Mitral stenosis	Diaphoretic Cyanotic	Progressive dyspnea Frothy blood-tinged sputum Prior thromboembolism	↑ (prominent A wave)	S_1 prominent or reduced (immobile valve leaflets) P_2 prominent Opening snap Diastolic rumbling murmur	Rales in > 50% of lung fields	Pulmonary edema Right ventricular prominence Left atrial enlargement	Tachyarrythmia (particularly atrial fibrillation) Right-axis deviation Right ventricular hypertrophy Atrial enlargement	Calcified, stenotic mitral valve
Pulmonary embolism	Anxious Cyanotic	Sudden pleuritic chest pain, dyspnea, cough, hemoptysis, or syncope Risk factors for pulmonary embolism Tachypnea (> 20 breaths/min)	↑ (prominent A wave)	S_2 (P_2) increased S_3, S_4 gallops (right sided) Holosystolic murmur (tricuspid regurgitation)	Clear	Oligemia Elevated hemidiaphragm Pleural effusion "Wedge-shaped" infiltrate Prominent hilar vessel	S_1, Q_3, T_3 pattern Nonspecific ST/T–wave changes Right bundle-branch block Sinus tachycardia	V/Q mismatch Abnormal pulmonary angiography Right ventricular prominence on echocardiogram
Cardiac tamponade	Pale Anxious Apprehensive	Hypotension Narrow pulse pressure Distended neck veins Pulsus paradoxus	↑↑ (absent Y descent)	Distant (if rapid pericardial fluid accumulation) ± Friction rub	Clear	Normal or enlarged cardiac silhouette	Low voltage T-wave flattening	Pericardial effusion Right atrial, right ventricular collapse on echocardiogram Abnormal Doppler flow patterns

L→R—left to right; MI—myocardial infarction; P_2—pulmonic second heart sound; S_1—first heart sound; S_2—second heart sound; S_3—third heart sound; S_4—fourth heart sound; ↔—normal; ↑—increased; ↑↑—markedly increased.

Evaluation of the Patient with Hypotension and Shock

coronary artery is also common. Severe multivessel coronary artery disease, prior infarction, or compromised collateral circulation may contribute to the development of shock in the absence of a large infarction.

DIAGNOSTIC EVALUATION

Following initial stabilization of the patient, the clinician must promptly begin a thorough diagnostic evaluation. In many instances, a diagnosis can be secured through a careful physical examination, chest radiography, electrocardiography, and routine blood tests. At times, vital historical

TABLE 5 KEY HEMODYNAMIC REFERENCE POINTS FOR PATIENTS WITH PULMONARY ARTERY CATHETERS

Cardiac chamber catheter site	Normal pressures, mm Hg
Right atrium	
Range	0–6
Mean	3
Right ventricle	
Systolic	15–30
Diastolic	0–6
Pulmonary artery	
Systolic	15–30
Diastolic	5–13
Mean	10–18
Pulmonary capillary bed	
Mean	2–12

information can be provided by friends, family members, and medical records. Specialized testing, including echocardiography (transthoracic/transesophageal), coronary angiography, computed tomography, magnetic resonance imaging, and pulmonary artery catheterization may be required to confirm a diagnosis. The checklist in Table 4 should be helpful in making a diagnosis.

EARLY MANAGEMENT

Whenever possible, patients with cardiogenic shock should be managed in an intensive care unit. Close observation is an absolute necessity, and both intra-arterial and hemodynamic monitoring should be considered strongly.

Intra-arterial Monitoring

Direct blood pressure measurement is more accurate than noninvasive, indirect measurement in patients with hemodynamic instability and shock. Intra-arterial monitoring allows careful titration of vasoactive drugs and provides immediate access for frequent blood sampling, including blood gas analysis. The preferred cannulation site is the radial artery; however, other sites (femoral artery, dorsalis pedis artery, brachial artery) may also be used. Potential complications of intra-arterial monitoring include bleeding, thrombosis, embolism, limb ischemia, pseudoaneurysm formation, infection, and peripheral neuropathy.

Hemodynamic Monitoring

Pulmonary artery catheterization for hemodynamic monitoring has four primary objectives (Table 5):
1. To assess left ventricular and right ventricular function,
2. To assess changes in hemodynamic status,

TABLE 6 HEMODYNAMIC PARAMETERS IN PATIENTS WITH HYPOTENSION AND SHOCK (GUIDELINES FOR DIAGNOSIS)

	RA, mm Hg	RV, mm Hg*	PA, mm Hg*	PWP, mm Hg	AO, mm Hg	CI, L/min/m²	SVR, dyne/sec/cm⁻⁵
Normal	0–6	25/0–6	25/6–12	6–12	120/80	≥2.5	1200–1500
Hypovolemia	0–2	15/0–2	15/2–6	2–6	< 90/60	< 2.0	> 1500
Cardiogenic shock	8	50/8	50/25	25	< 90/60	< 2.0	> 1500
Septic shock							
Early	0–2	25/0–2	25/0–6	0–6	< 90/60	> 2.5	< 1000
Late	0–4	25/4–10	25/4–10	4–10	< 90/60	< 2.0	> 1000
Massive PE	8–12	50/12	50/12	<12	< 90/60	< 2.0	> 1200
Tamponade	12–18	30/12–18	30/12–18	12–18	< 90/60	< 2.0	> 1200
Right ventricular infarction	12–20	30/12–20	30/12	<12	< 90/60	< 2.0	> 1200
Ventricular septal rupture	6	60/60–8	60/25	25	< 90/60	< 2.0	> 1500

*The first value represents the mean value; the second is the range.

AO—aortic pressure; CI—cardiac index; PA—pulmonary artery; PE—pulmonary embolism; PWP—pulmonary wedge pressure; RA—right atrium; RV—right ventricle; SVR—systemic vascular resistance.

3. To guide treatment with pharmacologic and nonpharmacologic agents, and
4. To gather prognostic information.

The hemodynamic information obtained from pulmonary arterial catheterization can be used directly in both patient management and diagnosis (Tables 6 and 7).

Potential complications of catheterization include balloon rupture, knotting, pulmonary infarction, arterial perforation, thromboembolism, heart block, arryhthmias (supraventricular or ventricular), myocardial perforation with tamponade, and infection.

Pharmacologic Therapy

Inotropic therapy should be used in the early stages of hypotension and/or hypoperfusion until the cause is determined and definitive therapy implemented. Although the concern regarding exacerbation of ischemia in patients with acute MI is a consideration, prolonged periods of hypotension often result in reduced oxygen delivery and compromised myocardial perfusion [7••].

Dopamine is an immediate precursor of norepinephrine. It has both α- and β-adrenergic agonist properties as well as dopaminergic-receptor agonism within the mesenteric and renal vascular beds. At doses required to increase mean arterial pressure and cardiac output (5 to 8 μg/kg/min), heart rate and myocardial oxygen demand may be increased [8]. In the presence of acidemia, higher doses (up to 10 μg/kg/min) may be required to produce a hemodynamic improvement; at this dose, atrial and ventricular tachyarrythmias may occur.

Dobutamine is a synthetic derivative of isoproterenol. It increases cardiac output at doses between 2.5 and 5.0 μg/kg/min without significantly increasing either heart rate or myocardial oxygen demand [9]. Therefore, in the setting of MI complicated by cardiogenic shock, dobutamine is considered the inotropic agent of choice.

Norepinephrine is a potent α-receptor antagonist (increases peripheral vascular resistance). It exhibits some myocardial β1-receptor agonism as well. Norepinephrine should be used in patients with hypotension refractory to other inotropic agents, and is the preferred agent in septic (vasodilatory) shock.

The efficacy of dopamine and dobutamine may decline with long-term administration. Tachyphylaxis may represent a downregulation of myocardial adrenergic receptors. Phosphodiesterase inhibitors increase cyclic AMP concentrations without relying directly on adrenergic receptors. Amrinone and milrinone have been used successfully in the treatment of cardiogenic shock [10].

The classic paradigm for cardiogenic shock, characterized by reduced myocardial contractility in a majority of responsible disorders and acute events, is accompanied by an increase in systemic vascular resistance. Observations from the SHOCK trial [11•] challenge traditional thinking and revealed variable degrees of systemic vascular resistance. This variation may be the result of triggered inflammatory responses that cause vasodilation, as well as myocardial depression. The importance of recent insights relates directly to potential therapies designed to inhibit inflammatory mediators or their end products (nitric oxide, for example).

Patients with increased left ventricular mass and diastolic dysfunction, hypertensive heart disease, or hypertrophic cardiomyopathy complicated by cardiogenic shock create a particularly complex clinical condition. Inotropic agents may be ineffective or worsen cardiac performance. Calcium channel blockers (verapamil, diltiazem) or β-blockers given as a continuous intravenous infusion can improve ventricular distensibility and diastolic filling. In refractory congestive heart failure accompanied by hypotension, a pure α-agonist such as phenylephrine hydrochloride (Neo-Synephrine, Winthrop Pharmaceuticals, New York, NY), used in combination with supportive care, may be beneficial. Caution is recommended when considering the administration of calcium channel blockers and/or β-blockers in the setting of hypotension.

Fibrinolytic therapy is useful in the treatment of massive pulmonary embolism. Intravenous tissue-plasminogen activator appears to be the agent of choice [12]. Unfortunately, while reducing the incidence of congestive heart failure and cardiogenic shock among patients with MI, fibrinolytic therapy has not been shown to improve survival when administered in the presence of cardiogenic shock [13•].

Antiarrhythmics (amiodarone, lidocaine, procainamide) or electrical cardioversion should be used as needed for patients with hemodynamically compromising supraventricular and ventricular tachyarrhythmias.

Mechanical Intervention

Intra-aortic balloon counterpulsation (IABP) should be considered with cardiogenic shock, particularly those with

---

TABLE 7 MEASURES CALCULABLE FROM HEMODYNAMIC DATA

Cardiac index = $\dfrac{\text{Cardiac output (L/min)}}{\text{Body surface area (m}^2)}$

Normal: 2.5–4.5 L/min/m^2

Mean arterial pressure = $\dfrac{(2 \times \text{Diastolic}) + \text{Systolic}}{3}$

Normal: 70–95 mm Hg

Systemic vascular resistance = $\dfrac{\text{MAP-RA}}{\text{CO}} \times 80$

Normal: 1200–1500 dyne/sec/cm^{-5}

CO—cardiac output; MAP—mean arterial pressure; RA—right atrial pressure.

global myocardial ischemia or MI complicated by papillary muscle rupture or ventricular septal rupture. It is contraindicated in patients with severe aortic insufficiency. The observed hemodynamic changes following IABP insertion include:

- 10% to 20% increase in cardiac output,
- A reduction in systolic and an increase in diastolic blood pressure (increased mean arterial pressure),
- A diminution in heart rate, and
- An increase in urine output.

In some patients, combined IABP and inotropic therapy is required to achieve and maintain an acceptable blood pressure (systolic > 90 mm Hg; mean, > 70 mm Hg) and cardiac index (> 2.2 L/min/m^2).

Coronary angiography and urgent coronary angioplasty may improve survival for patients with MI complicated by cardiogenic shock [14–16•]. Restoration of coronary arterial patency in retrospective studies and pooled series has been associated with a nearly 50% reduction in the mortality rate.

Alternative mechanical interventions include:

- Pericardiocentesis for patients with cardiac tamponade,
- Balloon valvuloplasty for those with critical aortic or mitral stenosis when surgical correction is not feasible, and
- Pacemaker placement for patients with severe bradyarrhythmias, conduction disturbances, or right ventricular infarction refractory to fluid administration and inotropic support (atrioventricular pacing may be required with some patients).

The International Shock Registry results support early revascularization as an important treatment modality for patients with MI complicated by cardiogenic shock [17•].

The SHOCK trial [5••] randomized patients who developed cardiogenic shock after ST segment elevation or bundle branch block MI to either a strategy of emergent revascularization (*n* = 152) or initial medical stabilization followed by delayed revascularization (*n* = 150), as clinically indicated. Intra-aortic balloon counterpulsation was recommended, as was fibrinolytic therapy (unless angiography was immediately available in the emergency revascularization group). The 30-day mortality rates for the emergent revascularization and medical stabilization groups were 47% and 56%, respectively (*P* = 0.11). The corresponding rates at 6 months were 50.3% and 63.1%, respectively (*P* = 0.027) (Fig. 3).

Surgical Intervention

Corrective surgery is most beneficial in patients with mechanical defects (papillary muscle rupture, ventricular septal rupture), critical valvular heart disease (aortic stenosis, aortic insufficiency, mitral stenosis), and severe coronary artery disease (three-vessel disease, left main disease). In a majority of cases, initial stabilization is achieved by inotropic support in combination with a circulatory assist device. Overall, the best results are achieved when surgical intervention is undertaken promptly [18,19].

Cardiac transplantation is a therapeutic alternative for a selective group of individuals with cardiogenic shock. Mechanical circulatory support as a "bridge" to cardiac transplantation includes a total artificial heart and ventricular assist devices [20,21] (Table 8).

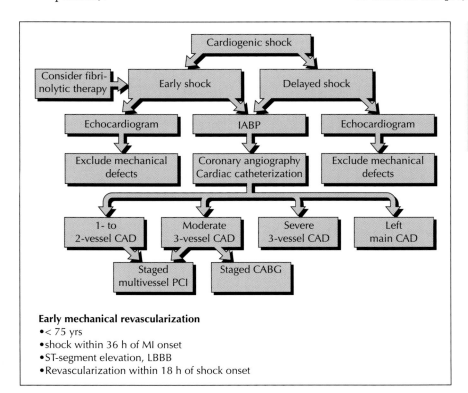

Early mechanical revascularization
- < 75 yrs
- shock within 36 h of MI onset
- ST-segment elevation, LBBB
- Revascularization within 18 h of shock onset

FIGURE 3 Diagnostic and early management algorithm for patients with cardiogenic shock. CABG—coronary artery bypass grafting; CAD—coronary artery disease; IABP—intra-aortic balloon pump; LBBB—left bundle branch block; MI—myocardial infarction; PCI—percutaneous coronary intervention. (*Adapted from* Hochman *et al.* [11•].)

TABLE 8 TREATMENT OPTIONS IN CARDIOGENIC SHOCK

Pharmacologic	Mechanisms of action
Dobutamine	Inotropic support
Dopamine	Inotropic support
Norepinephrine	Inotropic support, vasopressor
Phenylephrine	Vasopressor
Tissue-plasminogen activator	Fibrinolysis (pulmonary embolism ± MI)
Amiodarone, lidocaine, procainamide	Antiarrhythmic
Mechanical	
Intraaortic balloon pump	Improve cardiac output Increase coronary artery perfusion
Hemopump	Improve cardiac output
Percutaneous cardio-pulmonary support	Improve cardiac output Improve tissue perfusion
Pacemaker	Restore heart rate Restore atrioventricular synchrony
Percutaneous coronary intervention	Improve myocardial perfusion and ventricular performance
Pericardiocentesis	Improve preload, ventricular filling
Surgery	Correct mechanical defects

MI—myocardial infarction.

A ventricular assist device (VAD) can support a failing right ventricle (RVAD), left ventricle (LVAD), or both ventricles (BIVAD). The technology is approved as a bridge to cardiac transplantation in patients with refractory cardiogenic shock either before (precardiotomy) or after (postcardiotomy) surgical revascularization (when feasible). In the latter condition, VAD may be used as "destination therapy" pending recovery of the ischemic myocardium [22•]. These devices are typically placed at heart transplant centers and include Thoratec VAD system: Bridge to Transplant; TCI Heartmate: Bridge to Transplant; Abiomed: Post-cardiotomy support.

REFERENCES AND RECOMMENDED READING

Recently published papers of particular interest have been highlighted as:
• Of interest
•• Of outstanding interest

1.• Hasdai D, Califf RM, Thompson TD, et al. for the GUSTO-1 investigators: Predictors of cardiogenic shock after thrombolytic therapy for acute myocardial infarction. J Am Coll Cardiol 2000, 35:136–143.

2.•• Hochman JS, Buller CE, Sleeper LA, et al.: Cardiogenic shock complicating acute myocardial infarction: etiologies, management and outcome. A report from the SHOCK trial registry. Should we emergently revascularize occluded coronaries for cardiogenic shock? J Am Coll Cardiol 2000, 36:1063–1070.

3. Webb JG, Sleeper LA, Buller JE, et al.: Implications of the timing of onset of cardiogenic shock after acute myocardial infarction: a report from the SHOCK trial registry. J Am Coll Cardiol 2000, 36:1084–1090.

4.• Holmes DR, Berger PB, Hochman JS, et al.: Cardiogenic shock in patients with acute ischemic syndromes with and without ST segment elevation. Circulation 1999, 100:2067–2073.

5.•• Hochman JS, Sleeper LA, Webb JG, et al.: Early revascularization in acute myocardial infarction complicated by cardiogenic shock. N Engl J Med 1999, 341:625–634.

6. Page DL, Caulfield JB, Kastor JA, et al.: Myocardial changes associated with cardiogenic shock. N Engl J Med 1971, 285:133–137.

7.•• Stevenson LW: Clinical use of inotropic therapy for heart failure: looking backward or forward? Part 1: Inotropic infusions during hospitalization. Circulation 2003, 108:367–372.

8. Mueller HS, Evans R, Ayres SM: Effect of dopamine on hemo-dynamics and myocardial metabolism in shock following acute myocardial infarction in man. Circulation 1978, 57:361–365.

9. Francis GS, Sharma B, Hodges M: Comparative hemodynamic effects of dopamine and dobutamine in patients with acute cardiogenic circulatory collapse. Am Heart J 1982, 103:995–1000.

10. Klocke RK, Mager G, Kux A, et al.: Effects of a 24-hour milri-none infusion in patients with severe heart failure and cardiogenic shock as a function of the hemodynamic initial condition. Am Heart J 1991, 121:1965–1973.

11.• Hochman JS: Cardiogenic shock complicating acute myocardial infarction: expanding the paradigm. Circulation 2003, 107:2998–3002.

12.• Goldhaber SZ, Kessler CM, Heit JA, et al.: Recombinant tissue-type plasminogen activator versus a novel dosing regimen of urokinase in acute pulmonary embolism: a randomized controlled multicenter trial. J Am Coll Cardiol 1992, 20:24–31.

13.• Becker RC: Hemodynamic, mechanical and metabolic determi-nants of thrombolytic efficacy: a theoretic framework for assessing the limitations of thrombolysis in patients with cardio-genic shock. Am Heart J 1993, 125:919–929.

14. Abbottsmith CW, Topol EJ, George BS, et al.: Fate of patients with acute myocardial infarction with patency of the infarct-related vessel achieved with successful thrombolysis versus rescue angiography. J Am Coll Cardiol 1990, 16:770–778.

15. Lee L, Erbel R, Brown TM, et al.: Multicenter registry of angio-plasty therapy of cardiogenic shock: initial and long-term survival. J Am Coll Cardiol 1991, 17:599–603.

16.• Eltchaninoff H, Simpfendorfer C, Franco I, et al.: Early and 1-year survival rates in acute myocardial infarction complicated by cardiogenic shock: a retrospective study comparing coronary angioplasty with medical treatment. Am Heart J 1995, 130:459–464.

17.• Hochman JS, Boland J, Sleeper LA, et al.: Current spectrum of cardiogenic shock and effect of early revascularization on mortality: results of an international registry. Circulation 1995, 91:873–881.

18. Phillips SJ, Kongtahworn C, Slanner JR, Zeff MT: Emergency coronary artery reperfusion: a choice therapy for evolving myocardial infarction: results in 339 patients. J Thorac Cardiovasc Surg 1983, 86:679–688.

19. DeWood MA, Notske RN, Hensley GR, *et al.*: Intra-aortic balloon counterpulsation with or without reperfusion for myocardial shock. *Circulation* 1980, 61:1105–1112.

20. Joyce LD, Johnson KE, Pierce WS: Summary of the work experience with clinical use of total artificial hearts as heart support devices. *J Heart Transplant* 1986, 5:229–235.

21. Joyce LD, Kiser JC, Eales F, *et al.*: Experience with generally accepted centrifugal pumps. *Ann Thorac Surg* 1996, 61:287–290.

22.• Farrar D, Hill D, Pennington G, *et al.*: Preoperative and postoperative comparison of patients with univentricular and biventricular support with the Thoratec ventricular assist device as a bridge to cardiac transplantation. *J Thorac Cardiovasc Surg* 1997, 113:202–209.

SELECT BIBLIOGRAPHY

Hibbard MD, Holmes DR, Bailey KR, *et al.*: Percutaneous transluminal coronary angioplasty in patients with cardiogenic shock. *J Am Coll Cardiol* 1992, 19:639–646.

Hollenburg SM, Kavinsky CJ, Parrillo JE: Cardiogenic shock. *Ann Intern Med* 1999, 131:47–59.

Holmes DR Jr, Bates ER, Kleinman NS, *et al.* for the GUSTO-I Investigators: contemporary reperfusion therapy for cardiogenic shock. The GUSTO-I Trial experience. *J Am Coll Cardiol* 1996, 26:668–674.

Kleiman NS, Terrin M, Meuller HS, *et al.* for the TIMI Investigators: Mechanisms of early death despite thrombolytic therapy: experience from the TIMI II study. *J Am Coll Cardiol* 1992, 19:1129–1135.

McCallister BD, Christian TF, Gersh BJ, Gibbons RJ: Prognosis of myocardial infarctions involving more than 40% of the left ventricle after reperfusion therapy. *Circulation* 1993, 88(part 1):1470–1475.

Evaluation of the Patient with Palpitations and Non–life-threatening Cardiac Arrhythmias

Kelly Anne Spratt
Eric L. Michelson

8

Key Points
- Palpitations are a frequent but relatively nonspecific cardiac symptom.
- Palpitations are not a reliable indicator of any particular cardiovascular finding or arrhythmia.
- Palpitations are clinically important when there is associated functional incapacity or concern of the patient, when they cause severe hemodynamic sequelae, or serve as harbingers of life-threatening cardiac arrhythmias in selected patients.
- A thorough history, physical examination, and judicious use of laboratory testing usually guide management.
- Management must encompass the nature and severity of the palpitations, the patient's general medical and cardiac conditions, the mechanism of the arrhythmia, and an algorithm for risk stratification.

Palpitations are a common symptom and frequent cause of outpatient visits to generalists and cardiovascular subspecialists. This chapter emphasizes a holistic yet focused, practical, and cost-effective approach to evaluating patients with palpitations. It is a reference for initiating management strategies in most patients with palpitations and non–life-threatening cardiac arrhythmias.

PALPITATIONS

Definitions

In this discussion, *palpitation* is defined broadly as an uncomfortable or abnormal awareness of the heart beating. Symptoms vary and may be described as heavy beating of the heart, fluttering in the chest, skipped beats, rapid heart beating, "flip-flopping" sensation, irregular heart beating, pounding in the neck, or some other unpleasant sensation depending on the underlying cardiac rhythm and the patient. Palpitations are a relatively nonspecific symptom and are not a reliable indicator of any particular cardiovascular finding or arrhythmia.

Symptomatic Manifestations of Arrhythmias

Cardiac symptoms as a manifestation of arrhythmias can be very nonspecific. Patients may present with a variety of complaints. Among individuals with documented cardiac arrhythmias, some are completely asymptomatic, some have palpitations, and others have symptoms that may present as angina, dyspnea, fatigue, effort intolerance, dizziness, near-syncope or syncope, or even noncardiac symptoms such as gastrointestinal upset [1,2].

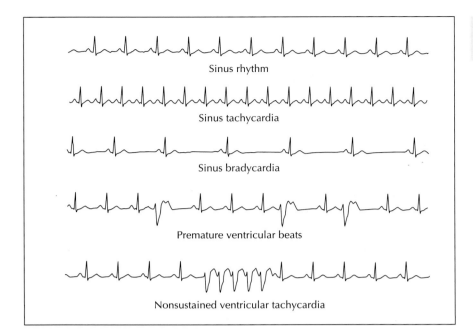

FIGURE 1 Electrocardiographic rhythms typically associated with palpitations.

Sinus rhythm

Sinus tachycardia

Sinus bradycardia

Premature ventricular beats

Nonsustained ventricular tachycardia

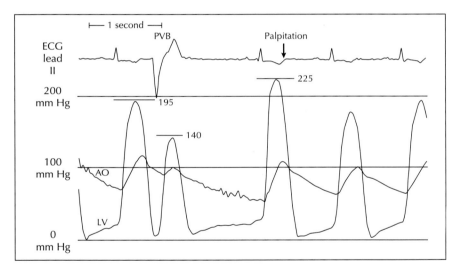

FIGURE 2 Increased left ventricular pressure (LV) after premature ventricular beat (PVB) in a patient with severe aortic stenosis and palpitations (*arrow*). AO—aortic pressure; ECG—electrocardiogram.

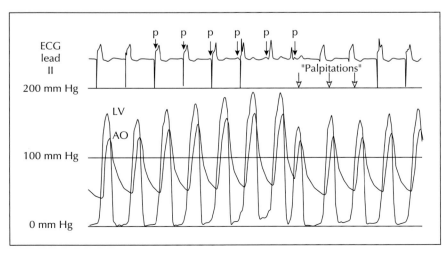

FIGURE 3 Pacemaker syndrome—the effects of atrioventricular dissociation on cardiac hemodynamics. There is a drop of 40 mm Hg in systemic blood pressure with atrioventricular asynchrony associated with palpitations (*open arrows*). *Arrows* indicate P waves. AO—aortic pressure; ECG—electrocardiogram; LV—left ventricular pressure.

Mechanisms

Arrhythmias can produce palpitations through multiple mechanisms. Arrhythmias can cause symptoms related to disorders of rhythm, disorders of rate, alterations in patterns of cardiac contractility, or alterations in cardiovascular hemodynamics. Intermittent disorders of rhythm such as paroxysmal supraventricular tachycardias, paroxysmal atrial fibrillation, atrial premature beats, and ventricular premature beats are frequent causes of palpitations. Disorders of rate also can be perceived as palpitations, and even sinus tachy- or bradycardia can cause symptoms (Fig. 1). In many cases, only normal sinus rhythm is found when using ambulatory electrocardiographic (ECG) recording

TABLE 1 PATIENT HISTORY

General medical history
Hypertension
Thyroid disease
Electrolyte disorder
Neuropsychiatric disorder
   Depression
   Anxiety
   Panic disorder
Diabetes mellitus
Sarcoidosis
Amyloidosis
Hemochromatosis
 	
Cardiovascular history
Ischemic heart disease
Hypertrophic heart disease
Mitral valve prolapse
Valvular heart disease
Preexcitation/Wolff-Parkinson-White syndrome
Long-QT syndrome
Rheumatic heart disease
Heart failure/cardiomyopathy
Congenital heart disease syncope and near syncope
 	
Social history
Ethanol use
Caffeine use
Tobacco use
Illicit drug use
Stress
Exercise
 	
Family history
Cardiovascular disease
Sudden cardiac death
Arrhythmias

techniques. This finding may suggest either a noncardiac origin or an awareness of increased contractility secondary to a surge in catecholamines (*eg*, before an interview, examination, or appearance on stage).

Inappropriate sinus tachycardia is an increasingly recognized cause of palpitations due to disorders of rate, especially in young women [3]. These patients often feel quite debilitated and have a sensitivity to intrinsic catecholamines that causes them to feel "on edge." Although more commonly associated with young women, this syndrome has also been noted in elderly women when carefully evaluated for this disorder. Of note, in at least one study of elderly women with inappropriate sinus tachycardia, all had concomitant anxiety disorder. Treatment for this disorder has included β-blockers, which may dissipate the catecholamine surges but also have an anxiolytic effect. Although sinus node modification has been attempted, the success rate is less than ideal. In patients with associated postural hypotension, the symptoms of hypotension and near syncope are not changed and the primary disorder may be an autonomic dysregulation [4].

The alterations in cardiac contractility and increased stroke volume that occur after premature ventricular beats also may be interpreted as palpitations (Fig. 2). Any arrhythmia associated with atrioventricular (AV) dissociation or varying patterns of AV conduction may cause symptoms related to a variety of mechanisms including altered atrial contribution to ventricular filling, which affects cardiac output, or atrial contraction against closed AV valves, which causes engorgement and regurgitation of blood into the pulmonary veins and venae cavae (Fig. 3) and venous pulsations in the neck. Characteristically, AV nodal reentrant tachycardia causes a regular, rapid "pounding in the neck" related to (right) atrial contraction against the closed (tricuspid) AV valve with each heartbeat [5].

The "neck pounding" has been noted in some symptomatic patients even during sinus rhythm, and subsequent electrophysiologic testing found a significant number to have dual atrioventricular nodal pathways with very long, slow pathway conduction times [6].

PATIENT EVALUATION

Initial Evaluation and Medical History

The ideal initial evaluation of the patient with palpitations is a thorough history and physical examination [7,8]. Most important to the general medical history is to determine the presence of common conditions (*eg*, hypertension or thyroid disease) that affect the cardiovascular system and possibly potentiate arrhythmias as well as to identify less common systemic disorders (*eg*, sarcoidosis) (Table 1). In adult noninsulin-dependent diabetic patients palpitations may be an indicator of poor glycemic control [9•]. Electrolyte abnormalities such as hypomagnesemia or hypokalemia may exacerbate the propensity for arrhythmias in both normal as well as structurally abnormal hearts. A thorough social history must be reviewed, and patients should be asked if they use tobacco, alcohol, caffeine or illicit drugs, as they will rarely volunteer this information. Family history should be reviewed regarding parents, siblings, and other family members with a history of cardiovascular disease, sudden cardiac death, or arrhythmias. As part of the initial history, it is also essential to determine the use of concomitant medications, whether prescription or over-the-counter drugs, that may affect the cardiovascular system (Table 2). Drugs associated with prolongation of the QT interval on the electrocardiogram in susceptible individuals may be associated with palpitations related to paroxysms of nonsustained ventricular tachyarrhythmias and may need to be discontinued to prevent the development of life-threatening torsade de pointes.

In women, palpitations may wax and wane with estrogen levels, often increasing in severity premenstrually. Also, the vasomotor symptoms associated with the perimenopausal and menopausal time frame may be associated with palpitations. Palpitations may precede the complete cessation of menses at the time of menopause.

It is also important to assess the patient's overall sense of well-being and probe thoroughly for clues to psychological illnesses such as depression and panic disorder as either may be the primary underlying affliction in many patients with palpitations. For example, patients with panic attacks are often exquisitely sensitive to heartbeat perception and an awareness of a change in heart rate may trigger further anxiety, which culminates in a vicious cycle of panic [10•]. The early identification of these patients is important as this can lead to avoidance of unnecessary testing and earlier initiation of treatment directed at the underlying problem. In such patients, recurrence of palpitations is frequent and may be associated with impaired work performance as well as a greater number of emergency medical visits [11•–13•].

Characteristics of Palpitations

Once a detailed, general medical history is obtained, the physician should characterize the patient's symptoms of palpitations qualitatively and quantitatively [14,15]. This includes establishing the frequency and duration of symptoms, the temporal pattern of symptoms, and the situations or circumstances that provoke or relieve symptoms (Table 3). The onset and termination of palpitations may help to identify the responsible arrhythmia. Symptoms that begin and terminate abruptly favor a reentrant or reciprocating tachycardia, such as AV reciprocating tachycardia or AV nodal reentrant tachycardia, whereas symptoms that begin abruptly but persist for days or recur several days in a row favor a diagnosis of paroxysmal atrial fibrillation [9•,14]. The rate and regularity, or irregularity, are also important characteristics. For example, even in patients with otherwise normal cardiac function, supraventricular tachycardias are frequently disabling [15•]. Exacerbating or ameliorating factors, associated symptoms (eg, dyspnea, lightheadedness, syncope, and angina), and response to prophylaxis, avoidance of potentiating factors, or interventions all may provide clues to an effective arrhythmia evaluation and management strategy.

Physical Examination

The physical examination should focus on the stigmata of structural heart disease including hypertensive heart disease. It should also focus on recognition of noncardiac disorders and the systemic manifestations of diseases (eg, thyroid disorder and alcohol or drug abuse) known to affect the heart and predispose patients to arrhythmias.

TABLE 2 NONCARDIAC DRUGS ASSOCIATED WITH PALPITATIONS*

α-Adrenergic agonist	**Endocrine**
Phenylpropanolamine	Thyroxine
Phenylephrine	
	Anticholinesterase
β-Adrenergic agonist	Physostigmine
Terbutaline	Neostigmine
Isoproterenol	
Albuterol	**Antimuscarinic**
	Atropine
Methylxanthine	Scopolamine
Theophylline	
	Illicit
Psychoactive	Amphetamine
Phenothiazines[†]	Cocaine
Tricyclics[†]	

*Partial listing of more commonly associated drugs.
[†]Associated with QT interval prolongation.

TABLE 3 CHARACTERISTICS OF PALPITATIONS

Frequency
Temporal pattern
Situations/circumstances
Positional changes
Onset/termination
Duration
Heart rate
Rhythm regularity/irregularity
Exacerbating factors
Ameliorating factors
Associated symptoms
Response to prophylaxis or interventions

Laboratory Testing

Initial routine laboratory testing should be limited to those tests likely to lead to a diagnosis or guide a management strategy. These may include a serum potassium or hemoglobin determination or an evaluation of thyroid function.

Electrocardiography is the cornerstone in the evaluation of patients with palpitations and is often useful in determining the mechanism of the responsible arrhythmia as well as the presence of underlying cardiac disease. The ECG can make the diagnosis of preexcitation syndrome, long-QT syndrome, Mobitz type I or type II heart block, or other conduction system disease. Supraventricular or ventricular premature beats also may be identified, but the modern, computerized, multilead ECG often records only 12 to 15 seconds of rhythm, which is usually insufficient to diagnose rhythms that are not clearly present clinically when the recording begins. If a diagnosis is not made, a form of ambulatory ECG monitoring is usually the next step. If symptoms are frequent (ie, daily), testing is often initiated with 24-hour ambulatory ECG recording. Unfortunately, this is nondiagnostic in many if not most cases. However, if symptoms are intermittent, the diagnostic test of choice is usually an external event recorder. Event recorders are generally used for 2 to 4 weeks and are very effective for adults who have palpitations lasting several minutes in duration and in whom there is the capacity to successfully initiate a recording. Recorders with memory loops and others with radiotransmitters allow the capture of briefer episodes. More recently introduced are implantable loop recorders that are implanted subcutaneously in the patient's chest wall and have a battery life of about 14 months. These devices have both patient-activated settings as well as automatically triggered settings that can be patient tailored to record brady- or tachycardias. This can be the best diagnostic option for some elderly and pediatric patients, for patients with incapacitating but infrequent episodes, as well as those for whom there is concern that there would not be the appropriate coordination of symptoms and activation such as for patients whose symptoms may awaken them from sleep [16–20].

Event recorders or implantable loop recorders are especially effective in patients in whom symptoms are debilitating but brief and may not be present by the time they reach a physician's office or the emergency department [21•,22•]. In either case, correlation of symptoms with ECG findings (or lack of findings) is essential [1]. It is generally not sufficient merely to identify an arrhythmia on ambulatory monitoring, but rather it is the close temporal relationship of a patient's typical symptom of palpitations with specific electrocardiographic findings that reveals the diagnosis. For example, the correlation of episodes of palpitations with normal sinus rhythm on the ambulatory or event recording despite the presence of premature ventricular contractions at other times would be helpful in suggesting the diagnosis of anxiety rather than an arrhythmia as the cause of the patient's symptoms. In addition, adequate time must be given to establish an arrhythmia or lack of arrhythmia. This has been the impetus for implantable loop recorders as a diagnostic option. Studies of these monitors indicate that there is a 50% to 80% diagnostic yield but this often takes 8 to 12 months.

Figure 1 shows single-lead ECG strips of various rhythms typically documented by ambulatory ECG recording or event monitoring. Often, at least two leads are recorded simultaneously to facilitate interpretation.

The optimal cost-effective duration of external event monitoring appears to be 2 weeks. In one study [23], the cost per new diagnosis increased from approximately $100 in week 1 to more than $5000 in week 3. Cost effectiveness of implantable loop recorders has been studied in patients with syncope and found to be competitively cost effective in patients willing to undergo such a procedure [24].

The initial thorough history, physical examination, and routine laboratory testing are usually within the purview of the generalist in the evaluation of patients with palpitations. Exceptions may include patients known to have more advanced or specific cardiovascular disorders or those having palpitations associated with more severe or potentially life-threatening sequelae. Recently, comprehensive consensus guidelines have been developed addressing the management of patients with atrial fibrillation and other forms of supraventricular tachycardia. These guidelines provide a useful framework and foundation for approaching patients in whom these diagnoses can be established [25,26].

Risk Stratification

Although palpitations are a relatively frequent cause of outpatient visits to physicians, they are associated with serious cardiac arrhythmias in only a minority of cases [27••]. Risk stratification is critical to the evaluation of patients who present with palpitations. The physician must stratify patients as to those with symptomatic but benign arrhythmias, those with prognostically important arrhythmias, and those with potentially life-threatening or hemodynamically important tachy- or bradyarrhythmia.

In patients with unremarkable history, physical examination, ECG, and routine laboratory results and who experience minor symptoms without significant arrhythmia on ambulatory monitoring, no further cardiovascular evaluation is usually necessary. Reassurance for the patient is appropriate. Conversely, in patients whose findings are more remarkable and symptoms more incapacitating, or for whom an increased risk of sudden death is clearly suspected, more aggressive diagnostic evaluation is warranted, in some cases including cardiac catheterization or electrophysiologic studies (Table 4). These cases are usually referred to a cardiovascular specialist, and some highly specialized invasive tests (eg, electrophysiologic studies) are done by subspecialists. The challenge to the clinician is to identify those individuals at increased risk for lethal or hemodynamically important arrhythmias from among those patients with intermediate findings and to choose the most appropriate diagnostic modality. In Table 5, low-risk patients are stratified as those who often require minimal evaluation, and high-risk patients are those who may require a more extensive work-up. Table 6 elaborates on several common rhythm abnormalities within these patient profiles, and based on this patient risk profile, Figure 4 presents an algorithm for the evaluation of patients with palpitations.

In managing patients with palpitations, cost-effectiveness of the evaluation must encompass several factors in

TABLE 4 DIAGNOSTIC MODALITIES

Noninvasive	**Clinical indication**
Electrocardiography*	Initial test for patients with palpitations or suspected arrhythmia
24-hour electrocardiographic monitoring*	Daily symptoms of palpitations or near-syncope
Ambulatory event recording*	Less frequent symptoms of palpitations or near-syncope
Echocardiography	Assessment of known or suspected structural heart disease and for evaluation of cardiac function or ischemic heart disease
Radionuclide studies	Assessment of known or suspected ischemic heart disease and less commonly for evaluation of cardiac function
Exercise stress testing*	Evaluation of exercise-induced arrhythmia or screening for ischemic heart disease
Head-up tilt testing	Evaluation of vasodepressor/vasovagal syncope
Invasive†	
Cardiac catheterization	Evaluation of cardiac/coronary anatomy and cardiac function in high-risk patients with known or suspected ischemic/structural or valvular heart disease
Electrophysiologic testing	Evaluation of patients with life-threatening or hemodynamically important arrhythmias
Implantable (subcutaneous) loop event recorders	Infrequent but incapacitating symptoms of palpitations, near-syncope, or syncope

*Initial testing modalities usually available to generalists.

†Invasive diagnostic modalities done by cardiovascular specialists and subspecialists.

TABLE 5 RISK STRATIFICATION OF PATIENTS WITH PALPITATIONS FOR LETHAL OR HEMODYNAMICALLY IMPORTANT ARRHYTHMIAS

Low risk
Patients without structural heart disease
Patients without a history of near-syncope or syncope
Patients without evidence of myocardial ischemia
Patients with preserved left ventricular function

High risk
Patients with structural heart disease
Patients with history of syncope
Patients with left ventricular ejection fraction < 40% or symptomatic heart failure
Patients with known coronary artery disease or myocardial infarction
Patients with conduction system disease
Patients with long-QT syndrome
Patients with Wolff-Parkinson-White syndrome

TABLE 6 EVALUATION OF ARRHYTHMIAS IN PATIENTS WITH PALPITATIONS

Benign arrhythmias that generally do not require extensive evaluation
Sinus bradycardia
Sinus arrhythmia
Isolated atrial premature beats
Isolated ventricular premature beats

Arrhythmias that may require more extensive evaluation
Tachy-brady syndrome
Atrioventricular nodal reentrant tachycardias
Atrioventricular reciprocating tachycardias
Nonsustained ventricular tachycardia
Inappropriate sinus tachycardia

Arrhythmias that generally require further invasive evaluation
Persistent atrial or sinus tachycardia
Preexcitation/Wolff-Parkinson-White syndrome
Atrial fibrillation/atrial flutter
Sustained ventricular tachycardia

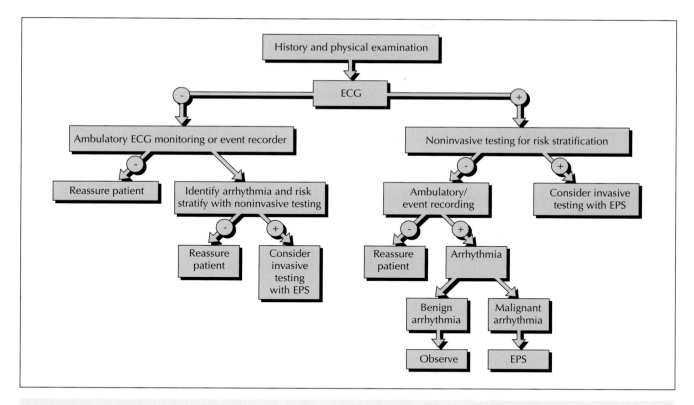

FIGURE 4 Diagnostic evaluation of palpitations. ECG—electrocardiography; EPS—electrophysiologic study.

addition to the direct cost of diagnostic testing. These include the adverse effect of palpitations on the patient's quality of life and productivity at work as well as the consequences of not recognizing a potentially lethal underlying cardiovascular problem.

Knowledgeable evaluation of patients with palpitations is mandatory as a prelude to appropriate management. Avoidance of precipitating factors, if readily identified, can be helpful, with the cooperation of the patient. Reassurance is of major importance after a benign condition has been confirmed. Only a minority of patients with palpitations are candidates for pharmacologic therapy. In some patients, prophylaxis is warranted; in others with infrequent bouts, it may be sufficient to use a "cocktail" of one or more drugs at the time of an episode.

Conventional antiarrhythmic drugs that are currently available have limitations in efficacy and tolerability [28]. In many cases, the propensity of these agents to cause more serious arrhythmias (*ie*, proarrhythmia) or other pulmonary, hematologic, or hepatic toxicity outweighs any potential benefit in suppressing the arrhythmia that is causing the palpitations. In some cases, beta-blockers can be used effectively to reduce the occurrence and severity of symptomatic episodes when a catecholamine component is a major factor.

For example, one not well-recognized cause of palpitations, especially in young women, is inappropriate sinus tachycardia. These patients often feel quite debilitated, and

their hypersensitivity to catecholamines may yield a feeling of being "on edge."

CONCLUSION

Palpitations are a common symptom that can be a source of distress for the patient and a challenge for the physician. An optimal approach to evaluating the patient with palpitations is holistic; systematic with respect to the history, physical examination, and selected laboratory testing; and must include risk stratification. The evaluation strategy must be practical, cost-effective, and relevant to a well-defined algorithm for patient management.

REFERENCES AND RECOMMENDED READING

Recently published papers of particular interest have been highlighted as:

• Of interest

•• Of outstanding interest

1. Zeldis SM, Levine BJ, Michelson EL, Morganroth J: Cardiovascular complaints: correlation with cardiac arrhythmias on 24-hour electrocardiographic monitoring. *Chest* 1980, 78:456–462.

2. Page RL, Wilkinson WE, Clair WK, *et al.*: Asymptomatic arrhythmia in patients with symptomatic paroxysmal atrial fibrillation and paroxysmal supraventricular tachycardia. *Circulation* 1994, 89:224–227.

3. Lopera G, Castellanos A, Moleiro F, *et al.*: Chronic inappropriate sinus tachycardia in elderly females. *Ann Noninvasive Electrocardiol* 2003, 2:139–143.

4. Shen WK, Low PA, Jahangir A, *et al.*: Is sinus node modification appropriate for inappropriate sinus tachycardia with features of postural orthostatic tachycardia syndrome? *Pacing Clin Electrophysiol* 2001, 24: 217–230.

5. Gursoy S, Steurer G, Brugada J, *et al.*: The hemodynamic mechanism of pounding in the neck in atrioventricular nodal reentrant tachycardia. *N Engl J Med* 1992, 327:772–774.

6. Geelen P, Primo J, Brugada J, *et al.*: Neck pounding during sinus rhythm: a new clinical manifestation of dual atrioventricular nodal pathways. *Heart* 1998, 79:490–492.

7. Lee TH: Chest discomfort and palpitation. In *Harrison's Principles of Internal Medicine*, edn 15. New York: McGraw-Hill; 2001:60–66.

8. Braunwald E: The history. In *Heart Disease: A Textbook of Cardiovascular Medicine*, edn 6. Philadelphia: WB Saunders; 2001:37–40.

9.• Karen JC, Curtis LG, Summerson JH: Symptoms and complications of adult diabetic patients in a family practice. *Arch Fam Med* 1996, 5:135–145.

10.• Ehlers A, Breuer P: How good are patients with panic disorder at perceiving their heartbeats? *Biol Psychol* 1996, 42:165–182.

11.• Barsky AJ, Cleary PD, Coeytaux RR, Ruskin JN: The clinical course of palpitations in medical outpatients. *Arch Intern Med* 1995, 55:1702–1708.

12.• Weber BE, Kapoor WN: Evaluation and outcomes of patients with palpitations. *Am J Med* 1996, 100:138–148.

13.• Barsky AJ, Ahern DK, Bailery ED, Delamates BA: Predictors of persistent palpitations and continued medical utilization. *J Fam Prac* 1996, 42:465–472.

14. Falk RH: Atrial fibrillation. *N Engl J Med* 2001, 344:1067–1077.

15.• Wood KA, Drew BJ, Scheinmann MM: Frequency of disabling symptoms in supraventricular tachycardia. *Am J Cardiol* 1997, 79:145–149.

16. Seidl K, Rameken M Breunung S, *et al.*: Diagnostic assessment of recurrent unexplained syncope with a new subcutaneously implantable loop recorder: Reveal Investigators. *Europace* 2000, 2:256–262.

17. Rossano J, Bloemerst B, Sreeram N, *et al.*: Efficacy of implantable loop recorders in establishing symptom-rhythm correlation in young patients with syncope and palpitations. *Pediatrics* 2003, 112:228–233.

18. Mason PK, Wood MA, Reese DB, *et al.*: Usefulness of implantable loop recorders in office-based practice for evaluation of syncope and palpitations in patients with and without structural heart disease. *Am J Cardiol* 2003, 92:1127–1129.

19. Ermis C, Zhu AX, Pham S, *et al.*: Comparison of automatic and patient-activated arrhymia recordings by implantable loop recorders in the evaluation of syncope. *Am J Cardiol* 2003, 92:815–819.

20. Benditt DG, Ermis C, Pham S, *et al.*: Implantable diagnostic monitoring devices for evaluation of syncope, tachy- and brady arrhythmias. *J Interv Card Electrophysiol* 2003, 9:137–144.

21.• Fogel RI, Evans JJ, Prystowsky EN: Utility and cost of event recorders in the diagnosis of palpitations, presyncope, and syncope. *Am J Cardiol* 1997, 79:207–208.

22.• Kinlay S, Leitch JW, Neil A, *et al.*: Cardiac event recorders yield more diagnoses and are more cost-effective than 48-hour Holter monitoring in patients with palpitations. *Ann Intern Med* 1996, 124:16–20.

23. Zimetbaum PJ, Kim KY, Josephson M, *et al.*: Diagnostic yield and optimal duration of continuous-loop event monitoring for the diagnosis of palpitations: a cost-effective analysis. *Ann Intern Med* 1998, 128:890–895.

24. Krahn AD, Klein GJ, Yee R, *et al.*: Cost implications of testing strategy in patients with syncope. *J Am Coll Cardiol* 2003, 42:495–501.

25. Fuster V, Ryden LE, Asinger RW, *et al.*: ACC/AHA/ESC guidelines for the management of patients with atrial fibrillation. *Eur Heart J* 2001, 22:1852–1923.

26. Blomstrom-Lindqvist C, Scheinman MM, Aliot EM, *et al.*: ACC/AHA/ESC guidelines for the management of patients with supraventricular arrhythmias. *J Am Coll Cardiol* 2003, 42:1493–1531.

27.•• Zimetbaum P, Josephson ME: Evaluation of patients with palpitations. *N Engl J Med* 1998, 338:1369–1373.

28. Sljapic TN, Kowey PR, Michelson EL: Antiarrhythmic Drugs. In *Cardiovascular Pharmacotherapeutics Manual*, edn 2. Edited by Frishman WH, Sonnenblick EH, Sica DA. New York: McGraw-Hill; 2004:213–262.

9

Evaluation of the Patient with Syncope

Charles M. Blatt
Thomas B. Graboys

Key Points

- Five percent to 10% of emergency visits and hospitalizations involve investigation and management of patients with syncope.
- Patient history is key in defining the cause of the syncopal event; a witness is often a critical historian.
- Patient history must focus on a detailed setting for the syncopal event and should define any situational relationships.
- The physical examination must assess orthostatic potential and focus on potential cardiac and carotid obstructive lesions.
- Multiple unwitnessed syncopal events under curious circumstances should be suspected as factitious.
- Over-the-counter medications may interact with prescribed medications, especially in the elderly, and must be considered as a cause of syncope.
- Referral to a specialist is warranted when either neurologic or cardiac brady- or tachyarrhythmic causes are suggested by preliminary testing.

Syncope accounts for 5% to 10% of emergency room visits and hospitalizations. Traditionally, syncope is viewed as either cardiac or neurologic in origin. These processes overlap, however, because of the dominant role of the vagus nerve and myocardial mechanoreceptors in the generation of neurocardiogenic syncope. Intense peripheral vasodilation followed by bradycardia is mediated by inhibition of sympathetic efferents and enhancement of parasympathetic efferent activity. Psychogenic syncope bridges the gap between cardiac and neurogenic syncope by many inadequately defined mechanisms. Causes of syncope are listed in Table 1; a diagnostic approach is shown in Figure 1.

HISTORY

Patient history is the key to determining the origin of the syncopal event. Physical examination and laboratory tests are important in a minority of events. The clinician should establish a clinical description of the syncopal event with questions such as the following:

Was the syncope witnessed or unwitnessed?
Does the patient have a memory of the event?
Was the event prodromal?
Was it a singular or recurrent episode?
Were injuries associated with the syncopal event?

Can a situational relationship be established?
  Did the patient rise abruptly [1]?
  Did the patient urinate (postmicturition) [2]?
  Did the patient defecate [3]?
  Did the patient eat a meal (postprandial) [4]?
  Did the patient cough?
  Did the patient swallow?
  Was the patient exposed to intense pain?
  Was the patient exposed to the sight of blood?
  Has the patient recently started a new drug regimen?
  Was the patient dehydrated and/or on vasodilating
    medications, such as angiotensin-converting enzyme
    (ACE) inhibitors, angiotensin receptor blockers, or
    calcium blockers?

The physician must first exclude potential polypharmaceutical drug–drug interactions that might induce either a brady- or tachycardiac event. For the elderly patient, beta-adrenergic and calcium-blocking agents may induce sinoatrial block. Aggravation of ventricular arrhythmia or "proarrhythmia" by antiarrhythmic drugs [5] and herbal preparations with untested effects, doses and potential for interaction, should also be excluded among patients with syncope who are receiving these agents.

Witnesses

The witness to the syncopal event fills in the history that the patient cannot provide. If episodes of syncope are multiple and all unwitnessed with curious circumstances in which a witness could not be present, factitious syncope must be considered. Witnesses should be located and interviewed to focus the inquiry and lead to a more cost-effective diagnostic approach. Panic attacks, anxiety episodes, and conversion reactions may be diagnosed with the aid of

a witness, thus eliminating the need for further testing that would delay introduction of therapy [6].

Patient Memory

The patient's memory of the syncopal event may be helpful, and the patient should be asked to recreate in detail the circumstances leading to the event. A postictal confusion, with or without evidence of urinary or fecal incontinence, clearly points to a neurologic cause, whereas clearheadedness immediately after the event points away from seizure as a cause. A completely nonprodromal event, independent of body position or activity, may focus diagnostic events to uncovering complete heart block, especially for the older patient for whom a sclerocalcific process may affect the cardiac conduction system. The nature of the prodrome, if witnessed or recalled, is likely to help define a vagally mediated event, including pallor, diaphoresis, nausea, and suggestive historical details.

Multiple Events

Multiple syncopal episodes may define a patient with a benign process or point to a psychogenic cause [7]. In general, the clinical history tends to be more valuable in distinguishing vasodepressor syncope from syncope caused by either atrioventricular block or ventricular tachycardia [8].

Setting the Stage

The history obtained from the patient and any witnesses should set the stage of the syncopal event in detail, with precise definition of the time of day; altitude; relation to meals; events of the preceding 24 hours; change in routine patterns of sleep, bowel movement, and food and fluid intake; coincident medication, including novel combinations of prescription and over-the-counter medication; and preceding breathlessness, palpitations, and chest discomfort. The witness must be questioned for evidence of seizure activity; was the patient postictal or incontinent? In addition to the obvious tonic-clonic grand mal activity, evidence of petit mal must be sought. Pulmonary embolism is often overlooked as a cause of syncope, and a conducive historical setting for this problem must be considered. This history includes recent inactivity, travel, or surgery.

PHYSICAL FINDINGS

Although a meticulous history is the cornerstone of defining the cause of syncope, physical findings also may contribute to the correct diagnosis (Table 2). Foremost is the demonstration of substantial positional changes in blood pressure. Blood pressure readings should be taken in both arms while the patient is supine, sitting, and standing. A normal response is a slight decrease in pressure when assuming the upright posture, but blood pressure is maintained within 30 to 60 seconds and a slight increase in heart rate occurs. Among older patients complaining of postural dizziness or

TABLE 1 CAUSES OF SYNCOPE	
Arrhythmia	Situational
Bradyarrhythmia	Coughing
Tachyarrhythmia	Defecation
Supraventricular	Eating
Ventricular	Micturition
Carotid sinus sensitivity	Swallowing
Cerebrovascular disease	Valvular
Drug induced	Aortic stenosis
Vasodilation	Pulmonic stenosis
Arrhythmogenic	Miscellaneous
Neurocardiogenic	Idiopathic hypertrophic
Orthostatic	subaortic stenosis
Pulmonary embolism	Atrial myxoma (right
Psychogenic	or left)
Anxiety	
Conversion	
Panic	

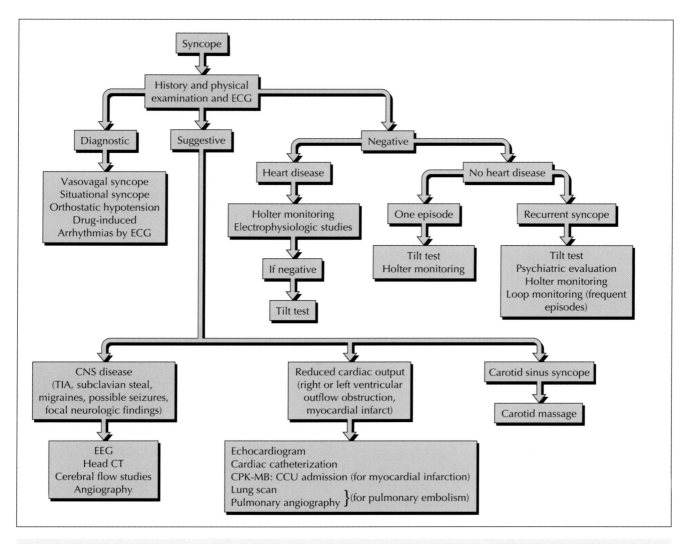

FIGURE 1 Diagnostic approach to syncope. CCU—coronary care unit; CNS—central nervous system; CPK-MB—creatine phosphokinase-muscle brain units; CT—computed tomography; ECG—electrocardiography; EEG—electroencephalography; TIA—transient ischemic attack. (*Adapted from* Kapoor [8].)

TABLE 2 PHYSICAL EXAMINATION FINDINGS
Orthostatic vital signs
Blood pressure
Supine, sitting, standing after 30 and 60 seconds
Heart rate
Appropriate rise
Persistent decline with standing
Cardiac bruits
Cardiac obstructive murmurs
Aortic stenosis
Mitral stenosis
Hypertrophic cardiomyopathy
Ectopy
Neurologic examination

near loss of consciousness, orthostatic hypotension induced by antihypertensive drugs is a frequent cause of postural dizziness of frank syncope. Potent antihypertensive drugs may induce a decrease of 20 to 30 mm Hg in blood pressure when assuming an upright posture. The postural change in blood pressure is accentuated in the dehydrated state.

Autonomic Dysfunction

While standing, patients with idiopathic orthostatic hypotension experience a gradual decrease in blood pressure without a commensurate increase in heart rate. This type of autonomic dysfunction also may be a sign of Shy-Drager's disease. Individuals with high vagal tone not only may demonstrate changes in heart rate while obtaining postural blood pressures but also profound sinus bradycardia. A slow heart rate may indicate the patient's predisposition to vasodepressor or vasovagal syncope.

Auscultation of the Carotid Vessels and Heart

Careful examination of the carotid vessels for bruits and auscultation of the heart may determine the presence of aortic stenosis or obstructive hypertrophic cardiomyopathy. The presence of a high density of ectopic beats also may help to define arrhythmia as a potential cause of syncope. Central nervous system examination can exclude evidence for focal neurologic deficit. In most patients, however, physical findings are not helpful and not nearly as critical to the diagnosis as a proper history.

LABORATORY EVALUATION

Ambulatory and Transtelephonic Electrocardiographic Monitoring

Laboratory evaluation of a patient with syncope (Table 3) should focus on where the diagnosis will most likely be found. Any historical suggestion of cardiac arrhythmia, either tachycardia or bradycardia, demands 48 to 72 hours of ambulatory monitoring. A transtelephonic device with loop memory capacity may help document a cardiac rhythm when events are infrequent [9]. The implantable loop recorder (ILR) can record and store ECG rhythm for a year or more. The device can be programmed to be activated by rapid heart rates or by pauses. The ILR has been shown to be more effective in determining the source of syncope [10] and more cost-effective when compared with conventional strategies of making a diagnosis [11]. The exercise tolerance test may provide invaluable information regarding underlying heart disease and the ability to provoke ventricular tachycardia of hemodynamic significance as well as bradycardia or advanced atrioventricular block [12].

Carotid Sinus Massage

The coincidence of coronary artery disease may be demonstrated by an exercise test, and the application of carotid sinus massage during the routine 12-lead electrocardiogram may provide information regarding carotid bulb sensitivity. A sensitive carotid may be stimulated by a tight collar when the neck is rotated thus generating a profound bradycardia leading to a syncopal event [13].

Electrophysiologic provocation studies [14] may provide clues regarding the ease of stimulating a brady- or tachyarrhythmia and help to define the sinoatrial recovery time, which may be helpful under well-defined circumstances [15]. The tachy-brady syndrome, wherein the abrupt termination of rapid supraventricular tachycardia (including atrial fibrillation or flutter) produces a prolonged sinus pause resulting in prolonged asystole and near or complete syncope. The pursuit of invasive studies depends on exclusion of the more obvious causes of syncope. Usually, an electrophysiologic study is deferred until a full noninvasive evaluation is completed [16].

Autonomic Testing

Autonomic testing using head-up tilt and an isoproterenol infusion has been studied in detail [17–19]. The appearance of intense bradycardia and hypotension during head-up tilt, with or without the infusion of isoproterenol, and the induction of near syncope or syncope suggestive of the clinical scenario are diagnostic of neurocardiogenic syncope. An increase in myocardial contractility and a coincidental decline in left ventricular end-diastolic dimension precede the onset of syncope [20]. A vagus-mediated slowing of the heart rate appears to play a secondary role to vasodepression in inducing a hypotensive syncopal episode. This appears to explain the inefficacy of cardiac pacing in the management of patients with neurocardiogenic syncope [21].

Echocardiography

Echocardiography occasionally supplements and clarifies issues raised on physical examination. Systolic murmurs may require further clarification regarding the potential for hemodynamically critical aortic stenosis, pulmonary stenosis, idiopathic hypertrophic subaortic stenosis (IHSS), or atrial myxoma to be the source of syncope. The patient with unsuspected IHSS receiving a diuretic may experience a syncopal episode; with rehydration the patient may have no further symptoms. Ventricular or atrial tachyarrhythmia in the setting of IHSS also may cause syncope.

MANAGEMENT

Single Event

Typically, the first episode of lost consciousness is based on a vasovagal event; however, this diagnosis is one of exclusion. Patient history is typical, with an absence of neuro-

TABLE 3 LABORATORY EVALUATION

By the generalist
Carotid sinus massage
Electrocardiography
Ambulatory electrocardiographic monitor
Transtelephonic "loop memory"
Exercise tolerance test
Electroencephalography
If indicated by physical examination:
    Echocardiography
    Carotid arterial noninvasive tests

By the specialist
Signal-averaged electrocardiography
Cardiac electrophysiologic study
Tilt-table autonomic testing

logic prodrome or sequelae and a spontaneous resumption of consciousness without the need for resuscitation. These features define the diagnosis and determine further management. In many cases, a solitary episode of lost consciousness suggests either cardiac or neurologic syncope and requires further evaluation.

Multiple Episodes

There is more concern if the patient experiences two or more syncopal episodes, particularly if they share historical characteristics. At times, several days of hospitalization are needed to define the syncope as neurologic, which may only be disclosed through a sleep-deprived electroencephalogram, for example, or a cardiac rhythm disorder that may either have been a brady- or tachycardiac event. Evaluation of the patient with syncope depends on the unique nature and frequency of the event and the clinical condition of the patient.

Pharmacologic Options

Dietary supplementation of salt and water to expand extracellular fluid volume has been a simple and common approach to the initial management of patients with presumed vasovagal or neurally mediated syncope. Because underhydration is common, it is appropriate to encourage all patients to increase their water and electrolyte-enriched fluid intake. The mineralocorticoid fludrocortisone is an effective agent for promoting renal retention of salt in water [22]. The adverse effects of excessive mineralocorticoid, including hypertension, acne, edema, and mood alteration, often limit its use.

The search for effective and well-tolerated pharmacologic interventions for the treatment of patients with vasovagal syncope has generated several candidate therapies, noted here.

Beta-adrenergic blockade

Beta-adrenoreceptor blocking agents have become the most common pharmacologic approach to managing patients with vasovagal syncope. Theoretically, the beta-blockers reduce the intensity of catecholamine stimulation of the cardiac mechanoreceptors induced by an underfilled left ventricle. Most assessments of beta-blockers have been conducted as nonrandomized trials, but a small placebo-controlled, randomized study [23] has confirmed the effectiveness of atenolol in preventing tilt-table–induced syncope, as well as the recurrence of syncope over several months.

Alpha-adrenergic agonists

A randomized, placebo-controlled trial [24] of an alpha-adrenergic receptor agonist, midodrine, has provided an alternative to the beta-blocking agents used for treating patients with vasovagal syncope. Midodrine activates alpha-adrenoreceptors in arterial and venous vessels, thereby increasing peripheral vascular tone and reducing peripheral vascular pooling.

Selective serotonin reuptake inhibitors

The beneficial effects of the selective serotonin reuptake inhibitor paroxetine in patients with vasovagal syncope enrolled in a randomized, placebo-controlled study were recently reported [25]. Paroxetine is hypothesized to have its beneficial effect by altering the central serotonergic regulation of sympathetic neural transmitters.

Other pharmacologic interventions

Disopyramide has been studied for its potential role in managing patients with vasovagal syncope. The negative inotropic, anticholinergic, and peripheral vasoconstricting properties suggested a potential for efficacy, but randomized trials do not support its use. Other anticholinergic agents such as scopolamine and propantheline bromide have not been studied in sufficiently large numbers of patients to recommend their routine use. Theophylline and clonidine have also been proposed as potential therapies, but inadequate data are available regarding their efficacy.

Orthostatic Training on the Tilt Table

An alternative to pharmacologic therapy has been tested in adolescents with recurrent syncope and positive tilt-table test results [26]. These patients adhered to a training regimen consisting of twice-a-day tilt table sessions lasting up to 40 minutes per session. Significant improvement in symptoms has been reported in this group of patients, who are often intolerant of or unresponsive to pharmacologic therapy.

Permanent Cardiac Pacing

The use of permanent transvenous cardiac pacing has been proposed as a management strategy for patients with recurrent vasovagal syncope. Cardiac pacing in this setting, however, remains controversial because of the often profound vasodilatation that occurs simultaneously with the bradycardia. Clinical observations of patients who have fainted despite adequate pacemaker response fuel this controversy. The North American Vasovagal Pacing Study [27] demonstrated fewer syncopal events in the patients randomly assigned to the dual chamber pacemaker therapy. The pacemaker was programmed to pace at a relatively high rate if a predetermined decrease in heart rate was detected. This study involved only 54 patients, but the results were judged to be statistically significant.

WHEN TO REFER

The generalist should maintain responsibility for the overall care of the patient and integration of the evaluation and therapy for syncope with the patient's preexisting medical and social problems. It is often the valued role of the generalist to maintain a critical perspective on results of the general and specialized testing. If one test does not fit a scenario that the bulk of the other diagnostic tests support, it may need to be discarded. One test result should not countermand the weight of clinical sensibility if the other objective tests lean away from the diagnosis supported by that single test.

Under most circumstances, the generalist proceeds with a thorough history and physical examination, including carotid sinus massage, an electrocardiogram, and a 24-hour ambulatory monitor. If the physical examination suggests an obstructive lesion of the carotid arteries, referral for carotid noninvasive testing is indicated. If the vascular obstruction is reported as significant, referral to a neurologist or vascular surgeon is warranted. The neurologist also should be consulted when the history suggests a seizure disorder.

Cardiac murmurs suggestive of valvular obstructive disease or hypertrophic obstructive cardiomyopathy require prompt referral. Consultation with a cardiologist is indicated if pathology is defined or the murmur remains enigmatic and the history suggests a cardiac source of syncope.

Referral to the cardiologist also is advised when the 24-hour ambulatory monitor provides various types of data. An unambiguous, complete atrioventricular block requires pacemaker implantation. Tachyarrhythmia, particularly ventricular, requires referral to the cardiologist to determine the need for further assessment with electrocardiographic signal averaging or arrhythmia provocation (electrophysiologic studies).

REFERENCES

1. Lipsitz LA: Orthostatic hypotension in the elderly. *N Engl J Med* 1989, 321:952–956.

2. Kapoor WN, Peterson JR, Karpf M: Micturition syncope. *JAMA* 1985, 253:796–798.

3. Kapoor WN, Peterson J, Karpf M: Defecation syncopes: a symptom with multiple etiologies. *Ann Intern Med* 1986, 146:2377–2423.

4. Lipsitz LA, Pluchino FC, Wei JY, *et al.*: Cardiovascular and norepinephrine responses after meal consumption in elderly (older than 75 years) persons with postprandial hypotension and syncope. *Am J Cardiol* 1986, 58:810–815.

5. Velebit V, Podrid PJ, Lown B, *et al.*: Aggravation and provocation of ventricular arrhythmias by antiarrhythmic drugs. *Circulation* 1982, 65:886–894.

6. Linzer M, Pontinen M, Gold DT, *et al.*: Impairment of physical and psychosocial health in recurrent syncope. *J Clin Epidemiol* 1991, 44:1037–1044.

7. Linzer M, Felder A, Hackel A, *et al.*: Psychiatric syncope: a new look at an old disease. *Psychosomatics* 1990, 31:181–188.

8. Kapoor WN: Diagnostic evaluation of syncope. *Am J Med* 1991, 90:91–106.

9. Sivakumaran S, Krahn AD, Klein GJ, *et al.*: A prospective randomized comparison of loop recorders versus Holter monitors in patients with syncope or presyncope. *Am J Med* 2003, 115:1–5.

10. Krahn AD, Klein GJ, Yee R, Skanes AC: Randomized assessment of syncope trial: conventional diagnostic testing versus a prolonged monitoring strategy. *Circulation* 2001, 104:46–51.

11. Krahn AD, Klein GJ, Yee R, *et al.*: Cost implications of testing strategy in patients with syncope: randomized assessment of syncope trial. *J Am Coll Cardiol* 2003, 42:495–501.

12. Podrid PJ, Graboys TB, Lampert S, Blatt CM: Exercise stress testing for exposure of arrhythmia. *Circulation* 1987, 75:60–65.

13. Lewis T: A lecture on vasovagal syncope and the carotid sinus mechanism. *BMJ* 1932, 1:873–876.

14. Krol RB, Morady F, Flaker CG, *et al.*: Electrophysiologic testing in patients with unexplained syncope: clinical and noninvasive predictors of outcome. *J Am Coll Cardiol* 1987, 10:358–363.

15. Linzer M, Prystowsky EN, Divine GW, *et al.*: Predicting the outcome of electrophysiologic studies in syncope: validation of a derived model. *J Gen Intern Med* 1991, 6:113–120.

16. Lown B: Management of patients at high risk of sudden death. *Am Heart J* 1982, 103:689–697.

17. Almquist A, Goldenberg IF, Milstein S, *et al.*: Provocation of bradycardia and hypotension by isoproterenol and upright posture in patients with unexplained syncope. *N Engl J Med* 1989, 320:346–351.

18. Grubb BP, Temesy-Armos P, Han H, Elliot L: Utility of upright tilt-table testing in the evaluation and management of syncope of unknown origin. *Am J Med* 1991, 90:6–10.

19. Kapoor WN, Brant N: Evaluation of syncope by upright tilt testing with isoproterenol: a nonspecific test. *Ann Intern Med* 1992, 116:358–363.

20. Shalev Y, Gal R, Tchou PJ, *et al.*: Echocardiographic demonstration of decreased left ventricular dimensions and vigorous myocardial contraction during syncope induced by head-up tilt. *J Am Coll Cardiol* 1991, 18:746–751.

21. Sra JS, Jazayeri MR, Avitall B, *et al.*: Comparison of cardiac pacing with drug therapy in the treatment of neurocardiogenic (vasovagal) syncope with bradycardia or asystole. *N Engl J Med* 1993, 328:1085–1090.

22. Scott WA, Pongiglione G, Bromberg BI, *et al.*: Randomized comparison of atenolol and fludrocortisone acetate in the treatment of pediatric neurally mediated syncope. *Am J Cardiol* 1995, 76:400–402.

23. Mahananda N, Bjuripanyo K, Kangagate C, *et al.*: Randomized double-blind, placebo-controlled trial of oral atenolol in patients with unexplained syncope and positive upright tilt table test results. *Am Heart J* 1995, 130:1250–1253.

24. Ward CR, Gray JC, Gilroy JJ, Kenny RA: Midodrine: a role in the management of neurocardiogenic syncope. *Heart* 1998, 79:45–49.

25. Girolamo ED, Iorio CD, Sabatini P, *et al.*: Effects of paroxetine hydrochloride syncope: a randomized, double-blinded, placebo-controlled study. *J Am Coll Cardiol* 1999, 33:1227–1230.

26. Girolamo ED, Iorio CD, Leonzio L, *et al.*: Usefulness of a tilt training program for the prevention of refractory neurocardiogenic syncope in adolescents: a controlled study. *Circulation* 1999, 100:1798–1801.

27. Connoly SJ, Sheldon RS, Roberts RS, Gent M: The North American vasovagal pacemaker study: a randomized trial of permanent cardiac pacing for the prevention of vasovagal syncope. *J Am Coll Cardiol* 1999, 33:16–20.

SELECT BIBLIOGRAPHY

Benditt DG, Ferguson DW, Grubb BP, *et al.*: Tilt table testing for assessing syncope: American College of Cardiology [review]. *J Am Coll Cardiol* 1996, 28:263–275.

Benditt DG, Fahy GJ, Luri KG, *et al.*: Pharmacotherapy of neurally mediated syncope. *Circulation* 1999, 100:1242–1248.

Bloomfield DM: A symposium: a common faint: tailoring treatment for targeted groups of patients with vasovagal syncope. *Am J Cardiol* 1999:84.

Kinlay S, Leitch JW, Neil A, *et al.*: Cardiac event recorders yield more diagnosis and are more cost-effective than 48 hour Holter monitoring in patients with palpitations: a controlled clinical trial. *Ann Intern Med* 1996, 124:16–20.

Low PA, Gilden JL, Freeman R, *et al.*: Efficacy of midodrine vs placebo in neurogenic orthostatic hypotension: a randomized, double-blind multicenter study. *JAMA* 1997, 277:1046–1051.

Martin TP, Hanusa BH, Kapour WN: Risk stratification of patients with syncope [comment]. *Ann Emerg Med* 1997, 29:459–466.

Ooi WL, Barrett S, Hossain M, *et al.*: Patterns of orthostatic blood pressure change and their clinical correlates in a frail, elderly population. *JAMA* 1997, 277:1299–1304.

Evaluation of the Patient Resuscitated from Cardiac Arrest

10

Peter Ott

Eric N. Prystowsky

Key Points

- Sudden cardiac death (SCD) is the most common cause of mortality in adults less than age 65 years of age.
- Coronary artery disease is the most common cause of cardiac arrest.
- Survivors of cardiac arrest should undergo a complete history and physical examination as well as cardiac catheterization and electrophysiologic evaluation.
- Clinical trials have shown superior efficacy of implantable cardioverter defibrillators (ICDs) in preventing SCD.
- Antiarrhythmic drug therapy alone or catheter ablation therapy may have a role in selected patients.
- Survivors of cardiac arrest are at a high risk for a recurrent episode if not treated properly, so referral to a clinical electrophysiologist is suggested.

Sudden cardiac death (SCD) is the most common cause of mortality in adults less than 65 years of age [1]. It is estimated that sudden cardiac death claims a patient approximately every 1 to 2 minutes [2]. There are various cardiac causes for sudden death (Table 1). In a relatively small percentage of patients, bradycardia may be the first arrhythmia identified in the cardiac arrest victim, but ventricular fibrillation (VF) or rapid sustained ventricular tachycardia (VT-S) is more common (Fig. 1) [3–7].

Cobb *et al.* [8] were pioneers in establishing community-based intervention for cardiac arrest victims. They developed a rapid response system for emergency services in Seattle using the Seattle Fire Department. Approximately 60% of Seattle residents 12 years of age and older have had some training in cardiopulmonary resuscitation. Even in such an emergency care system, only approximately 30% of cardiac arrest victims are discharged from the hospital alive. Most communities, especially in more rural areas of the United States, have far fewer successful resuscitations. In Memphis, approximately 10% to 13% of patients with cardiac arrest and out-of-hospital ventricular tachycardia or ventricular fibrillation who are given emergency care are discharged from the hospital alive [9]. Because survival rates are so poor in patients with out-of-hospital cardiac arrest caused by ventricular fibrillation or VT-S, physicians should determine who is at greatest risk for these arrhythmias in order to prevent the first episode and decrease sudden death.

Recently, the automatic external defibrillator (AED) has been introduced. This device can be applied by first responders or lay people and automatically directs and delivers therapy, such as defibrillation for ventricular fibrillation. Experience with this therapy in casinos, in airports, and on board airliners has been extremely encouraging. It is expected that this technology will be applied more widely in the future [10].

Causes of Sudden Cardiac Death

Heart Disease

Sudden cardiac death because of ventricular fibrillation occurs most commonly in patients with heart disease. By far, coronary artery disease is the most common condition associated with sudden cardiac death [11,12], and it is important to identify whether cardiac arrest occurred at the time of acute myocardial infarction (MI) (Fig. 2). Cobb *et al.* [13] reported a 1-year mortality rate of 2% in patients with an acute MI at the time of cardiac arrest compared with 22% in patients without acute MI. Coronary artery spasm can cause ventricular fibrillation, but it has been documented as the cause of cardiac arrest in only a small percentage of patients [14].

Some patients with hypertrophic or dilated cardiomyopathy as well as those with certain forms of congenital heart disease (*eg*, postoperative tetralogy of Fallot) also can be at risk for sudden cardiac death [15]. There is sometimes a familial pattern of sudden cardiac death, especially in certain idiopathic dilated cardiomyopathies or in hypertrophic cardiomyopathy.

Electrophysiologic Abnormalities

Patients with the Wolff-Parkinson-White (WPW) syndrome rarely have cardiac arrest [16]. The most common form of tachycardia in this syndrome is paroxysmal supraventricular tachycardia, which is usually a regular, narrow QRS-complex tachycardia. In some patients, atrial fibrillation may cause a rapid ventricular rate because of conduction from the atrium to the ventricle over the accessory pathway; this can subsequently degenerate into ventricular fibrillation (Fig. 3) [16].

Patients with the idiopathic long-QT syndrome are at risk for syncope and cardiac arrest [17]. Typically, these patients have torsades de pointes, a polymorphic ventricular tachycardia, which can degenerate into ventricular fibrillation. Long-QT syndrome has a strong familial pattern, with autosomal dominant and recessive modes of inheritance. The hallmark is a prolonged QT interval and T-wave abnormalities, although this is not present in every electrocardiogram. Therapy can usually prevent cardiac arrest. It is important to make an accurate diagnosis and to evaluate other family members who may be at risk.

Infrequently, patients with no evidence of structural heart disease can have ventricular fibrillation. In a recent series of 19 patients with idiopathic ventricular fibrillation, six had a history of syncope and two had presyncope before cardiac arrest [18]. However, ventricular tachyarrhythmias are an uncommon cause for syncope in patients with no identifiable structural heart disease. Thus, it is not advisable to pursue aggressively this cause for syncope in most patients, unless a strong suspicion exists for the presence of ventricular tachycardia.

In 1992 [19], a group of patients with syncope, cardiac arrest, or both but no documented heart disease was characterized by a peculiar pattern on the resting ECG: ST-segment elevation in leads V_1 to V_3 and a right bundle branch morphology in lead V_1 (Fig. 4). This pattern is now

TABLE 1 COMMON CAUSES OF CARDIAC ARREST
Heart disease
Coronary artery disease
Cardiomyopathy
Congenital heart disease
Electrophysiologic abnormalities
Wolff-Parkinson-White syndrome
Long-QT syndrome
Idiopathic ventricular fibrillation
Iatrogenic
Proarrhythmia with drugs
Electrolyte derangements

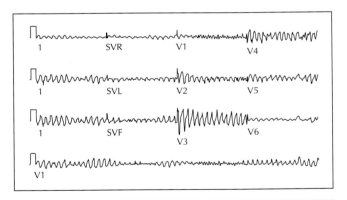

FIGURE 1 Twelve-lead electrocardiogram of ventricular fibrillation recorded during electrophysiologic study of a patient in whom arrhythmia was induced with programmed ventricular stimulation.

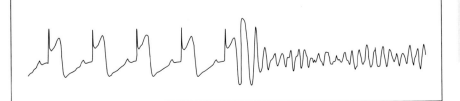

FIGURE 2 Emergence of ventricular fibrillation during the first hour of acute myocardial infarction. (*Adapted from* Prystowsky [22].)

called Brugada syndrome, after the original authors. ECG recordings during symptoms show abrupt onset of rapid polymorphic VT, which can degenerate into VF. Recent genetic studies have linked this disorder to abnormalities of the cardiac sodium channel in some families. This ion channel abnormality leads to an abnormal right ventricular epicardial action potential, which results in an endocardial-to-epicardial transmural voltage gradient. This voltage gradient explains the ST-segment elevation in the anterior chest leads and can set the stage for so-called phase 2 reentry resulting in polymorphic VT or VF [20]. This syndrome is frequently familial, and asymptomatic patients may be identified with routine ECG recordings. If left untreated, patients with this disease have a high risk of recurrent syncope of cardiac arrest. After initial diagnosis, the risk of syncope or sudden death is 30% to 40% at 2-year follow-up, regardless of whether the patient presented with symptoms or was asymptomatic [21]. The ECG features can fluctuate or may be seen only after exposure to class Ia, Ic, or III antiarrhythmic drugs. This latter feature appears to confer a lower risk for SCD. Currently only the implantable cardioverter defibrillator (ICD) has been successful in preventing sudden death in this otherwise healthy but high-risk patient population. Thus, the recognition of this syndrome and screening of family members are of the utmost importance.

Iatrogenic Causes

Aggressive diuresis with subsequent marked hypokalemia can lead to cardiac arrest because of ventricular fibrillation. A more common iatrogenic cause of cardiac arrest is proarrhythmia resulting from drug use, especially antiarrhythmic drugs. Several types of ventricular proarrhythmias exist, including drug-associated ventricular fibrillation, new-onset VT-S, incessant ventricular tachycardia, and torsades de pointes. Patients with depressed left ventricular function and those with a history of VT-S are more likely to develop proarrhythmia during antiarrhythmic drug treatment.

An example of torsades de pointes ventricular proarrhythmia is shown in Figure 5. This patient had heart disease and atrial fibrillation. Intravenous procainamide failed to terminate atrial fibrillation, and electrical cardioversion restored sinus rhythm. The QT interval was markedly prolonged immediately after cardioversion. Approximately 10 minutes later, the patient developed torsades de pointes and required resuscitative efforts. Because ventricular proarrhythmia often occurs during the first few days of therapy, we recommend starting antiarrhythmic drugs in-hospital under heart rhythm monitoring for patients with heart disease.

APPROACH TO SURVIVORS OF CARDIAC ARREST

Evaluation

Survivors of cardiac arrest should undergo a complete history and physical examination. The history may reveal data suggesting a long-term problem with cardiac dysfunction, such as exertional shortness of breath. Alternatively, the patient may relate a history of chest pain that has increased in severity over several weeks before cardiac arrest. In our experience, patients almost always have some degree of retrograde amnesia when they awaken after cardiac arrest. This usually precludes any useful information regarding events that immediately preceded the cardiac arrest, unless an observer can provide these data. It should be ascertained

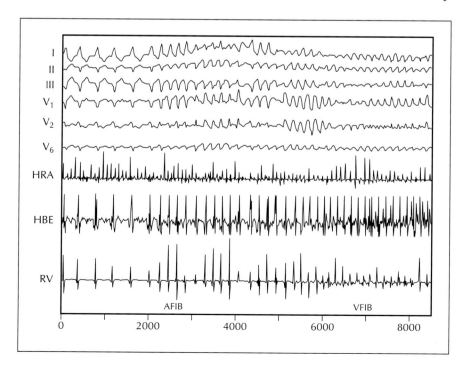

FIGURE 3 Atrial fibrillation (AFIB) initiated during electrophysiologic study of a patient with anterograde conduction over the accessory pathway. Simultaneous tracings are from electrocardiographic leads I, II, III, V_1, V_2, and V_6 as well as from intracardiac leads in the high right atrium (HRA), His bundle area (HBE), and right ventricle (RV). Atrial fibrillation is evidenced by the rapid, irregular rhythm recorded on the HRA lead. At the left, the wide, grossly irregular QRS complexes are caused by conduction over the accessory pathway. At the right, ventricular fibrillation (VFIB) has occurred. (*Adapted from* Prystowsky *et al.* [23].)

whether the patient took any new prescription or over-the-counter drugs. Some aggressive diets (*eg*, liquid protein diets) can lead to marked abnormalities in electrolytes and development of ventricular tachyarrhythmias. When appropriate, one should investigate and screen for use of illicit drugs, especially cocaine.

Physical examination may reveal the presence of atherosclerosis, detected by findings of peripheral vascular disease such as a decreased arterial pulse or the presence of xanthomas or xanthelasma. Cardiac examination may disclose a ventricular (S_3) or atrial gallop (S_4), suggesting the possibility of systolic or diastolic dysfunction. Significant cardiac murmurs may be heard, and evidence for systemic diseases (*eg*, thyrotoxicosis) that affect the heart also may be present.

Extensive laboratory investigation is required. Serial cardiac enzymes and electrocardiograms are necessary to diagnose an acute myocardial infarction. The electrocardiogram also may uncover the long-QT syndrome, a previous MI, nonspecific findings that suggest cardiomyopathy, or the presence of ventricular preexcitation. Serum electrolyte testing may diagnose severe hypokalemia. Other blood tests are usually unrevealing but are occasionally helpful; for example, a substantially elevated erythrocyte sedimentation rate may suggest acute myocarditis or vasculitis.

Echocardiography is a requisite part of the work-up. Myocardial size and function as well as valvular abnormalities are easily evaluated with this technique. Cardiac catheterization should be performed in all patients unless the cause of cardiac arrest is obvious, *eg*, an acute MI [24•]. Treadmill exercise testing may be useful in patients with suspected coronary artery disease to evaluate functional status or in those who had cardiac arrest during exertion. In my

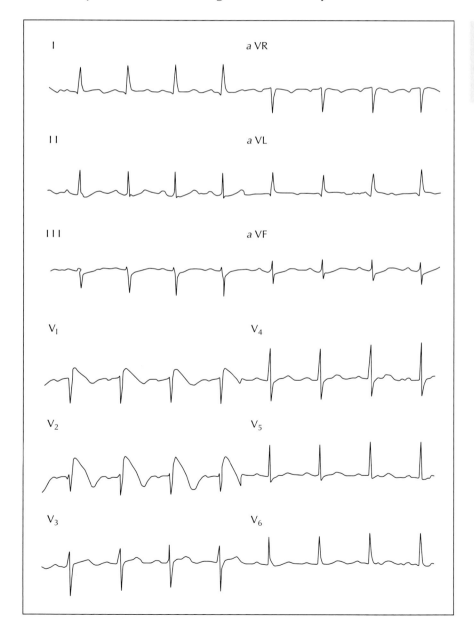

FIGURE 4 The Brugada syndrome. A peculiar pattern on the resting electrocardiogram: ST-segment elevation in leads V_1 to V_3 and a right bundle branch morphology in lead V_1 [19].

experience, VT-S rarely emerges during the exercise test in patients who are referred for cardiac arrest [25].

A complete electrophysiologic evaluation should be done for patients in whom an unequivocal precipitating cause of cardiac arrest has not been identified. Atrial pacing tests sinus node function and atrioventricular (AV) conduction, as well as evaluates the inducibility of supraventricular tachycardia. Most importantly, pacing the ventricle with introduction of premature beats may initiate VT-S or ventricular fibrillation [26] (Fig. 6). Sustained monomorphic ventricular tachycardia is induced more commonly in patients with coronary artery disease compared with other forms of heart disease or idiopathic ventricular fibrillation [21]. In a review of 1233 survivors of cardiac arrest who underwent electrophysiologic evaluation, 42% had sustained monomorphic ventricular tachycardia initiated, whereas 16% had sustained polymorphic ventricular tachycardia or ventricular fibrillation induced [26].

Treatment

An approach to therapy is summarized in Figure 7. Patients with a clearly reversible etiology for cardiac arrest are given specific therapy for that condition. An example is routine post-MI care for patients with ventricular fibrillation that occurred within the first 48 hours after MI. Most patients do not have an obvious cause for the cardiac arrest, and treatment depends on the type of heart disease present. The overwhelming majority of patients have either coronary artery disease or cardiomyopathy. Data are sparse on patients with idiopathic ventricular fibrillation, however, but early defibrillator implantation should be considered in these cases [18]. The accessory pathway should be ablated in cardiac arrest survivors with Wolff-Parkinson-White syndrome and rapid preexcited ventricular rates during atrial fibrillation induced at electrophysiologic study [24•]. This is accomplished with endocardial catheter ablation techniques.

Recently two randomized, multicenter clinical trials have clarified the role of the ICD versus antiarrhythmic drug therapy (predominantly amiodarone) in patients with high-risk ventricular arryhthmias. The AVID (Antiarrhythmics Versus Implantable Defibrillators) trial [27•] enrolled 1013 patients after sustained VF or sudden death as well as patients with sustained VT associated with syncope or poor LV function (EF<40%) to therapy with an ICD or empirical amiodarone. After a 3-year follow-up, the total mortality (primary endpoint) was reduced from 74% in patients randomized to amiodarone to 64% in patients randomized to the ICD (P<0.02), resulting in a statistically significant and clinically relevant relative risk reduction of 35%, 27%, and 30% at 1, 2, and 3 years' follow-up, respectively. A similar study, CIDS (Canadian Implantable Defibrillator Study; n=659) [28•] produced a qualitatively similar, though statistically borderline, result (20% reduction of total mortality; 33% reduction of arrhythmic mortality). Post-hock analyses [29,30] of these two trials suggest that the ICD survival benefit is limited to patients with severe left ventricular dysfunction (ejection fraction [EF] <35%) and advanced heart failure.

Thus, in patients resuscitated from potentially life-threatening ventricular arrhythmias, the ICD has been shown to improve survival and should be considered as the therapy of first choice. In addition, the underlying cardiac disease process requires comprehensive therapy such as coronary artery bypass surgery if appropriate, aggressive heart failure management, or both. Given the enormous advances in transvenous device implantation, the ICD is usually implanted after bypass surgery, and the use of epicardial patch electrodes has largely been abandoned. The role of electrophysiologic study in these patients is changing from guiding antiarrhythmic drug therapy to assessing the arrhythmic substrate, its response to anti-tachycardia pacing, and evaluation of other (mainly supraventricular) tachycardia substrates. Although some omit an electrophysiologic study altogether, citing the inevitable ICD therapy,

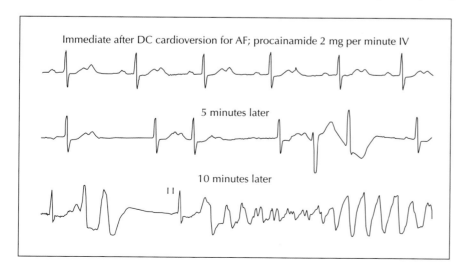

FIGURE 5 Development of torsades de pointes ventricular proarrhythmia in a patient treated with procainamide for atrial fibrillation (AF). DC—direct current; IV—intravenous. (Adapted from Prystowsky and Klein [24•].)

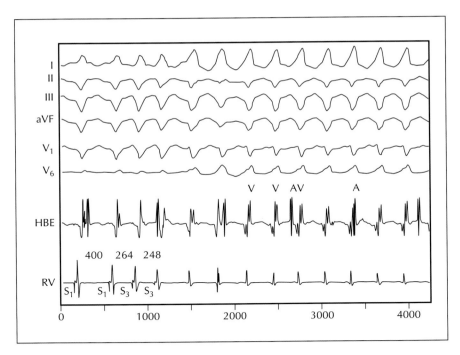

FIGURE 6 Initiation of sustained rapid ventricular tachycardia during programmed ventricular stimulation. Simultaneous tracings are electrocardiogram leads I, II, III, aVF, V₁, V₆, and intracardiac electrograms from the His bundle (HBE) and right ventricle (RV). The RV is paced at cycle length 400 msec (150/min) for eight beats, and two premature stimuli (S₂, S₃) are introduced with coupling of intervals of 264 and 248 msec, respectively. After the second premature stimulus, sustained ventricular tachycardia occurs and ventriculoatrial dissociation is noted on the HBE lead, with more ventricular (V) than atrial (A) electrograms.

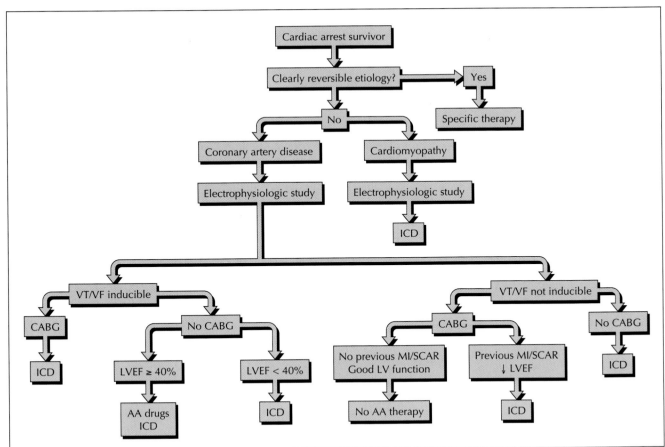

FIGURE 7 Approach to therapy for cardiac arrest survivors. AA—antiarrhythmic; CABG—coronary artery bypass graft surgery; ICD—implantable cardioverter defibrillator; LVEF—left ventricular ejection fraction; MI—myocardial infarction; SCAR— myocardial scar; VF—ventricular fibrillation; VT—sustained ventricular tachycardia.

the authors believe a comprehensive evaluation of these patients should include a complete electrophysiologic study.

PREVENTION OF CARDIAC ARREST

Patients often have symptoms that are possibly related to an arrhythmia. These include palpitations, presyncope, dizziness, and syncope. The aggressiveness of the work-up depends not only on the symptom but also on the underlying cardiac condition; an approach to these patients is demonstrated in Figure 8. Patients without any structural heart disease and no electrocardiographic abnormalities should undergo ambulatory electrocardiographic monitoring, usually with a handheld or loop event recorder, to evaluate palpitations. Syncope or presyncope in patients without heart disease is often caused by neurally mediated syncope, which is best uncovered during tilt-table evaluation. Patients with a prolonged QT interval and potential arrhythmic symptoms should undergo electrocardiographic monitoring to correlate symptoms with an electrocardiographic tracing. Electrophysiologic study is usually not helpful in these individuals; causes other than arrhythmias for dizziness or syncope should be sought. Therapy should be initiated if any suspicion exists that the symptoms relate to a ventricular arrhythmia. β-blockers are the initial treatment of choice.

Patients with WPW syndrome, cardiomyopathy, or coronary artery disease likely have an arrhythmic cause for their symptoms. Presyncope, dizziness, or syncope in these individuals requires electrophysiologic evaluation. If palpitations are present, either a noninvasive or invasive work-up may be done, depending on the characteristics of the palpitations. For example, if the patient relates a rapid, long-lasting episode of palpitations, electrophysiologic study is recommended. Alternatively, a patient may report skipped beats, in which case ambulatory electrocardiographic recordings are the initial recommendation. Therapy is directed by the findings of the work-up. In clinical practice, the infrequency of symptoms and difficulties handling the external recording device may limit the yield of such an approach. Recently, the implantable loop recorder has been introduced. This device, about the size of a pack of chewing gum, is easily implanted subcutaneously in the prepectoral region. The loop monitor can be either activated by the patient (at the time of the symptoms) or activates automatically on detection of programmable bradycardia and tachycardia parameters. Clinical trials with this device have shown a high diagnostic yield in patients with infrequent yet potentially serious conditions [31].

Few patients with out-of-hospital cardiac arrest are resuscitated early enough to allow survival and discharge from the hospital with minimal brain damage. Thus, risk stratification is a reasonable attempt to prevent the first cardiac arrest event in asymptomatic individuals; an approach to risk stratification is shown in Figure 8. The concept of risk stratification is to determine which individuals most closely resemble patients who have already had a cardiac arrest because of VT-S or VF [32]. Factors considered are the arrhythmia, heart disease, and left ventricular dysfunction. Asymptomatic patients without heart disease are at minimal risk for sudden cardiac death. Survivors of cardiac arrest and patients with a history of VT-S are at high risk for sudden cardiac death. Heart disease, often with marked left ventricular dysfunction, is usually present. Individuals having either premature ventricular complexes or nonsustained ventricular tachycardia with variable degrees of heart disease and left ventricular dysfunction are at intermediate risk for sudden cardiac death. This is the group for which risk stratification is suggested. In this intermediate group, the risk for sudden cardiac death increases as left ventricular dysfunction worsens, as shown by the shift from the left to the right in Figure 9. On the righthand side of the column, the patients have similar characteristics to individuals who have already suffered a VT-S or VF.

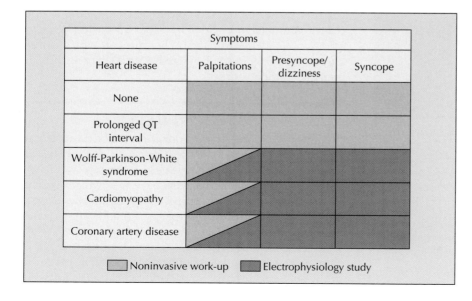

FIGURE 8 Initial work-up of patients with possible arrhythmic symptoms.

The primary prevention of cardiac arrest has been greatly advanced with the completion of three randomized, multicenter clinical trails targeting patients with prior myocardial infarction, reduced left ventricular function (EF <35%), with or without asymptomatic nonsustained VT on a Holter recording [33•,34]. This patient population has an increased risk of sudden death caused by VT or VF. In two trials, electrophysiologic study was used for risk stratification. In the MADIT trial [32] (*n*=196), patients with inducible sustained VT were randomized to ICD versus antiarrhythmic therapy (primarily amiodarone). After an average of 27 months' follow-up, the total mortality was reduced by 54% in patients randomized to the ICD arm (15% vs 38%; *P*=0.009). The MUSTT trial [33•] randomized patients with inducible VT (*n*=704) to either electrophysiologic-guided antiarrhythmic drug therapy (an ICD was implanted if at least one drug failed to suppress VT inducibility) or no antiarrhythmic drug therapy. After a follow-up of 5 years, when compared with the nontreated inducible group, arrhythmic mortality was significantly reduced only in patients treated with the ICD but not the group treated with supposedly "effective" antiarrhythmic drugs (9% vs 37%; *P* < 0.001). In a similar fashion, total mortality was reduced only in the ICD-treated group and not in patients treated with antiarrhythmic drugs (24% vs 55%; *P* < 0.001). Of interest, this study also shed considerable doubt on the utility of electrophysiologic study as a risk-stratifying tool in this patient population. Indeed, in the electrophysiologic study "negative" registry group, the rates of cardiac arrest or death from arrhythmia were considerable [35•]. The MADIT II trial [36••] randomly assigned patients with CAD, prior MI, and low EF (LV EF < 30%) to ICD versus no ICD therapy. Of note, no arrhythmia qualifier or electrophysiologic study was

required. After a mean follow-up of 20 months, the ICD group showed a significantly reduced total mortality (14.2% vs 19.8%; *P* = 0.016).

Thus, at present, patients with coronary artery disease, prior MI, and low ejection fraction (EF < 35%) should be strongly considered for ICD therapy as primary prophylaxis. Whether the same strategy is applicable to patients with underlying dilated cardiomyopathy (DCMP) is unclear, and this patient population remains a clinical challenge. The AMIOVIRT Trial [37] randomly assigned patients (*n* = 103) with a DCMP (EF < 35%) and nonstained VT to ICD therapy or amiodarone therapy. At 1 and 3 years follow-up, survival rates were identical between these groups. Similarly, the CAT trial [38] enrolled patients (*n* = 104) with recently diagnosed (< 9 months) DCMP (EF < 30%) to ICD versus no ICD. After a mean follow-up period of 5.5 years, no difference in mortality was seen.

Although in these two small studies patients did not benefit from ICD therapy, two recent larger trials show data suggesting that patients with DCMP may benefit from an ICD just as do those with an ischemic cardiomyopathy. The DEFINITE trial [39] randomized 458 patients with a DCMP (EF < 35%, nonsustained VT, or frequent premature ventricular contractions on Holter monitoring) to optimal medical therapy with or without ICD. The 2-year total mortality was 14.1% in the non-ICD group versus 7.9% in the ICD group (*P* = 0.08). While not statistically significant, this is indeed an encouraging and clinically important finding. A highly significant reduction in arrhythmic mortality (three versus 14 deaths, *P* = 0.006) was seen in the ICD group.

Reported in meetings only, the SCD-HeFT (Sudden Cardiac Death in Heart Failure) trial enrolled 2521 patients with class II/III heart failure on optimal medication and randomized to amiodarone, ICD, or placebo. One-half of patients had heart failure due to a DCMP. Over a 5-year follow-up, there was no difference in total mortality between placebo-treated and amiodarone-treated patients. However, the ICD group had an important 23% reduction in total mortality. These results were independent of the etiology of heart failure. Thus, patients with a nonischemic cardiomyopathy benefited as well as those with an ischemic cardiomyopathy.

Arrhythmia	PVCs, VT-NS	PVCs / VT-NS		VT-S,VF
Heart disease	Absent	Present		Present
LV dysfunction	Absent	Absent	Present	Present
Potential risks for SCD	Minimal	Intermediate		High

FIGURE 9 Risk stratification to identify patients most likely to have cardiac arrest. The first column (*light*) includes patients with premature ventricular complexes (PVCs) and nonsustained ventricular tachycardia (VT-NS) who have no heart disease. Patients in the far righthand column (*dark*) have a history of sustained ventricular tachycardia (VT-S) or ventricular fibrillation (VF). Risk stratification involves the patients in the middle column (*shaded*). LV—left ventricular; SCD—sudden cardiac death. (*Adapted from* Prystowsky [32].)

WHEN TO REFER

If not treated properly, survivors of cardiac arrest are usually at high risk for a recurrent episode. These individuals should be referred to a clinical electrophysiologist. Patients with long-QT syndrome may be evaluated initially by a cardiologist, but they also may require input from a clinical electrophysiologist, especially if defibrillator therapy is contemplated. Patients with syncope or presyncope who have heart disease or WPW syndrome should be referred to an electrophysiologist. Palpitations thought to be primarily extrasystoles can be evaluated by the primary care physician or cardiologist. If the clinician is concerned about a more serious arrhythmia, the patient should be referred to an electrophysiologist.

REFERENCES AND RECOMMENDED READING

Recently published papers of particular interest have been highlighted as:
- Of interest
- Of outstanding interest

1. Cupples LA, Gagnon DR, Kannel WB: Long- and short-term risk of sudden coronary death. *Circulation* 1992, 85:11–18.

2. Gillum FR: Sudden coronary death in the United States, 1980–1985. *Circulation* 1989, 79:756–765.

3. Prystowsky EN, Heger JJ, Zipes DP: The recognition and treatment of patients at risk for sudden death. In *Cardiac Emergencies*. Edited by Eliot RS, Saenz A, Forker AD. Kisco, NY: Futura Publishing; 1982:353–384.

4. Cobb LA, Werner JA, Trobaugh GB: Sudden cardiac death. I. A decade's experience with out-of-hospital resuscitation. *Mod Concepts Cardiovasc Dis* 1980, 49:31–36.

5. Liberthson RR, Nagel EL, Hirschman JC, Nussenfeld SR: Pre-hospital ventricular defibrillation. Prognosis and follow-up course. *N Engl J Med* 1974, 291:317–321.

6. Myerburg RJ, Conde CA, Sung RJ, *et al.*: Clinical, electrophysiologic and hemodynamic profile of patients resuscitated from pre-hospital cardiac arrest. *Am J Med* 1980, 68:568–576.

7. Luu M, Stevenson WG, Stevenson LW, *et al.*: Diverse mechanisms of unexpected cardiac arrest in advanced heart failure. *Circulation* 1989, 80:1675–1680.

8. Cobb LA, Weaver WD, Fahrenbruch CE, *et al.*: Community-based interventions for sudden cardiac death. Impact, limitations, and changes. *Circulation* 1992, 85(I):98–102.

9. Kellermann AL, Hackman BB, Somes G, Kreth TK: Impact of first-responder defibrillation in an urban emergency medical services system. *JAMA* 1993, 270:1708–1713.

10. Valenzuela TD, Denise JR, Nichol G, *et al.*: Outcome of rapid defibrillation by security officers after cardiac arrest in casinos. *N Engl J Med* 2000, 343:1206–1209.

11. Liberthson RR, Nagel EL, Hirschman JC, *et al.*: Pathophysiologic observations in pre-hospital ventricular fibrillation and sudden cardiac death. *Circulation* 1974, 49:790–798.

12. Reichenbach DD, Moss NS, Meyer E: Pathology of the heart in sudden cardiac death. *Am J Cardiol* 1977, 39:865–872.

13. Cobb LA, Werner JA, Trobaugh GB: Sudden cardiac death. II. Outcome of resuscitation; management, and future directions. *Mod Concepts Cardiovasc Dis* 1980, 49:37–42.

14. Myerburg RJ, Kessler KM, Mallon SM, *et al.*: Life-threatening ventricular arrhythmias in patients with silent myocardial ischemia due to coronary artery spasm. *N Engl J Med* 1992, 326:1451–1455.

15. Maron BJ, Roberts WC, Epstein SE: Sudden death in hypertrophic cardiomyopathy: a profile of 78 patients. *Circulation* 1982, 65:1388–1394.

16. Klein GJ, Prystowsky EN, Yee R, *et al.*: Asymptomatic Wolff-Parkinson-White. Should we intervene? *Circulation* 1989, 80:1902–1905.

17. Moss AJ, Robinson J: Clinical features of the idiopathic long QT syndrome. *Circulation* 1992, 85(I):140–144.

18. Wever EFD, Hauer RNW, Oomen A, *et al.*: Unfavorable outcome in patients with primary electrical disease who survived an episode of ventricular fibrillation. *Circulation* 1993, 88:1021–1029.

19. Brugada P, Brugada J: Right bundle-branch block, persistent ST segment elevation and sudden cardiac death: a distinct clinical and electrocardiographic syndrome: a multicenter report. *J Am Coll Cardiol* 1992, 20:1391–1396.

20. Gussak I, Antzelevitch C, Bjerregaard P, *et al.*: The Brugada syndrome: clinical electrophysiologic and genetic aspects. *J Am Coll Cardiol* 1999, 33:5–15.

21. Brugada J, Brugada R, Brugada P: Right-bundle branch block and ST segment elevation in leads VI through V3: a marker for sudden death in patients without demonstrable structural heart disease. *Circulation* 1998, 97:457–460.

22. Prystowsky EN: Tachyarrhythmias: the role of antiarrhythmic drugs in the therapeutic hierarchy. In *Tachycardias: Mechanisms and Management*. Edited by Josephson ME, Wellens HJJ. 1993, 375–389.

23. Prystowsky EN, Knilans TK, Evans JJ: Diagnostic evaluation and treatment strategies for patients at risk for serious cardiac arrhythmias. Part 2: Ventricular tachyarrhythmias and Wolff-Parkinson-White syndrome. *Mod Concepts Cardiovasc Dis* 1991, 60:55–59.

24.• Prystowsky EN, Klein GJ: *Cardiac Arrhythmias: An Integrated Approach for the Clinician*. New York: McGraw-Hill; 1994.

25. Evans JJ, Skale BT, Windle JR, *et al.*: Comparison of ventricular tachycardia induction between exercise and electrophysiologic testing in patients with ventricular tachycardia [abstract]. *Circulation* 1984, 70:423.

26. Knilans TK, Prystowsky EN: Antiarrhythmic drug therapy in the management of cardiac arrest survivors. *Circulation* 1992, 85:118–124.

27.• The Antiarrhythmics Versus Implantable Defibrillators (AVID) Investigators: A comparison of anti-arrhythmic drug therapy with implantable defibrillators in patients resuscitated from near fatal ventricular arrhythmias. *N Engl J Med* 1997, 337:1576–1583.

28.• Connolly SJ, Gent M, Roberts RS, *et al.*: Canadian Implantable Defibrillator Study (CIDS): A randomized trial of the implantable cardioverter defibrillator against amiodarone. *Circulation* 2000, 101:1279–1302.

29. Domanski MJ, Sakseena S, Epstein AE, *et al.*: Relative effectiveness of the implantable cardioverter-defibrillator and antiarrhythmic drugs in patients with varying degrees of left ventricular dysfunction who have survived malignant ventricular arrhythmias. *J Am Coll Cardiol* 1999, 34:1090–1095.

30. Sheldon R, Connolly S, Krahn A, *et al.*: Identification of patients most likely to benefit from implantable cardioverter defibrillator therapy: The Canadian Implantable Defibrillator Study. *Circulation* 2000, 101:1660–1664.

31. Krahn AD, Klein GJ, Yee R, *et al.*: Randomized assessment of syncope trial: conventional diagnostic testing versus a prolonged monitoring strategy. *Circulation* 2001, 104:46–51.

32. Prystowsky EN: Antiarrhythmic therapy for asymptomatic ventricular arrhythmias. *Am J Cardiol* 1988, 61:102A–107A.

33.• Moss AJ, Hall WJ, Cannom DS, *et al.*: Improved survival with an implantable defibrillator in patients with coronary disease at increased risk for ventricular arrhythmias. *N Engl J Med* 1996, 335:1933–1940.

34.• Buxton EA, Lee KL, Fisher JD, *et al.*: A randomized study of the prevention of sudden death in patients with coronary artery disease. *N Engl J Med* 1999, 341:1882–1920.

35.• Buxton AE, Lee KL, DiCarlo L, *et al.*: Electrophysiologic testing to identify patients with coronary artery disease who are at risk for sudden death. *N Engl J Med* 2000, 342:1937–1945.

36.•• Moss AJ, Zareba W, Hall J, *et al.*: Prophylactic implantation of a defibrillator in patients with myocardial infarction and reduced ejection fraction. *N Engl J Med* 2002, 346:877–883.

37. Strickenberger SA, Hummel JD, Bartlett TG, *et al.*: Amiodarone versus implantable cardioverter defibrillator randomized trial in patients with nonischemic dilated cardiomyopathy and asymptomatic nonsustained ventricular tachycardia: AMIOVIRT. *J Am Coll Cardiol* 2003, 41:1707–1712.

38. Bansch D, Antz M, Boczor S, *et al.*: Primary prevention of sudden cardiac death in idiopathic dilated cardiomyopathy. The Cardiomyopathy Trial (CAT). *Circulation* 2002, 105:1453–1458.

39. Kadish A, Dyer A, Daubert JP, *et al.*: Prophylactic defibrillator implantation in patients with nonischemic dilated cardiomyopathy. *N Engl J Med* 2004, 350:2151–2158.

SELECT BIBLIOGRAPHY

Cummins RO, Ornato JP, Thies WH, Pepe PA: Improving survival from sudden cardiac arrest: the "chain of survival" concept. *Circulation* 1991, 83:1832–1847.

Mirowski M, Reid PR, Mower MM, *et al.*: Termination of malignant ventricular arrhythmias with an implanted automatic defibrillator in human beings *N Engl J Med* 1980, 303:322–324.

Maron BJ, Shirani J. Poliac LC, *et al.*: Sudden death in young competitive athletes: clinical, demographic and pathological profiles. *JAMA* 1996, 276:199–204.

Gilman JK, Naccarelli GV: Evaluation and management of sudden death survivors. *J Intensive Care Med* 1997, 12:1–11.

11

Evaluation of the Patient with Edema

Michael H. Humphreys
Joy L. Logan

Key Points

- Edema formation occurs from localized causes such as inflammation or lymphatic or venous obstruction, or in a generalized manner, usually in the setting of cardiac, liver, or renal disease.

- In cardiac and liver disease, edema is the result of sodium retention because of sensed arterial underfilling.

- Nephrotic edema usually results from primary renal sodium retention, usually without any evidence of arterial underfilling.

- The management of generalized edema is directed at the underlying disease as well as at the edema itself.

- General measures useful in the management of generalized edema include restriction of dietary salt intake and administration of diuretics.

- Specific measures such as abdominal paracentesis in patients with cirrhotic ascites may also be useful.

- The therapeutic approach to the treatment of generalized edema should be based on the severity of the edema and the symptoms it causes.

Edema comes from the Greek word for swelling. Rather than being a disease process itself, edema is a reflection of some underlying condition; its management must therefore be placed in the larger context of the management of this condition [1•].

EDEMA FORMATION

Edema is the accumulation of excess extravascular, extracellular fluid. The filtration of plasma, water, and electrolytes occurs across virtually all capillaries in the body. The rate of filtration is determined by the magnitude of the Starling forces, the differences in hydrostatic and oncotic pressures between the capillary lumen and the interstitium, and by the permeability and surface area of the capillary wall. This filtered fluid is returned to the circulation by the lymphatics, so that the overall constancy of plasma volume is maintained. Edema results when the rate of capillary filtration exceeds the rate of lymphatic return. This can occur with a large increase in capillary hydrostatic pressure, with a large reduction in oncotic pressure, or with increased capillary permeability or surface area. Different types of edema can thus be characterized by one or more of these abnormalities; to a limited extent, recognition of the primary abnormality may offer a rationale for specific therapeutic interventions, such as the infusion of hyperoncotic albumin solutions to patients with hypoalbuminemia.

TYPES OF EDEMA

Edema may be classified as localized edema, which is confined to a specific region or extremity of the body, or as generalized edema, which reflects a widespread increase in extracellular fluid. Generalized edema usually has a dependent component; ankle and leg edema may be only mild after overnight recumbency, when the edema fluid has redistributed to the trunk, but it becomes much more noticeable after prolonged standing. Anasarca is generalized edema so severe that it can be detected in nearly all regions of the body by the indentation caused by the pressure of an applied finger (pitting edema).

EVALUATION AND TREATMENT OF THE PATIENT WITH LOCALIZED EDEMA

Localized edema results from a disturbance in the balance of fluid filtration and return that is confined to a localized region or vascular bed. Localized edema is readily recognized: it is restricted to a discrete area of the body, is asymmetric, and may be accompanied by other features such as pigmentary changes, redness, heat, and pain. Causes of localized edema are listed in Figure 1. Inflammatory edema results from localized tissue injury, usually from infection. Signs of inflammation, including erythema, heat, and pain, are present. The tissue edema results from a cytokine-mediated increase in capillary permeability and from hyperemia, which increases the capillary surface area by opening previously nonperfused capillaries. Angioneurotic edema is a special case of inflammatory edema.

Lymphatic obstruction leads to localized edema by blocking the route of return of normally filtered capillary fluid. The mechanism of the edema accumulation relates to an increase in tissue compliance as tissue hydrostatic pressure increases. Lymphatic obstruction typically occurs from tumor blockade or after lymph node dissection or irradiation. Venous obstruction increases capillary hydrostatic

pressure, leading to a rate of capillary filtration that exceeds the rate of lymphatic return. Chronic venous insufficiency in the lower extremities leads to hyperpigmentation and venous stasis ulcers. When thrombophlebitis is the cause of the venous obstruction, the characteristic inflammatory signs of this condition are present.

The recognition of localized edema generally poses no problem for the clinician. For the most part, its management rests with the management of the underlying condition.

EVALUATION OF THE PATIENT WITH GENERALIZED EDEMA

Generalized edema may prove to be more vexing. The major conditions leading to generalized edema are also listed in Figure 1. Unlike localized edema, generalized edema reflects a widespread disturbance in sodium metabolism whereby the kidneys retain sodium, which leads to a positive sodium balance. This is true even in the absence of structural renal disease, as is generally the case in cirrhosis of the liver and congestive heart failure.

The initial evaluation of the patient with generalized edema, like that of the patient with localized edema, is straightforward. The goal at this stage is to define the disease process responsible for the edema formation—the standard database obtained from the history taking, the physical examination, and screening laboratory studies is usually sufficient for this purpose.

Cardiac Edema

Cardiac edema occurs in patients with a history of heart disease; these patients usually have orthopnea, shortness of breath, dyspnea on exertion, and other symptoms of left ventricular failure. Peripheral edema in such patients is accompanied by elevated venous pressure, passive hepatic congestion, hepatojugular reflux, and other signs of right ventricular failure, as well as by cardiac findings of ventricular gallop rhythm; occasional patients with severe chronic lung disease and cor pulmonale exhibit signs of right-sided heart failure alone.

Laboratory studies in patients with cardiac edema should determine whether renal insufficiency coexists with the heart failure. If renal insufficiency, manifested by elevated blood urea nitrogen and serum creatinine concentrations, is present, the clinician must determine if it reflects renal hypoperfusion resulting from severe left ventricular failure or structural renal disease resulting from some related condition (*eg*, hypertensive nephrosclerosis or diabetes) or an unrelated process. Urinalysis is the best way to make this determination. Patients with prerenal azotemia usually have only modest proteinuria (trace to 1+) and a bland urinary sediment, whereas patients with structural renal disease are likely to have higher-grade proteinuria and formed elements (cells, casts, and oval fat bodies) in the sediment. The distinction is important because the management of heart failure in the setting of chronic renal

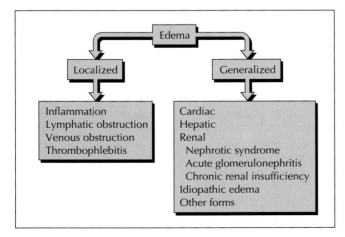

FIGURE 1 Causes of localized and generalized edema.

disease becomes more complicated, and consultation with a nephrologist may be necessary.

The renal and hormonal responses to heart failure are similar to the responses in true hypovolemic situations leading to a low urinary sodium and water excretion. The sympathetic nervous system is activated, antidiuretic hormone is released, and the renin-angiotensin-aldosterone axis is stimulated [1•,2]. Plasma levels of the natriuretic hormone, atrial natriuretic peptide (ANP) and brain natriuretic peptide (BNP), are elevated in heart failure. Myocardial expression of ANP occurs predominantly in the atria and BNP in the ventricles [3]. ANP counterregulates the vasoconstrictor and antinatriuretic actions of the heightened sympathetic and renin-angiotensin-aldosterone systems. The actions of BNP resemble those of ANP, but measurement of circulating levels of BNP has emerged as a potentially useful aid in the diagnosis of congestive heart failure [4].

Hepatic Edema

Generalized edema resulting from chronic liver disease likewise poses few diagnostic difficulties. This edema typically occurs in patients who exhibit signs of chronic liver disease, such as spider angiomata and palmar erythema, and jaundice is often present as well (Table 1).

Most patients with cirrhosis of the liver and moderate to severe ascites have reduced creatinine clearance even if the serum creatinine level is normal. This is because the muscle wasting that accompanies chronic liver disease reduces daily creatinine production so that diminished renal clearance may not be reflected in a rise in the serum concentration [5]. It follows that cirrhotic patients should have their creatinine clearance determined directly if nephrotoxic or renally excreted drugs are prescribed. Functional renal insufficiency in patients with hepatic cirrhosis exists along a continuum of progressive renal hypoperfusion that culminates ultimately in the pattern of functional renal failure called the hepatorenal syndrome; although these patients are universally edematous, management is directed at preserving renal function rather than at treating the edema. Urinalysis findings in uncomplicated cirrhosis with ascites

are indicative of a lack of structural renal disease: proteinuria is minimal, and the sediment is usually bland. However, in jaundiced patients who have bile in the urine, renal epithelial cells can be observed in the urinary sediment. This finding does not indicate tubular toxicity, as it does in other settings.

The pathogenesis of cirrhotic ascites involves arterial vasodilation leading to renal hypoperfusion and activation of the same antinatriuretic systems that occurs in congestive heart failure [1•,2]. Recent studies suggest that increased production of the potent vasodilator nitric oxide may be responsible for the arterial underfilling that results in sodium retention [6•]. Although the treatment of hepatic edema would logically involve interruption of these antinatriuretic systems, this approach has not been very successful in management (see later discussion).

Renal Edema

Generalized edema resulting from intrinsic renal disease occurs in three different settings (Fig. 1). In patients with nephrotic syndrome, edema is one of the hallmarks, as it is in acute glomerulonephritis, in which proteinuria is usually present but may not be of nephrotic magnitude (> 3.5 g/24 h). Finally, edema is often present in patients with chronic renal insufficiency, which usually but not always results from chronic glomerular disease. The mechanisms underlying sodium retention in these conditions may differ, but growing evidence suggests that "nephrotic" sodium retention resulting from hypovolemia and renal hypoperfusion due to reduced serum albumin concentration and plasma volume is actually quite rare. Additionally, evidence suggests that "nephritic" edema arising from primary sodium retention may be a common mechanism in proteinuric renal disease [7•]. Sodium retention in chronic renal insufficiency is a special case of nephritic edema resulting from impaired sodium excretion caused by the renal disease.

The evaluation of the patient with renal edema involves the development of the clinical database from the history taking and physical examination. Clues from the physical examination include the distribution of the edema: whereas cardiac and hepatic edema are dependent, renal edema has a special predilection for facial and periorbital areas, as well as a dependent component. Narrow, pale transverse bands appear in the nail beds of hypoalbuminemic patients (Muehrcke's lines); although these bands are not specific for nephrotic syndrome, they are most prominent in nephrotic patients. Urinalysis invariably reveals the presence of proteinuria (3+ to 4+), and the urine sediment provides clues as to the nature of the underlying renal disease.

Findings of nephrotic syndrome include hyaline casts, oval fat bodies, and lipid; the last can appear in several forms, including free lipid droplets, lipid-laden casts, and cholesterol esters viewed as "Maltese crosses" with the aid of polarizing filters on the microscope stage and eyepiece and often seen in oval fat bodies. Evidence of glomerular

TABLE 1 DIAGNOSIS OF HEPATIC EDEMA
Evidence of chronic liver disease
Spider angiomata
Palmar erythema
Jaundice
Presence of portal hypertension and ascites
Prominent venous pattern on abdominal wall
Esophageal varies
Peripheral edema (usually, but not always, present)

inflammation is indicated by hematuria, particularly if the bulk of the erythrocytes have a characteristic dysmorphic appearance, and erythrocyte casts. Occasionally, glomerulonephritis with a marked exudative component may cause pyuria and leukocyte casts to be present. Chronic renal insufficiency is suggested by broader, waxy casts. The evaluation should also include a 24-hour urine collection for the measurement of creatinine clearance and the quantitation of proteinuria. These data should enable the renal edema to be characterized as belonging to one of these three broad categories. Renal imaging with diagnostic ultrasonography is usually carried out to identify renal size and echodensity: kidneys from patients with acute glomerulonephritis and many forms of nephrotic syndrome are swollen and enlarged and have normal echodensity, whereas kidneys from patients with chronic renal insufficiency are characteristically reduced in size and have increased echodensity.

Table 2 summarizes some of the major characteristics of edema in cardiac, hepatic, and renal disease.

Idiopathic Edema

A fourth form of generalized edema has been termed *idiopathic edema* [8]. This puzzling and controversial entity is observed solely in women, nearly all of whom are of childbearing age. Many of these women view themselves as overweight even when this view is not shared by others, and the condition has been associated with eating disorders. Clinical identification of this entity rests with complaints of edema (usually dependent but also involving the face), abdominal bloating, and in many women, a dependency on diuretics. The patient's description of the severity of the edema often appears exaggerated, and the abdominal bloating is more likely to be related to bowel distention than to ascites. The standard clinical database is adequate to rule out other forms of generalized edema. The pathophysiology of this condition has remained enigmatic, and no agreement exists about the separate roles of the renin-angiotensin system, altered capillary permeability, estrogen and progesterone production, and several other factors that have sometimes been thought to participate in idiopathic edema formation. Many women who complain of this disorder take diuretics, and it has been suggested that edema can be reproduced in susceptible individuals by the combination of diuretic withdrawal and "binge" eating of carbohydrate and sodium after a period of near-fasting [9].

Other Forms of Edema

Other forms of generalized edema occur. These forms, which are usually mild in severity and often warrant no specific treatment, are listed in Table 3.

TREATMENT OF THE PATIENT WITH GENERALIZED EDEMA

In patients with generalized edema, a goal of therapy is often the management of the edema itself, even though edema is only a sign of an underlying condition. This section focuses on some of the measures that have been used in managing generalized edema.

TABLE 2 MAJOR FINDINGS IN THREE FORMS OF EDEMA			
	Cardiac	**Hepatic**	**Renal**
Dependent edema	++++	+++	++
Facial edema	-	-	Present
Ascites	+	++++	+
Hypoalbuminemia	-	++	++++
Proteinuria	0–Trace	0–Trace	++++

TABLE 3 OTHER FORMS OF GENERALIZED EDEMA	
Type	**Comments**
Cyclic edema	Can develop in women of childbearing age just before the monthly menstrual period; is self-limited and does not require treatment other than counseling; can be confused with idiopathic edema
Myxedema	Is the characteristic brawny edema that resists pitting; develops in patients with hypothyroidism
Edema due to the use of vasodilators	Results from sodium retention (with agents such as minoxidil and hydralazine) and may also result from altered capillary permeability (with nifedipine and possibly other calcium channel blockers of the dihydropyridine class); usually requires the addition of a diuretic to the therapeutic regimen
Edema of pregnancy	Is rarely a problem for the general internist, but its treatment often benefits from a nephrology consultation
Capillary leak syndrome	Develops in critically ill patients who are usually septic
Inferior vena cava obstruction	Rarely causes generalized edema
Protein-losing enteropathy	Rarely causes generalized edema

Indications

In the management of edema, as in the management of any other condition, the physician must determine that the benefits of therapy outweigh its risks and complications. In many patients, generalized edema is mild and poses no major difficulty for the patient; in such cases, its management need not be a major therapeutic focus. In other patients, edema is so severe and disabling that it must be addressed as a major target of therapy, particularly if complications directly attributable to the edema itself are present. Table 4 lists some of these complications.

General Measures

Because generalized edema indicates a disturbance in sodium metabolism reflecting an underlying primary disease (usually cardiac, liver, or renal disease), the management of edema must be regarded as only symptomatic therapy, and the physician must direct attention toward the management of the underlying disease itself in an effort to get at the root cause of the edema formation. Often, this requires consultation with the appropriate specialist; a full discussion of this management is beyond the scope of this chapter.

In cardiac failure, the main pharmacologic tools for improving left ventricular function are angiotensin-converting enzyme (ACE) inhibitors and β-blockers [10]. The benefit of ACE inhibitors in this setting reflects the activation of the renin-angiotensin-aldosterone system in heart failure: in addition to exerting favorable effects on preload and afterload, ACE inhibitors improve renal hemodynamics and may thereby potentiate the effect of diuretics in heart failure [11]. Aldosterone blockade with spironolactone or eplerenone also is an important treatment for patients with severe congestive heart failure [10,12]. The benefit effects of these drugs in congestive heart failure are

probably not solely the result of their diuretic and antikaliuretic effects, but may also be due to reduced inflammation, fibrosis, oxidative stress, and platelet aggregation within the cardiovascular system [12].

The management of chronic liver disease offers fewer options, and the major goal of therapy is to stabilize this condition, chiefly by behavioral modification to eliminate alcohol intake in patients with alcoholic cirrhosis. Promising therapies for chronic hepatitis are being developed. The management of nephrotic edema offers a wider array of approaches, including disease-specific interventions such as the administration of glucocorticoids, immunosuppressive agents, and antiplatelet drugs, and nonspecific measures such as a modest restriction of dietary protein intake (0.8 g/kg/24 h) and the use of ACE inhibitors. These latter measures reduce the severity of the proteinuria and may thereby facilitate the management of the edema; they may also arrest or retard the progressive renal insufficiency that accompanies many forms of nephrotic syndrome [13].

In addition to the management of the underlying disease, several other measures have general applicability in the management of edema. Bed rest has long been recognized as an adjunctive treatment of edema, presumably because of the reduction in antinatriuretic stimuli associated with upright posture and, in patients with heart failure, the lowered demand on cardiac output. However, in most cases, it is too impractical to be very useful. Restriction of dietary sodium intake is another measure of general utility in the management of edema. Theoretically, if sodium intake could be reduced to a level below the prevailing rate of sodium excretion, a negative sodium balance would ensue and the edema would clear. In practice, this is usually impossible to achieve. Most patients in the phase of avid sodium retention associated with edema formation excrete less than 10 mEq/d of sodium. Reducing sodium intake to this level can be accomplished only on a metabolic ward with strict supervision of dietary intake. More modest degrees of sodium restriction (30–50 mEq/d, which is equivalent to roughly 1.5–2 g of sodium) can be achieved in the outpatient setting by motivated, compliant patients, and this intake may be adequate to balance excretion in edematous patients with less avid sodium retention. However, in most patients, dietary restriction to this level retards but does not prevent further edema formation, and other measures are necessary to reduce its severity.

Diuretic administration is the mainstay of edema management and is used in virtually all forms of generalized edema. The three groups of diuretics most commonly used in the management of edema are presented in Table 5. In clinical practice, the milder-acting thiazide diuretics are usually the agents of first choice in approaching the management of edema with diuretics. It is rational to initiate therapy in cirrhosis with spironolactone because of the hyperaldosteronism that is usually associated with cirrhotic edema. The effective dose can be determined by monitoring urine sodium and potassium concentrations: when the

TABLE 4 COMPLICATIONS OF EDEMA AND ASCITES

Peripheral edema
Cellulitis
Venous thrombosis
Impaired vision from periorbital edema
Pain
Unacceptable cosmetic impact
Scrotal and penile edema
Limitation of physical activity
Pleural effusions

Ascites
Impaired intestinal absorption
Esophageal reflux
Dyspnea from impaired diaphragmatic excursion
Umbilical or inguinal hernias
Spontaneous bacterial peritonitis

sodium-to-potassium ratio rises above 1, inhibition of aldosterone's tubular action has been achieved [14]. Doses of up to 400 mg/d may be required. Spironolactone has also been shown to be effective in some nephrotic patients [15].

The potassium-sparing diuretics should not be used in patients with moderate to advanced renal insufficiency, nor should potassium supplements be administered with them, in order to reduce the risk of producing potentially serious hyperkalemia. However, the response to diuretic therapy varies from patient to patient depending on the stage of the disease and the pattern of tubular sodium reabsorption. Many patients with moderate to severe edema are unresponsive to thiazides or potassium-sparing agents and require more potent high-ceiling diuretics or combinations of agents acting at different nephron sites [11].

Because the renal sodium retention leading to edema formation may reflect the normal renal compensation to sensed circulatory inadequacy, diuretic therapy can be viewed as a pharmacologic interruption of a normal compensatory response. This contributes to the complications of diuretic administration on the one hand and to "escape" from the action of the diuretics on the other. Resistance to the diuretic's effects can occur for various reasons, including inadequate or ineffective treatment of the primary disease, delayed drug absorption (which may result from edematous gastrointestinal mucosa), and inadequate dosage [16]. However, escape most commonly reflects intravascular volume depletion with a decreased glomerular filtration rate and increased reabsorption of sodium at nephron sites proximal to the site of action of the diuretic.

Excess circulating antidiuretic hormone, aldosterone, or both may also contribute to enhanced tubular reabsorption of sodium and water. If renal plasma flow is sufficiently impaired, an inadequate amount of diuretic may be transported to the tubular cell. An older study indicated that reabsorption of up to 900 mL of ascites per day is possible in patients with liver disease undergoing diuretic treatment without causing an impairment in renal function [17]. Consequently, diuresis of the cirrhotic patient with no peripheral edema should not exceed this rate in order to avoid plasma volume depletion and worsened renal hypoperfusion. In nephrosis, the binding of furosemide by protein in the tubular fluid may interfere with its action; consequently, higher doses may be required [16].

A continuous intravenous infusion of furosemide has been shown to have greater diuretic efficacy and less ototoxicity in patients with severe heart failure than does the same total dose of drug given in intermittent intravenous injections [18]. Resistance to loop diuretics may occur because of hypertrophy of thiazide-sensitive sodium reabsorptive sites that are distal to the site of action of furosemide. Therefore, combination therapy consisting of a loop diuretic such as furosemide and thiazide may help to restore natriuresis in patients who have developed resistance to the loop agent alone [19].

Specific Measures

The plethora of treatments in addition to those outlined previously is testimony to the fact that general measures are not always effective in treating edema. Some of these additional treatments are listed in Table 6. Pleurocentesis and paracentesis can be used for the direct removal of edema fluid accumulated in thoracic and abdominal cavities. If no other treatment is provided at the same time, the fluid usually reaccumulates. The indications for these procedures are related to symptoms caused by them, although small volumes may be removed for diagnostic purposes.

TABLE 5 SELECTED DIURETICS IN THE TREATMENT OF EDEMA

Class	Initial dose, *mg*	Maximum daily dose, *mg*	Duration of action, *h*
Thiazides			
Chlorothiazide	250	1000	6–12
Hydrochlorothiazide	25	100	6–12
Chlorthalidone	25	100	48
Metolazone	2.5	20	12–24
Loop diuretics			
Bumetanide	0.5	10	4–6
Ethacrynic acid	25	200	6–8
Furosemide	20	400	6–8
Torsemide	10	200	12–16
Potassium-sparing agents			
Amiloride	5	20	24
Spironolactone	25	400	48
Triamterene	50	300	6–12

Pleurocentesis should be undertaken when the pleural effusion is large and compromises respiration, either through the sense of dyspnea or through impairment of gas exchange by the compression of lung parenchyma. Paracentesis may be carried out for relief of tense ascites, which can also interfere with respiratory function by limiting diaphragmatic excursion. In the cirrhotic patient, paracentesis may have the added benefit of improving systemic hemodynamics. The elevated intra-abdominal pressure from tense ascites compresses the inferior vena cava and limits venous return to the heart. Removal of as little as 500 mL of ascites is sufficient to obviate this problem and improve cardiac filling pressures and output [20]. In recent years, large-volume paracentesis has gained favor in the management of intractable cirrhotic ascites [20,21]. With careful monitoring and aseptic technique, this approach does not lead to deteriorating renal function, particularly if it is accompanied by the concurrent infusion of albumin. However, because the fluid usually reaccumulates, paracentesis must be repeated periodically.

A number of plasma volume expansion maneuvers have been tried for the management of cirrhotic and nephrotic edema in an effort to correct the renal hypoperfusion state that may characterize these conditions. Plasma and hyperoncotic albumin infusions preferentially expand the plasma compartment while maintaining or increasing plasma oncotic pressure, and they may transiently improve renal

function, even to the point of increasing sodium excretion. Administration of albumin has been shown to modestly potentiate the natriuretic effect of furosemide in patients with nephrotic syndrome [22]. In the case of liver disease, fresh frozen plasma infusions may also provide depleted clotting factors. However, this approach has limited utility in the management of edema. The infusions are expensive, and their effects on renal function are at best transient; moreover, they have no effect on the underlying disease process. In addition, the portal pressure in cirrhotic patients is higher after volume expansion [23], increasing the risk for gastrointestinal bleeding, and the infused protein is rapidly excreted into the urine in nephrotic patients. For these reasons, alternative approaches to volume expansion therapy have been advocated.

In cirrhotic patients, ascitic fluid reinfusion reduces the volume of ascites and restores it to the plasma compartment. This technique has improved renal function and promoted natriuresis in the short term, particularly if it is accompanied by the administration of high-ceiling diuretics. However, this cumbersome procedure, which has a high risk of infection and sepsis, air embolism, and activation of the clotting system, is no longer carried out, particularly because large-volume paracentesis is an acceptable alternative in the management of intractable ascites. A method of chronic ascitic fluid infusion is achieved with the surgical insertion of a peritoneovenous (LeVeen) shunt. Tubing containing a one-way valve is placed with one end in the peritoneal cavity. It is tunneled subcutaneously, and the other end is inserted into the right atrium through the internal jugular vein. Whenever intra-abdominal pressure exceeds right atrial pressure, ascitic fluid is delivered by this route into the bloodstream.

Although the initial, uncontrolled experience with this technique was favorable in the management of intractable ascites, data from controlled studies have not indicated a clear-cut utility of the technique, particularly in view of the high percentage of shunt failure, sepsis, and activation of the clotting cascade. A controlled trial comparing shunting with repeated paracentesis found no differences in the morbidity and survival rates between these two approaches to the management of ascites [24].

Head-out water immersion, in which the patient is immersed to the neck in a tub of thermoindifferent water for 4 or 5 hours, is another form of central blood volume expansion that has been used in treating cirrhotic and nephrotic edema. The water pressure redistributes blood volume from the periphery to the great veins of the thorax, thereby correcting sensed underfilling and reflexly acting on the kidneys to lead to natriuresis. Although the increase in sodium excretion during immersion is impressive, patients revert to their avid sodium-retaining state after they come out of the immersion tub. The benefit is thus only transitory, and no report to date has commented on the use of this technique in the long-term management of edema. Rather, its utility lies in the ability to explore some

TABLE 6 TREATMENT OF EDEMA

General measures
Treatment of the primary disease
Bed rest
Sodium restriction
Diuretic administration

Specific measures
Fluid removal
  Pleurocentesis (heart failure, cirrhosis, nephrosis)
  Paracentesis (heart failure, cirrhosis, nephrosis)
Plasma volume expansion
  Infusion of plasma or hyperoncotic albumin solutions
    (cirrhosis, nephrosis)
  Ascitic fluid reinfusion (cirrhosis)
  Insertion of a peritoneovenous shunt (cirrhosis)
  Head-out water immersion (cirrhosis, nephrosis)
Pharmacologic therapy
  Vasodilators (heart failure)
  Angiotensin-converting enzyme inhibitors (heart failure,
    nephrosis)
  Vasoconstrictors (cirrhosis)
Continuous arteriovenous hemofiltration (heart failure,
  nephrosis)

of the pathophysiologic mechanisms that lead to sodium retention and edema formation in these conditions.

Pharmacologic therapy (in addition to diuretic use) has been used in the management of edema. The agents used include both vasocontrictor and vasodilator compounds, as well as agents to inhibit renin secretion or angiotensin II production. With the notable exception of the use of after-load- and preload-reducing agents in the treatment of congestive heart failure, this approach has resulted in only limited benefit in the management of edema [11].

The technique of continuous arteriovenous hemofiltration affords a means of fluid removal over the short term in patients with congestive heart failure. Extracorporeal circulation is used, and arterial blood pressure provides the force for the ultrafiltration of plasma water through a semipermeable membrane contained in a small cartridge. Ultrafiltration rates can be extremely high with this system. Its major drawback is the requirement for an extracorporeal circuit, but it can be used to assist volume control until other measures improve cardiac function sufficiently to allow the native kidneys to resume their homeostatic function. It has also been advocated in the management of severe nephrotic edema. It is obviously reserved for desperate situations and is carried out, usually in the critical care setting, by an experienced nephrologist.

REFERENCES AND RECOMMENDED READING

Recently published papers of particular interest have been highlighted as:

- • Of interest
- •• Of outstanding interest

1.• Gines P, Humphreys MH, Schrier RW: Edema. In *Textbook of Nephrology*, edn 3. Edited by Massry SG, Glassock RJ. Baltimore: Williams & Wilkins; 1995: 582–589.

2. Schrier RW: Pathogenesis of sodium and water retention in high-output and low-output cardiac failure, nephrotic syndrome, cirrhosis, and pregnancy. *N Engl J Med* 1988, 319:1065–1072, 1127–1134.

3. Humphreys MH: Natriuretic Peptides. In *Textbook of Nephrology*, edn. 4. Edited by Massry SG, Glassock RJ. Philadelphia: Lippincott Williams & Wilkins; 2001:194–200.

4. Shapiro BP, Chen HH, Burnett JC, *et al.*: Use of brain natriuretic peptide concentration to aid in the diagnosis of heart failure. *Mayo Clin Proc* 2003, 78:481–486.

5. Papadakis MA, Arieff AI: Unpredictability of clinical evaluation of renal function in cirrhosis. *Am J Med* 1987, 82:945–952.

6.• Martin P-Y, Schuer RW: Pathogenesis of water and sodium retention in cirhosis. *Kidney Int* 1997, 51:(suppl 59):S-43-S-49.

7.• Humphreys MH: Mechanisms and management of nephrotic edema. *Kidney Int* 1994, 45:266–281.

8. MacGregor GA, de Wardener HE: Idiopathic edema. In *Diseases of the Kidney*, edn 6. Edited by Schrier RW, Gottschalk CW. Boston: Little, Brown; 1997:2343–2351.

9. Macgregor GA, Roulston JE, Markandu ND, *et al.*: Is "idiopathic" oedema idiopathic? *Lancet* 1979, i:397–400.

10. Klein L, O'Connor CM, Gattis WA, *et al.* Pharmacologic therapy for patients with chronic heart failure and reduced systolic function: review of trials and practical considerations. *Am J Cardiol* 2003, 91(suppl):18F–40F.

11. Abraham WT, Schrier RW: Edematous disorders: pathophysiology of renal sodium and water retention and treatment with diuretics. *Curr Opin Nephrol Hypertens* 1993, 2:798–805.

12. Pitt B, Remme W, Zannad F, *et al.*: Eplerenone, a selective aldosterone blocker in patients with left ventricular dysfunction after myocardial Infarction. *N Engl J Med* 2003, 348:1302–1321.

13. Orth SR, Ritz E: The nephrotic syndrome. *N Engl J Med* 1998, 338:1202–1211.

14. Eggert RC: Spironolactone diuresis in patients with cirrhosis and ascites. *Br Med J* 1970, 4:401–403.

15. Shapiro M, Hasbargen J, Hensen J, Schrier RW: Role of aldosterone in the sodium retention of patients with nephrotic syndrome. *Am J Nephrol* 1990, 10:44–48.

16. Brater DC: Resistance to diuretics: mechanisms and clinical implications. *Adv Nephrol* 1993, 22:349–369.

17. Shear L, Ching S, Gabuzda GJ: Compartmentalization of ascites and edema in patients with hepatic cirrhosis. *N Engl J Med* 1970, 282:391–396.

18. Dormans T, van Meuel J, Gerlag P, *et al.*: Diuretic efficacy of high dose furosemide in severe heart failure: bolus injection vs constant infusion. *J Am Coll Cardiol* 1996, 28:376–382.

19. Wood AJ: Diuretic therapy. *N Engl J Med* 1998, 339:387–395.

20. Simon DM, McCain JR, Bonkovsky HL, *et al.*: Effects of therapeutic paracentesis of systemic and hepatic hemodynamics and on renal and hormonal function. *Hepatology* 1987, 7:423–429.

21. Kellerman PS, Linas SL: Large-volume paracentesis in treatment of ascites [editorial]. *Ann Intern Med* 1990, 112:889–891.

22. Fliser D, Zurbrüggen I, Mutschler E, *et al.*: Coadministration of albumin and furosemide in patients with the nephrotic syndrome. *Kidney Int* 1999, 55:629–634.

23. Boyer JL, Chatterjee C, Iber FL, Basu AK: Effect of plasma-volume expansion on portal hypertension. *N Engl J Med* 1966, 275:750–755.

24. Gines P, Arroyo V, Vargas V, *et al.*: Paracentesis with intravenous infusion of albumin as compared with peritoneovenous shunting in cirrhosis with refractory ascites. *N Engl J Med* 1991, 325:829–835.

SELECT BIBLIOGRAPHY

DeSanto NG, Capasso G, Papalia T, De Napoli N: Edema: pathophysiology and therapy. *Kidney Int* 1997, 51(59).

Seldin DW, Giebisch G: *Diuretic Agents: Clinical Physiology and Pharmacology*. Academic Press; 1997.

Seldin DW, Giebisch G, eds.: *The Regulation of Sodium and Chloride Balance*. New York: Raven Press; 1990.

Staub NC, Taylor AE, eds.: *Edema*. New York: Raven Press; 1984.

Risk Factors for and Prevention of Atherosclerotic Cardiovascular Disease

12

Pantel S. Vokonas
William B. Kannel

Key Points

- Atherosclerotic cardiovascular disease (CVD), in all its clinical manifestations, represents the leading cause of disability and mortality throughout much of the industrialized world.
- Epidemiologic studies have identified several important risk factors for CVD including hypertension, hyperlipidemia, cigarette smoking, diabetes, obesity, and physical inactivity.
- Cardiovascular risk is assessed in the outpatient setting using standard clinical procedures and simple laboratory tests followed by appropriate measures to modify relevant factors.
- Information available from intervention studies has already validated the efficacy and safety of preventive management of several risk factors in reducing the toll of CVD in the population.

Atherosclerotic cardiovascular disease (CVD) encompasses a broad spectrum of disease conditions of the heart and circulation that include coronary heart disease (CHD), cerebrovascular disease, and peripheral vascular disease (PVD). Because congestive heart failure often shares antecedents of atherosclerotic and hypertensive heart disease, it is also included under the heading of CVD.

The incidence of almost all cardiovascular events increases dramatically with advancing age (Fig. 1), serving to emphasize the heavy toll of disability and death attributable to CVD throughout life as well as the need for preventive attention for persons of all ages.

Because these conditions represent leading causes of morbidity and mortality in the United States and throughout much of the industrialized world, a working knowledge of risk factors for CVD and potential benefits of their modification on the part of primary care physicians and other health care professionals would make an important contribution to the future clinical and preventive management of this constellation of diseases.

RISK FACTORS FOR CARDIOVASCULAR DISEASE

Evidence from epidemiologic investigations indicates that a number of identifiable factors are associated with enhancement or acceleration of the underlying athero-sclerotic process [1••] and thus, contribute to the development of clinical manifestations of CVD. This represents the central concept of the so-called risk-factor hypothesis, which constitutes the mainstay of modern cardiovascular prevention.

In this context, advanced age and male gender are two of the most important such risk factors; however, both factors are considered irremediable. Attention, therefore, focuses on attributes that can be potentially modified. These factors can be broadly classified in two categories: 1) atherogenic personal traits such as hypertension, hyperlipidemia, and glucose intolerance; or 2) lifestyle influences such as smoking, physical inactivity, and dietary patterns. Several well-established risk factors for CVD are considered in detail below.

Blood Pressure and Hypertension

Although conventional clinical wisdom emphasizes hypertensive risk related to elevations of diastolic blood pressure (diastolic hypertension), evidence from Framingham and other studies indicates an equal if not more potent risk for CVD associated with elevations of systolic blood pressure [2]. This is particularly relevant in older persons in whom progressive vascular stiffening results in significant elevations of systolic blood pressure and high prevalence of isolated systolic hypertension.

Relations between CVD occurrence and systolic and diastolic components of blood pressure are illustrated in Figures 2 and 3, respectively. Absolute risk, based on CVD incidence rates, is usually two to three times higher in older persons at corresponding levels of blood pressure, and tends to be higher in men than in women.

Risk gradients for CVD are generally similar in direction and magnitude when individuals are classified according to hypertensive status instead of absolute levels of blood pressure (Table 1). Overall risk of CVD tends to be two to three times higher in subjects with definite hypertension than in normotensive subjects, whereas risk is intermediate for those patients with mild hypertension. Similar patterns of risk attributable to hypertension have been documented specifically for CHD, stroke, congestive heart failure, and PVD (Table 2). When considered alone, isolated systolic hypertension also confers substantial risk of CVD events.

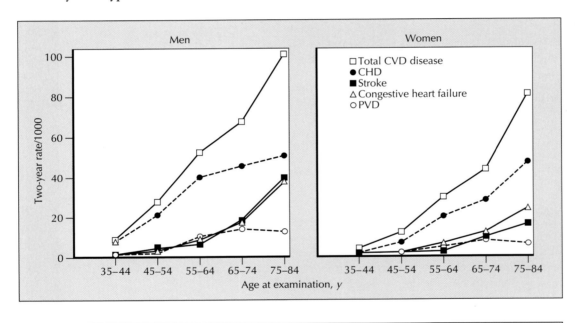

FIGURE 1 Age trends in incidence of total cardiovascular disease (CVD) and component CVD outcomes including coronary heart disease (CHD), stroke, congestive heart failure, and peripheral vascular disease (PVD) for men and women. Framingham Study, 26-year follow-up.

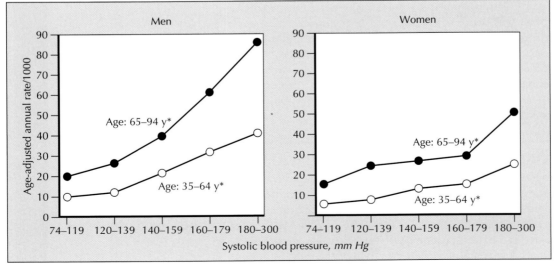

FIGURE 2 Risk of cardiovascular disease by age, sex, and level of systolic blood pressure. Framingham Study, 30-year follow-up. *$P<0.001$ (age-adjusted Wald statistic for logistic regression analysis). (*Adapted from* Vokonas et al. [2].)

Previous data from randomized clinical trials have established a strong case for the efficacy of treating combined elevations of systolic and diastolic blood pressure in hypertensive patients at all ages, although considerable uncertainty remained regarding the treatment of isolated systolic hypertension. The findings of the Systolic Hypertension in the

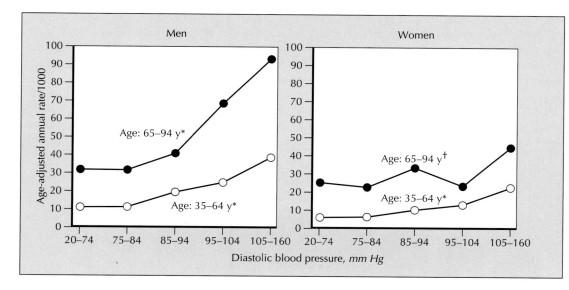

FIGURE 3
Risk of cardiovascular disease by age, sex, and level of diastolic blood pressure. Framingham Study, 30-year follow-up. *P< 0.001, †P< 0.05 (age-adjusted Wald statistic for logistic regression analysis.) *Adapted from Vokonas et al. [2].*

TABLE 1 RISK OF CARDIOVASCULAR DISEASE BY HYPERTENSIVE STATUS ACCORDING TO AGE AND SEX: FRAMINGHAM STUDY, 30-YEAR FOLLOW-UP

Hypertensive status	Average annual age-adjusted rate per 1000, CVD			
	35–64 y*		65–94 y*	
	Men	Women	Men	Women
Normal (<140/90 mm Hg)	11	5	22	19
Mild (140–160/90–95 mm Hg)	20	10	40	26
Definite (>160/95 mm Hg)	31	17	73	35

*All trends significant at P<0.001.
CVD—cardiovascular disease.

TABLE 2 RISK OF CARDIOVASCULAR EVENTS BY HYPERTENSIVE STATUS: FRAMINGHAM STUDY, 30-YEAR FOLLOW-UP

Cardiovascular event	Age-adjusted risk ratio*			
	35–64 y		65–94 y	
	Men	Women	Men	Women
Coronary heart disease	2.6§	3.3§	2.9§	2.0§
Stroke	6.0§	3.0§	3.1§	3.0§
Peripheral vascular disease	2.5§	3.0§	1.50	1.7‡
Congestive heart failure	3.0§	3.0§	3.8§	2.0§
CVD†	2.8§	3.4§	3.3§	1.8§

*Ratio of definite hypertension; normotension; hypertension defined as blood pressure greater than 160/95 mm Hg.
†In persons free of any CVD at the initial visit: ‡P<0.05, §P<0.001, hypertensives versus normotensives.
CVD—cardiovascular disease.

Elderly Program (SHEP) [3] and other studies [4,5,6••], however, have served to dispel much of this uncertainty.

In addition to substantial reductions in cerebrovascular events and congestive heart failure, the majority of such studies performed in older persons to date have consistently demonstrated beneficial trends or significant reductions in CHD events and mortality. Such results appear to be considerably less apparent in clinical therapeutic trials in predominantly middle-aged hypertensive patients [4].

Blood Lipids

Abnormalities of blood lipids represent well-established risk factors for at least two components of CVD, namely CHD and PVD. Regarding CHD, evidence from population studies indicates that overall incidence rates for CHD correlate well with serum total cholesterol levels [7–10]. The character of this relation further suggests that a change in serum cholesterol of 1% corresponds to a directionally similar change in CHD incidence of approximately 2%. Data from the Framingham Study that illustrate this relation for men and women at varying ages are shown in Figures 4 and 5.

Although useful in screening large populations for dyslipidemias, serum cholesterol cannot be considered the sole measure of risk for CHD attributable to serum lipids. This is based on our current understanding of lipoprotein

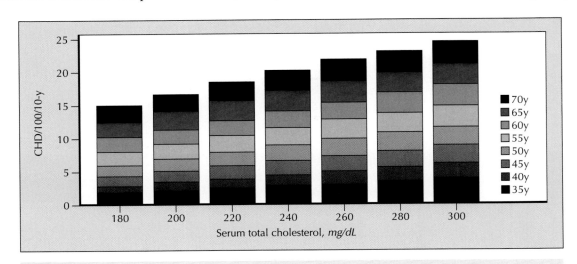

FIGURE 4 Relation of serum cholesterol to coronary heart disease (CHD) in men who have systolic blood pressures of 120 mm Hg or less, no diabetes, no left ventricular hypertrophy as determined by electrocardiogram, no cigarette smoking, and average high-density lipoprotein cholesterol levels at 45 mg/dL. (*Adapted from* Castelli *et al.* [9].)

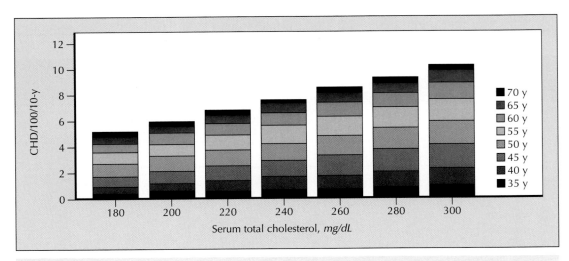

FIGURE 5 Relation of serum cholesterol to coronary heart disease (CHD) in women with systolic blood pressures of 120 mm Hg or less, no diabetes, no left ventricular hypertrophy as determined by electrocardiogram, no cigarette smoking, and average high-density lipoprotein cholesterol levels at 55 mg/dL. (*Adapted from* Castelli *et al.* [9].)

cholesterol subfractions and the availability of standardized laboratory methods to measure them in clinical practice [10]. Serum total cholesterol tends to index low-density-lipoprotein (LDL) cholesterol, which varies directly with CHD risk (Fig. 6) and is considered atherogenic. High-density-lipoprotein (HDL) cholesterol varies inversely with CHD incidence (Fig. 7) and is considered anti-atherogenic or protective. This lipid moiety adds substantial precision in assessing coronary risk at limited additional cost. Construction of a serum cholesterol–to-HDL ratio provides a highly accurate characterization of CHD risk in subjects of the Framingham Study, as illustrated in Figure 8. Indeed, addi-

tional data from Framingham and other studies confirm the overall reliability of the cholesterol/HDL ratio in assessing CHD risk in younger and older persons, and also in men and women. The rationale for this approach is that the ratio reliably captures the effect of a dynamic equilibrium of lipid transport into and out of body tissues, possibly including the intima of blood vessels.

Data from several studies, including the Framingham Study, suggest that serum triglycerides may be important predictors for CHD in men or women, but not consistently in both sexes. Despite these observations, the current consensus holds that elevated levels of serum triglycerides represent a risk marker for obesity, glucose intolerance, and low HDL levels, all of which confer risk for CHD and, to the extent possible, deserve preventive attention [11].

Data from intervention studies using dietary or drug therapy demonstrate the benefit of lipid alteration in reducing risk of initial CHD events [10,12,13••]. Because nearly all such investigations have been conducted in middle-aged men, considerable uncertainty remains regarding the efficacy and safety of such measures in women and in older persons of both sexes [13••]. Information from four large clinical trials, however, makes a compelling case for reducing elevated or even average levels of LDL cholesterol with drugs in patients with established angina pectoris or following myocardial infarction (MI) [14–16,17••]. These effects of drug therapy in the secondary prevention of CHD events, *ie*, in persons with pre-existing CHD, appear to be beneficial irrespective of age in both sexes. Nearly all such recent clinical trials have also demonstrated the benefit of statin drug therapy in reducing the subsequent incidence of stroke events in treated patients [18]. Current management of hyperlipidemia in a person considered to be at risk therefore should consist of a highly individualized approach beginning with appropriate dietary measures and weight control before initiating a trial of specific drug therapy to achieve a carefully monitored lipid-lowering effect. Details regarding the treatment of dyslipidemias appear in Chapter 13.

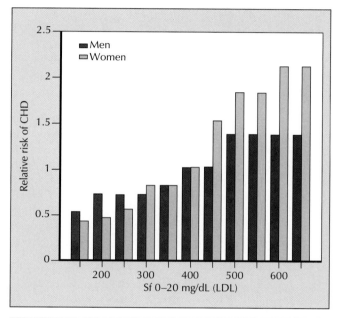

FIGURE 6 Relation of low-density-lipoprotein (LDL) cholesterol to relative risk of coronary heart disease (CHD) occurrence. Framingham Study, 30-year follow-up. (*From* Castelli *et al.* [7].) Sf—Svedberg flotation units.

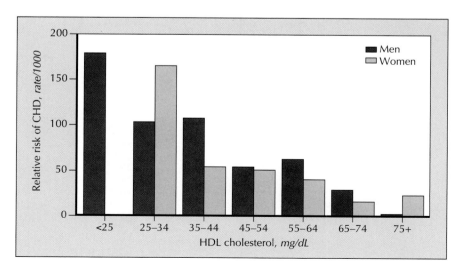

FIGURE 7 Relation of high-density-lipoprotein (HDL) cholesterol to coronary heart disease (CHD) incidence in 4 years. Framingham Study. *Adapted from* Castelli *et al.* [7].)

Cigarette Smoking

Carbon monoxide derived from cigarette smoke reduces the oxygen-carrying capacity of hemoglobin. In addition, nicotine and other substances are known to exert potent effects on vascular smooth muscle and blood platelets, possibly initiating thrombotic events in persons whose circulation has already been compromised by underlying atherosclerosis [19]. Smoking is also suspected of triggering ventricular arrhythmias, resulting in sudden death in vulnerable persons presumably by enhancing sympathetic tone and reducing the threshold to ventricular fibrillation.

Data from Framingham and other studies are quite consistent with the effects of such mechanisms and actually document strong risk associations between cigarette smoking and an array of CVD outcomes including CHD (Fig. 9), stroke, PVD, and death [20,21].

Glucose Tolerance and Diabetes Mellitus

A number of clinical measures are employed in the Framingham Study to identify impaired glucose tolerance, nearly all of which demonstrate significant risk associations with CVD [20]. These measures include blood glucose levels, glycosuria, and the composite risk categories designated as glucose intolerance and diabetes mellitus. Although diabetes mellitus confers enhanced risk in men, overall risk increases dramatically for younger and older women. Similar patterns of risk are noted specifically for CHD, stroke, and PVD as well as coronary

and cardiovascular mortality. Diabetes also emerges as an important risk factor in the development of congestive heart failure, particularly in older women with insulin-dependent diabetes mellitus. Presumably, the microvascular disease unique to diabetes, as well as other mechanisms, serves to produce progressive damage to heart muscle, ultimately resulting in compromised ventricular function and heart failure.

There is limited evidence that control of hyperglycemia by oral hypoglycemic agents or insulin effectively forestalls the development or complications of CVD, although encouraging trends in this regard were identified in the Diabetes Control and Complications Trial [22]. Available information would, therefore, continue to support the concept that there is more to be gained in reducing risk by correcting associated cardiovascular risk factors in persons with diabetes than by attention confined to early detection and control of hyperglycemia [23].

Left Ventricular Hypertrophy

Left ventricular hypertrophy (LVH) as determined by the electrocardiogram emerges as a strong risk factor for CHD in both sexes. Modest increases in CHD incidence are noted for voltage criteria for LVH alone with marked additional risk conferred by definite LVH which, in addition to voltage criteria, includes repolarization (ST and T wave) abnormalities consistent with LVH. These ECG findings presumably reflect derangements of myocardial structure and function related to early compromise of the underlying

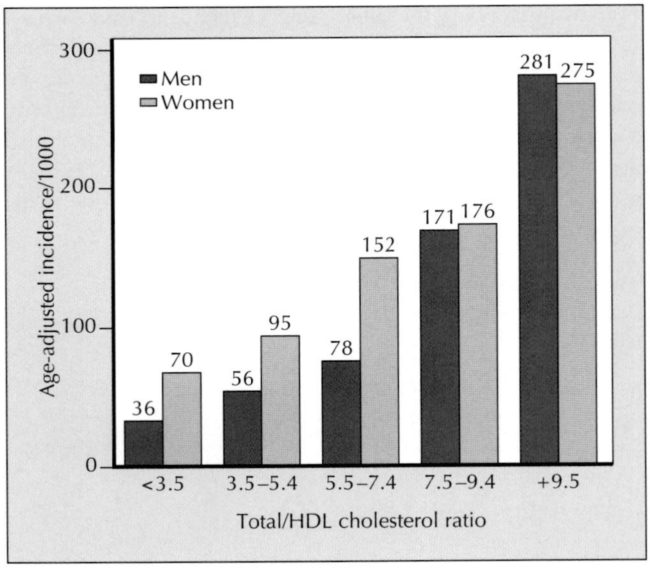

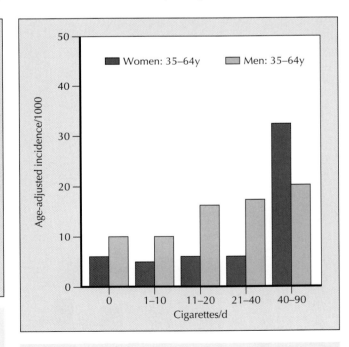

FIGURE 8 Risk of coronary heart disease (CHD) by total to high-density lipoprotein (HDL) cholesterol ratios among men and women 50 to 90 years of age. Framingham Study, 26-year follow-up.

FIGURE 9 Risk of coronary heart disease based on cigarette consumption, age-adjusted incidence rates. Framington Study, 30-year follow-up. (*Adapted from* Cupples and D'Agostino [20].)

coronary circulation that appear before the development of clinical manifestations of CHD [24].

In this context, LVH (LV mass) as determined by cardiac echocardiography has emerged as an extremely potent independent predictor of CHD as well as other CVD events, especially in older persons [25].

Body Weight

Progressive increases in body weight resulting in obesity represent important risk factors for CVD in men and women at all ages. Increases in body weight translate into directionally similar changes in several risk factors considered to be more directly related to the pathogenesis of atherosclerosis than obesity [26]. These include increases in blood pressure, serum cholesterol and triglycerides, and blood glucose. The exception is HDL cholesterol, which varies inversely with body weight. Data from Framingham and other studies, however, document the independent contribution of obesity in the development of CVD and its component outcomes [20,27]. Such observations serve to emphasize the need to incorporate measures ultimately designed to control or, if necessary, to gradually reduce body weight as part of comprehensive risk management. When coupled with appropriate dietary measures, weight control is particularly useful in the initial management of patients with hypertension, dyslipidemia, and diabetes or combinations of these conditions.

Studies also indicate that character of fat distribution is as important as total adiposity in conferring risk for developing CVD. Thus, the pattern of increased abdominal or truncal obesity is often also associated with hypertension, hyperlipidemia, and glucose intolerance, collectively termed the *metabolic syndrome* [28,29]. This constellation of clinical findings is closely related to the phenomenon of insulin resistance that contributes to enhanced CVD risk.

Physical Activity

Accumulating evidence now suggests that lifetime vigorous physical activity may forestall CHD in men, although similar evidence is not yet available for women [30,31]. Previously reported data from the Framingham Study indicating that overall mortality (including coronary mortality) was inversely related to level of physical activity in middle-aged men support these findings. Although a program of regular physical activity coupled with appropriate dietary and weight-control measures should be strongly encouraged for persons of all ages, it would be unwise to place undue emphasis on this approach alone in attempting to reduce the risk for CVD.

Other Risk Factors

Several hematologic or hemostatic factors are described as risk variables in the Framingham Study. Hematocrit appeared to contribute to CVD in middle-aged men and women, but not in older persons [20]. White blood cell count—which is strongly correlated with the number of cigarettes smoked per day, hematocrit, and vital capacity—is also associated with enhanced risk for CVD in men (both smokers and nonsmokers), but only in women smokers [32]. These data are consistent with reports from other studies. Plasma fibrinogen showed strong risk associations for CVD in men similar to findings from other studies [33]. Significant risk associations, however, are not apparent in women.

Elevated blood levels of homocysteine appear to be an independent risk factor for CVD, a finding confirmed in Framingham and other studies [34]. Homocysteine has multiple deleterious effects on vascular endothelium ultimately leading to thrombosis [35]. Factors that may increase homocysteine levels include advancing age, renal insufficiency, vitamin-deficient diets, and drugs that interact with folic acid and vitamins B_6 and B_{12}. Although there is a paucity of data from large controlled clinical trials documenting the benefits of lowering homocysteine on subsequent atherothrombotic events, many clinicians screen for and treat hyperhomocysteinemia in patients with established CVD. Combinations of folic acid and vitamins B_6 and B_{12} are usually employed for therapy.

Inflammatory phenomena are now recognized as playing a central role in the extended pathophysiologic processes resulting in atherosclerosis and its thrombotic complications [1••]. Levels of high-sensitivity C-reactive protein (CRP), a marker of systemic inflammation, represent a strong predictor of both initial and recurrent CHD events [36]. Because drugs such as aspirin and statins can attenuate this inflammatory process, CRP may have an important role in identification and treatment of certain apparently healthy individuals at enhanced risk for CHD (*eg*, patients with normal lipid patterns) for primary prevention. CRP levels can also serve as a clinically useful guide for an array of cardioprotective therapies already validated in the secondary prevention of CVD events in patients with established CHD.

An extensive array of psychosocial, occupational, dietary, and other factors are described as putative risk parameters for CVD in the Framingham Study; however, limited information is available regarding specific associations of these factors with CVD in young or older persons. A report characterized the independent contribution of parental history as a risk factor for CHD in the Framingham Study [37].

CARDIOVASCULAR RISK PROFILES

Although associations between a specific risk factor and CVD can be considered in isolation as a single relation, in many instances combinations of several risk factors may constitute the observed risk profile. In such instances, risk of CVD can be reliably estimated by synthesizing a number of

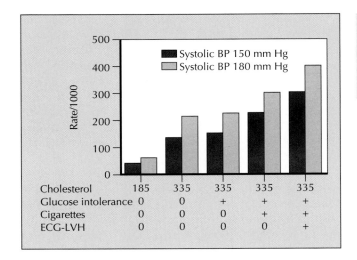

Figure 10 Risk of coronary heart disease in 8 years at systolic blood pressures (BPs) of 150 and 180 mm Hg according to the intensity of other factors, men 45 years of age. Framingham Study, 26-year follow-up. ECG-LVH—left ventricular hypertrophy as determined by electrocardiogram.

risk factors into a composite score, based on a multiple logistic function [38]. Risk factors are assessed by standard clinical procedures (smoking history, blood pressure, and ECG) and by routine laboratory studies (serum total cholesterol, HDL cholesterol, and blood glucose). This type of composite index permits detection of individuals at relatively high risk on the basis of marked elevation of a single factor or because of marginal abnormalities of several risk factors.

This multivariate risk scenario is illustrated in Figure 10, which characterizes the risk of CHD at two predefined levels of systolic blood pressure and then considers changes in the levels or values of other risk factors toward worsening risk. Note that CHD incidence increases progressively with the additional impact of other risk factors for both categories of blood pressure.

Specially prepared charts incorporating this multivariate approach can be used to assess risk in the clinical setting; Figures 11 and 12 are used to predict the probability of CHD [39].

PERSPECTIVES FOR PRIMARY PREVENTION OF CARDIOVASCULAR DISEASE

Effective prevention of a specific disease or cluster of diseases such as CVD often requires two basic approaches, and primary care physicians can play important roles in implementing both. The first approach focuses on individuals identified to be at risk for CVD. These persons usually require additional assessment of risk factors, extensive counseling, and the initiation of appropriate measures to reduce the probability of CVD outcomes. Continued medical surveillance is necessary to maintain long-term control of operative risk factors. The objective is to delay or prevent the development of disease in that individual.

The second approach addresses a defined population. In this approach, community-based screening programs focusing on risk factors such as hypertension or hyperlipidemia are used to identify susceptible persons for individualized

medical attention. Public education efforts and other techniques are employed to curb cigarette smoking and to encourage less atherogenic diets, regular exercise, and other beneficial measures. The objective with this approach is to shift the overall distribution of risk factors to one favoring a lower rate of occurrence of CVD in the population.

Such considerations are more relevant today than ever before. Recently, a marked and progressive decline in mortality due to CHD and CVD has occurred in the United States and several other industrialized nations. Age-specific trends indicate decreasing mortality due to CVD, including CHD and stroke, across the entire age span. Similar trends in cardiovascular mortality have been identified in the Framingham population [40]. At the same time, the prevalence of several CVD risk factors such as untreated hypertension, elevated serum cholesterol levels, and cigarette smoking has diminished in the general population, while impressive improvements have occurred in the diagnosis and treatment of CVD. Although the available information supports the contention that both of these potentially beneficial effects have contributed to the observed decline in mortality from CVD, the current consensus gives greater weight to the success of widespread primary preventive strategies, resulting in lowered levels of major risk factors that contribute to disease, rather than to improved diagnosis and treatment of established disease [41].

ACKNOWLEDGMENT

The authors thank Ms. Claire Chisholm for her invaluable assistance in preparing this manuscript. This work was supported by the Cooperative Studies Program/ERIC of the Department of Veterans Affairs, the Massachusetts Veterans Epidemiology Research and Information Center (MAVERIC), the Visiting Scientist Program of the Framingham Heart Study and grant nos. N01-HV-92922, N01-HV52971, and 5T32-HL-07374-13 of the National Institutes of Health.

CHD Score Sheet for Men

(sum from steps 1-6)

Step 1

Age		
Years	LDL pts	Chol pts
30–35	1	[-1]
35–39	0	[0]
40–44	1	[1]
45–49	2	[2]
50–54	3	[3]
55–59	4	[4]
60–64	5	[5]
65–69	6	[6]
70–74	7	[7]

Step 2

LDL-C		
(mg/dL)	(mmol/L)	LDL pts
<100	<2.59	-3
100–129	2.60–3.36	0
130–159	3.37–4.14	0
160–190	4.15–4.92	1
≥190	≥4.92	2

Cholesterol		
(mg/dL)	(mmol/L)	Chol pts
<160	<4.14	[-3]
160–199	4.15–5.17	[0]
200–239	5.18–6.21	[1]
240–279	6.22–7.24	[2]
≥280	≥7.25	[3]

Step 3

HDL-C			
(mg/dL)	(mmol/L)	LDL pts	Chol pts
<35	<0.09	2	[2]
35–44	0.91–1.16	1	[1]
45–49	1.17–1.29	0	[0]
50–59	1.30–1.55	0	[0]
≥60	≥1.56	-1	[-2]

Step 4

Blood pressure					
Systolic (mm Hg)	Diastolic (mm Hg)				
	<80	80–84	85–89	90–99	≥100
<120	10 [0] pts				
120–129		0 [0] pts			
130–139			1 [1] pts		
140–159				2 [2] pts	
≥160					3 [3] pts

Note: When systolic and diastolic pressures provide different estimates for point scores, use the higher number.

Step 5

Diabetes		
	LDL pts	Chol pts
No	0	[0]
Yes	2	[2]

Step 6

Smoker		
	LDL pts	Chol pts
No	0	[0]
Yes	2	[2]

Step 7

Adding up the points	
Age	_____
LDL-C or chol	_____
HDL-C	_____
Blood pressure	_____
Diabetes	_____
Smoker	_____
Point total	_____

Key
Relative risk:
- Very low
- Low
- Moderate
- High
- Very high

(determine CHD risk from point total)

Step 8

CHD risk			
LDL pts total	10-y CHD risk	Chol pts total	10-y CHD risk
>-3	1%		
-2	2%		
-1	3%	[>1]	[2%]
0	4%	[0]	[3%]
1	5%	[1]	[3%]
2	6%	[2]	[4%]
3	7%	[3]	[5%]
4	8%	[4]	[7%]
5	9%	[5]	[8%]
6	10%	[6]	[10%]
7	14%	[7]	[13%]
8	18%	[8]	[16%]
9	22%	[9]	[20%]
10	27%	[10]	[25%]
11	33%	[11]	[31%]
12	40%	[12]	[37%]
13	47%	[13]	[45%]
≥14	≥56%	[≥14]	[≥53%]

(compare to average person your age)

Step 9

Comparative Risk			
Age (years)	Average 10-y CHD risk	Average 10 y hard* CHD risk	Low† 10-y CHD risk
30–34	3%	1%	2%
35–39	5%	4%	3%
40–44	7%	4%	4%
45–49	11%	8%	4%
50–54	14%	10%	6%
55–59	16%	13%	7%
60–64	21%	20%	9%
65–69	25%	22%	11%
70–74	30%	25%	14%

*Hard CHD events exclude angina pectoris.

†Low risk was calculated for a person the same age, optimal blood pressure, LDL-C 100–129 mg/dL or cholesterol 160–199 mg/dL, HDL-C 45 mg/dL for men or 55 mg/dL for women, non-smoker, no diabetes.

Risk estimates were derived from the experience of the Framingham Heart Study, a predominantly Caucasion population in Massachusetts, USA.

FIGURE 11 Coronary heart disease (CHD) score sheet for men. HDL-C—HDL cholesterol; HDL—high density lipoprotein; LDL—low-density lipoprotein; LDL-C—LDL cholesterol.

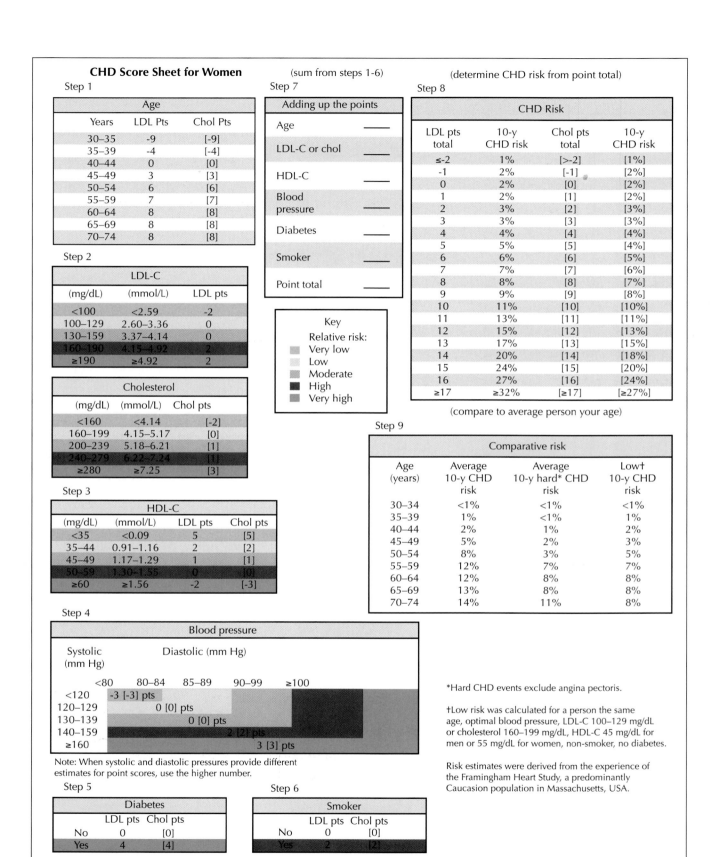

FIGURE 12 Coronary heart disease (CHD) score sheet for women. HDL-C—HDL cholesterol; LDL—low-density lipoprotein; LDL-C— LDL cholesterol.

KEY REFERENCES

Recently published papers of outstanding interest, as identified in *References and Recommended Reading*, have been annotated.

•• Ross R: Atherosclerosis-an inflammatory disease. Review article. Mechanisms of disease. *N Engl J Med* 1999, 340:115-126.

This review highlights the critical role of endothelial dysfunction, leukocyte-endothelial interactions, and coronary risk factors in the early phases of atherogenesis. These events precede the more familiar processes of atherosclerosis described under the "response to injury" hypothesis previously promulgated by Dr. Ross. Based on this constellation of information, the author reconceptualizes atherosclerosis as an inflammatory disease unique to arteries but otherwise analagous to chronic inflammatory conditions in other tissues and organ systems throughout the body.

•• The ALLHAT Officers and Coordinators for the ALLHAT Collaborative Research Group. Major outcomes in high-risk hypertensive patients randomized to angiotensin-converting enzyme inhibitor or calcium channel blocker vs diuretic: the Antihypertensive and Lipid-Lowering Treatment to Prevent Heart Attack Trial (ALLHAT). *JAMA* 2002, 288:2981–2997.

This was a very large, practice-based, randomized clinical trial that compared the effects of a diuretic (chlorthalidone) on CHD morbidity and mortality with three newer antihypertensive drugs: amlodipine, a calcium channel blocker; lisinopril, an angiotensin-converting enzyme inhibitor; and doxazosin, an alpha-adrenergic blocker (discontinued before the end of the trial). A large, ethnically diverse hypertensive population of 33,357 men and women participated in the trial, and 36% had a history of type 2 diabetes mellitus. The 6-year rate for the primary outcome of combined CHD and nonfatal MI was approximately 11% in the three treatment groups. The rate for all-cause mortality was also similar among treatment groups. Several conclusions made by the authors of the study report suggesting that the diuretic chlorthalidone was superior in some respects to the other two antihypertensive drugs—such as in providing protection from subsequent development of congestive heart failure—were widely criticized within the clinical community.

•• Heart Protection Study Collaborative Group: MRC/BHF Heart Protection Study of cholesterol lowering with simvastatin in 20,536 high-risk individuals: a randomised placebo-controlled trial. *Lancet* 2003, 360:7–22.

This large clinical trial randomized 20,536 men and women, ages 40 to 80 years with baseline total cholesterol levels greater than 135 mg/dL and considered to be at high risk for death from CHD (prior MI or other CHD, diabetes, hypertension, or occlusive disease of noncoronary arteries) to either simvastatin (40 mg/d) or placebo. After a 5-year follow-up period, there was a significant reduction in all-cause mortality (13%, $P < 0.001$) in patients randomized to simvastatin compared with placebo. The primary component of this effect was a significant reduction (17%, $P < 0.0001$) in the overall risk of vascular death (CHD and other vascular death). Of interest, there appeared to be similar cardioprotective effects of simvastatin therapy in this patient population across the entire distribution of baseline cholesterol (or LDL cholesterol) levels from high to well below average levels.

REFERENCES AND RECOMMENDED READING

Recently published papers of particular interest have been highlighted as:
•• Of outstanding interest

1.•• Ross R: Atherosclerosis-an inflammatory disease. Review article. Mechanisms of disease. *N Engl J Med* 1999, 340:115-126.

2. Vokonas PS, Kannel WB, Cupples LA: Epidemiology and risk of hypertension in the elderly: the Framingham Study. *J Hypertens* 1988, 8(suppl I):53-59.

3. SHEP Cooperative Research Group:Prevention of stroke by antihypertensive drug treatment in older persons with isolated systolic hypertension: final results of the Systolic Hypertension in the Elderly Program (SHEP). *JAMA* 1991,265:3255-3264.

4. Mulrow CD, Cornell JA, Herrera CR, *et al.*: Hypertension in the elderly: implications and generalizability of randomized trials. *JAMA* 1994, 272:1932-1938.

5. Dahlof B, Devereux R, Kjeldsen SE, *et al.*: Cardiovascular morbidity and mortality in the Losartan Intervention For Endpoint reduction in hypertension study (LIFE): a randomized trial against atenolol. *Lancet* 2002, 359:995–1003.

6.•• The ALLHAT Officers and Coordinators for the ALLHAT Collaborative Research Group: Major outcomes in high-risk hypertensive patients randomized to angiotensin-converting enzyme inhibitor or calcium channel blocker vs diuretic: the Antihypertensive and Lipid-Lowering Treatment to Prevent Heart Attack Trial (ALLHAT). *JAMA* 2002, 288:2981–2997.

7. Castelli WP, Wilson PW, Levy D, Anderson K: Cardiovascular risk factors in the elderly. *Am J Cardiol* 1989, 63:12H-19H.

8. Pikkanen J, Linn S, Heiss G, *et al.*: Ten-year mortality from cardiovascular disease in relation to cholesterol level among men with and without preexisting cardiovascular disease. *N Engl J Med* 1990, 322:1700-1707.

9. Castelli WP, Anderson K, Wilson PWF, *et al.*: Lipids and risk of coronary heart disease. The Framingham Study. *Ann Epidemiol* 1992, 2:23-28.

10. Levine GN, Keaney JF Jr, Vita JA: Cholesterol reduction in cardiovascular disease: clinical benefits and possible mechanisms. *N Engl J Med* 1995, 332:512-519.

11. Rubins HB: Triglycerides and coronary heart disease: implications of recent clinical trials. *J Cardiovasc Risk* 2000, 7:339–345.

12. Shepherd J, Cobbe SM, Ford I, *et al.*: for the West of Scotland Coronary Prevention Study Group:Prevention of coronary heart disease with pravastatin in men with hypercholesterolemia. *N Engl J Med* 1995, 333:1301-1307.

13.•• Downs JR, Clearfield M, Weis I, *et al.*: Primary prevention of acute coronary events with lovastatin in men and women with average cholesterol levels: Results of AFCAPS/Tex CAPS. *JAMA* 1998, 379:1615-1622.

14. Scandinavian Simvastatin Survival Study Group: Randomized trial of cholesterol lowering in 4444 patients with coronary heart disease: The Scandinavian Simvastatin Survival Study (4S). *Lancet* 1994, 344:1383-1389.

15. Sacks FM, Pfeffer MA, Moye LA, *et al.*: for the Cholesterol and Recurrent Events Trial Investigators. The effects of pravastatin on coronary events after myocardial infarction in patients with average cholesterol levels. *N Engl J Med* 1996, 335:1001-1009.

16. The Long-Term Intervention with Pravastatin in Ischemic Disease (LIPID) Study Group: Prevention of cardiovascular events and death with pravastatin in patients with coronary heart disease and a broad range of initial cholesterol levels. *N Engl J Med* 1998, 339:1349-1357.

17.•• Heart Protection Study Collaborative Group: MRC/BHF Heart Protection Study of cholesterol lowering with simvastatin in 20,536 high-risk individuals: a randomised placebo-controlled trial. *Lancet* 2002, 360:7–22.

18. Herbert PR, Gaziano JM, Chan KS, *et al.*: Cholesterol lowering with statin drugs, risk of stroke, and total mortality: an overview of randomized trials. *JAMA* 1997, 278:313-321.

19. Muller JE, Abela GS, Nesto RW, *et al.*: Triggers, acute risk factors and vulnerable plaques: the lexicon of a new frontier. *J Am Coll Cardiol* 1994, 23:809-813.

20. Cupples LA, D'Agostino RB: Some risk factors related to the annual incidence of cardiovascular disease and death using pooled repeated biennial measurements: Framingham Heart Study, a 30-year follow-up. In *The Framingham Study: An Epidemiological Investigation of Cardiovascular Disease.* Edited by Kannel WB, Wolf PA, Garrison RJ: National Heart, Lung and Blood Institute; NIH Publication No.1987:87-2703.

21. Burns DM: Epidemiology of smoking-induced cardiovascular disease. *Prog Cardiovasc Dis* 2003, 46:11-29.

22. Diabetes Control and Complications Trial Research Group: The effect of intensive treatment of diabetes in the development and progression of long-term complications in insulin-dependent diabetes mellitus. *N Engl J Med* 1993, 329:997-986.

23. Gaede P, Vedel P, Larsen N, *et al.*: Multifactorial intervention and cardiovascular disease in patients with type 2 diabetes. *N Engl J Med* 2003, 348:383-393.

24. Levy D, Salomon M, D'Agostino RB, *et al.*: Prognostic implications of baseline electrocardiographic features and their serial changes in subjects with left ventricular hypertrophy. *Circulation* 1994, 90:1786-1793.

25. Levy D, Garrison RJ, Savage DD, *et al.*: Prognostic implications of echocardiographically determined left ventricular mass in the Framingham Heart Study. *N Engl J Med* 1990, 322:1561-1566.

26. Borkan GA, Sparrow D, Wisnieski C, *et al.*: Body weight and coronary risk: patterns of risk factor change associated with long-term weight change. The Normative Aging Study. *Am J Epidemiol* 1986, 124:410-419.

27. Manson JE, Colditz GA, Stampfer MJ, *et al.*: A prospective study of obesity and risk of coronary heart disease in women. *N Engl J Med* 1990, 322:882-889.

28. Haffner SM: Lipoprotein disorders associated with type 2 diabetes mellitus and insulin resistance. *Am J Cardiol* 2002, 90:55i-61i.

29. McLaughlin T, Abbasi F, Cheal K, *et al.*: Simple metabolic markers identify overweight persons who are insulin resistant. *Ann Intern Med* 2003, 139:802-809.

30. Berlin JA, Colditz GA: A meta-analysis of physical activity in the prevention of coronary heart disease. *Am J Epidemiol* 1990, 132:612-628.

31. Paffenbarger RS Jr, Hyde RT, Wing AL, *et al.*: The association of changes in physical activity level and other lifestyle characteristics with mortality among men. *N Engl J Med* 1993, 328:533-537.

32. Kannel WB, Anderson K, Wilson PWF: White blood cell count and cardiovascular disease. *JAMA* 1992, 267:1253-1256.

33. Lowe GD, Rumley A: Fibrinogen and its degradation products as thrombotic risk factors. *Ann NY Acad Sci* 2001, 936:560-565.

34. Bostom AG, Rosenberg IH, Silbershatz H, *et al.*: Nonfasting plasma total homocysteine levels and stroke incidence in elderly persons: the Framingham Study. *Ann Intern Med* 1999, 131:352-355.

35. Haynes WG: Hyperhomocysteinemia, vascular function and atherosclerosis: effects of vitamins. *Cardiovasc Drugs Ther* 2002, 16:391-399.

36. Ridker PM: Clinical application of C-reactive protein for cardiovascular disease detection and prevention. *Circulation* 2003, 107:363-369.

37. Myers RH, Kiely DK, Cupples LA, *et al.*: Parental history is an independent risk factor for coronary artery disease: The Framingham Study. *Am Heart J* 1990, 120:963-969.

38. Chambless LE, Dobson AJ, Patterson CC, *et al.*: On the use of a logistic risk score in predicting risk of coronary heart disease. *Stat Med* 1990, 9:385-396.

39. Wilson PWF, D'Agostino RB, Levy D, *et al.*: Prediction of coronary heart disease using risk factor categories. *Circulation* 1998, 97:1837-1847.

40. Sytkowski PA, Kannel WB, D'Agostino RB: Changes in risk factors and the decline in mortality from cardiovascular disease. The Framingham Heart Study. *N Engl J Med* 1990, 322:1635-1641.

41. Goldman L: Cost-effectiveness perspectives in coronary heart disease. *Am Heart J* 1990, 119:733-739.

SELECT BIBLIOGRAPHY

Adult Treatment Panel III: Executive Summary of the Third Report of the National Cholesterol Education Program (NCEP) Expert Panel on Detection, Evaluation, and Treatment of High Blood Cholesterol in Adults. *JAMA* 2001, 285:2486-2497.

American Heart Association/American College of Cardiology Consensus Panel Statement on Preventive Cardiology for Women. *Circulation* 1999, 99:2480-2484.

Chobanian AV, Bakris GL, Blaock HR, *et al.*: The Seventh Report of the Joint National Committee on Prevention, Evaluation, and Treatment of High Blood Pressure: The JNC 7 Report. *JAMA* 2002, 289:2534-2573.

Gotto AM Jr: Management of dyslipidemia. *Am J Med* 2002, 112(Suppl 8A):10S-18S.

Smith SC Jr, Blair SN, Bonow RD, *et al.*: AHA/ACC guidelines for preventing heart attack and death in patients with atherosclerotic cardiovascular disease:2001 update. *Circulation* 2001, 104:1577-1579.

The Effect of Exercise on the Heart and the Athlete's Heart

13

Barry A. Franklin
J. Norman Patton
Gerald F. Fletcher

Key Points

- The maximal oxygen consumption or aerobic capacity is considered the best single index of cardiorespiratory fitness or conditioning.

- Exercise training reduces the rate-pressure product at any given submaximal work rate; however, the effects of regular exercise on myocardial perfusion, regional wall motion abnormalities, and ejection fraction are less clear but probably beneficial.

- Exercise may benefit the heart by favorably modifying many of the risk factors that are associated with the development of coronary artery disease.

- A low level of aerobic fitness has been shown to be a powerful and independent risk factor for cardiovascular and all-cause mortality.

- Pathophysiologic evidence suggests that the increased myocardial demands of vigorous exercise may precipitate cardiac arrest or acute myocardial infarction in persons with known or occult cardiovascular disease, especially if they are habitually sedentary.

- Endurance-trained athletes often demonstrate enhanced left ventricular dimension and performance, a significantly higher aerobic capacity compared with similarly aged control subjects, and electrocardiographic anomalies that are generally considered normal variants.

Exercise training appears to play an important role in the primary and secondary prevention of coronary artery disease (CAD). The salutary effects of chronic exercise training are well documented. Recent studies also suggest that exercise, when incorporated as part of an intensive multifactorial intervention, can stabilize or even reverse the progression of atherosclerotic CAD [1••,2].

There are, however, limitations to the benefits that exercise offers relative to the prevention and rehabilitation of patients with CAD. Contrary to the speculation of some observers [3], regular exercise training, regardless of the intensity, duration, or both, does not confer "immunity" to CAD [4]. Moreover, recent reports [5–7] suggest that vigorous physical activity may actually trigger cardiovascular events in persons with a diseased or susceptible heart.

This chapter reviews the physiologic effects of endurance exercise on the heart, with specific reference to cardiorespiratory fitness, cardiac function and pathophysiology, coronary risk factors, all-cause mortality, cardiovascular events, and the athlete's cardiovascular system.

CARDIORESPIRATORY FITNESS

Aerobic capacity, which is physiologically defined as the highest rate of oxygen transport and utilization achieved at peak effort, may be expressed in terms of a modification of the Fick equation: $\dot{V}O_2 = HR \times SV \times (CaO_2 - C\bar{v}O_2)$, where

$\dot{V}O_2$ is somatic oxygen consumption in mL per minute, HR is heart rate in beats per minute, SV is stroke volume in mL per beat, and ($CaO_2 - C\bar{v}O_2$) is the arteriovenous (AV) oxygen difference in mL of oxygen per dL of blood. All three increase with exercise but the AV oxygen difference does not improve further with training.

Within physiologic limits, enhanced venous return increases the heart's end-diastolic volume, stretching cardiac muscle fibers and increasing their force of contraction. During exercise there is an increase in ejection fraction resulting from both this increase in end-diastolic volume

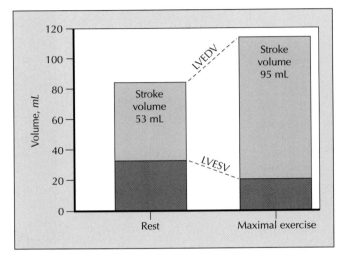

FIGURE 1 Changes in stroke volume from rest to maximal upright exercise are shown in young, healthy men. LVEDV—left ventricular end-diastolic volume; LVESV—left ventricular end-systolic volume. (*Adapted from* Poliner *et al.* [8].)

and a decreased end-systolic volume (Fig. 1) [8]. The latter is due to increased ventricular contractility, secondary to catecholamine-mediated sympathetic stimulation.

Typical circulatory data at rest and during maximal exercise in a healthy sedentary man, a patient with CAD, and a world-class endurance athlete are shown in Table 1. The 10-fold increase in oxygen consumption at maximal exercise ($\dot{V}O_2$max) in the sedentary man is intermediate to the six- and 23-fold increases in the cardiac patient and endurance athlete, respectively. Interindividual variations in aerobic capacity are primarily due to marked differences in maximal cardiac output rather than the peripheral extraction of oxygen. Because there is little variation in maximal systemic arteriovenous oxygen difference with training, $\dot{V}O_2$max virtually defines the pumping capacity of the heart. Therefore, it is of major importance in the evaluation of cardiovascular disease.

Most exercise studies in persons with and without heart disease have demonstrated 10% to 30% increases in preconditioning values of $\dot{V}O_2$max, with the greatest improvements among the most unfit [9•]. The enhancement in $\dot{V}O_2$max is achieved by both central and peripheral, but mainly the latter, adaptations; the latter also provides a distinct hemodynamic advantage at submaximal and maximal exercise (Table 2). Because a given submaximal task or work rate requires a relatively constant aerobic requirement (mL/kg/min), the cardiac patient who has undergone an exercise training program works at a lower percentage of $\dot{V}O_2$max, with greater reserve.

For most deconditioned adults and patients with CAD, the threshold intensity for exercise training probably lies between 40% and 60% $\dot{V}O_2$max; however, considerable evidence suggests that it increases in direct proportion to

TABLE 1 HYPOTHETICAL CIRCULATORY DATA AT REST AND DURING MAXIMAL EXERCISE FOR A SEDENTARY MAN, A PATIENT WITH HEART DISEASE, AND A WORLD-CLASS ENDURANCE ATHLETE

Condition	Oxygen consumption, L/min	mL/kg/min	Cardiac output, L/min	Heart rate, bpm	Stroke volume, mL/beat	Arteriovenous oxygen difference, mL/dL blood
Sedentary man (70 kg)						
Rest	0.25	3.5*	6.1	70	87	4.0
Maximal exercise	2.50	35.0	17.7	190	93	14.0
Cardiac patient (70 kg)						
Rest	0.25	3.5*	6.1	82	74	4.0
Maximal exercise	1.50	21.5	10.4	165	66	13.6
World-class endurance athlete (70 kg)						
Rest	0.25	3.5*	6.1	45	136	4.0
Maximal exercise	5.60	80.0	35.0	190	184	16.0

*3.5 mL/kg/min = 1 metabolic equivalent; average resting metabolic rate expressed per unit body weight.

the pretraining $\dot{V}O_2$max or level of habitual physical activity [10]. The interrelationship among the training intensity, frequency, and duration may permit a low to moderate training intensity to be quite effective through increases in the exercise frequency, duration, or both. Although it is widely believed that aerobic benefits from exercise accrue only from continuous workouts of 30 minutes or more, recent studies have shown similar improvements in cardiorespiratory fitness in subjects who completed three discontinuous 10-minute bouts of moderate exercise on a workout day [11]. Thus, it appears that the improvement in $\dot{V}O_2$max may depend more on the total amount of exercise accomplished or kilocalories expended than on the specific exercise frequency, intensity, or duration.

CARDIAC FUNCTION: PATHOPHYSIOLOGY

The effects of chronic aerobic exercise training on the autonomic nervous system reduce myocardial demands at rest and during exercise, even when low-to-moderate training intensities are used [12]. Vagal tone appears to be increased at rest, whereas sympathoadrenergic drive (circulating catecholamines, particularly norepinephrine) is decreased during exercise [13]. The result is a reduction in the rate-pressure product at any given oxygen uptake or submaximal work rate, especially when the muscle groups used during training are employed (Fig. 2) [14]. Myocardial demand is largely a function of maximal heart rate and blood pressure

---

TABLE 2   MECHANISMS RESPONSIBLE FOR THE INCREASE OF VO₂MAX WITH PHYSICAL CONDITIONING

Central

Increased cardiac output and stroke volume at maximal exercise (predominantly normal patients)

Increased central blood volume and total hemoglobin

Peripheral

Increased size and number of skeletal muscle mitochondria

Increased myoglobin (increased O_2 storage)

Increased oxidative enzymes (*eg*, succinic dehydrogenase, cytochrome oxidase)

Increased skeletal muscle capillary density

The above peripheral mechanisms lead to:

Decreased cardiac output (decreased muscle blood flow) at a given submaximal workload

Increased CaO_2 - CvO_2 at submaximal and maximal work rates

CaO_2 – CvO_2—arteriovenous oxygen difference in mL O_2/dL blood; VO_2max—maximal oxygen consumption.

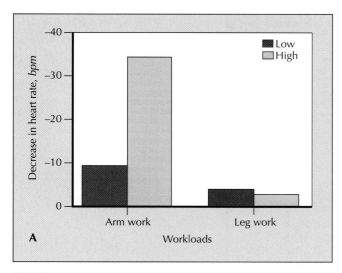

FIGURE 2   **A**, Arm training using a cycle ergometer markedly decreased the heart rate response during arm exercise at low and high workloads, whereas the heart rate reduction during leg work was small. **B**, Similarly, leg training markedly decreased the heart rate during leg work, whereas the heart rate reduction during arm work was minimal. (*Adapted from* Clausen *et al.* [14].)

while $\dot{V}O_2$ is related to heart rate times its stroke volume times $\dot{V}O_2$ difference. Reduced myocardial demands presumably allow the cardiac patient to perform at a higher "symptom-limited" workload before reaching the reproducible rate-pressure product that evokes ischemic ST-segment depression, anginal symptoms (Fig. 3), or both.

The effects of physical conditioning on myocardial perfusion, regional wall motion abnormalities, and ejection fraction are less clear. However, limited data support the benefit of high-intensity exercise training in improving left ventricular (LV) ejection fraction in men with CAD [15•]. Studies describing changes in ventricular arrhythmias following exercise rehabilitation have also produced inconsistent results [1••]. Some investigators have used thallium exercise testing and multiple-gated image acquisition scans on subjects before and after exercise training programs to assess changes in cardiac function. Although the findings have been generally unimpressive, modest improvements have been reported with and without vigorous exercise training regimens [10]. In contrast, angiographic studies in group trials have failed to confirm the appearance of new coronary collateral vessels following exercise training [16]. Today it is widely believed that the proliferation of collaterals often stems, at least in part, from a compromised coronary circulation secondary to the progression of CAD [17].

Improvements, if any, in coronary blood flow may perhaps be related to the conditioning bradycardia or reduced norepinephrine release at submaximal exercise. Because coronary blood flow predominates during diastole, coronary perfusion time is increased (Fig. 4). Thus, decreased heart rate with exercise training appears to play a critical role in patients with ischemic heart disease in view of the potential for increased coronary blood flow and reduced oxygen demands on the myocardium.

Exercise training as a sole intervention does not necessarily halt the progression of CAD or, for that matter, prevent restenosis or reinfarction. However, intensive multifactorial intervention (including exercise) can result in regression or limitation of progression of angiographically documented coronary atherosclerosis [1••]. One study [2], which included a low-fat, low-cholesterol diet (fat < 20% of energy; cholesterol < 200 mg/d) showed that a minimum of 1600 kcal per week of physical activity may halt the progression of CAD, whereas regression may be achieved with an energy expenditure of 2200 kcal per week (Fig. 5). For many patients, these goals would require walking 15 and 20 miles per week, respectively.

CORONARY RISK FACTORS

Regular exercise may indirectly benefit the heart by favorably modifying many of the risk factors that are associated with the development of CAD [9•,10,18••,19•]. Aerobic exercise training can promote modest decreases in body weight, fat stores, blood pressure (particularly in hypertensive patients) [20], total blood cholesterol, serum triglycerides, and low-density lipoprotein (LDL) cholesterol, and increases in the "antiatherogenic" high-density lipoprotein (HDL) cholesterol subfraction. Exercise-mediated reductions in total cholesterol and LDL cholesterol occur primarily when concomitant body weight losses occur [21]. Diabetes mellitus may also be favorably affected by regular physical activity [9•,19•].

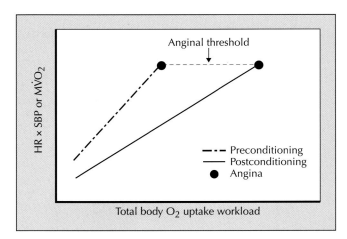

FIGURE 3 Effect of physical conditioning on the heart rate times systolic blood pressure product (HR x SBP) and myocardial oxygen consumption ($M\dot{V}O_2$) at submaximal and peak exercise. Peak body oxygen uptake and workload are augmented by exercise training. Myocardial oxygen requirements are reduced at a given workload or oxygen uptake, but angina occurs at the same HR x SBP product, indicating that the major mechanism of beneficial action of exercise therapy is reduction of $M\dot{V}O_2$ rather than an increased myocardial oxygen supply.

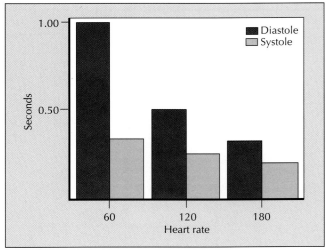

FIGURE 4 Relationship of systolic and diastolic time to heart rate. Since coronary blood flow predominates during diastole, with increased heart rate, as during exercise, diastolic (perfusion) time is disproportionately shortened. Reduction of heart rate at rest and during exercise becomes critical to the prevention of ischemia in patients with coronary artery disease.

FITNESS AND MORTALITY

Recent studies [22,23•,24••,25•,26–28,29•] have shown that a low level of aerobic fitness is an independent risk factor for all-cause mortality. In one investigation [22] researchers prospectively studied 10,224 men and 3120 women who were given a preventive medical examination and a maximal treadmill exercise test to assess their aerobic fitness. Over an average follow-up period of slightly more than 8 years, 240 men and 43 women died. In general, the higher the initial level of fitness, the lower was the subsequent death rate from cancer and heart disease (Fig. 6). This was so even after statistical adjustments were made for age, coronary risk factors, and family history of heart disease. Moreover, there appeared to be no additional benefit (ie, lower mortality) associated with fitness levels higher than 9 to 10 metabolic equivalents (METs). For men, the greatest reduction in risk occurred as one progressed from the lowest level of fitness (≤ 6 METs) to the next lowest level (7 METs), suggesting that even a modest improvement in fitness among the most unfit confers a substantial health benefit. The investigators concluded that the fitness levels associated with a plateau in death rates, 9 to 10 METs, can be attained by most men and women who walk briskly on a regular basis (for example, an 18–20 minute mile pace) [18••,19•,20].

Subsequently, these investigators examined the relationship between changes in aerobic fitness and the risk of death in men [23•]. Participants were 9777 men (20 to 82 years of age) who were given two preventive medical examinations, which included an assessment of aerobic fitness by maximal exercise testing, about 5 years apart. Approximately 5 years after the second examination, deaths from all causes and from cardiovascular disease were determined. The highest death rate occurred in men who were unfit at both examinations (122.0/10,000 man-years); the lowest death rate was in men who were physically fit at both examinations (39.6/10,000 man-years). Men who improved from the *untrained* to the *trained* category between the first and second examinations had an intermediate death rate (67.7/10,000 man-years), even after adjustments were made for age, health status, and other risk factors. For each minute increase in treadmill test time between examinations, there was a corresponding 7.9% decrease in risk of mortality.

A more recent study [24••] reported the relative risk for all-cause mortality for several mortality predictors (Table 3), including low fitness (20% least trained). Untrained men and women were approximately twice as likely to die during an 8-year follow-up period compared with their exercised-trained counterparts. Moreover, the protective effect of training held for smokers and nonsmokers as well as for those

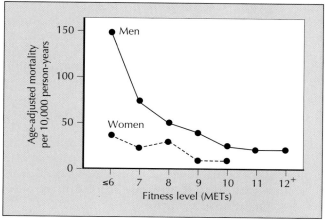

FIGURE 6 Age-adjusted, all-cause mortality rates per 10,000 person-years of follow-up by physical fitness (measured in metabolic equivalents [METs]) achieved during maximal treadmill exercise testing. (*Adapted from* Blair *et al.* [22].)

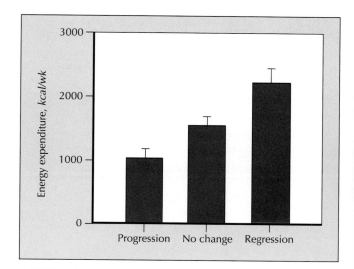

FIGURE 5 Effects of physical activity on coronary morphology in patients with coronary artery disease (CAD). The lowest activity level was noted in patients with progression of CAD (1022 ± 142 kcal/wk) compared with patients with no change (1533 ± 122 kcal/wk) or regression (2204 ± 237 kcal/wk) (*P* < 0.005). (*Adapted from* Hambrecht *et al.* [2].)

TABLE 3 RELATIVE RISK FOR ALL-CAUSE MORTALITY FOR SELECTED MORTALITY PREDICTORS, MEN AND WOMEN, AEROBICS CENTER LONGITUDINAL STUDY, 1970–1989

Mortality predictor	Relative risk*	
	Men	Women
Low fitness (20% less fit)	2.03	2.23
Current or recent cigarette smoker	1.89	2.12
Systolic blood pressure ≥ 140 mm Hg	1.67	0.89
Cholesterol ≥ 240 mg/dL	1.45	1.16
Body mass index ≥ 27 kg/m²	1.33	1.18

*Adjusted for age and examination year.

with and without elevated cholesterol levels or hypertension. In a related analyses [30•], moderate-to-high trained men with a body mass index (BMI) greater than 30 kg/m² had approximately one third the age-adjusted death rate of lean (< 27 BMI) untrained men. Collectively, these findings and other recent reports [25•–27,29•] support the hypothesis that regular physical activity improves health and delays death in persons with and without documented CAD. This effect seems to be especially important in those who exercise more vigorously and achieve higher levels of training capacity as evidenced by greater levels of V̇O₂max [27].

More current studies support the benefits of physical activity and fitness in decreasing morbidity and mortality. Another evaluation [31] of the Harvard alumni study of 7337 men assessed the relative intensity of physical activity and risk of coronary disease. An inverse association between relative intensity of activity (an individual's perceived exertion) and risk of coronary disease was found among men who did not satisfy current activity guidelines. These findings provide encouragement for older persons who may not be willing or physically able to follow current recommendations. In a large study, 9518 white women aged 65 years who increased activity over the 5.7-year study period had lower mortality from all causes [32]. These changes in mortality, however, were weaker among women 75 years or older, and among those with overall poor health status. In the specific area of stroke, a meta-analysis was used to study the relation between physical activity and stroke incidence or mortality [33]. Twenty-three studies (18 cohorts) met inclusion criteria. It was concluded that both moderate and high-level activity are associated with reduced risk of total, ischemic, and hemorrhagic stroke. Therefore, data continues to evolve supporting the many benefits of regular physical activity.

CARDIOVASCULAR EVENTS

Pathophysiologic evidence suggests that the increased myocardial demands of vigorous exercise may precipitate cardiovascular events in persons with known or occult CAD. By increasing myocardial oxygen consumption and simultaneously shortening diastole and coronary perfusion time, exercise may evoke a transient oxygen deficiency in the subendocardial tissue, which may be exacerbated by a decrease in venous return secondary to an abrupt cessation of exercise. In addition to symptomatic or silent myocardial ischemia [34], sodium-potassium imbalance, increased catecholamine excretion, and circulating free fatty acids may all be arrhythmogenic. The additional risk of cardiac arrest during vigorous exercise, compared with that at other times, may be more than 100-fold during or soon after heavy physical exertion [5].

The critical question, however, is whether or not the cardiovascular benefits of regular exercise outweigh the transient, additional risk. The relative risk of cardiac arrest during exercise compared with that at other times is 56 times greater among sedentary men but only 5 times greater among men with high levels of habitual physical activity [35]. However, the total risk of cardiac arrest among habitually active men was only 40% of that for sedentary men. Thus, these findings agree with the hypothesis that vigorous physical activity both protects against but may provoke sudden cardiac death under certain conditions [36].

The notion that strenuous physical exertion can precipitate acute myocardial infarction, particularly in persons who are habitually sedentary (Table 4), has been supported by two recent studies [6,7]. This may occur with abrupt increases in heart rate and blood pressure that disrupt vulnerable atherosclerotic plaque and lead to thrombotic occlusion of a coronary vessel [37]. An increase in platelet activation and hyperreactivity, which could contribute to (or even initiate) coronary thrombosis, has also been reported in inactive subjects but not in physically trained ones who engaged in sporadic high-intensity exercise [38].

THE ATHLETE'S HEART

Certain electrocardiographic findings are common and usually "normal" in athletes or those who are "endurance trained." These include sinus bradycardia (heart rate < 60 bpm), sinus arrhythmia, sinus pauses, first-degree atrioventricular (AV) block, second-degree AV block (Mobitz type I), wandering atrial pacemaker, AV junctional rhythms, incomplete right bundle branch block, rightward QRS axis, ventricular hypertrophy, minor ST segment depression or elevation (early repolarization), and altered T waves [39–41]. The amplitude of the QRS complex may also be at or above the upper limit of normal. Such anomalies in highly trained athletes likely result from changes in sympathetic or parasympathetic tone, increases in LV mass, dimensions, or both, rather than from pathologic alterations in the cardiovascular system. Most atrial and ventricular premature complexes and atrial tachycardias are

TABLE 4 RELATIVE RISK OF EXERTION-RELATED MYOCARDIAL INFARCTION ACCORDING TO THE USUAL FREQUENCY OF STRENUOUS PHYSICAL EXERTION*

Study	Frequency of exertion, times/wk	Relative risk
German [7]	< 4	6.9
	≥ 4	1.3
United States [6]	< 1	107
	1–2	19.4
	3–4	8.6
	≥ 5	2.4

*≥ 6 metabolic equivalents (METs) (1 MET = 3.5 mL O₂/kg/min).

also considered normal variants and are nonspecific for heart disease [42]. However, complex ventricular ectopy, including runs of ventricular tachycardia, may require extensive cardiologic evaluation before medical clearance for athletic participation.

The cardiac profile of individuals who participate regularly in vigorous, isotonic exercise is characterized by LV volume overload with increased LV internal dimension, end-diastolic volume, stroke volume, and myocardial mass [43]. These changes are associated with enhanced LV performance and a significantly higher aerobic capacity compared with similarly aged control subjects. $\dot{V}O_2$max values in national class and championship athletes vary from a high of 94 mL/kg/min, now reported in a cross-country skier, to values between 40 and 45 mL/kg/min for athletes participating in anaerobic-type sports. Although intense physical training may increase the $\dot{V}O_2$max by 25% or more, it has become increasingly apparent that natural endowment (*ie*, genetics or family history) rather than training per se, plays a major role in producing a gold medal winner in an Olympic endurance event [44]. The increase in cardiac mass in athletes may be similar from an imaging perspective to that seen in disease. However, in most cases, diastolic LV function is normal in the athletic heart.

Fortunately, sudden death events in athletes are extremely rare occurrences. The prevalence of athletic-related deaths appears to be about one in 200,000 high school-age athletes and is higher in older athletes [45••,46]. CAD is the most frequent autopsy finding in athletes over the age of 35 years who die during competition or training [47]. In contrast, inherited structural cardiovascular abnormalities, including hypertrophic cardiomyopathy, idiopathic LV hypertrophy, myocardial bridging, and anomalous origin of the left coronary artery, are the major causes of sudden death during exercise in younger athletes [48•].

The primary goal of cardiac preparticipation screening should be to determine whether the athlete has a history of syncope or chest pain. This information can be economically assessed with a questionnaire [49] designed to specifically identify a family history of sudden cardiac death, hypertrophic cardiomyopathy, Marfan's syndrome, or premature CAD. In such cases, additional studies are clinically warranted. Recently, an expert panel appointed by the American Heart Association issued the US's first set of standardized recommendations for the screening of young athletes for potentially fatal cardiovascular disease [50••]. When cardiac abnormalities are diagnosed, physicians should use established guidelines to formulate recommendations for continued participation or disqualification from competitive sports [51•].

ACKNOWLEDGMENT

The authors thank Brenda White and Darlene Gunsolus for their assistance in preparing this manuscript.

KEY REFERENCES

Recently published papers of outstanding interest, as identified in *References and Recommended Reading*, have been annotated.

•• Wenger NK, Froelicher ES, Smith LK, *et al.*: *Clinical Practice: Guideline: Cardiac Rehabilitation.* Rockville, MD: U.S. Department of Health Service, Agency for Health Care Policy and Research and National Heart, Lung, and Blood Institute; 1995.

The definitive reference on the physiologic and psychosocial outomes that are associated with an exercise-based cardiac rehabilitation program.

•• Fletcher GF, Balady GJ, Amsterdam EA, *et al.*: Exercise standards for testing and training: a statement for healthcare professionals from the American Heart Association. *Circulation* 2001, 104:1694-1740.

This document represents a major update on the role of exercise testing and prescription in the primary and secondary prevention of cardiovascular disease.

•• Blair SN, Kampert JB, Kohl HW III, *et al.*: Influences of cardiorespiratory fitness and other precursors on cardiovascular disease and all-cause mortality in men and women. *JAMA* 1996, 276:205-210.

A classic study highlighting the important role of physical inactivity (low aerobic fitness) as a major, independent risk factor for heart disease.

•• Maron BJ, Thompson PD, Puffer JC, *et al.*: Cardiovascular pre-participation screening of competitive athletes. *Circulation* 1996, 94:850-856.

The first definitive US guidelines and recommendations for the appropriate preparticipation screening of competitive athletes.

REFERENCES AND RECOMMENDED READING

Recently published papers of particular interest have been highlighted as:

• Of interest

•• Of outstanding interest

1.•• Wenger NK, Froelicher ES, Smith LK, *et al.*: *Clinical Practice Guideline: Cardiac Rehabilitation.* Rockville, MD: U.S. Department of Health Service, Agency for Health Care Policy and Research and National Heart, Lung, and Blood Institute; 1995.

2. Hambrecht R, Niebauer J, Marburger C, *et al.*: Various intensities of leisure time physical activity in patients with coronary artery disease: effects on cardiorespiratory fitness and progression of coronary atherosclerotic lesions. *J Am Coll Cardiol* 1993, 22:468-477.

3. Bassler TJ: Marathon running and immunity to heart disease. *Physician Sportsmed* 1975, 3:77-80.

4. Noakes TD, Opie LH, Rose AG, *et al.*: Autopsy-proved coronary atherosclerosis in marathon runners. *N Engl J Med* 1979, 301:86-89.

5. Cobb LA, Weaver WD: Exercise: a risk for sudden death in patients with coronary heart disease. *J Am Coll Cardiol* 1986, 7:215-219.

6. Mittleman MA, Maclure M, Tofler GH, *et al.*: Triggering of acute myocardial infarction by heavy physical exertion: protection against triggering by regular exertion. *N Engl J Med* 1993, 329:1677-1683.

7. Willich SN, Lewis M, Löwel H, *et al.*: Physical exertion as a trigger of acute myocardial infarction. *N Engl J Med* 1993, 329:1684-1690.

8. Poliner LR, Dehmer GJ, Lewis SE: Left ventricular performance in normal subjects: a comparison of the responses to exercise in the upright and supine position. *Circulation* 1980, 62:528–534.

9.• Balady GJ, Fletcher BJ, Froelicher ES, *et al.*: Cardiac rehabilitation programs. A statement for healthcare professionals from the American Heart Association. *Circulation* 1994, 90:1602–1610.

10. Franklin BA, Gordon S, Timmis GC: Amount of exercise necessary for the patient with coronary artery disease. *Am J Cardiol* 1992, 69:1426–1431.

11. DeBusk RF, Stenestrand U, Sheehan M, *et al.*: Training effects of long versus short bouts of exercise in healthy subjects. *Am J Cardiol* 1990, 65:1010–1013.

12. Franklin BA, Besseghini I, Golden LH: Low intensity physical conditioning: effects on patients with coronary heart disease. *Arch Phys Med Rehabil* 1978, 59:276–280.

13. Ferguson RJ, Taylor AW, Côté P, *et al.*: Skeletal muscle and cardiac changes with training in patients with angina pectoris. *Am J Physiol* 1982, 24:H830–H836.

14. Clausen JP, Trap-Jensen J, Lassen NA: The effects of training on the heart rate during arm and leg exercise. *Scand J Clin Lab Invest* 1970, 26:295–301.

15.• Oberman A, Fletcher GF, Lee J, *et al.*: Efficacy of high-intensity exercise training on left ventricular ejection fraction in men with coronary artery disease (the training level comparison study). *Am J Cardiol* 1995, 76:643–647.

16. Franklin BA: Exercise training and coronary collateral circulation. *Med Sci Sports Exerc* 1991, 23:648–653.

17. Price SA, Wilson LM. *Pathophysiology: Clinical Concepts of Disease Processes*, edn 6. St. Louis: Mosby; 2003.

18.•• Fletcher GF, Balady GJ, Amsterdam EA, *et al.*: Exercise standards for testing and training: a statement for healthcare professionals from the American Heart Association. *Circulation* 2001, 104:1694–1740.

19.• Thompson PD, Buchner D, Pina IL, *et al.*: Exercise and physical activity in the prevention and treatment of atherosclerotic cardiovascular disease: a statement from the Council on Clinical Cardiology (Subcommittee on Exercise, Rehabilitation, and Prevention) and the Council on Nutrition, Physical Activity, and Metabolism (Subcommittee on Physical Activity). *Circulation* 2003, 107:3109–3116.

20. Franklin BA, Gordon S, Timmis GC: Exercise prescription for hypertensive patients. *Ann Med* 1991, 23:279–287.

21. Vu Tran Z, Weltman A: Differential effects of exercise on serum lipid and lipoprotein levels seen with changes in body weight: a meta-analysis. *JAMA* 1985, 254:919–924.

22. Blair SN, Kohl HW III, Paffenbarger RS, *et al.*: Physical fitness and all-cause mortality: a prospective study of healthy men and women. *JAMA* 1989, 262:2395–2401.

23.• Blair SN, Kohl HW III, Barlow CE, *et al.*: Changes in physical fitness and all-cause mortality: a prospective study of healthy and unhealthy men. *JAMA* 1995, 273:1093–1098.

24.•• Blair SN, Kampert JB, Kohl HW III, *et al.*: Influences of cardiorespiratory fitness and other precursors on cardiovascular disease and all-cause mortality in men and women. *JAMA* 1996, 276:205–210.

25.• Paffenbarger RS, Jr., Hyde RT, Wing AL, *et al.*: The association of changes in physical-activity level and other lifestyle characteristics with mortality among men. *N Engl J Med* 1993, 328:538–545.

26. Sandvik L, Erikssen J, Thaulow E, *et al.*: Physical fitness as a predictor of mortality among healthy, middle-aged Norwegian men. *N Engl J Med* 1993, 328:533–537.

27. Lee IM, Hsieh CC, Paffenbarger RS Jr.: Exercise intensity and longevity in men. The Harvard Alumni Health Study. *JAMA* 1995, 273:1179–1184.

28. Vanhees L, Fagard R, Thijs L, *et al.*: Prognostic significance of peak exercise capacity in patients with coronary artery disease. *J Am Coll Cardiol* 1994, 23:358–363.

29.• Ehsani AA, Martin WH III, Heath GW, Coyle EF: Cardiac effects of prolonged and intense exercise training in patients with coronary artery disease. *Am J Cardiol* 1982, 50:246–254.

30.• Barlow CE, Kohl HW III, Gibbons LW, Blair SN: Physical fitness, mortality and obesity. *Int J Obes Relat Metab Disord* 1995, 19 Suppl 4:S41–S44.

31. Lee IM, Sesso HD, Oguma Y, Paffenbarger RS Jr.: Relative intensity of physical activity and risk of coronary heart disease. *Circulation* 2003, 107:1110–1116.

32. Gregg EW, Cauley JA, Stone K, *et al.*: Relationship of changes in physical activity and mortality among older women. *JAMA* 2003, 289:2379–2386.

33. Lee CD, Folsom AR, Blair SN: Physical activity and stroke risk: a meta-analysis. *Stroke* 2003, 34:2475–2481.

34. Hoberg E, Schuler G, Kunze B, *et al.*: Silent myocardial ischemia as a potential link between lack of premonitoring symptoms and increased risk of cardiac arrest during physical stress. *Am J Cardiol* 1990, 65:583–589.

35. Siscovick DS, Weiss NS, Fletcher RH, Lasky T: The incidence of primary cardiac arrest during vigorous exercise. *N Engl J Med* 1984, 311:874–877.

36. Thompson PD, Mitchell JH: Exercise and sudden cardiac death: protection or provocation. *N Engl J Med* 1984, 311:914–915.

37. Richardson PD, Davies MJ, Born GV: Influence of plaque configuration and stress distribution on fissuring of coronary atherosclerotic plaques. *Lancet* 1989, 2:941–944.

38. Kestin AS, Ellis PA, Barnard MR, *et al.*: Effect of strenuous exercise on platelet activation state and reactivity. *Circulation* 1993, 88:1502–1511.

39. Knowlan DM. The electrocardiogram in the athlete. In *Cardiovascular Evaluation of Athletes: Toward Recognizing Athletes at Risk of Sudden Death*. Edited by Waller BF, Harvey WP. Newton, NJ: Laennec Publishing; 1993:43.

40. Huston TP, Puffer JC, Rodney WM: The athletic heart syndrome. *N Engl J Med* 1985, 313:24–32.

41. Lichtman J, RA OR, Klein A, Karliner JS: Electrocardiogram of the athlete. Alterations simulating those of organic heart disease. *Arch Intern Med* 1973, 132:763–770.

42. Pantano JA, Oriel RJ: Prevalence and nature of cardiac arrhythmias in apparently normal well-trained runners. *Am Heart J* 1982, 104:762–768.

43. Kaimal KP, Franklin BA, Moir TW, Hellerstein HK: Cardiac profiles of national-class race walkers. *Chest* 1993, 104:935–938.

44. Bouchard C, Lesage R, Lortie G, *et al.*: Aerobic performance in brothers, dizygotic and monozygotic twins. *Med Sci Sports Exerc* 1986, 18:639–646.

45.•• Maron BJ, Thompson PD, Puffer JC, *et al.*: Cardiovascular preparticipation screening of competitive athletes: addendum: an addendum to a statement for health professionals from the Sudden Death Committee (Council on Clinical Cardiology) and the Congenital Cardiac Defects Committee (Council on Cardiovascular Disease in the Young), American Heart Association. *Circulation* 1998, 97:2294.

46. Maron BJ, Poliac LC, Roberts WO: Risk for sudden cardiac death associated with marathon running. *J Am Coll Cardiol* 1996, 28:428–431.

47. Waller BF, Roberts WC: Sudden death while running in conditioned runners aged 40 years or over. *Am J Cardiol* 1980, 45:1292–1300.

48.• Maron BJ, Shirani J, Poliac LC, *et al.*: Sudden death in young competitive athletes. Clinical, demographic, and pathological profiles. *JAMA* 1996, 276:199–204.

49. Ades PA: Preventing sudden death: Cardiovascular screening of young athletes. *Physician Sportsmed* 1992, 20:75–89.

50.•• Maron BJ, Thompson PD, Puffer JC, *et al.*: Cardiovascular preparticipation screening of competitive athletes. A statement for health professionals from the Sudden Death Committee (clinical cardiology) and Congenital Cardiac Defects Committee (cardiovascular disease in the young), American Heart Association. *Circulation* 1996, 94:850–856.

51.• Maron BJ, Mitchell JH: 26th Bethesda Conference: recommendations for determining eligibility for competition in athletes with cardiovascular abnormalities. *J Am Coll Cardiol* 1994, 24:845–899.

SELECT BIBLIOGRAPHY

Fletcher GF: Holter recording in athletes: purposes and indication. In *Cardiovascular Evaluation of Athletes*. Edited by Walter BF, Harvey WP. Newton: Laennec Publishing; 1993:87.

Franklin BA, Almany SL, Hauser AM: Cardiovascular evaluation of the athlete. In *Sports Injuries: Mechanisms, Prevention, and Treatment*. Edited by Fu FH, Stone DA. Baltimore: Williams & Wilkins Co.; 1994:111–121.

Approach to the Patient with Hyperlipidemia

Neil J. Stone

14

Key Points

- Endothelial damage in the setting of risk factors sets the stage for the complex process of atherosclerosis. Plaque rupture is more common in hyperlipidemic patients. Vulnerable plaques have a large accumulation of core liquid and a high density of macrophages at the margins of its thinned fibrous plaque. Plaque rupture occurs more frequently in men with coronary artery disease (CAD) who have abnormal lipids.

- Lipids are transported on lipoproteins. Cholesterol-rich lipoproteins are low-density lipoprotein (LDL) and high-density lipoprotein (HDL). Triglyceride-rich lipoproteins include very low-density lipoprotein (VLDL) and chylomicrons, as well as remnant particles. VLDL and remnant particles are important as increased levels are shown to indicate increased risk of progression of CAD in angiographic trials. Non-HDL cholesterol (non-HDL-C) is a measure of both LDL cholesterol (LDL-C) and triglyceride-rich lipoproteins and is a secondary target after LDL-C.

- Both total cholesterol and HDL-C should be measured in all adults older than 19 years at least once every 5 years.

- Intervention focuses on not only LDL-C calculated by measurement of fasting total cholesterol, triglycerides, and HDL-C, but also non-HDL-C as a secondary target. For those with coronary disease, HDL-C may be a third target.

- Risk factors include age, menopausal status, hypertension, cigarette smoking, and family history of premature cardiovascular disease (before 65 years of age in female relatives and 55 years of age in male relatives). Diabetes mellitus is now considered a coronary risk equivalent along with noncoronary forms of atherosclerotic vascular disease or a 10-year risk of a coronary event that exceeds 20%. Those patients who have a "coronary risk equivalent" have LDL-C goals similar to those with CAD.

- Sedentary lifestyle and obesity can lead to the metabolic syndrome. The metabolic syndrome is diagnosed empirically when a patient has three or more of the following: increased waist circumference, low HDL-C, high triglycerides, abnormal fasting glucose, and blood pressure above 130/85 mm Hg. Recognition of the metabolic syndrome not only indicates increased CAD risk, but also that of type 2 diabetes mellitus.

- Secondary causes of hyperlipidemia should always be ruled out before treatment begins. Important causes to remember include hypothyroidism, nephrosis, liver disease, excess alcohol and/or diet, and medications such as female hormones, steroids, or beta-blockers.

- Diet is important in reducing LDL-C, and along with regular exercise helps combat weight gain and insulin resistance. Fruits and vegetables, fiber, and fish (omega 3 fatty acids) have all been shown to reduce coronary event rates.

- Primary prevention trials have shown the value of statin therapy in middle-aged subjects characterized by low HDL-C or having a high-risk profile.

- Secondary prevention trials have shown the ability of statins over a wide range of LDL-C values to produce enhanced survival, fewer cardiovascular events, and fewer revascularization procedures.

- Successful drug therapy must consider both liver-active drugs and intestinally active drugs alone or in combination. Examples of the former include statins, niacin, and fibrates such as gemfibrozil or fenofibrate. Examples of the latter include cholestyramine, colestipol, colesevelam, and ezetimibe. Guidelines for their successful use alone or in combination are given.

INTRODUCTION

Convincing evidence now shows that aggressive lipid and lipoprotein treatment in those at high risk for coronary artery disease (CAD) events can positively influence the complex process of atherosclerosis. Often initiated with endothelial damage, atherosclerosis is facilitated by hypercholesterolemia and other risk factors. A decrease in plaque cholesterol due to a reduction in modified lipoproteins, local inflammatory and immune responses, and even improvement in abnormal endothelial regulation occur with successful therapy. This is important because harmful disruption of atherosclerotic plaque is most likely to occur in hypercholesterolemic patients with a large accumulation of core lipid and a high density of lipid-laden macrophages at the margins of its thinned fibrous cap [1]. Lesions with these characteristics comprise only 10% to 20% of the overall lesion population but account for 60% to 90% of the acute clinical events [2].

In those with elevated cholesterol values, lipid-lowering with simvastatin [3] or pravastatin [4] after myocardial infarction (MI) or unstable angina (UA) improves clinical outcomes with enhanced survival, fewer cardiovascular events, and fewer revascularization procedures. This beneficial effect (although not reduced total mortality) extends to post-MI patients with normal cholesterol values given pravastatin [5] or high-risk groups without prior CAD given pravastatin or lovastatin [6,7]. Four recent statin trials have extended these observations. In the Heart Protection Study (HPS), simvastatin 40 mg reduced total mortality as well as coronary and stroke endpoints in a high-risk population that included those with CAD, noncoronary forms of atherosclerosis, and diabetics [8••]. This striking decrease in event rates occurred in those with low-density lipoprotein cholesterol (LDL-C) above and below 116 mg/dL. In the Prosper Study, pravastatin 40 mg reduced coronary, but not stroke event rates in an older population that extended up to 83 years of age [9]. The lack of effect on stroke may have been related to the short duration of the trial (3.2 years) and/or the low rate of stroke in the placebo group. Finally, the Anglo-Scandinavian Cardiac Outcomes Trial (ASCOT) showed the benefit of atorvastatin 10 mg in a high-risk primary prevention group of subjects with hypertension and three CAD risk factors[10]. The trial was stopped due to achievement of the main endpoints after only 3 years. The lipid arm of the Antihypertensive and Lipid-Lowering Treatment to Prevent Heart Attack Trial (ALLHAT) had serious design flaws that prevented firm conclusions about statin use [11]. In the control group, there was a substantial use of statins such that the difference in LDL-C lowering between the treatment group on pravastatin 40 mg and the control group was only about 18%. No significant effect of this amount of LDL-C lowering on event rates was seen.

Although the above studies used the statin class of lipid lowering agents, improvement in CAD event rates has been seen in randomized clinical trials using diet, bile acid sequestering drugs (such as cholestyramine and colestipol), niacin, gemfibrozil, fenofibrate, and partial ileal bypass surgery. Beneficial effects on endothelial function can occur after a single treatment of apheresis [12]. Thus, the contemporary approach to the prevention and treatment of atherosclerosis requires a detailed understanding of lipid and lipoprotein metabolism.

Cholesterol

Cholesterol is vital for animal life because of its key role in cell membranes and in the production of adrenal and sex hormones and vitamin D. It is a waxy, tasteless substance derived from acetate. The major production is in the liver cell. 3-Hydroxy-3-methylglutaryl-coenzyme A (HMG-CoA) reductase regulates the rate-limiting step of cholesterol synthesis as mevalonate is produced from HMG-CoA. Competitive inhibitors of this step reduce hepatic cholesterol pools, increase LDL cell surface receptors, and lower blood levels of LDL-C. Cholesterol is degraded into bile acids. Interruption of the enterohepatic circulation causes a depletion of the bile acid supply such that the liver cholesterol pool is depleted. This results in an increase in liver cell receptors for LDL, the lipoprotein that carries most of the cholesterol in plasma. A genetic deficiency of normally functioning receptors leads to increased levels of LDL-C in the blood and an enhanced risk for coronary heart disease (CHD) that can lead to fatal outcomes early in life in the most severe cases.

Triglycerides

Triglycerides (TGs) are sources of dietary fat. They have a glycerol backbone to which is attached fatty acids. TGs are stored in adipose tissue and can be converted into fatty acids for energy (Table 1). Those fatty acid chains without double bonds are called saturated. Those with a single double bond are called monounsaturated, and those with multiple double bonds are called polyunsaturated. Increased ingestion of saturated fats raises serum cholesterol by their action on the LDL receptor. When unsaturated fats replace saturated fats in the diet, serum cholesterol values fall. Polyunsaturated fats are subdivided into two classes—omega 6 and omega 3—depending on the position of the first double bond. Omega 3 fatty acids affect platelet function and are particularly useful in severe hypertriglyceridemia. Diets with an increase in omega 3 fatty acids in contrast to omega 6 fatty acids may reduce sudden death independent of their effect on lipids [13].

Lipids

Lipids are transported in the blood as part of large macromolecules called lipoproteins. Chylomicrons carry dietary fat, and very low-density lipoprotein (VLDL) from the liver carries endogenously produced TG. Normally, VLDLs are converted to cholesterol-rich LDL in the plasma. High-density lipoproteins (HDLs) function in reverse cholesterol transport to return cholesterol to the liver and aid in the metabolism of TG-rich lipoproteins. Additional mechanisms that may explain why high HDL levels lower risk of CAD include 1) helping to reduce oxidation of LDL through associated paroxonase activity [14], 2) inhibiting cytokine-induced expression of adhesion molecules [15], and 3) enhancing the fibrinolytic process [16].

Each lipoprotein class (chylomicrons, VLDL, LDL, HDL) has specific proteins called apolipoproteins (apo) that serve either as ligands or links to specific receptors or as needed cofactors in metabolic reactions. VLDL and LDL carry one molecule of apo B on each particle. Thus, an elevated apo B level indicates an increased number of atherogenic particles and is associated with enhanced coronary risk even when LDL-C levels are not raised. Apo A-I is carried on HDL cholesterol (HDL-C). Levels of apo A-I are inversely related to CAD risk. Indeed, an exciting new frontier was suggested by the provocative results of treating coronary patients with infusions of apo A-I milano, a special form of HDL that is associated with a reduced risk of CAD [17••].

Special lipoproteins are not routinely measured, but may provide useful information in selected cases. Issues such as standardization, availability, cost, and incremental value must be resolved before they are measured routinely. Lipoprotein (a), or Lp(a) is an LDL particle bound to apo a (pronounced "little a"). It is a large, water soluble glycoprotein and has a sequence similarity to plasminogen. This carries the potential for impaired thrombolysis. It is a common, heritable risk factor for premature atherosclerosis, although its predictive value is not confirmed in all studies [18]. It is an acute-phase reactant and should not be measured at the time of an acute event. High serum levels of L(a) are associated with both apo (a) and increased apo B in the vessel wall. There are clear-cut, black-white differences in Lp(a), with the distribution in whites skewed to the left. A meta-analysis showed that Lp(a) was not correlated well with traditional risk factors and there was a significant difference in risk between the upper and lower thirds of the distribution [19].

Niacin and estrogen lower Lp(a), whereas resins, fibrates, and HMG CoA reductase inhibitors (statins) do not. In the Familial Atherosclerosis Treatment Study (FATS), Lp(a) correlated strongly with baseline severity of atherosclerosis and subsequent progression, but its predictive power was not seen in the treatment groups where LDL-C was lowered to below 100 mg/dL [20].

Small dense LDL are atherogenic particles that are more easily oxidized. When a coronary prone individual has plasma TG over 150 and low HDL-C, an increase should be suspected. More sophisticated analysis shows elevations in intermediate density lipoproteins, reduction in large LDL, and reductions in HDL, especially HDL2. There are genetic and environmental determinants: investigators have described an inherited trait called "pattern B" in contrast to the large, buoyant LDL seen in pattern A. Pattern B is expressed maximally in men over 20 years of age and postmenopausal women. In the Framingham Offspring study, as the body mass index increased, the proportion of those with small dense LDL increased [21]. Elevated levels occur in familial combined hyperlipidemia, hyperapobetalipoproteinemia, and type 2 diabetes. A clinical clue to a patient with small dense LDL (along with elevated apo B and high insulin) is a TG value above 180 mg/dL and an increased waist circumference [22].

High-sensitivity C-reactive protein (hs-CRP) predicts increased cardiac risk in men and women, and most important, the prediction by hs-CRP is beyond that provided by cholesterol and HDL-C measurements [23]. Moreover, hs-CRP predicts elevated risk in subjects without overt hyperlipidemia, and adds prognostic information to risk scoring, LDL-C, and even the metabolic syndrome [24]. The more risk factor components of the metabolic syndrome, the higher the hs-CRP. Benefits from aspirin and statins are more likely in those with elevated hs-CRP. While awaiting

TABLE 1 DIETARY FATTY ACIDS		
Class	**Fatty acids**	**Foods**
Saturated	Lauric, myristic, palmitic; stearic is saturated but converted to monosaturates	Animal and vegetable fats; examples: fatty meats, butter, coconut oil, palm kernel oil
Monounsaturated; n-9	Oleic acid	Not essential as synthesized; examples: olive and canola oil; peanut oil
Trans-fatty acids	Elaidic acid	Stick margarines, french fries, commercial baked goods
Polyunsaturated; n-6	Linoleic acid	Essential as not synthesized; examples: corn, safflower, walnut, sunflower oils
Polyunsaturated; n-3	Linoleic acid (plant sources), eicosapentaenoic acid and docosahexanoic acid (marine sources)	Marine oils; examples: mackerel, cod liver oil; vegetable sources include tofu and canola oil

an ongoing clinical trial, hs-CRP values would appear to influence management most in those with an intermediate risk of a coronary event.

DIAGNOSIS

Laboratory Studies

Measurement of lipids and lipoproteins

The Adult Treatment Panel III (ATP III) report for the recognition, evaluation, and treatment of hypercholesterolemia in adults provides an evidence-based platform on which to base clinical decisions in this field. LDL-C is still the major target of cholesterol-lowering therapy [25]. Major risk factors are tallied to determine a patient's global risk (Table 2). Those at very high risk are called "CHD risk equivalents." ATP III defined inclusion in this category as those without overt CHD who had a 10-year Framingham risk of more than 20%. Included in this group are those with noncoronary forms of atherosclerosis, such as carotid atherosclerosis, peripheral vascular disease, or an abdominal aortic aneurysm, and diabetics (Table 3). Although the latter may not always have a short-term risk greater than 20%, they have a substantial long-term risk that must be recognized. The report also puts emphasis on triglycerides and HDL-C in lipid management. Most important, the report underscored the importance of recognizing and treating those who acquired multiple, metabolic risk factors or the metabolic syndrome in response to an atherogenic diet, sedentary lifestyle, and weight gain.

Serum cholesterol may be obtained in the nonfasting state. Values of 200 mg/dL or greater are elevated and require further work-up. However, a cholesterol level under 200 mg/dL is not completely reassuring. Low serum HDL-C (< 40 mg/dL) is seen frequently in those with CAD and may be associated with a total cholesterol under 200 mg/dL. This combination is particularly noted in men with a family history of premature CAD [26]. Thus, a nonfasting sample that measures total cholesterol and HDL-C can be very useful in determining if further work-up is needed. If abnormal values are found (total cholesterol >200 mg/dL or HDL-C < 40 mg/dL), it is important to repeat them and obtain a fasting lipoprotein profile. This should be done in the fasting state, 9 to 12 hours after the meal. This allows for reliable measurement of TGs (TGs are so highly variable that to minimize variability, the patient should be fasting and at a steady weight). A nonfasting TG value is useful only in the patient with abdominal pain and suspected pancreatitis; here, values over 1000 mg/L suggest chylomicronemia as a cause of the pancreatitis.

For most patients, however, a fasting lipid panel that measures total cholesterol, TGs, and HDL-C allows calcu-

TABLE 2 RISK FACTORS AND ADULT TREATMENT PANEL III		
Major risk factors (other than LDL-C)	**Details**	**Comments**
Age	Male ≥ 45 years of age; female ≥ 55 years of age	Age is a strong determinant of risk in the Framingham Risk Score
Family history of premature CHD	Definite myocardial infarction or sudden death before age 55 years in father or other male first-degree relatives; or before age 65 years in mother or other female first-degree relatives	The Framingham Study felt family history was explained in great part by the associated risk factors; others hold that family history is a strong and independent risk factor in its own right
Current cigarette smoking	Within the past month	Always offer to assist the patient in quitting when you obtain this information
Hypertension	≥ 140/90 mm Hg or on antihypertensive medication	Although latest Joint National Committee goal is 120/80 mm Hg, for purposes of risk assesment this cutpoint is used
Low HDL-C	< 40 mg/dL	A high HDL-C ≥ 60 mg/dL is considered a "negative" or protective risk factor and reduces the tally or risk factors by one; those with high HDL-C can still get coronary disease, however, so the entire risk picture must be considered

CHD—coronary heart disease; HDL-C—high-density-lipoprotein cholesterol; LDL-C—low-density-lipoprotein cholesterol.

lation of LDL-C and non-HDL-C. An optimal LDL-C is below 100 mg/dL (Table 4). This is the goal for those with CAD or those with "coronary risk equivalents."

For those with two or more risk factors, the LDL-C goal is less than 130 mg/dL. For those with zero to one risk factor, the LDL-C goal is less than 160 mg/dL. In those with two or more risk factors, the goals may be modified by calculating the 10-year Framingham risk or looking at emerging risk factors such as hs-CRP. For example, a 50-year-old nonsmoking man with treated hypertension and a cholesterol of 250 mg/dL and an HDL-C of 42 mg/dL has a 10-year Framingham CAD risk of 10%. Here an elevated hs-CRP (> 3.0) may influence the decision to start a statin sooner than the clinician might have based on these numbers. Those at very high risk (CAD or CAD equivalents) or very low risk (few risk factors especially in a young person) don't require further testing as it will not likely affect any treatment decisions. In older patients, some clinicians prefer to look at either ankle-brachial index, carotid imaging, or coronary calcium to help them more precisely risk stratify.

An HDL-C below 40 mg/dL increases CAD risk and is a major risk factor. Clinicians must remember that the mean HDL-C for women is 55 mg/dL and 45 mg/dL for men. Thus, an HDL-C in the 40 to 50 range is still low for women. For primary prevention efforts, behavioral changes to raise HDL-C should be stressed. Reducing excess body weight, stopping cigarette smoking, lowering elevated TG values, and replacing sedentary habits with regular exercise can lead to increased HDL-C. These behavioral changes are most likely to show effects when the TGs are also elevated. Exercise must be regular and sustained over many months before an elevation of HDL-C is seen. Alcohol raises HDL-C, but it cannot be recommended for this purpose because of the negative aspects associated with excess usage (especially in women and younger persons). High HDL-C (over 60 mg/dL) is linked to longevity syndromes and, at any level of LDL-C, suggests a more conservative approach to drug therapy than would be the case if the HDL-C were low. For those who require secondary prevention efforts

TABLE 3 CHD RISK EQUIVALENTS*

Risk equivalents	Comments
Diabetes mellitus: fasting blood sugar > 125 mg/dL or on diabetic therapy	Although diabetics can have a wide range of near-term risk, all have long-term risk of CHD
Noncoronary forms of atherosclerosis: 1) abdominal aortic aneurysm, 2) carotid artery disease (symptomatic or > 50% carotid narrowing, 3) peripheral arterial disease	Studies show a high 10-year risk of CHD death in these subgroups
Multiple risk factors such that global risk is > 20%: use Framingham score to determine this	Examples: 66-year-old woman with total cholesterol of 260 mg/dL, high-density lipoprotein of 35 mg/dL, treated blood pressure with systolic 145 mm Hg, and a smoker; 37-year-old man with same risk factors

*Those adults without established CHD who have an absolute, 10-year risk greater than 20% for developing major coronary events (myocardial infarction and coronary death). This is "equivalent" risk to those with established CHD.
CHD—coronary heart disease.

TABLE 4 LDL-C DECISION CUTOFFS: ATP III REPORT*

LDL-C	Criteria for "goal" level	Comment
< 100 mg/dL	This is "goal" for those at highest risk	Considered "optimal" LDL-C
< 130 mg/dL	This is "goal" for those with 2 or more risk factors and a 10-year risk of ≤ 20%	If global risk 10%–20%, consider drug therapy after 3 months of TLC if LDL-C ≥ 130 mg/dL; if global risk < 10%, consider drug therapy after 3 months of TLC if LDL-C ≥ 160 mg/dL
< 160 mg/dL	This is "goal" for those with 0–1 risk factors	If LDL-C > 190 mg/dL after TLC, consider drug therapy

*These are guidelines, and clinical judgment is required in all categories.
ATP III—Adult Treatment Panel III; LDL-C—low-density lipoprotein cholesterol; TLC—therapeutic lifestyle change.

due to existing CAD or equivalent high-risk states, drug therapy often raises HDL-C and this can be additive to behavioral changes.

Hypertriglyceridemia drops out as an independent risk factor in multivariate analysis. However, TGs are a valuable indicator of associated metabolic abnormalities. Those with levels above 150 mg/dL are more likely to have small, dense LDL. A clue to elevated fasting TG values is turbid serum (Fig. 1). If TGs exceed 1000 mg/dL, the serum is usually creamy, indicating chylomicronemia. The cream means that the patient is either not fasting (TG mildly elevated) or has a major TG removal disorder with an increased risk of pancreatitis (TG over 1000 mg/dL). A current classification is given in Table 5.

Accuracy of Measurements

Most labs can now show a precision and accuracy level of 5% or less for cholesterol. Table 6 shows some of the factors that must be considered when the clinician evaluates lipid measurements. Screening values can be nonfasting because simultaneous determination of cholesterol and HDL-C can determine the need for further testing. For detailed evaluation or for determining response to therapy, it is mandatory to sample individuals who have not eaten for 12 to 14 hours and have not had alcohol within the preceding 24 hours. The individual should also be at a level of stable weight without intercurrent illness or stress. In a study of adolescents at a boarding school, HDL-C was lower during and after infection [27].

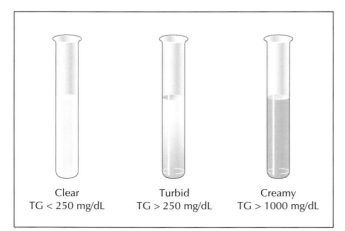

Clear
TG < 250 mg/dL

Turbid
TG > 250 mg/dL

Creamy
TG > 1000 mg/dL

FIGURE 1 Visual inspection and triglyceride (TG)-rich lipoproteins.

	TABLE 5 TRIGLYCERIDE DECISION LIMITS	
Triglyceride values	**Details**	**Comment**
< 150 mg/dL	Normal range	Nonetheless, if triglycerides < 100, likelihood of small dense LDL is much less
150–199 mg/dL	Borderline high	This is the range where lifestyle change can help greatly
200–499 mg/dL	High	If triglycerides in this range after LDL-C is at goal, calculate non-HDL-C as a secondary target; goal is 30 more than LDL-C goals
500 mg/dL or higher	Very high	These patients are at risk for pancreatitis; usually a genetic component and either alcohol, estrogen, poorly controlled diabetes, or hypothyroidism to cause high triglycerides that can lead to pancreatitis

HDL-C—high-density lipoprotein cholesterol; LDL-C—low-density lipoprotein cholesterol.

TABLE 6 SOURCES OF LABORATORY VARIATION IN LIPID MEASUREMENTS	
Behavioral	**Sampling sources**
Diet: fats raise TC, HDL; saturated fats raise LDL	Fasting: essential for accurate determination of TG
Obesity: increases TG, lowers HDL	Nonfasting: after eating, see increase in VLDL and lower LDL; TC changes to a small degree
Smoking: decreases HDL, *eg*, 11% in one study	Posture: About 9% higher for TC, LDL, and 10% higher for HDL-C with lying down compared with standing
Exercise: lowers cholesterol, TG; increases HDL	Fingerstick: can see unreliable values if technician not well trained or machine not calibrated regularly
Alcohol: increases TG, raises HDL	

HDL—high-density lipoprotein; HDL-C—high-density lipoprotein cholesterol; LDL—low-density lipoprotein; TC—total cholesterol; TG—triglycerides; VLDL—very low-density lipoprotein.

Sources of Error in Hospitalized Patients

It appears that cholesterol measured within the first 24 hours after MI reflects pre-event lipid values [28]. Yet cholesterol values fall markedly in the week after MI and TG levels rise. In one carefully done study, cholesterol fell 31% and LDL-C fell 48% in the week after an MI [29]. Because statin therapy has been so successful in post-MI patients, most cardiologists now start statin therapy at discharge along with dietary and activity counseling. This is shown to be a strong and independent positive predictor of subsequent use [30].

Risk Factors

Every patient evaluated for hyperlipidemia should have a checklist of risk factors on his or her chart. Not only are risk factors associated with dyslipidemia (lipid abnormalities are more likely in diabetics, hypertensives, and obese patients, for example), but the presence of multiple risk factors increases CAD risk.

Nonmodifiable risk factors include age and gender (men and postmenopausal women with increased risk). As the Framingham risk prediction model shows, age is a potent risk factor. In models where absolute risk is the basis for drug therapy, men over 45 years of age and women over 55 years of age are more likely to qualify due to their enhanced CAD risk.

Modifiable risk factors include excess LDL, low HDL, hypertension (including systolic hypertension in the elderly), type 2 diabetes mellitus (T2DM), cigarette smoking, and targets such as sedentary lifestyle and abdominal or male pattern obesity. Femoral-gluteal obesity is primarily a cosmetic problem, whereas abdominal obesity is a marker for the stigmata of insulin resistance. These include hypertension, hyperglycemia, low HDL-C, and hypertriglyceridemia [31]. This clustering of risk factors causes an increased risk of CAD. Most of this clustering is due to the effects of sedentary lifestyle and obesity and it is a major

problem for family physicians, internists, and specialists alike. This was denoted by ATP III as the metabolic syndrome. The metabolic syndrome is diagnosed empirically when a patient has three or more of the following: increased waist circumference, low HDL-C, high TGs, abnormal fasting glucose, and blood pressure above 130/85 mm Hg (Table 7). Recognition of the metabolic syndrome not only indicates increased CAD risk, but also increases the risk for T2DM.

Secondary causes of elevated blood lipids

Secondary causes of elevated blood lipids should always be determined. A useful mnemonic is to think of the three Ds: diet, drugs, and diseases (Table 8). If secondary causes are not seen, primary hyperlipidemia should be considered and the family is screened.

Familial hyperlipidemia and coronary artery disease

Hyperlipidemia in survivors of MI was determined in a classic study in Seattle using spouse controls and defining hyperlipidemia as elevations of cholesterol and TG above the 95th percentile [32]. With this definition, hyperlipidemia was seen in 33% of survivors under age 60 years with familial forms accounting for over 20% of cases (Table 9). In clinical practice, those with a family history of premature CAD and an LDL-C over 190 mg/dL or a low HDL-C (< 40 mg/dL) should be considered for drug therapy.

Lipid abnormalities in men with angiographically documented CAD were quantified by Genest *et al.* [33] who examined 321 men and used age- and body mass index–matched subjects from the Framingham Offspring Study who were free of CAD (Table 10). They found that the most frequent dyslipidemias (used 90th percentile values for LDL-C and TGs and 10th percentile values for HDL) involved HDL-C. Even after correcting for use of

TABLE 7 CLINICAL CRITERIA FOR THE METABOLIC SYNDROME*

Risk factors	Defining level	Comments
Abdominal obesity (waist circumference)	Men: > 40 inches (102 cm); women: > 35 inches (88 cm)	In our clinic, we empirically use cutoffs 10% lower for Asian populations
Hypertriglyceridemia	TG ≥ 150 mg/dL	Patients should be fasting 9–12 hours and at stable weight
Low HDL-C	Men: < 40 mg/dL; women: < 50 mg/dL	When a low HDL-C is associated with high TG, insulin resistance should be considered
Hypertension	Blood pressure ≥ 130/85 mm Hg	Measure after patient has been seated for 5 minutes
Impaired fasting glucose	Fasting blood sugar ≥ 110 mg/dL	A 2-hour glucose tolerance test may be useful as well

*For diagnosis, choose any three of the criteria in this table. Clinical note: all of these criteria are improved with small amounts of weight loss achieved with increased exercise and decreased caloric intake.

HDL-C—high-density-lipoprotein cholesterol; TG—triglycerides.

beta-blockers, sampling bias, and diet effects, they noted 35% of patients with CAD with a total cholesterol level under 200 mg/dL. In this group, almost 75% had a low HDL-C (under 35 mg/dL in that study; now a low HDL-C is under 40 mg/dL). Elevated Lp(a) was also commonly seen. Many lipid experts hold that Lp(a) measurements are particularly useful in those with a personal or family history of premature CAD.

Women and risk of coronary artery disease

Among menopausal women, hormone replacement therapy can reverse the menopausal changes of raised LDL-C and lowered HDL-C. Estrogen treatment may lower LDL-C by 10% to 19% and raise HDL-C 16% to 18% in a dose-dependent fashion with oral therapy, but with little effect with transdermal estrogen [34]. Since estrogen patches do not raise TGs like their oral counterparts, they can be useful

TABLE 8 SECONDARY CAUSES OF HYPERCHOLESTEROLEMIA AND HYPERTRIGLYCERIDEMIA

Secondary causes of hypercholesterolemia	Rule out by performing
Diet	Dietary history; focus on saturated fats, dietary cholesterol
Drugs*	Diuretics, steroids, anabolic steroids, venlafaxine
Hypothyroidism	TSH test
Nephrotic syndrome	Urine analysis, serum albumin
Obstructive liver disease	Abnormal alkaline phosphatase and enzymes
Diabetes mellitus	FBS, glycated hemoglobin
s/p transplantation	Multiple causes including drugs such as steroids; weight gain
Secondary causes of hypertriglyceridemia	**Rule out by performing**
Diet	Dietary history; focus on calorie excess, alcohol
Drugs*	Steroids, estrogens, retinoic acid, beta-blockers, protease inhibitors, diuretics, tamoxifen
Hypothyroidism	TSH test
Nephrotic syndrome (severe)	Urine analyis, serum albumin
Chronic renal disease	BUN, creatinine
Diabetes mellitus	FBS, glycated hemoglobin

*Drugs listed are examples; this is not a complete list.
BUN—blood urea nitrogen; FBS—fasting blood sugar; s/p—status post; TSH—thyroid-stimulating hormone.

TABLE 9 GENETIC FORMS OF HYPERCHOLESTEROLEMIA

Name	Diagnosis	Comments
Familial hypercholesterolemia	Elevated LDL-C; heterozygotes: TC 325–500 mg/dL; homozygotes: TC 500–1000 mg/dL; tendon xanthomas (in childhood in homozygous cases)	Defective or absent LDL receptors
Familial combined hyperlipidemia	Elevated apolipoprotein B levels in muliple family members with varying lipid profiles	Increased secretion of apo B
Severe primary polygenic elevation of LDL-C	Elevated LDL levels without evidence of tendon xanthomas	Clearance of LDL usually retarded; E4 allele of apo E may play a role
Rare forms 　Familial defective apo B 　Autosomal recessive hypercholes-terolemia 　Beta-sitosterolemia	These are rare conditions that require special lipid testing	

apo—apolipoprotein; LDL-C—low-density-lipoprotein cholesterol; TC—total cholesterol.
Adapted from Stone and Blum [78].

in women with high TGs in whom unopposed estrogen can lead to marked hypertriglyceridemia. Progestins tend to counter lipid changes caused by estrogens, but newer progestins may not have the adverse effects on HDL-C as seen with older formulations. The Heart and Estrogen Replacement Study (HERS) trial showed an increase in 1-year mortality in older women with CAD and failed to show an improvement in CAD mortality with hormone replacement over the course of the trial [35]. The Women's Health Initiative (WHI) examined the value of hormone therapy in postmenopausal women. The WHI investigators stopped the estrogen-plus-progestin study after finding that the associated health risks outweighed the benefits [36]. Thus, for women with hypercholesterolemia, lifestyle change and drug therapy employing the principles noted in this chapter should be used as the first steps in treating hyperlipidemia noted in the postmenopausal woman. This is in contrast to the older recommendation that suggested hormone therapy should be the first option.

THERAPY

Therapeutic Lifestyle Change

The ATP III emphasized the need to consider lifestyle change rather than focusing narrowly on just dietary change. Its concept of therapeutic lifestyle change (TLC) involves diet and exercise and a more healthy way of living. The three elements of this approach can be thought of as directed to the various risk components.

Behaviors to lower low-density lipoprotein cholesterol

The ATP III dietary recommendations continue to emphasize a diet low in saturated fats (and trans-fatty acids) to lower LDL-C. In addition, ATP III suggested the use of higher fiber diets and plant stanol/sterol esters to augment dietary attempts at lowering LDL-C to goal. Soluble fiber is a useful adjunct to cholesterol-lowering therapy and can be obtained in the form of oats (they have a greater proportion of soluble fiber than any other grain) or in vegetables and pectin-rich fruits. Using a combination of psyllium,

fiber, almonds, and soy protein, LDL-C lowering comparable to lovastatin 20 mg/day can be obtained [37].

The rationale for dietary change to lower LDL-C and hence coronary events is supported by large-scale studies as well as angiographic trials. Worthy of mention is the St. Thomas Atherosclerosis Regression Trial (STAR) that showed a remarkable improvement with diet in British men with angina pectoris [38]. After 39 months, the proportion of subjects who showed an increase in luminal diameter was 4% for usual care, 38% for the dietary group, and 33% for the diet and resin group. The authors showed that change in the angiographic appearance of the coronary segments was independently and significantly correlated with LDL-C change during the trial.

Behaviors to improve the metabolic syndrome

The ATP III wished to focus on increased caloric intake and sedentary habits. Its dietary recommendations did not focus on a specific number for total fat in the diet, but recommended a range of 25% to 35% due to the observation that total fat intake below 25% often aggravated the low HDL and high TGs seen in these patients [39]. The allowed higher fat intake was designed to permit carbohydrate intakes to fall below 60% for those with T2DM and the metabolic syndrome who have been shown to benefit from diets with more unsaturated fat and lower carbohydrate intake [40]. The ATP III also suggested regular exercise as recommended by the Surgeon General's report and found to be important for maintenance of weight loss.

The Finnish Diabetes Prevention Trial [41] and the Diabetes Prevention Program [42••] employed regimens that embrace the TLC concept of increased exercise, weight loss, and a diet high in fiber and low in saturated fat. Both studies focused on those subjects with impaired fasting glucose. In striking fashion, the nondrug intervention groups in these trials reduced the likelihood of subsequent T2DM by 60%!

Regular exercise was a strong component in both of these trials. In addition to helping maintain weight loss, regular exercise can help raise HDL-C and control TG levels.

Ornish *et al.* [43] reported on a small group of motivated individuals who were given a very low fat diet (less than 10%

TABLE 10 LIPID ABNORMALITIES IN CORONARY DISEASE		
Lipid abnormalities	**Coronary artery disease, %**	**Controls, %**
Low HDL alone	19.3	4.4
High TG/low HDL-C	9.7	4.4
High HDL-C	12.1	9.0
High TG/high LDL/low HDL	3.4	0.2
Lp(a) excess	15.8	10.0

HDL-C—high-density-lipoprotein cholesterol; LDL—low-density lipoprotein; Lp(a)—lipoprotein (a); TG—triglycerides.
Adapted from Genest *et al.* [33].

calories of fat) as well as a program of exercise, cigarette cessation, and stress reduction. At 1 year, the intervention group had a marked weight loss (10 kg), achieved an LDL-C below 100 mg/d, and showed, in contrast to the control group, improvement on serial coronary angiography. Thus, clinicians need to emphasize to patients the value of diet and exercise together to promote a gradual, sustained weight loss.

Behaviors to promote a more healthy overall diet

The ATP III endorsed diets that emphasize fruits, vegetables, fiber, and fish rich in omega 3 fatty acids (Table 11). Most recently diets high in fiber have been shown to reduce both LDL-C and hs-CRP. The American Heart Association (AHA) has issued an advisory recommending increased omega 3 fatty acids in the diet for all patients, with 1 g of omega 3 fatty acids/d for those with CAD [44••]. This recommendation was influenced by secondary prevention trials using fish and fish oils (Diet and Reinfarction Trial [DART] [45], Gruppo Italiano per lo Studio della Sporavvivenza nell'Infarto Miocardico [GISSI] [46] as well as the Lyon trial that utilized the Mediterranean diet supplemented with a plant-based source of omega 3 fatty acids) [47]. All three of these trials have demonstrated a striking reduction in CAD deaths that appears not to be related to improvement in blood lipids. Taken together, this suggests that a "Mediterranean-style" diet with a variety of fruits and vegetables, grains, unsaturated oils, and fish is more heart healthy than the typical American fare of high calories with large servings of animal and dairy fats.

The AHA's latest recommendations for a therapeutic diet are divided into differing components [48]. They recommend an overall healthy eating pattern emphasizing a variety of fruits, vegetables, grains, low-fat or nonfat diary products, fish, legumes, poultry, and lean meats. More individualized approaches involving medical nutrition therapy for specific subgroups such as those who wish to improve body weight, cholesterol, or blood pressure are also given. The Dietary Approach to Stop Hypertension (DASH) diet that emphasized fruits, vegetables, low or nonfat dairy products, and lowered salt intake has been shown to be very effective in lowering blood pressure in men and women with hypertension. No discussion of nonpharmacologic approaches would be complete without mentioning that epidemiologic data show that modest alcohol consumption appears to protect against CHD. Most physicians are not aware that critical analysis of this observational data set does not support an advantage of red versus white wine or beer. Nor does it even prove that there is a causal connection between wine drinking and reduced risk of CAD [49]. The protective effect of alcohol is mediated chiefly through raised HDL-C. Owing to the effects of higher intakes of alcohol in promoting cardiac arrhythmia like atrial fibrillation, heart failure, stroke, liver disease, and fatal accidents, physicians should discuss the benefits as well as the risks and negative aspects with their patients.

Practical advice

Attitude, knowledge, and skills are important prerequisites to behavioral change. Dietary assessment is required to determine progress and can be used in such a way to involve the patient in this behavioral change. Ask the patient if he or she has the specific skills needed to be on a therapeutic diet, such as knowing how to read labels, how to order when eating out, and how to prepare modified fat foods that fit into the diet. Referral to a dietitian is invaluable in helping patients develop the necessary knowledge

TABLE 11 THERAPEUTIC LIFESTYLE CHANGE (ADULT TREATMENT PANEL III)		
Goal	**Features**	**Examples**
Lower LDL-C	Saturated fat < 7% and dietary cholesterol < 200 mg/d; also keep trans-fatty acids low; total fat intake between 25% and 35%	Keep fatty cuts of meats low and use low fat or nonfat dairy products; use higher fiber foods in diet; supplement with plant stanol ester–enriched products for further LCL-C lowering
Treat features of metabolic syndrome	Intensified weight management; increase physical activity; avoid total fat above 25% as this can raise triglycerides and lower HDL-C	Enlist help of registered dieticians for medical nutrition therapy; encourage programs such as Weight Watchers
Eat a healthy diet	More fruits, vegetables, fatty fish approximately two meals/week; high-fiber foods such as breakfast cereals (oatmeal, oatbran, etc.)	See above; talk about healthy substitutes for meals; avoid excess alcohol if patient drinks; for those with CHD, the American Heart Association has endorsed 1 g of omega 3 fatty acids a day

CHD—coronary heart disease; HDL-C—high-density-lipoprotein cholesterol; LDL-C—low-density-lipoprotein cholesterol.

and skills needed for meaningful change. Also programs such as Weight Watchers can be useful in teaching valuable skills about portion control and calorie counting. Two useful means for giving the patient immediate feedback (the equivalent of home glucose monitoring) include keeping a daily food intake diary and wearing a pedometer.

Drug Treatment

When to start and which drug to use?

Drug therapy for abnormal blood lipids/lipoproteins should begin when a patient's risk of CAD is such that lifestyle change is inadequate to reduce the excessive risk. The basis for this treatment is a large number of primary and secondary prevention trials employing a randomized, double-blind, placebo-controlled design.

For primary prevention, careful risk assessment is needed. Since drug therapy entails side effects, potential toxicity, and cost, the decision to begin lifetime treatment needs to be an informed one.

Before beginning drug therapy, it is useful to review with the patient the benefits as contrasted with the negative aspects or risks of such therapy. A young man or woman without other risk factors and an elevated cholesterol and LDL-C with a normal HDL-C may be better managed with lifestyle change. On the other hand, a 60-year-old hypertensive, dyslipidemic diabetic needs agressive treatment of lipid abnormalities without the need for further testing. To help clinicians gauge how to best do this, ATP III believes that determining risk factors, global risk through the Framingham risk score, and then setting LDL-C and non-HDL-C goals is the best way to proceed (Table 4). Some believe that evidence-based treatment with a "polypill" containing a statin, three antihypertensive drugs, aspirin, and folic acid would greatly reduce the coronary burden if given to those over age 55 years [50].

Primary prevention trials

Primary prevention clinical trials have shown that a significant reduction in CAD events can be achieved with cholesterol lowering therapy. The first large-scale trial, the Lipid Research Clinics Primary Prevention Trial, used cholestyramine resin to show that for every 1% the cholesterol was lowered, there was a 2% lowering of coronary risk [51]. The Helsinki Heart Trial used gemfibrozil, a fibrate that raised HDL-C as much as it lowered LDL-C [52]. This too showed a significant reduction in fatal and non-fatal MI. In this trial, most of the benefit occurred in men with a lipid profile characterized by high cholesterol, high TGs, and low HDL-C. These trials were followed by statin primary prevention trials such as the West of Scotland (WOSCOPS) trial [6] that used pravastatin, and the Air Force/Texas Coronary Atherosclerosis Prevention Study (AFCAPS-TEXCAPS) trial [7] that used lovastatin. The former trial used high-risk men whose mean age was 55 years. The latter trial used men older than 45 years and women older than 55 years with low HDL-C and elevated

ratios of cholesterol/HDL-C. Both trials significantly lowered the incidence of fatal and non-fatal MI and the need for revascularization procedures. In the WOSCOPS trial, there was a trend toward improved total mortality ($P = 0.051$). In the ASCOT trial, atorvastatin 10 mg was contrasted to placebo in hypertensive subjects with three or more risk factors and shown to reduce coronary events, such that the trial was halted by a data and safety monitoring committee after 3 years [10]. Taken together, these clinical trial data suggest the benefit of statins in primary prevention subsets with high absolute risks. Of note, in these trials as well as in secondary prevention trials, those subjects with low HDL-C derived more benefit from treatment (as compared with placebo) than those with high HDL-C [53].

Secondary prevention trials

The large size (20,000 subjects) of the HPS study showed convincingly that simvastatin 40 mg/d reduced total mortality, cardiovascular, coronary, and stroke endpoints in high-risk and CAD subjects both above and below the LDL-C goal of 100 mg/dL [8••]. This suggests that in those at very high risk (more than 20% for 10 years) of CAD, statin therapy should be given irrespective of the starting LDL-C level. The ATP III goal of less than 100 mg/dL still is important because the literature taken as a whole supports getting LDL-C down to less than 100 mg/dL even if this requires more than one drug. Based on HPS, however, some hold that there should be an optional goal for LDL-C of 70 mg/dL in this high-risk group. The negative results from the large ALLHAT trial [11], where the difference in LDL-C between treated and controls was only 18%, suggests that effective statin therapy lowers LDL-C by 38.8 mg/dL or more (1 mmol/L) as noted in HPS and in ASCOT [10].

The Veterans Affairs HDL Invervention Trial (VA HIT) trial was a randomized, double-blind trial of gemfibrozil therapy in 2531 men with CAD whose LDL-C was under 140 mg/dL and HDL-C under 40 mg/dL. Despite no lack of significant change in LDL-C between treatment and experimental groups, there was a 22% reduction in relative risk for nonfatal or fatal MI [54,55]. The gemfibrozil group had an HDL-C 6% higher and TG 31% lower than the control group. Of note, there were no significant differences in the rates of coronary revascularization, hospitalization for unstable angina, death from any cause, and cancer. Subsequent studies suggested that the benefit from gemfibrozil was most likely in those whose clinical characteristics suggested the metabolic syndrome [55].

Drug studies using coronary status on serial angiography as an endpoint have shown that aggressive lipid lowering therapy can reduce progression, cause apparent regression, and markedly reduce rates of symptomatic CAD. These angiographic trials have looked at hyperlipidemic, male coronary artery bypass graft (CABG) survivors, men with a family history of CAD and elevated apo B (probably a form

Drug class	Available agents and dose ranges		Lipid/lipoprotein effects	Side effects and practical points	Contraindications and cautions
	Drug	**Dosage**			
3-Hydroxy-3-methylglutaryl-coenzyme A reductase inhibitors (statins)	Lovastatin	20–80 mg/d	Most potent agents to lower LDL-C	Increased liver transaminases (stop statin if > 3 times upper limit of normal)	Absolute: active or chronic liver disease
	Pravastatin	20–80 mg/d	Raise HDL-C 5%–15%		Relative: use carefully with drugs that elevate blood levels (cyclosporine, coumadin); consider P450 interactions; P450: statins; 34A: lovastatin, pravastatin, simvastatin, atorvastatin; 2C9: fluvastatin, rosuvastatin; none: pravastatin
	Simvastatin	20–80 mg/d	Lower TG in proportion to LDL lowering	Myopathy: obtain baseline CK; if muscle weakness and pain, check CK; must stop if CK > 10 upper limit of normal	
	Fluvastatin	20–80 mg/d			
	Atorvastatin	10–80 mg/d			
	Rosuvastatin	5–40 mg/d			
Bile acid sequestrants (resins)	Cholestyramine	4–16 g/d	Lower LDL-C in the 15%–25% range	Gastrointestinal, including bloating, belching, aggravation of hemorrhoids, and constipation; decreased absorption or other drugs	Absolute: TG > 400 mg/dL or type III dysbetalipoproteinemia (first lower TG then add resins)
	Colestipol	5–20 g/d	HDL raised mildly TG are unchanged or can increase		
	Colesevelam	2.6–3.8 g/d			
Selective cholesterol absorption inhibitors	Ezetimibe	10 mg/d	Lower LDL-C an additional 18%–20% when added to statins; HDL may rise slightly; TG may fall slightly	Few side effects; Very rarely angioedema has been reported	Absolute: do not use in severe hypertriglyceridemia; Relative: can't recommend with fibrates until more data available
Niacin or nicotinic acid (not niacinamide)	Immediate release	1.5–3 g/d	Best agents for raising HDL-C (up to 30%–35%)	Prostaglandin-mediated flush, itching, redness	Absolute: chronic liver disease; severe gout
	Extended release	1–2 g/d	Lowers TG and LDL (latter at higher doses)	Hyperglycemia; Hyperuricemia/gout; Gastritis; Hepatotoxicity	Relative: hyperuricemia, peptic ulcer disease
	Sustained	1–2 g/d			
Fibrates	Gemfibrozil	1200 mg (in divided doses of 600 mg)	Major action on TG; up to 50% HDL raised 10%–20%; LDL-C variable (can go up in patients with combined hyperlipidemia)	Gastrointestinal distress; Gallstones (more likely with clofibrate, now rarely used); Myopathy	Absolute: severe renal or hepatic disease (avoid gemfibrozil with statins; fenofibrate is better tolerated)
	Fenofibrate	160 mg/d			

CK—creatine kinase; HDL-C—high-density-lipoprotein cholesterol; LDL-C—low-density-lipoprotein cholesterol; TG—triglycerides.

of combined hyperlipidemia) [56], and both male and female subjects with severe cholesterol elevations due to familial hypercholesterolemia [57]. In these trials, combination therapy with niacin and resin [55], statin and resin or niacin and resin [56], or triple therapy [58] were used. In the Program on the Surgical Control of Hyperlipidemia (POSCH), the use of partial ileal bypass to lower LDL in MI survivors also showed significant results compared with controls [59].

Another angiographic study looked at the value of lowering LDL-C below 100 mg/dL in CABG survivors [60]. In the Post CABG trial, a high-dose lovastatin group that had LDL-C lowered to less than 100 mg/dL had fewer new lesions and the need for revascularization as compared with those treated less aggressively to a much higher average LDL-C.

The Atorvastatin Versus Revascularisation Treatment (AVERT) trial [61] used men with either stage I or II angina who could complete 4 or more minutes on treadmill testing to test the hypothesis that medical treatment with atorvastatin, a potent agent to reduce LDL-C, would result in better outcomes than immediate referral to angioplasty. Twenty-two (13%) of the patients randomized to the atorvastatin group (with a 46% reduction in mean LDL-C to 77 mg/dL) had CAD events, as compared with 37 (21%) of the patients who underwent angioplasty (with an 18% reduction in mean LDL-C to 119 mg/dL.) The incidence of CAD events was thus 36% lower in the atorvastatin group over an 18-month period, but this did not reach statistical significance owing to the "multiple looks" performed during the study. Importantly, the reduction in events was caused by a smaller number of angioplasty procedures, coronary-artery bypass operations, and hospitalizations for worsening angina. As compared with the patients who were treated with angioplasty and usual care, the patients who received atorvastatin had a significantly longer time to the first ischemic event ($P = 0.03$). The Myocardial Ischemia Reduction with Aggressive Cholesterol Lowering (MIRACL) trial examined the benefits of statin therapy in the acute coronary syndrome [62]. In this trial, atorvastatin 80 mg/d was given to subjects on average about 63 hours after admission for an acute coronary syndrome and

lowered LDL-C from 124 mg/dL to 72 mg/dL. Compared with placebo, this aggressive statin treatment significantly reduced the likelihood of readmission for a coronary event in this short-term trial. A new generation of angiographic trials employing intravascular ultrasound is beginning and these should extend our understanding of how lipid therapy benefits the coronary patient.

Drugs that lower low-density lipoprotein cholesterol

The HMG CoA reductase inhibitors (statins) are the most powerful drugs for lowering LDL-C (Table 12). For the patient with multiple risk factors or coronary disease, they may be the most cost-effective because a low dose may allow the LDL-C goal to be met. With increasing dosage, there is less incremental lipid lowering. The older statins (lovastatin, pravastatin, simvastatin) are fungal derived. The newer statins (fluvastatin, atorvastatin, rosuvastatin) are synthetic. All statins lower LDL-C, TGs, and apo B, and raise HDL-C. In addition, there are significant effects on the atherothrombotic process that involve nonlipid mechanisms to varying degrees [63]. Statin therapy can modify endothelial function and inflammatory responses as well as affect determinants of plaque stability and thrombus formation.

Differences exist among statins as well [64] (Table 13). For example, rosuvastatin and atorvastatin have the longest half-lives, which accounts for their pronounced LDL-C lowering [64]. Some are more lipophilic than others. Pravastatin and rosuvastatin are the least lipophilic. Statins are well absorbed, but lovastatin should be taken with food for best results. As a rule, statins should be given at night. All statins lower TG in a constant relationship to their LDL lowering. Thus, the most potent statins to lower LDL-C will lower TG significantly as well (Table 12). Clinicians are cautioned that statins are generally ineffective in lowering TGs in patients with severe hypertriglyceridemia (TG concentrations exceeding 1000 mg/dL).

As a class, these drugs are well tolerated. Side effects include rash, sleep disturbance, gastrointestinal symptoms, and myalgia. Two infrequent, but serious side effects are an

---

TABLE 13 COMPARISON OF 3-HYDROXY-3-METHYLGLUTARYL-COENZYME A REDUCTASE INHIBITORS (STATINS)

Name	Half-life, h	Metabolism	Lipophilic	Renal excretion, %
Atorvastatin	Long, 15–30	CYP3A4	Yes	2
Fluvastatin	Short, 0.5–2.3	CYP2C9	Yes	6
Fluvastatin XL	Short, 4.7	CYP2C9	Yes	Not applicable
Lovastatin	Short, 2.9	CYP3A4	Yes	10
Pravastatin	Short, 1.3–2.8	No P450 metabolism	No	20
Rosuvastatin	Long, 19	CYP2C9	No	28
Simvastatin	Short, 2–3	CYP3A4	Yes	13

Adapted from **Ballantyne** *et al.* [79].

increase in liver transaminases and myositis. There is a low likelihood of liver transaminase rise (< 1%) with initial dosing and liver toxicity was not a significant problem in any of the large-scale statin trials. Low-level liver transaminase rise occurs often, but rises less than 1.5 times the upper limit of normal should not be the basis for cessation of statin therapy. Indeed, with time, the transaminase elevation may recede to the normal range. If liver transaminases exceed two times the upper limit of normal, the value is repeated and attention to causes of transaminase rise is sought. If values for liver transaminases exceed three times the upper limit of normal, they should be repeated; if confirmed, the statin should be stopped. Most often, the reason for a rise in liver enzymes is an interaction with another drug, alcohol, or other causes such as fatty liver. Statins do not increase the risk of gallstones.

Muscle problems with statins can range from nonspecific muscle aches and pains with normal creatine kinase (CK) values to full-blown myositis with prolonged or severe muscle weakness, elevated creatinine progressing to renal failure, and even death [65]. The risk of such a reaction can be exacerbated by abnormal liver, renal, or thyroid function and particularly in the presence of other medications that have been shown under certain circumstances to have an adverse interaction with statins. Drugs that should be used carefully are cyclosporine, fibrates, and niacin. The P450 interaction is discussed below. When confirmed CK values exceed 10 times the upper limit of normal, statin therapy should be stopped and the patient hydrated. When CK values are between three and 10 times the upper limit of normal, clinical judgment is required as to whether the therapy should be reduced, switched to another statin, or whether to avoid statins entirely. For those with muscle aching and only borderline CK elevations, attention to muscular trauma (very common), hypothyroidism, or even a rheumatologic evaluation can be useful in distinguishing whether a reason to change medication is present. Weakness and progressive elevations in CK are important clinical signals that the patient needs careful scrutiny to determine exactly whether this is a muscle, drug, or systemic problem.

There are several types of drug interactions. First, some drugs must be used cautiously with all statins. These are cyclosporine and warfarin. Statins can be used in those on cyclosporine, but it is wise to start at a low statin dose and increase carefully since statin concentrations are raised by cyclosporine. Likewise, when any statin is added to a patient on warfarin, a protime should be check within 2 to 3 days to see how this affects the international normalized ratio (INR). Second, an increasingly important interaction is that of statins with drugs that are also metabolized by the P450 cytochrome system. For example, lovastatin, simvastatin, and atorvastatin are metabolized by P450 3A4, the predominant P450 system in the liver. Levels of these drugs would be significantly affected by clarithromycin, erythromycin, ketoconazole, certain protease inhibitors, and even large amounts of grapefruit juice, which are inhibitors

of this pathway. Fluvastatin rosuvastatin (although minimally so) are metabolized by the cytochrome P450 2C9 system. Fluconazole is an inhibitor of this pathway and so should be avoided with these drugs. If the P450 interaction is not considered, the higher statin concentrations produced make side effects more likely [63]. Conversely, drugs that are inducers of this system, like barbiturates and carbamazepine, can reduce statin concentrations Pravastatin is not metabolized by the P450 cytochrome system and has no penetration of the central nervous system. Finally, gemfibrozil competes with statins for a glucuronidation pathway. This does not occur with fenofibrate [66].

The most important rule for avoiding toxicity with statin drugs is to be observant for "high-risk" patients who are more likely to get into trouble with drug toxicity or interactions. This means particular care must be taken with the elderly; women, particularly if frail or of small stature; those on complex, multidrug regimens; those with multiple illnesses; and statin use at the time of surgery or acute medical crises.

Gastrointestinal-active drugs such as bile acid sequestrants or resins bind bile acids in the intestine, prevent their ileal absorption, and thereby shrink the hepatic cholesterol pool as more bile acid production from cholesterol is required. This produces a beneficial increase in LDL receptors. These drugs may be particularly useful in two situations. First, they augment statins in lowering LDL-C and are a mainstay of the combined treatment of those with familial hypercholesterolemia. Second, due to their enviable safety record because they are not absorbed and hence nonsystemic, they are the drugs of choice for patients with diet-resistant high LDL-C for whom statin therapy may be problematic (those with statin intolerance, young women who wish to avoid statins due to the pregnancy risks, and young patients who want to avoid a systemic drug due to their young age). The available resins are the older cholestyramine and colestipol, dry powders that are mixed with fluids, and a gel capsule called colesevelam. They raise TG and should not be started if TG values are over 300 mg/dL. Patient tolerability can be a problem due to gastrointestinal side effects such as constipation, bloating, and aggravation of hemorrhoids. Resins should be started at low dosage and increased in gradual fashion to optimize patient tolerance. Mixing psyllium powder with a resin amplifies the LDL-C-lowering effect of the resin. They can bind other drugs (particularly digoxin and thyroid) and must be taken at least 60 minutes after or 3 to 4 hours before other drugs. Particular care must be taken if the patient is on warfarin.

A gastrointestinal-active drug that selectively impairs cholesterol absorption and so does not increase TG or bind other drugs is ezetimibe. It is taken once daily in a single dose of 10 mg/d and can augment lowering of LDC-C by statins by 18% to 20% [67]. This is substantial because it is equivalent to three doublings of the statin dosage (each doubling of a statin only lowers LDL-C by an additional 6%–7%).

Drugs that raise high-density lipoprotein cholesterol

Nicotinic acid preparations (niacin) offer excellent lipid lowering alternatives because they raise HDL, lower LDL-C, and lower TGs. These are the best drugs for raising HDL-C, and gains of 30% can be realized. Unlike statins, niacin lowers Lp(a). Niacinamide is another form of the vitamin, but it is not a lipid-lowering drug and should not be substituted for niacin. At low dosages, the effects of niacin on HDL-C and TGs are more readily seen than effects on LDL-C, which often require higher dosages. Niacin dosage should be increased in a scheduled manner to allow for patient acceptance of the vasodilator side effects. The flushing, redness, warmth, and even itching that can occur are prostaglandin mediated and alleviated by either taking an aspirin about 1 hour before or using an extended or sustained release. Immediate release niacin has the advantage of low cost, but must be taken two to three times daily with meals. The sustained release forms have had more hepatotoxicity compared with the immediate release. A newer time-release form given at bedtime appears to be well tolerated. In a study comparing 500 mg three times daily of unmodified niacin with 1.5 grams of this newer formulation, there was comparable efficacy, fewer episodes of flushing, a lesser uric acid rise, and an equivalent liver enzyme rise [68].

Monitoring of blood sugar, uric acid, and a liver panel every 3 to 4 months is prudent on niacin therapy. Marked lowering of total cholesterol and LDL-C that seems too good to be true should alert the clinician to underlying niacin-induced hepatotoxicity [69]. Patients should never switch from a dose of unmodified niacin to a long-acting niacin without beginning the titration sequence at a low niacin dosage, because toxicity can occur when an equivalent dose of long-acting niacin is substituted for a dose of unmodified niacin. Niacin can cause gout in those prone to hyperuricemia. It increases hepatic glucose output and can aggravate diabetic control. It is best avoided in those with borderline blood sugars not yet at the diabetic range. In those on diabetic medications, however, crystalline niacin and the time-release form of niacin are shown to be well tolerated and effective in improving lipids. Finally, niacin can raise homocysteine, although the significance is uncertain.

Niacin was shown in the Coronary Drug Project almost 30 years ago to reduce coronary morbidity in long-term follow-up, and even total mortality [70]. It has helped reduce angiographic as well as clinical endpoint rates when added to resins or simvastatin in two carefully done angiographic trials [71,72]. In the latter trial, antioxidant vitamins blocked the beneficial effects of niacin on HDL due to the interference with niacin's beneficial effects on HDL [73••].

Drugs that lower triglycerides

Fibric acid derivatives, such as gemfibrozil and fenofibrate, are drugs of choice in those with severe TG elevations (over 800 mg/dL) that could lead to acute pancreatitis. Fibrates are effective in coronary prevention in those with the metabolic syndrome or T2DM who do not have increased LDL-C. The beneficial effects of fibrates are likely due to their effect on the peroxisome proliferator activator receptors (PPAR) alpha system [74]. These ligand-activated transcription factors lead to increased synthesis of lipoprotein lipase (key enzyme that metabolizes TGs), apo A-I, A-II (major proteins of HDL), and reduction in apo CIII (inhibitor of lipoprotein lipase). These actions lower TG and raise HDL-C, but the effects on LDL-C are variable. Fenofibrate lowers LDL-C more than gemfibrozil in those with high LDL-C and normal TGs, but in those with elevated TGs, the shift from small to large LDL particles may cause the LDL-C to rise.

An emerging role in coronary prevention is developing. Gemfibrozil proved better than placebo in preventing first CAD events in men with high cholesterol and TGs in the Helsinki Heart Primary Prevention trial [52] and in preventing recurrent events in VA HIT [54]. In these studies, men who benefited from fibrate therapy had low HDL-C and high TGs. While the drugs proved safe in the above clinical trials, they should not be given if there is impaired renal or hepatic function. Both gemfibrozil and fenofibrate are not as lithogenic as clofibrate, but a small increased risk for gallstones appears to remain. An important difference in gemfibrozil and fenofibrate pertains to their ability to affect the glucuronidation of statins. Thus, fenofibrate is the fibrate of choice if combination with a statin is deemed desirable. Gemfibrozil is given as 600 mg tablets taken twice daily. Fenofibrate is available as a 54 mg pill and a maximal dose pill of 160 mg.

Fish oils (omega 3 fatty acids) lower TGs and are useful as adjunctive therapy when the patient presents with severe hypertriglyceridemia [68]. The dose is usually 3 to 4 g per day. In those with combined hyperlipidemia, fish oil can increase LDL-C levels similar to that seen with fibrate therapy. For those who have survived an MI, fish oil capsules (about 1 g of eicosapentaenoic acid [EPA] and docosahexanoic acid [DHA]) have been shown to lower CHD death rates in two large-scale trials.

Combination therapy is most valuable in three situations. The first situation is when LDL-C is so high that very large dosages of a single drug would be needed, possibly increasing toxicity. Here the addition of a resin (and occasionally niacin as well) may be required to control the marked LDL-C excess seen in familial hypercholesterolemia. The second situation is when lower doses of two drugs would minimize cost or side effects. An example would be adding a gastrointestinal-active drug to an initial dose of a statin. And the third situation is when multiple lipid abnormalities prevent a single lipid-lowering drug from sufficing. This is seen often in familial combined hyperlipidemia (FCHL). Statin therapy in hypertriglyceridemic patients decreases LDL-C and remnant lipoproteins [75]. However, statin therapy does not normalize LDL apo B metabolism or depressed HDL-C. Therefore, in high-risk patients with FCHL, there may be a therapeutic advantage to combining a statin with a drug that improves TG and HDL metabolism such as niacin or a fibrate. Since there is some increased risk from either liver toxicity or myositis with these combinations, these patients must be chosen and monitored carefully. Since a trial of diet and regular exercise designed to lose excess weight can improve HDL-C and TGs, this should be recommended prior to such therapy. In one small trial comparing lovastatin and gemfibrozil in FCHL patients, target LDL-C levels were achieved only in 11% of patients given gemfibrozil alone and target TG levels were achieved in 22% after lovastatin alone, whereas combined therapy normalized both lipid fractions in 96% of patients [76].

Treatment of low high-density lipoprotein cholesterol

Treatment of isolated low HDL-C is a controversial subject. Essentially, those with low HDL-C can be divided into three groupings based on global CAD risk. Life-long vegetarians with low HDL-C, LDL-C, and blood pressure are at low risk of near-term CAD events and do not require drug therapy. On the other hand, in those with risk factors, after behavioral therapy (quitting smoking, losing excess weight, avoiding excessive carbohydrates in the diet, and exercising regularly), statin therapy should be strongly considered. In middle-aged and older subjects with low HDL-C, lovastatin therapy reduced risk of first CAD event in the AFCAPS/TEXCAPS trial that selected subjects on the basis of a low HDL-C [7]. In an analysis of many of the recent statin trials, treatment with statins in those with low HDL-C lowers their risk to comparable subjects in the placebo group without low HDL-C [53]. The third group, those with CAD, also requires attention to HDL-C. In this group, treating elevated LDL-C and non-HDL-C are the first two goals of therapy. This usually involves a statin. Clinical trial data suggest that if HDL-C is still low, adding niacin or a fibrate would be beneficial. In coronary patients with low LDL-C to begin, the VA HIT trial showed beneficial effects of gemfibrozil (fibrate) therapy [46].

WHEN TO REFER

Primary care physicians as well as cardiologists should initiate drug therapy to lower LDL-C in patients who have documented atherosclerotic disease in the coronary, cerebral, or peripheral vascular circulation. Referral to a lipid specialist may be useful in cases where LDL-C goals are not met due to the severity of the hyperlipidemia or where a combination of therapies is required due to abnormalities in TGs and HDL-C as well. Lipid specialists can be particularly useful in cases where genetic abnormalities have made either diagnosis or successful treatment difficult to achieve. LDL apheresis, for example, may be indicated in those with CAD and LDL above 200 mg/dL despite ther-

apy. This requires a center with special experience in this technique. In those patients with TG values over 800 mg/dL, the concern is also for preventing acute pancreatitis. Indeed, hyperlipidemic pancreatitis can be difficult to treat and referral may be useful in this setting as well.

CURRENT CONTROVERSIES

How to define high-risk patients who require primary prevention with drug therapy is still controversial. Primary care physicians can take a careful family history and review the tally of risk factors. The roles of risk factor scores, measures of inflammation such as ultrasensitive C-reactive protein, carotid artery imaging, electron beam computed tomography, and ultrasonic evaluation of brachial artery endothelial function are still being determined. The ideal technique will be priced reasonably, add to the prediction of CAD beyond that of the lipid panel (cholesterol, TG, HDL-C, and LDL-C), and have acceptable precision and accuracy. The other controversy relates to drug therapy. Should statins be given to an ever wider circle of patients that includes younger as well as elderly patients? More information as to the benefits and risks is needed before this can be determined accurately.

A continuing controversy has been whether to start statins in-hospital and how big a statin dose should be given to those with acute coronary syndrome. The large-scale Pravastatin or Atorvastatin Evaluation and Infection Therapy (PROVE-IT) trial selected approximately 4000 subjects with recent hospitalization for an acute coronary syndrome and a median LDL-C of 108 mg/dL measured within 10 days of admission. During a mean follow-up of 24 months, the subjects receiving the intensive therapy with atorvastatin 80 mg achieved a median LDL-C of 62 mg/dL. The subjects treated with "standard" therapy with pravastatin 40 mg reached a median LDL-C of 95 mg/dL. The primary composite outcome (death from MI or any cause, revascularization need, and stroke) was reduced by 26.3% in the pravastatin group and 22.4% in the atorvastatin group, reflecting a highly significant 16% reduction in the hazard ratio in the atorvastatin arm. While awaiting other studies on acute coronary syndrome that are currently under way, aggressive treatment with a statin dose designed to lower LDL-C levels substantially in the coronary care unit seems reasonable based on these data. For those with a particularly heavy burden of risk (eg, diabetics with heart disease, heavy smokers with peripheral vascular disease), a lower optional LDL-C goal of about 70 mg/dL would be reasonable.

PREVENTION

Primary care physicians can stress diet and exercise and smoking cessation at each primary care visit. As part of the vital signs, the nurse or assistant can ask if the patient has thought about improving their lifestyle and is prepared to change. Poor diet, tobacco usage, and sedentary behavior can be noted along with blood pressure, pulse, and weight. Physicians can reinforce their willingness to help the patient change when he or she is ready. Although the advances in secondary prevention have been notable, prevention of obesity, marked diminution in smoking rates, and a healthier overall diet are achievable and desirable goals for the patient with hyperlipidemia.

CONCLUSION

This chapter has stressed the important strides that have been made in controlling CAD through lipid-lowering strategies. Primary care physicians should focus on elucidation and control of treatable risk factors. The endorsement of a healthier diet and regular exercise can help reduce obesity and strongly impact the risk factor profile by reducing hypertension, hyperlipidemia, and glucose intolerance. Lowering LDL-C deserves the highest priority in the patient shown to have CAD. The benefit of lipid lowering has been shown to extend to both women and men, patients both older and younger than 65 years, and patients with diabetes as well. Diabetics, with their multitude of risk factors, are prime examples that CAD is indeed a multifactorial disease [77].

KEY REFERENCES

Recently published papers of outstanding interest, as identified in *References and Recommended Reading*, have been annotated.

•• MRC/BHF Heart Protection Study of cholesterol lowering with simvastatin in 20,536 high-risk individuals: a randomised placebo-controlled trial. *Lancet* 2002, 360:7–22.

Blockbuster clinical trial showing that in high-risk subjects (CAD or CAD risk equivalents essentially) there is great clinical benefit in using simvastatin 40 mg whether the LDL-C was above or below 116 mg/dL.

•• Nissen SE, Tsunoda T, Tuzcu EM, *et al.*: Effect of recombinant Apo A-I Milano on coronary atherosclerosis in patients with acute coronary syndromes: a randomized controlled trial. *JAMA* 2003, 290:292–300.

Provocative study that raises the question as to whether acute intervention with HDL-raising therapies may be of value in the coronary syndrome. Larger scale, adequately controlled studies are needed before firm conclusions can be made as to the value of this therapy.

•• Diabetes Prevention Program Research Group: Reduction in the incidence of type 2 diabetes with lifestyle intervention or metformin. *N Engl J Med* 2002, 346:393–403.

A landmark trial that emphasizes the importance of lifestyle change in preventing progression to diabetes in those with impaired glucose tolerance.

•• Cheung MC, Zhao XQ, Chait A, *et al.*: Antioxidant supplements block the response of HDL to simvastatin-niacin therapy in patients with coronary artery disease and low HDL. *Arterioscler Thromb Vasc Biol* 2001, 21:1320–1326.

Demonstrates the value of obtaining clinical trial data before empirically recommending therapy. In this carefully done angiographic trial of subjects with CAD and low HDL-C, an antioxidant vitamin combination was shown to block niacin's beneficial action on HDL-C and cause less angiographic and clinical improvement in the niacin-simvastatin combination group.

•• Cannon CP, Braunwald E, McCabe CH, *et al.*: Comparison of intensive and moderate lipid lowering with statins after acute coronary syndromes. *N Engl J Med* 2004, 350:1495–1504.

Important study to read in the entirety. Established that in high-risk, acute coronary syndrome subjects, getting all to values for LDL-C under 100 mg/dL (and if possible to 70 mg/dL) is associated with greater benefit than a statin intervention that does not lower LDL-C as substantially.

REFERENCES AND RECOMMENDED READING

Recently published papers of particular interest have been highlighted as:
• Of interest
•• Of outstanding interest

1. Burke AP, Farb A, Malcolm GT, *et al.*: Coronary risk factors and plaque morphology in patients with coronary disease dying suddenly. *N Engl J Med* 1997, 336:1276–1282.

2. Brown BG, Zhao XQ, Sacco DE, Albers JJ: Arteriographic view of treatment to achieve regression of coronary atherosclerosis and to prevent plaque disruption and clinical cardiovascular events. *Br Heart J* 1993, 69(suppl 1):S48–S53.

3. Scandinavian Simvastatin Survival Study Group: Randomized trial of cholesterol lowering in 4444 patient with coronary heart disease: the Scandinavian Simvastatin Survival Study (4S). *Lancet* 1994, 269:3015–3023.

4. The Long-Term Intervention with Pravastatin in Ischaemic Disease (LIPID) Study Group: Prevention of cardiovascular events and death with pravastatin in patients with coronary heart disease and a broad range of initial cholesterol levels. *N Engl J Med* 1998, 339:1349–1357.

5. Sacks FM, Pfeffer MA, Moye LA, *et al.*: The effect of pravastatin on coronary events after myocardial infarction in patients with average cholesterol levels. *N Engl J Med* 1996, 335:1001–1009.

6. Shepherd J, Cobbe SM, Ford I, *et al.*, for the West of Scotland Coronary Prevention Study Group: Prevention of coronary heart disease with pravastatin in men with hypercholesterolemia. *N Engl J Med* 1995, 333:1301–1307.

7. Downs JR, Clearfield M, Weis S, *et al.*: Primary prevention of acute coronary events with lovastatin in men and women with average cholesterol levels: results of AFCAPS/TexCAPS. Air Force/Texas Coronary Atherosclerosis Prevention Study. *JAMA* 1998, 279:1615–1622.

8.•• MRC/BHF Heart Protection Study of cholesterol lowering with simvastatin in 20,536 high-risk individuals: a randomised placebo-controlled trial. *Lancet* 2002, 360:7–22.

9. Shepherd J, Blauw GJ, Murphy MB, *et al*, on behalf of the PROSPER study group: Pravastatin in elderly individuals at risk of vascular disease (PROSPER): a randomised controlled trial. *Lancet* 2002, 360:1623–1630.

10. Sever PS, Dahlof B, Poulter NR, *et al.*: Prevention of coronary and stroke events with atorvastatin in hypertensive patients who have average or lower-than-average cholesterol concentrations, in the Anglo-Scandinavian Cardiac Outcomes Trial–Lipid Lowering Arm (ASCOT-LLA): a multicentre randomised controlled trial. *Lancet* 2003, 361:1149–1158.

11. Writing Group: Major outcomes in moderately hypercholesterolemic, hypertensive patients randomized to pravastatin vs usual care: The Antihypertensive and Lipid-Lowering Treatment to Prevent Heart Attack Trial (ALLHAT-LLT). *JAMA* 2002, 288:2998–3007.

12. Tamai O, Matsuoka H, Itabe H, *et al.*: Single LDL apheresis improves endothelium-dependent vasodilatation in hypercholesterolemic humans. *Circulation* 1997 95:76–82.

13. de Lorgeril M, Salen P, Martin J-L, *et al.*: Mediterranean diet, traditional risk factors and the rate of cardiovascular complications after myocardial infarction. *Circulation* 1999, 99:779–785.

14. Aviram M, Rosenblat M, Bisgaier CL, *et al.*: Paraoxonase inhibits high-density lipoprotein oxidation and preserves its functions. A possible peroxidative role for paroxonase. *J Clin Invest* 1998, 101:1581–1590.

15. Cockerill GW, Saklatvala J, Ridley SH, *et al.*: High-density lipoproteins differentially modulate cytokine-induced expression of E-selectin and cyclooxygenase-2. *Arterioscler Thromb Vasc Biol* 1999, 19:910–917.

16. Saku K, Ahmad M, Glas-Greenwalt P, Kashyap ML: Activation of fibrinolysis by apolipoproteins of high density lipoproteins in man. *Thromb Res* 1985, 39:1–8.

17.•• Nissen SE, Tsunoda T, Tuzcu EM, *et al.*: Effect of recombinant ApoA-I Milano on coronary atherosclerosis in patients with acute coronary syndromes: a randomized controlled trial. *JAMA* 2003, 290:292–300.

18. Hackam DG, Anand SS. Emerging risk factors for atherosclerotic vascular disease: a critical review of the evidence. *JAMA* 2003, 290:932–940.

19. Danesh J, Collins R, Peto R: Lipoprotein(a) and coronary heart disease: meta-analysis of prospective studies. *Circulation* 2000,102:1082–1085.

20. Maher VM, Brown BG, Marcovina SM, *et al.*: Effects of lowering elevated LDL cholesterol on the cardiovascular risk of lipoprotein(a). *JAMA* 1995, 274:1771–1774.

21. Lamon-Fava S, Wilson PW, Schaefer EJ: Impact on body mass index on coronary heart disease in men and women in the Framingham Offspring Study. *Arterioscler Thromb Vasc Biol* 1996, 16:1509–1515.

22. Lemieux I, Pascot A, Couillard C, *et al.*: Hypertriglyceridemic waist: a marker of the atherogenic metabolic triad (hyperinsulinemia; hyperapolipoprotein B; small, dense LDL) in men. *Circulation* 2000, 102:179–184.

23. Ridker PM: High-sensitivity C-reactive protein and cardiovascular risk: rationale for screening and primary prevention. *Am J Cardiol* 2003, 92:17K–22K.

24. Ridker PM, Buring JE, Cook NR, Rifai N: C-reactive protein, the metabolic syndrome, and risk of incident cardiovascular events: an 8-year follow-up of 14 719 initially healthy American women. *Circulation* 2003, 107:391–397.

25. Executive Summary of the Third Report of the National Cholesterol Education Program (NCEP) Expert Panel on Detection, Evaluation, and Treatment of High Blood Cholesterol in Adults (AdultTreatment Panel III). *JAMA* 2001, 285:2486–2497.

26. Ginsburg GS, Safran C, Pasternak RC: Frequency of low serum high-density lipoprotein cholesterol levels in hospitalized patients with "desirable" total cholesterol levels. *Am J Cardiol* 1991, 68:187–192.

27. Gidding SS, Stone NJ, Bookstein LC, *et al.*: Month-to-month variability of lipids, lipoproteins, and apolipoproteins and the impact of acute infection in adolescents. *J Pediatr* 1998, 133:242–246.

28. Gore JM, Goldberg RJ, Matsumoto AS, *et al.*: Validity of serum total cholesterol level obtained within 24 hours of acute myocardial infarction. *Am J Cardiol* 1984, 54:722–725.

29. Avogaro P, Bon GB, Cazzolato G, *et al.*: Variations in apolipoproteins B and A1 during the course of myocardial infarction. *Eur J Clin Invest* 1978, 8:121–129.

30. Aronow HD, Novaro GM, Lauer MS, *et al.*: In-hospital initiation of lipid-lowering therapy after coronary intervention as a predictor of long-term utilization: a propensity analysis. *Arch Intern Med* 2003, 163:2576–2582.

31. Kaplan NM: The deadly quartet. Upper-body obesity, glucose intolerance, hypertriglyceridemia, and hypertension. *Arch Intern Med* 1989, 149:1514–1520.

32. Goldstein JL, Hazzard WR, Schrott HG, *et al.*: Hyperlipidemia in coronary heart disease. I. Lipid levels in 500 survivors of myocardial infarction. *J Clin Invest* 1973, 52:1533–1543.

33. Genest J, McNamara JR, Ordovas JM, *et al.*: Lipoprotein cholesterol, apolipoprotein A-I and B and lipoprotein (a) abnormalities in men with premature coronary disease. *J Am Coll Cardiol* 1992, 19:792–802.

34. Walsh BW, Schiff I, Rosner B, *et al.*: Effects of postmenopausal estrogen replacement on the concentrations and metabolism of plasma. *N Engl J Med* 1991, 325:1196–1204.

35. Hulley S, Grady D, Bush T, *et al.*, for the Heart and Estrogen/Progestin Replacement Study (HERS) Research Group: Randomized trial of estrogen plus progestin for secondary prevention of coronary heart disease in postmenopausal women. *JAMA* 1998, 280:605–613.

36. Writing Group for the Women's Health Initiative Investigators: Risks and benefits of estrogen plus progestin in healthy postmenopausal women. *JAMA* 2002, 288:321–333.

37. Jenkins DJ, Kendall CW, Marchie A, *et al.*: Effects of a dietary portfolio of cholesterol-lowering foods vs lovastatin on serum lipids and C-reactive protein. *JAMA* 2003, 290:502–510.

38. Watts GF, Lewis B, Brunt JN, *et al.*: Effects on coronary artery disease of lipid-lowering diet, or diet plus cholestyramine, in the St. Thomas' Atherosclerosis Regression Study (STARS). *Lancet* 1992, 339:563–569.

39. Knopp RH, Walden CE, Retzlaff BM, *et al.*: Long-term cholesterol-lowering effects of 4 fat-restricted diets in hypercholesterolemic and combined hyperlipidemic men. The Dietary Alternatives Study. *JAMA* 1997, 278:1509–1515.

40. Garg A: High-monounsaturated-fat diets for patients with diabetes mellitus: a meta-analysis. *Am J Clin Nutr* 1998, 67(suppl 3):577S–582S.

41. Tuomilehto J, Lindstrom J, Eriksson JG, *et al.*, the Finnish Diabetes Prevention Study Group: Prevention of type 2 diabetes mellitus by changes in lifestyle among subjects with impaired glucose tolerance. *N Engl J Med* 2001, 344:1343–1350.

42.•• Diabetes Prevention Program Research Group: Reduction in the incidence of type 2 diabetes with lifestyle intervention or metformin. *N Engl J Med* 2002, 346:393–403.

43. Ornish D, Brown SE, Scherwitz LW, *et al.*: Can lifestyle changes reverse coronary heart disease? The Lifestyle Heart Trial. *Lancet* 1990, 336:129–133.

44.•• Kris-Etherton PM, Harris WS, Appel LJ: Fish consumption, fish oil, omega-3 fatty acids, and cardiovascular disease. *Circulation* 2002,106:2747–2757.

45. Burr ML, Fehily AM, Gilbert JF, *et al.*: Effects of changes in fat, fish, and fibre intakes on death and myocardial reinfarction: diet and reinfarction trial (DART). *Lancet* 1989, 2:757–761.

46. Marchioli R, Barzi F, Bomba E, *et al.*: Early protection against sudden death by n-3 polyunsaturated fatty acids after myocardial infarction: time-course analysis of the results of the Gruppo Italiano per lo Studio della Sopravvivenza nell'Infarto Miocardico (GISSI)-Prevenzione. *Circulation* 2002, 105:1897–1903.

47. de Lorgeril M, Salen P, Martin JL, *et al.*: Mediterranean diet, traditional risk factors, and the rate of cardiovascular complications after myocardial infarction: final report of the Lyon Diet Heart Study. *Circulation* 1999, 99:779–785.

48. Krauss RM, Eckel RH, Howard B, *et al.*: AHA Dietary Guidelines: revision 2000: a statement for healthcare professionals from the Nutrition Committee of the American Heart Association. *Circulation* 2000, 102:2284–2299.

49. Goldberg IJ, Mosca L, Piano MR, Fisher EA; Nutrition Committee, Council on Epidemiology and Prevention, and Council on Cardiovascular Nursing of the American Heart Association: AHA Science Advisory: wine and your heart: a science advisory for healthcare professionals from the Nutrition Committee, Council on Epidemiology and Prevention, and Council on Cardiovascular Nursing of the American Heart Association. *Circulation* 2001, 103:472–475.

50. Wald NJ, Law MR: A strategy to reduce cardiovascular disease by more than 80%. *BMJ* 2003, 326:1419–1423.

51. Lipid Research Clinics Program: The Lipid Research Clinics Coronary Primary Prevention Trial Result. I. Reduction in incidence of coronary heart disease. *JAMA* 1984, 251:351–364.

52. Frick MH, Eto O, Haapa K, *et al.*: Helsinki Heart Study: Primary prevention trial with gemfibrozil in middle-aged men with dyslipidemia. *N Engl J Med* 1987, 317:1237–1245.

53. Ballantyne CM, Herd JA, Ferlic LL, *et al.*: Influence of low HDL on progression of coronary artery disease and response to fluvastatin therapy. *Circulation* 1999, 99:736–743.

54. Rubins HB, Robins SJ, Collins D, *et al.*: Gemfibrozil for the secondary prevention of coronary heart disease in men with low levels of high-density lipoprotein cholesterol. *N Engl J Med* 1999, 341:410–418.

55. Robins SJ, Rubins HB, Faas FH, *et al.*: Insulin resistance and cardiovascular events with low HDL cholesterol: the Veterans Affairs HDL Intervention Trial (VA-HIT). *Diabetes Care* 2003, 26:1513–1517.

56. Cashin-Hemphill L, Mack WJ, Pogoda JM, *et al.*: Beneficial effects of colestipol-niacin on coronary atherosclerosis. A 4-year follow-up. *JAMA* 1990, 264:3013–3017.

57. Brown G, Albers JJ, Fisher LD, *et al.*: Regression of coronary artery disease as a result of interim lipid-lowering therapy in men with high levels of apolipoprotein B. *N Engl J Med* 1990, 323:1289–1298.

58. Kane JP, Malloy MJ, Ports TA, *et al.*: Regression of coronary atherosclerosis during treatment of familial hypercholesterolemia with combined drug regimens. *JAMA* 1990, 264:3007–3012.

59. Buchwald H, Varco RL, Matts JP, *et al.*: Effect of partial ileal bypass surgery on mortality and morbidity from coronary heart disease in patients with hypercholesterolemia. *N Engl J Med* 1990, 323:946–955.

60. The Post Coronary Artery Bypass Graft Trial Investigators: The effect of aggressive lowering of low-density lipoprotein cholesterol levels and low-dose anticoagulation on obstructive changes in saphenous-vein coronary artery bypass grafts. *N Engl J Med* 1997, 336:153–162.

61. Pitt B, Waters D, Brown WV, *et al.*: Aggressive lipid-lowering therapy compared with angioplasty in stable coronary artery disease. *N Engl J Med* 1999, 341:70–76.

62. Schwartz GG, Olsson AG, Ezekowitz MD, *et al.*, Myocardial Ischemia Reduction with Aggressive Cholesterol Lowering (MIRACL) Study Investigators: Effects of atorvastatin on early recurrent ischemic events in acute coronary syndromes: the MIRACL study: a randomized controlled trial. *JAMA* 2001, 285:1711–1718.

63. Rosenson RS, Tangney CC: Antiatherothrombotic properties of statins: implications for cardiovascular event reduction. *JAMA* 1998, 279:1643–1650.

64. Knopp RH: Drug treatment of lipid disorders. *N Engl J Med* 1999, 341:498–511.

65. Thompson PD, Clarkson P, Karas RH: Statin-associated myopathy. *JAMA* 2003, 289:1681–1690.

66. Prueksaritanont, T, Subramanian R, Fang X, *et al.*: Glucuronidation of statins in animals and humans: a novel mechanism of statin lactonization. *Drug Metab Dispos* 2002, 30:505–512.

67. Stone N: Combination therapy: its rationale and the role of ezetimibe. *Eur Heart J Suppl* 2002, 4(suppl J): J19–J22.

68. Knopp RH, Alagona P, Davidson M, *et al.*: Equivalent efficacy of a time-release form of niacin (Niaspan) given once-a-night versus plain niacin in the management of hyperlipidemia. *Metabolism* 1998, 47:1097–1104.

69. Tato F, Vega GL, Grundy SM: Effects of crystalline nicotinic acid-induced hepatic dysfunction on serum low-density lipoprotein cholesterol and lecithin cholesteryl acyl transferase. *Am J Cardiol* 1998, 81:805–807.

70. Canner PL, Berge KG, Wenger NK, *et al*: Fifteen year mortality in Coronary Drug Project patients: long-term benefit with niacin. *J Am Coll Cardiol* 1986, 8:1245–1255.

71. Brown G, Albers JJ, Fisher LD, *et al.*: Regression of coronary artery disease as a result of intensive lipid-lowering therapy in men with high levels of apolipoprotein B. *N Engl J Med* 1990, 323:1289–1298.

72. Brown BG, Zhao XQ, Chait A, *et al.*: Simvastatin and niacin, antioxidant vitamins, or the combination for the prevention of coronary disease. *N Engl J Med* 2001, 345:1583–1592.

73.•• Cheung MC, Zhao XQ, Chait A, *et al.*: Antiioxidant supplements block the response of HDL to simvastatin-niacin therapy in patients with coronary artery disease and low HDL. *Arterioscler Thromb Vasc Biol* 2001, 21:1320–1326.

74. Barbier O, Torra IP, Duguay Y, *et al.*: Pleiotropic actions of peroxisome proliferator-activated receptors in lipid metabolism and atherosclerosis. *Arterioscler Thromb Vasc Biol* 2002, 22:717–726.

75. Vega GL, Grundy SM: Effect of statins on metabolism of apo-B-containing lipoproteins in hypertriglyceridemic men. *Am J Cardiol* 1998, 81:36B–42B.

76. Vega GL, Grundy SM: Comparison of lovastatin and gemfibrozil in normolipidemic patients with hypoalphalipoproteinemia. *JAMA* 1989, 262:3148–3153.

77. Badimon JJ, Fuster V, Chesebro JH, Badimon L: Coronary atherosclerosis. A multifactorial disease. *Circulation* 1993, 87(suppl 2):2-3–2-16.

78. Pathophysiology of hyperproteineimia. In *Management of Lipids in Clinical Practice*, edn 4. Edited by Stone NJ, Blum CB. Caddo, OK: Professional Communications, Inc.; 2002.

79. Ballantyne CM, Corsini A, Davidson MH, *et al.*: Risk for myopathy with statin therapy in high-risk patients. *Arch Intern Med* 2003, 163:553–564.

Evaluation and Management of the Patient with Hypertension
Robert G. Luke

15

> ### Key Points
> - The primary care physician plays the key role in the detection, assessment, and treatment of essential (primary) hypertension. Screening is cost effective.
> - Ninety percent of all hypertension is primary; 5% to 10% is secondary.
> - Secondary hypertension mainly results from renal or renovascular disease. Clinical features identify a minority of patients for work-up for these and other causes.
> - High normal blood pressures and stage 1 hypertension respond well to nonpharmacologic measures such as dietary modifications and exercise.
> - Pharmacologic intervention is usually lifelong.
> - Many patients can now be treated with a single daily dose of a single drug with no or minimal side effects.
> - Antihypertensive drugs are currently underutilized, but are safe, effective, and can substantially reduce cardiovascular events and progressive renal disease.

This chapter deals with the diagnosis, initial work-up, and approach to treatment of patients with hypertension. A more detailed discussion of antihypertensive drug therapy and of the diagnosis of secondary causes of hypertension is provided in Chapter 28. This chapter alone, however, should facilitate the initial management of hypertension in the ambulatory setting.

ROLE OF THE GENERALIST

About 30% of adults in the United States have hypertension, which is defined as blood pressure of greater than or equal to 140/90 mm Hg. Hypertension is the major risk factor for stroke, cardiac failure, and nephrosclerosis, and one of the most important risk factors for atherosclerosis. Two thirds of those over 60 years of age are hypertensive and preventative treatment is especially effective and necessary in this group, including patients with isolated systolic hypertension [1,2••] (diastolic blood pressure [DBP] < 90 mm Hg and systolic blood pressure [SBP] > 150–160 mm Hg). The generalist must screen for, diagnose, and treat hypertension in all patients. In addition, the generalist selects 5% to 10% of such patients to undergo detailed study for secondary causes of high blood pressure, some of which cause curable high blood pressure. Treatment of hypertension in the past three decades has reduced the prevalence of fatal stroke by 60% and that of fatal myocardial infarction by about 40%, and it has very much reduced the prevalence of hypertensive heart failure and malignant hypertension. Although this effect has not yet been documented, it is likely that the prevalence of hypertensive nephrosclerosis, which causes 30% of all end-stage renal disease, will also be reduced considerably. Surveys show that only two thirds of patients are being

TABLE 1 CLASSIFICATION OF BLOOD PRESSURE FOR ADULTS AGED 18 YEARS AND OLDER

Category	Systolic pressure, *mm Hg*	Diastolic pressure, *mm Hg*
Normal	120 and	80
Prehypertension	120–130 or	80–89
Hypertension		
Stage 1	140–159 or	90–99
Stage 2	≥ 160	≥ 100
Isolated systolic hypertension	≥ 160	< 90

Adapted from Chobanian *et al.* [2••].

TABLE 2 ASSOCIATED RISK FACTORS FAVORING ANTIHYPERTENSIVE DRUG THERAPY

Hyperlipidemia
Diabetes mellitus
Renal disease; microalbuminuria
Black race
Coronary artery disease
Left ventricular hypertrophy
Cerebrovascular disease
Family history of premature cardiovascular events or renal replacement therapy
Smoking

treated, and only half of those have a blood pressure of 140/90 mm Hg or less [3•].

Thus, the role of the generalist in hypertension is important and clear in detection, prevention, and treatment. Lifestyle [4•] and pharmacologic treatments are cost effective, and with patience and skill, the primary care physician can manage hypertension, when indicated, with antihypertensive drugs in the majority of patients. This is true preventive therapy mainly in asymptomatic patients. With the large array of efficacious medications now available, the physician's goal can be control of blood pressure within the indicated range, with virtually no side effects, and even improvement in quality of life [5].

EPIDEMIOLOGY OF ESSENTIAL HYPERTENSION

Hypertension is either primary (essential) or, in approximately 10% of patients, secondary. Secondary hypertension mainly results from renal disease or renovascular hypertension. The latter condition, and the small number of cases (about 1%) due to endocrine causes, are potentially curable. Essential hypertension usually develops between 35 and 55 years of age and is associated with a family history of the condition.

Screening for hypertension is cost effective for all adults. Blood pressure should be measured at all initial contacts with the physician. Healthy adults with normal blood pressure should have their blood pressure rechecked in the absence of other reasons for medical visits perhaps every 2 to 3 years. Patients with prehypertensive blood pressures (Table 1), however, should have at least yearly blood pressure measurements thereafter and should have a screen for other cardiovascular risk factors (Table 2).

High blood pressure is more common in men. Both its prevalence and untreated hypertension in individual

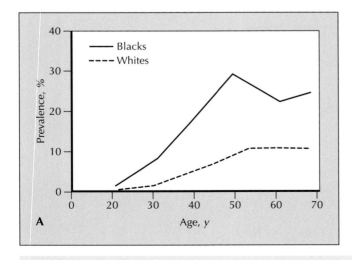

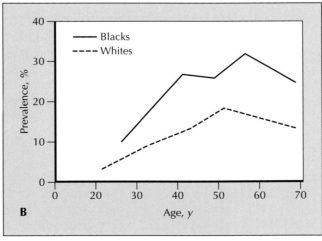

FIGURE 1 Percent prevalence of diastolic blood pressure greater than 95 mm Hg in black and white women (**A**) and men (**B**). (*Adapted from* Troyler [26].)

patients increases with age. In blacks, hypertension is more common, develops at an earlier age, is more severe, and more often causes target organ damage (especially stroke and renal failure) (Fig. 1).

TABLE 3 DECISION POINTS IN EVALUATING THE HYPERTENSIVE PATIENT
Does the patient
Have sustained hypertension?
Take relevant drugs?
Have hypertensive disease (effects on target organs)?
Have other risk factors for cardiovascular disease?
Have sleep apnea?
Have hypothyroidism? [23]
Need lifestyle modifications?
Need antihypertensive drugs? Is therapy emergent or urgent? Which drug or drugs?
Need the minimum work-up or a more extensive search for a secondary cause or causes?

TABLE 4 TARGET ORGAN DAMAGE
Cardiac
Paroxysmal nocturnal dyspnea
Exertional dyspnea
Angina
History of myocardial infarction
Left ventricular hypertrophy
Increased pulse pressure* (if over 65 years of age)
Central nervous system
Transient ischemic attack
Stroke
Retinal
Severe vasospasm
Exudates
Hemorrhages
Papilledema
Renal
Proteinuria
Microalbuminuria
Hematuria
Serum creatinine level of > 1.4 mg/dL
Vascular
Peripheral vascular disease
*Systolic blood pressure minus diastolic blood pressure.

Systolic blood pressure correlates best with risk for cardiovascular events [6]. Hypertension in children less than 16 years of age (> 140/90 mm Hg) is usually secondary [7]. Drug treatment for essential hypertension in this age group is rarely indicated, except in children with associated type 1 or type 2 diabetes mellitus or in controlled prospective trials.

DIAGNOSTIC APPROACH

The physician's initial goal is to attempt to answer the questions raised in Table 3. Hypertension cannot be diagnosed based on a single blood pressure reading or in a single visit, unless severe hypertension (≥ 160/100 mg Hg) or target organ damage is present (Table 4).

Blood pressure should be taken carefully and according to protocol (Fig. 2) [2••]. A diagnosis of hypertension should not be made until a mean blood pressure of more than (or equal to) 140/90 mm Hg is confirmed on at least two further visits.

This judicious approach to diagnosis is important. Labeling a patient "hypertensive" is not without some potentially negative effects [8]. The patient's concept of himself or herself may change from one of being well to one of being ill, leading, for example, to absenteeism from work. Similarly, many nonspecific symptoms (*eg*, headache

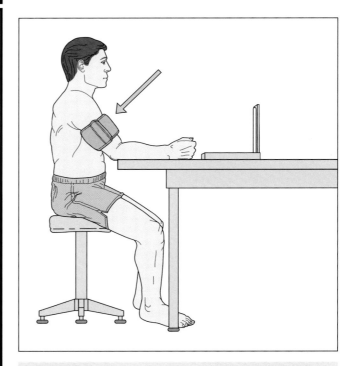

FIGURE 2 Protocol for measuring blood pressure. Patient seated, resting 5 minutes. Arm supported by table, unrestricted by tight clothing. Cuff bladder at least 80% of arm circumference. Take blood pressure twice in the same arm 2 minutes apart. Check blood pressure in other arm and also with the patient standing.

and dizziness) are often wrongly blamed on mild to moderate hypertension—by both patients and physicians [9]! Only severe essential hypertension is associated with symptoms, and essential hypertension usually evolves over many years before becoming severe.

With secondary hypertension, however, it is the rate of rise of the blood pressure rather than the actual blood pressure level itself that determines severity. For example, a patient with acute glomerulonephritis and a previously normal blood pressure may become ill with target organ damage at a blood pressure of approximately 160/100 mm Hg. The same is true in preeclampsia.

The history and physical examination findings will aid greatly in answering all of the issues in Table 3 (Fig. 3). Symptoms and signs of hypertensive disease should be sought (Table 4). Discontinuance of therapy with certain drugs may ameliorate or correct high blood pressure (Table 5). At the first visit, even if the patient's blood pressure is only prehypertensive [2••] (120–140/80–89 mm Hg), a minimum work-up should be considered. This work-up consists of urinalysis; measurement of serum levels of creatinine, potassium, calcium, glucose, and lipids (low-density lipoprotein, high-density lipoprotein, and triglycerides); and electrocardiography. Even slight hypertension may be an initial presentation of underlying primary renal disease, such

as adult dominant polycystic disease or chronic glomerulonephritis. The presence of diabetes mellitus or renal disease or other risk factors (Table 2) usually indicates treatment even at prehypertensive levels of blood pressure [2••,10•].

An electrocardiogram may reveal left atrial or left ventricular hypertrophy (an independent risk factor for cardiovascular events) or evidence of ischemic heart disease. Clinical, radiologic, and electrocardiographic findings (Fig. 4) are less sensitive indicators of left ventricular hypertrophy than is echocardiography. The latter is still too expensive for routine assessment of hypertension but can be a useful test when it is difficult to determine the need for drug therapy [11]. Microalbuminuria, best measured in the morning urine as albumin/creatinine ratio, is directly and positively correlated with cardiovascular risk even in nondiabetics [12,13•].

CLASSIFICATION OF PATIENT'S HYPERTENSION

After one or several visits, as described previously, the physician should be able to answer the questions in Table 3 and to classify the patient's condition tentatively according to the guidelines in the seventh report of the Joint National Committee on Detection, Evaluation and Treatment of High Blood Pressure, and by evidence of target organ

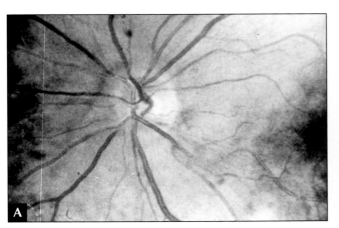

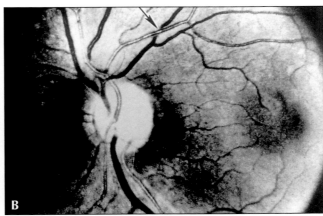

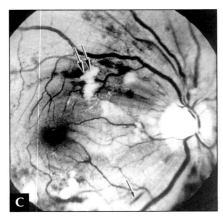

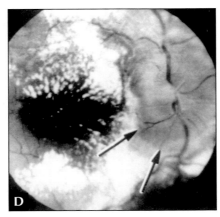

FIGURE 3 Physical examination findings in patients with hypertensive disease. **A,** Moderate narrowing of retinal arteries. **B,** Moderate arteriovenous crossing changes as shown by *arrow.* **C,** Grade III hypertensive retinopathy with flame-shaped hemorrhage (*single arrow*) and cottonwood spot (*double arrow*) exudates. **D,** Grade IV hypertensive retinopathy with papilledema (*arrows*), hard exudates, and macular star. (*From* Tso and Jampol [27]; with permission.)

damage, the need for a more extensive search for secondary causes, and the important but unusual requirement for immediate drug treatment, admission to the hospital, or both (Tables 1, 4, 6, 7) (Fig. 5) [2••].

TABLE 5 DRUGS THAT CAUSE OR INTERFERE WITH THERAPY FOR HYPERTENSION
Excess alcohol* and caffeine†
Oral contraceptive agents
Nonsteroidal antiinflammatory drugs
Cyclosporine, tacrolimus
Steroids
Nasal decongestants
Amphetamines, cocaine, ephedra
Erythropoietin
Monoamine oxidase inhibitors

*More than two drinks per day.
†Five cups per day [24].

INITIATION OF TREATMENT

Lifestyle Modifications

Lifestyle modifications (nonpharmacologic therapy) can be implemented in all patients with prehypertensive levels of blood pressure and above (Table 8). All of these interventions, including weight loss, salt restriction, increased dietary potassium (fruits and vegetables) (Table 9), and exercise have been documented to have beneficial and independent effects on blood pressure [4•]. The physician should persist with them in the compliant patient for 3 to 6 months before concluding that they are ineffective.

Both patients and physicians must understand that drug treatment is a lifelong commitment unless lifestyle modifications are subsequently more effective. Occasional drug samples taken intermittently when the patient believes his

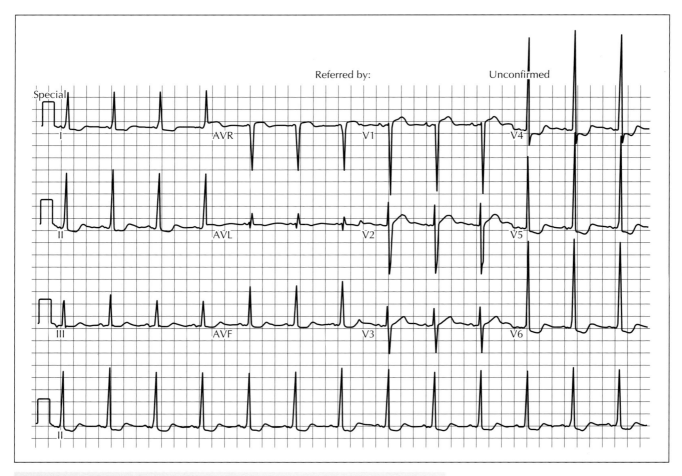

FIGURE 4 Electrocardiogram showing left ventricular hypertrophy by voltage criteria (SV_1 plus RV_5 or $RV_6 \geq 35$ mm) with secondary ST- and T-wave changes.

TABLE 6 INDICATIONS OF THE NEED TO SEARCH FOR SECONDARY CAUSES OF HYPERTENSION

General

Age of onset at < 30 or > 55 years

Severe hypertension (systolic pressure > 180 mm Hg; diastolic pressure > 110 mm Hg)

Abrupt onset, rapid increase in severity, or development of resistance to previously effective therapy

Specific

Symptoms of pheochromocytoma

Unexplained hypokalemia (primary aldosteronism)

Signs of Cushing's syndrome

Palpable kidneys, renal bruit, or abnormal urinalysis results (renal or renovascular hypertension)

Delayed or absent femoral pulses (coarctation)

TABLE 7 INDICATIONS FOR IMMEDIATE OR EARLY TREATMENT IN PATIENTS WITH HYPERTENSION*

Hypertensive emergency (immediate treatment)

Hypertensive encephalopathy

Acute left ventricular failure

Severe pre eclampsia

Deteriorating renal function

Cerebral hemorrhage

Hypertension with dissecting aortic aneurysm

Unstable angina

Myocardial infarction

Hypertensive urgency (early treatment)

Hypertensive grade III or IV retinal changes

Severe preoperative or perioperative hypertension

*Immediate means within 1 hour; early, within 24 hours.

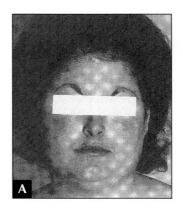
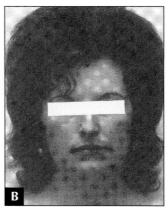
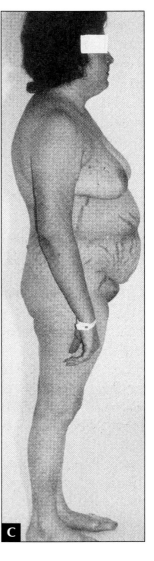

FIGURE 5 Patient with Cushing's disease (**A** and **C**) and 1 year after removal of an adrenal adenoma (**B**). (*From* Tyrrell [28]; with permission.)

TABLE 8 LIFESTYLE MODIFICATIONS FOR PATIENTS WITH HIGH-NORMAL AND HIGHER BLOOD PRESSURE

Modification	Comments
Stop smoking*	Might allow avoidance of antihypertensive drug therapy in mild hypertension if smoking is the only associated cardiovascular risk factor
Restrict daily alcohol intake	< 2 oz of liquor, 8 oz of wine, or 24 oz of beer
Moderately restrict daily salt intake	6 g (100 mmol) of sodium chloride
Eat a diet high in potassium	Beneficial in the absence of renal insufficiency or hyperkalemia; pleasant because high in vegetables and fresh fruit; salt substitutes containing potassium may be useful
Reduce weight by at least 10 lbs (obese patients)	Often reduces blood pressure significantly
Engage in moderate, regular isotonic exercise	For example, walking briskly at least three times per week for 30 to 45 minutes

*Smoking does not cause chronic hypertension but is an important associated risk factor for cardiovascular disease and progressive renal disease.

risks are additive (Table 2). Patients with type 1 diabetes mellitus or renal disease should be treated for even slight elevations in blood pressure, especially if microalbuminuria is present or blood pressure is progressively rising in prehypertensive ranges [13•]. If all risk factors listed in Table 2 are absent, it is reasonable to observe the patient for 6 to 12 months, especially if readings are in the lower blood pressure range of prehypertension (Fig. 6). Semiautomatic home and work blood pressure measuring devices cost in the $50 to $100 range and are quite useful with careful calibration and instruction in their use.

Significant errors in blood pressure measurement and therefore in the classification of hypertension can be caused by very stiff vessels in elderly arteriosclerotic patients (pseudohypertension); by "white coat" hypertension, in which ambulatory at-home blood pressure measurements are much lower than blood pressure measurements obtained at the physician's office (although this finding is not necessarily always benign); and by cuff inflation hypertension [14–16]. Discrepancies between target organ damage and blood pressure levels or unexpected hypotensive reactions to antihypertensive therapy should bring these possible errors to mind. Ambulatory blood pressure monitoring may help to elucidate the situation.

Drug Selection and Goals of Treatment

A total of 75% of patients with mild to moderate hypertension can be managed by a single drug if moderate (not maximal, to minimize side effects) doses of the five classes of drugs suitable for initial therapy (Table 10) are tried sequentially [17]. Absent specific indications (Table 10), one would usually initially try a thiazide, then either a beta-blocker, angiotensin-converting enzyme (ACE) inhibitor, or angiotensin 2 receptor blocker or a long-acting calcium channel blocker. In diabetics, patients with renal disease, and other patients with increased cardiovascular risks, ACE inhibitors are preferred for initial therapy. Combination tablets (calcium channel blocker and ACE inhibitor, beta-blocker and diuretic, and ACE inhibitor and diuretic) are also available for therapy, especially when more than one drug is required to reach target levels, and may improve compliance. Other than for men with prostatism and hypertension, alpha$_1$-blockers such as doxazosin are no longer suitable for initial therapy [18].

Target blood pressure should be 140/90 mm Hg or less. If the patient has diabetes or renal disease, target blood pressure should be 130/80 mm Hg [2••,10•]. Especially if 24-hour protein excretion exceeds 1 g, target blood pressure should be 120 to 130 mm Hg systolic and 75 to 80

TABLE 9 EQUIVALENT POTASSIUM RATIONS*	
Legumes	**Vegetables**
Beans (dry): 40 g	Greenhouse asparagus: 200 g
Broad beans (dry): 50 g	String beans: 200 g
Peas (fresh): 260 g	Mushrooms: 100 g
Canned beans: 230 g	Peppers: 450 g
Frozen peas: 160 g	Turnip: 200 g
Lentils (dry): 70 g	Squash: 300 g
Chick peas (dry): 60 g	Carrots: 250 g
Broad beans (fresh): 160 g	Fennel: 200 g
Canned lentils: 250 g	Potatoes: 100 g
	Radicchio: 300 g
Fresh fruit	Cabbage: 200 g
Apricots: 160 g	Artichoke globe: 150 g
Cherries: 180 g	Cauliflower: 150 g
Peaches: 200 g	Eggplant: 300 g
Oranges: 200 g	Green tomatoes: 250 g
Pears: 400 g	Spinach: 100 g
Grapes: 200 g	Broccoli: 150 g
Orange juice: 250 g	Chicory: 150 g
Apples: 450 g	Lettuce: 200 g
Plums: 170 g	Green peppers: 400 g
Bananas: 150 g	Prickly lettuce: 200 g
Grapefruit: 200 g	
	Dairy
	Milk (skimmed): 350 g

*Each ration contains approximately 10–12 mmol of potassium; patients in the intervention group were advised to eat three to six rations per day. The amount of each ration is reported as "net weight."

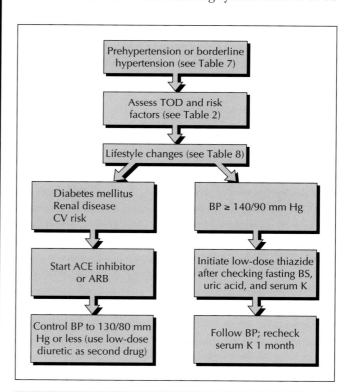

FIGURE 6 Algorithm for prehypertension. ACE—angiotensin-converting enzyme; ARB—angiotensin 2 receptor blocker; BP—blood pressure; BS—blood sugar; CV—cardiovascular; K—vitamin K; TOD—target organ damage.

Drug class*	Indications	Contraindications/problems
Thiazide diuretic (chlorthalidone)	Very cheap, long-term efficacy established, potentiate other drug groups, isolated systolic hypertension, CHF, older and black patients	Gout; hypokalemia, diminished glucose tolerance and hyperlipidemia—minimal clinical importance if dose does not exceed 25 mg
Loop diuretic (furosemide)	Serum creatinine level > 2 mg/dL; resistant edema	Readily cause extracellular fluid volume depletion
Beta-blocker (atenolol)	CAD, younger whites, CHF,[†] perioperative[‡]	Asthma, RD, PVD, CHF, IDDM
ACE inhibitor (enalapril)	RD, LVH, CHF,[†] increased CV risk; diabetes mellitus; whites	Renal artery stenosis, hyperkalemia
Angiotensin II blocker (losartan)	Same as ACE inhibitor (use if cough prevents use of ACE inhibitor)	Same as ACE inhibitor
Calcium channel blockers	CAD, RD, PVD; blacks	CHF[†]
Dihydropyridine (amlodipine)	Cyclosporine-induced CAD, RD, PVD; blacks	Use long-acting only
Other (diltiazem)		Bradycardia, heart block

*The examples in parentheses are prototypes.

[†]ACE inhibitors are used for CHF with systolic dysfunction; calcium channel blockers like diltiazem are being used for patients with CHF due to diastolic dysfunction (normal LV ejection fraction), as in some hypertensives; carvedilol is the beta-blocker of choice in patients with CHF.

[‡]See Fleisher [25].

ACE—angiotensin-converting enzyme; CAD—coronary artery disease; CHF—congestive heart failure; CV—cardiovascular; IDDM—insulin-dependent diabetes mellitus; LV—left ventricular; LVH—left ventricular hypertrophy; PVD—peripheral vascular disease; RD—renal disease.

Condition	Specialist referred to	Comments
Suspected renal disease	Nephrologist	
Suspected renal artery stenosis	Renovascular group*	Clinical and angiographic study by this group offers the most cost-effective outcome
Renovascular renal failure (ischemic renal failure)[†]	Renovascular group*	This problem is seen with increasing frequency; it should be suspected in elderly patients who often smoke and who have diffuse evidence of atherosclerotic disease, hypertension, or "flash" pulmonary edema, and an elevated serum creatinine level without evidence of another primary renal disease[‡]
Unexplained hypokalemia; symptoms suggestive of pheochromocytoma, elevated urinary catecholamine levels, or clinical findings suggestive of Cushing's syndrome	Specialist in hypertension (nephrologist, cardiologist, or endocrinologist)	Use a "hypertensologist" with experience in cost-effective work-up

*Ideally, a nephrologist, a vascular radiologist, and a vascular surgeon.

[†]Bilateral severe renal artery stenosis with renal atrophy or an absent or atrophic kidney plus contralateral severe renal artery stenosis.

[‡]Renal function may deteriorate acutely with an angiotensin-converting enzyme inhibitor.

mm Hg diastolic [18]. Diastolic blood pressure, however, should not be lowered below 85 mm Hg in patients with ischemic coronary artery disease or cerebrovascular disease to avoid worsening ischemia of the heart or brain. In patients with postural hypotension (*eg*, from diabetic autonomic neuropathy and in the elderly), the standing blood pressure must be targeted.

A single daily dose is most convenient for the patient. Care must be taken, however, to ensure that blood pressure control is still adequate in the awakening period between 6:00 and 10:00 AM, because this is a period of increased sudden death from stroke and myocardial infarction [19].

Thiazide diuretics have been used for over 40 years and remain cheap and effective drugs, either as initial therapy or as an addition to other medications, especially ACE inhibitors, angiotensin 2 receptor blockers or beta-blockers [20••]. Many trials have demonstrated their effectiveness in isolated systolic hypertension and in elderly persons with hypertension [1]. Before these agents are prescribed, fasting blood glucose, serum potassium, and uric acid levels should be checed as a baseline; the serum potassium levels should be checked again in about 1 month. Unless the patient is receiving digoxin or has another cause of potassium loss, the use of routine potassium supplements or a potassium-sparing diuretic is not necessary. Prospective control studies have now established the benefits, independent of blood pressure level achieved in most instances, for ACE inhibitors or angiotensin 2 receptor blockers (most believe that their mechanisms of action and effects are quite similar) for hypertensive nephrosclerosis [21•], diabetes mellitus [10•], and for patients at increased cardiovascular risk [22•]. Vasodilators such as hydralazine and minoxidil may cause reflex tachycardia and edema and are not suitable for initial therapy.

In the case of a hypertensive medical emergency or urgency in the office, oral captopril, clonidine, or labetalol are rapidly acting and useful while the physician arranges admission to a hospital special care unit, which is usually necessary in such patients (Table 7). Overly rapid correction of blood pressure in these circumstances can precipitate ischemic events, and the immediate goal of treatment should not be to restore normal levels but rather to reduce diastolic blood pressure initially by about 15 to 20 mm Hg or to the 160 to 170/100 to 110 mm Hg range. Very high blood pressure alone is not a reason to treat emergently in the absence of symptoms or target organ damage. Restarting therapy with previously effective medications in noncompliant patients may be all that is necessary: blood pressure may increase markedly after sudden cessation of central alpha$_2$-blockers (*eg*, clonidine), but this rise usually responds to the restarting of therapy. In patients with severe hypertension but no emergent or urgent indication to treat, reasonable regimens are a beta-blocker plus a thiazide diuretic, or an ACE inhibitor (or angiotensin 2 receptor blocker) plus a thiazide or a calcium channel blocker.

SECONDARY HYPERTENSION

Routine screening of all hypertensive patients for secondary causes of hypertension is not cost effective, except for performing urinalysis and measuring serum creatinine levels to screen for primary renal disease, by far the most common cause of secondary hypertension. Proteinuria before hypertension usually indicates primary renal disease. Hypertensive nephrosclerosis is associated with only modest proteinuria (< 2 g/24 h), and only after many years of hypertension. It is more frequent in the fourth and fifth decades of life in blacks, and it usually only occurs in whites older than 60 years of age in the absence of malignant hypertension.

Renovascular hypertension is the most common cause of correctable hypertension. Urinalysis and serum creatinine levels are of no value in screening for renovascular hypertension; indeed, no single screening test is adequate, and if clinical suspicion warrants a search for it, the gold standard remains renal arteriography, which is, unfortunately, an expensive and invasive procedure. In the age group of 35 to 55 years for whites and 25 to 55 for blacks, a search is required only for patients with initially severe hypertension, those with a renal bruit, or those whose hypertension is resistant to therapy with two or three concurrently used antihypertensive agents. An imperfect but reasonable screening test for functional renal artery stenosis is the captopril isotope renogram. If structural renal disease (polycystic kidneys, obstruction, reflux nephropathy) is suspected, renal ultrasound is indicated.

Table 11 provides information on referring patients with secondary causes of hypertension.

KEY REFERENCES

Recently published papers of outstanding interest, as identified in *References and Recommended Reading*, have been annotated.

•• Chobanian A, Bakris G, *et al.*: The Seventh Report of the Joint National Committee on Prevention, Detection, Evaluation, and Treatment of High Blood Pressure, The JNC 7 Report. *JAMA* 2003, 289:2560–2580.

This paper is required reading. The category of prehypertension is justified in JNC 7 as being an indication for lifestyle modification to prevent the likely progression to hypertension with increasing age; blood pressures even at this level are associated with a doubling of cardiovascular risk [29]. The designation, however, includes millions of patients and some may, unless we are careful, change their self-image from being well to being ill.

•• The ALLHAT officers and coordinators for the ALLHAT Collaborative Research Group: Major outcomes in high-risk hypertensive patients randomized to angiotensin-converting enzyme inhibitor or calcium channel blocker vs diuretic, the Antihypertensive and Lipid-Lowering Treatment to Prevent Heart Attack Trial (ALLHAT). *JAMA* 2002, 288:2981–2996.

This paper is also required reading. The findings of ALLHAT have markedly influenced the recommendations of JNC 7. The recommendation that a low-dose thiazide is the best first agent for treating uncomplicated hypertension is clear. However, there are many exceptions especially for the initial use of ACE inhibitors or angiotensin receptor blockers as discussed previously in this chapter. In either case, diuretics are usually the second agent added if not used initially. The "first use" issue for low-dose diuretics has engendered controversy [30,31], has been supported by meta-analysis [32], but is contradicted by a recent paper from Australia [33] in which ACE inhibitors "bested" diuretics. This author agrees with Frohlich [30] that we should carefully individualize our therapy rather than argue about which of a series of effective drugs is best.

REFERENCES AND RECOMMENDED READING

Recently published papers of particular interest have been highlighted as:
- Of interest
- •• Of outstanding interest

1. SHEP Cooperative Research Group: Prevention of stroke by anti-hypertensive drug treatment in older persons with isolated systolic hypertension. *JAMA* 1991, 265:3255–3264.

2.•• Chobanian A, Bakris G, *et al.*: The Seventh Report of the Joint national Committee on Prevention, Detection, Evaluation, and Treatment of High Blood Pressure, The JNC 7 Report. *JAMA* 2003, 289:2560–2580.

3.• Hajjar I, Kotchen T: Trends in Prevalence, Awareness, Treatment, and Control of Hypertension in the United States. 1988 – 2000. *JAMA* 2003, 290:199–206.

4.• Whelton P, He J, *et al.*: Primary prevention of hypertension, clinical and public health advisory from the National High Blood Pressure Education Program. *JAMA* 2002, 288: 1882–1883.

5. Grimm RJ, Grandits GA, Cutler MA, *et al.*: Relationships of quality-of-life measures to long-term lifestyle and drug treatment in the treatment of mild hypertension study. *Arch Intern Med* 1997, 157:638–648.

6. Pastor-Barriuso R, Banegas J, *et al.*: Systolic blood pressure, diastolic blood pressure, and pulse pressure, an evaluation of their joint effect on mortality. *Ann Intern Med* 2003, 139:731–739.

7. Task Force on Blood Pressure Control in Children: Report of the second task force on blood pressure control in children—1987. *Pediatrics* 1987, 79:1–25.

8. Haynes RB, Sackett DL, Taylor DW, *et al.*: Increased absenteeism from work after detection and labeling of hypertensive patients. *N Engl J Med* 1978, 299:741–744.

9. Weiss NA: Relation of high blood pressure to headache, epistaxis, and selected other symptoms. *N Engl J Med* 1972, 287:631–633.

10.• Vijan S, Hayward R: Treatment of hypertension in type 2 diabetes mellitus: blood pressure goals, choice of agents, and setting priorities in diabetes care. *Ann Intern Med* 2003, 138:593–602.

11. Frolich ED, Chobanian AV, Devereau RB, *et al.*: The heart in hypertension [review article] . *N Engl J Med* 1992, 327:998–1008.

12. Pontremoli R: Microalbuminuria in essential hypertension—its relation to cardiovascular risk factors. *Nephrol Dial Transplant* 1996, 11:2113–2134.

13.• Gerstein H, Mann J, *et al.*: Albuminuria and risk of cardiovascular events, death, and heart failure in diabetic and nondiabetic individuals. *JAMA* 2002, 286:421–426.

14. Mejiia AD, Egan BR, Schork NJ, *et al.*: Artefacts in measurement of blood pressure and lack of target organ involvement in the assessment of patients with treatment-resistant hypertension. *Ann Intern Med* 1990, 112:270–277.

15.• Pickering TG, James GD, Boddie C, *et al.*: How common is white coat hypertension? *JAMA* 1988, 259:225–228.

16. Cardillo C, De Felice F, Campia U, *et al.*: Psychophysiological reactivity and cardiac end-organ changes in white coat hypertension. *Hypertension* 1993, 21:836–844.

17. Dickerson JE, Hingorani AD, Ashby MJ, *et al.*: Optimisation of antihypertensive treatment by crossover rotation of four major classes. *Lancet* 1999, 353:2008–2013.

18. The ALLHAT Officers and Coordinators for the ALLHAT Collaborative Research Group: Major cardiovascular events in hypertensive patients randomized to doxazosin versus chlorthalidone. *JAMA* 2000, 283:1967–1975.

19. Quyyumi AA: Circadian rhythms in cardiovascular disease. *Am Heart J* 1990, 130:726–733.

20.•• The ALLHAT Officers and Coordinators for the ALLHAT Collaborative Research Group: Major outcomes in high-risk hypertensive patients randomized to angiotensin-converting enzyme inhibitor or calcium channel blocker vs diuretic, the Antihypertensive and Lipid-Lowering Treatment to Prevent Heart Attack Trial (ALLHAT): *JAMA* 2002, 288: 2981–2996.

21.• Wright J, Bakris G, *et al.*: Effect of blood pressure lowering and antihypertensive drug class on progression of hypertensive kidney disease: result from the AASK trial. *JAMA* 2002, 288:2421–2467.

22.• Yusuf S, Sleight P, Pogue J, *et al.*: Effects of an angiotensin-converting enzyme inhibitor, ramipril, on cardiovascular events in high-risk patients. *N Engl J Med* 2000, 342:145–153.

23. Fletcher AK, Weetman AP: Hypertension and hypothyroidism. *Hum Hypertens* 1998, 12:79–82.

24. Rakic V, Burke V, Beilin LJ: Effects of coffee on ambulatory blood pressure in older men and women. *Hypertension* 1999, 33:869–873.

25. Fleisher L: Preoperative evaluation of the patient with hypertension. *JAMA* 2002, 287:2043–2046.

26. Troyler H: Socioeconomic status, age, and sex in the prevalence and prognosis of hypertension in blacks and whites. In *Hypertension: Pathophysiology, Diagnosis, and Management*, vol. 1. Edited by Laraugh JH, Brenner BM. New York: Raven Press; 1990:159–174.

27. Tso O, Jampol L: Hypertensive retinopathy, choroidopathy, and optic neuropathy of hypertensive ocular disease. In *Hypertension: Pathophysiology, Diagnosis, and Management*, vol. 1. Edited by Laragh JH, Brenner BM. New York: Raven Press; 1990:433–465.

28. Tyrrell JB: Cushing's syndrome. In *Cecil Textbook of Medicine*, edn 19. Edited by Wyngaarden JB, Smith LH, Bennett JC. Philadelphia: WB Saunders; 1992:1284–1288.

29. Vasan R, Larson M, *et al.*: Impact of high-normal blood pressure on the risk of cardiovascular disease. *N Engl J Med* 2001, 345:1291–1298.

30. Frohlich E: treating hypertension—what are we to believe? *N Engl J Med* 2003, 348:639–641.

31. Messerli F: ALLHAT, or the soft science of the secondary end point. *Ann Intern Med* 2003, 139:777–780.

32. Psaty B, Lumley T, *et al.*: Health outcomes associated with various antihypertensive therapies used as first-line agents, a network meta-analysis. *JAMA* 2003, 289:2534–2544.

33. Wing L, Reid C, *et al.*: A Comparison of outcomes with angiotensin-converting-enzyme inhibitors and diuretics for hypertension in the elderly. *N Engl J Med* 2003, 348:583–592.

SELECT BIBLIOGRAPHY

Kaplan NM: *Clinical Hypertension*, edn 8. Edited by Collins N. Baltimore: Lippincott: Williams & Wilkins; 2002.

Oparil S, Zaman M, Calhoun D: Pathogenesis of hypertension. *Ann Intern Med* 2003, 139:761–776.

16

Secondary Hypertension

Thomas G. Pickering
Norman K. Hollenberg

Key Points

- Secondary hypertension occurs in less than 5% of cases, but its diagnosis is important because of the possibility of a permanent cure.

- Routine screening of all hypertensive patients is not recommended and should be reserved for those in whom clinical clues are present.

- Renovascular hypertension is the commonest type and should be suspected in two populations: young women with severe or recent hypertension, and older patients with evidence of atherosclerotic disease.

- Captopril renography is one of the best noninvasive tests for diagnosing renovascular hypertension.

- Although both aldosterone-secreting tumors and pheochromocytomas may be diagnosed biochemically, an anatomic diagnosis may be difficult to make because aldosteronomas may be very small, and pheochromocytomas occur outside the adrenal glands.

In about 5% of cases, hypertension can be attributed to a secondary cause, such as a renal or endocrine disorder. The diagnosis of such cases is important not only because of the potential for a permanent cure but also because, if untreated, the underlying disorder may cause other problems, such as renal failure [1]. Hypertension may be the presenting manifestation of these conditions, or it may be one of a variety of signs and symptoms in patients with systemic disease (Table 1).

WHEN TO SCREEN FOR SECONDARY HYPERTENSION

Routine screening of all hypertensive patients for secondary causes is not recommended because the expense and unreliability of the available screening tests make it uneconomical. Two general indications for screening are the severity of the hypertension and the presence of clinical clues detected during routine examination. Renovascular hypertension has a prevalence of less than 5% in the general hypertensive population but is as high as 30% in patients with accelerated hypertension [2]. Essential hypertension occurs rarely before the age of 15 years, and young hypertensive children should be investigated thoroughly for a secondary cause.

Renovascular Hypertension

Renovascular hypertension is by far the most common secondary cause of hypertension and is often difficult to diagnose. It has two main causes: fibromuscular dysplasia and atheromatous stenosis. In younger patients (< 50 years of age), fibromuscular dysplasia of the renal arteries predominates, and in older patients reno-

TABLE 1 CAUSES OF SECONDARY HYPERTENSION

Causes presenting as hypertension	Causes presenting as systemic disease
Renal artery stenosis (fibromuscular dysplasia or atheroma)	Cushing's disease
Renal parenchymal disease	Scleroderma
Aldosterone-secreting tumor	Collagen disease (systemic lupus erythematosus, polyarteritis)
Glucocorticoid-remediable aldosteronism	Hypothyroidism
Pheochromocytoma	
Coarctation of the aorta	
Drug-induced hypertension	

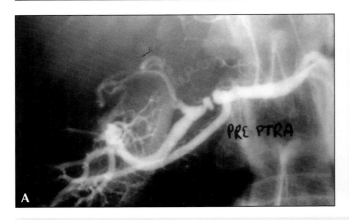

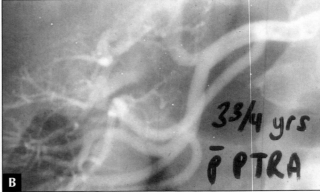

FIGURE 1 Renal angiogram showing fibromuscular dysplasia before (**A**) and after (**B**) renal angioplasty, which in this case cured the hypertension.

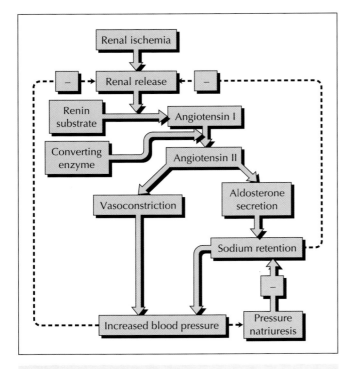

FIGURE 2 The renin-angiotensin-aldosterone system in renovascular hypertension.

vascular hypertension usually results from atheroma [3,4•]. Fibromuscular dysplasia is usually confined to the renal arteries, where it is characterized by one or more fibrous bands that partly occlude the lumen (Fig. 1). Its etiology is unknown, although smoking may contribute. Most patients do not have a family history of hypertension. Atheromatous stenoses commonly are bilateral and associated with stenosis in other arteries. Because essential hypertension accelerates the development of atheroma, lesions in the renal arteries could be both a cause and a consequence of the hypertension.

To cause hypertension, a renal artery stenosis must be of sufficient severity to impair blood flow to the kidney, which responds by increasing renin secretion. This response activates angiotensin and aldosterone and hence raises blood pressure (Fig. 2). When the stenosis is limited to one renal artery, there is no accompanying sodium retention because the increased arterial pressure in the unaffected kidney results in a pressure natriuresis (Fig. 3A). When only one kidney is present and its artery is stenosed, the renin is normal and the hypertension largely results from sodium retention (Fig. 3B). When both arteries are stenosed, there also may be sodium retention because both kidneys are protected from the high systemic pressure as a result of the stenosis, and no pressure natriuresis occurs (Fig. 3C) [5].

Clinical clues suggestive of renovascular hypertension are shown in Table 2. If these clues are present, further work-up of the patient may be appropriate. The only viable office screening tests are renin-sodium profiling and an oral captopril test. Renin-sodium profiling is performed by relating the plasma renin activity to the 24-hour urinary sodium excretion. A high or normal renin level is compatible with renovascular hypertension, whereas a low renin level excludes it. The captopril test is performed by taking blood for plasma renin activity before and 1 hour after the administration of captopril, 25 mg, by mouth [6]. In patients with normal renin levels, an increase of renin of more than 150% is very suggestive of renovascular disease (Fig. 4); however, false-positive results are common in high-renin patients [7•].

When there is a moderate level of suspicion that renovascular disease is present, the best screening test is probably a renal scan performed with mercaptoacetyl triglycine (MAG$_3$) (Fig. 5) after a single oral dose of captopril [8]. This test is more reliable than a conventional scan because the captopril reduces the glomerular filtration rate in the presence of a renal artery stenosis. If the index of suspicion is very high, or if the captopril scan results are positive, arteriography is indicated. The sensitivity and specificity of diagnostic studies for renovascular hypertension is listed in Table 3.

Revascularization is the preferred form of treatment. If possible, this should be done by angioplasty or, alternatively, by surgery (*eg*, by a hepatorenal artery bypass for the right kidney or a splenorenal artery bypass for the left). In younger patients with fibromuscular disease, angioplasty often cures the hypertension [5]; in older patients, the cure rates are lower no matter which form of revascularization is used [1]. If the ischemic kidney is small and functionless, nephrectomy may be indicated. Medical treatment is reserved generally for patients who are judged to be ineligible for one of these procedures.

Aldosteronoma

In patients whose serum potassium level is low in the absence of thiazide diuretics, an aldosterone-secreting tumor should be suspected [9]. A 24-hour urine collection for electrolytes and aldosterone should be obtained; high urine potassium, high aldosterone, and low plasma renin activity are characteristic. Differentiation from bilateral adrenal hyperplasia is obtained by CT scan of the adrenal

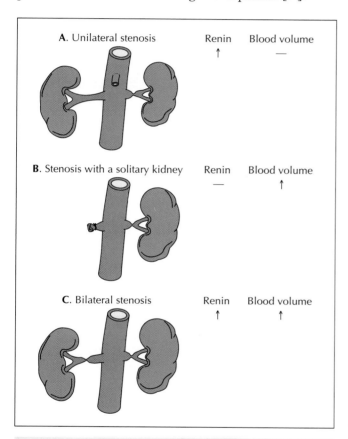

FIGURE 3 Three models of renovascular hypertension: **A**, Unilateral renal artery stenosis. **B**, Stenosis with a solitary kidney. **C**, Bilateral stenoses.

TABLE 2 CLINICAL CLUES SUGGESTIVE OF RENOVASCULAR HYPERTENSION
Severe or refractory hypertension in any patient
Moderate or severe hypertension in a young white woman
Vascular bruits
Azotemia; high renin; hypokalemia; proteinuria
Sudden onset of hypertension

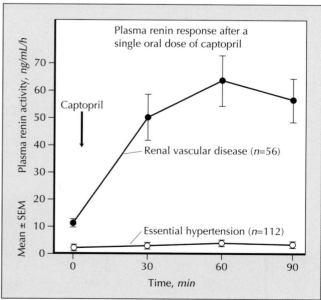

FIGURE 4 The increase of plasma renin activity after a single oral dose of captopril may distinguish patients with essential hypertension from patients with renovascular hypertension.

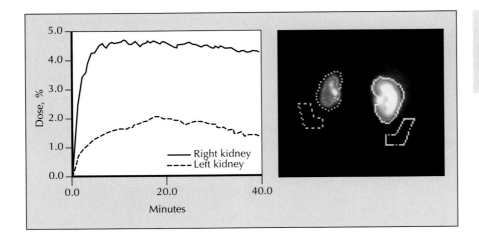

Figure 5 Renal scan in an azotemic patient suggests renal artery stenosis of the left kidney. Note the asymmetry of kidney size and delayed uptake of isotope by the left kidney. (*See* Color Plate.)

TABLE 3 DIAGNOSTIC STUDIES FOR RENOVASCULAR HYPERTENSION

	Senstivity, %	Specificity, %
Rapid sequence IVP	74	86
Isotope renography with ACE inhibition test	93	95
Peripheral vein PRA with ACE inhibition test (captopril test)	74	89
Renal vein ratio of PRA test (stenotic/contralateral):		
>1.3	85	40
>1.9	78	60
Peripheral vein PRA	92	96
Intravenous digital subtraction angiography	88	89
Doppler ultrasonography	86	93
MRI	97	95
Renal artery angiography	100	100

ACE—angiotensin-converting enzyme; IVP—intravenous pyelography; PRA—plasma renin activity.

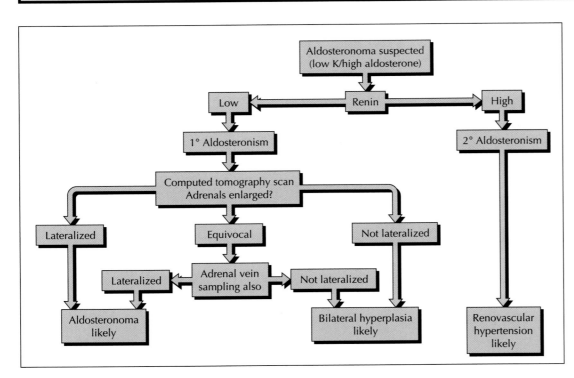

Figure 6 Approach to the diagnosis of aldosterone-secreting tumor.

Cardiology for the Primary Care Physician

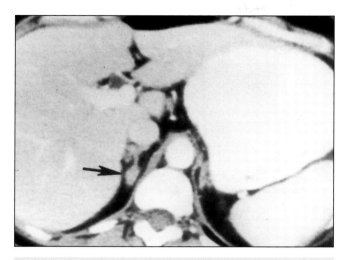

FIGURE 7 Computed tomography scan showing aldosterone-secreting tumor (*arrow*).

glands (Fig. 6). Aldosteronomas may be difficult to localize because of their small size (Fig. 7). Adrenalectomy usually is curative.

Glucocorticoid-remediable Aldosteronism

Although exceedingly rare, this condition is of great interest because it represents the only form of hypertension for which a specific genetic mutation has been identified [10]. Its inheritance is autosomal dominant and the condition clinically presents in the same way as aldosterone-secreting tumor, with hypertension and hypokalemia. However, the increased aldosterone secretion is corticotropin-dependent and hence reversible by administration of glucocorticoids (dexamethasone, which suppresses corticotropin).

Medical management of aldosterone-producing adenomas using potassium-sparing diuretics led to maintained blood pressure reduction and correction of hypokalemia in 24 patients who had documented aldosterone-producing adenomas for 5 years or more [11] (Table 4).

| | | | | | | Electrolyte levels at time of diagnosis (last follow-up) | | | |
| | | | | Blood pressure at presentation,* *mm Hg* | Most recent blood pressure measurement,* *mm Hg* | Sodium, *mmol/L* | Potassium, *mmol/L* | Chloride, *mmol/L* | Carbon dioxide, *mmol/L* |
Patient	Age, *y*	Sex	Follow-up, *y*						
1	65	M	5	170/94	120/80	145 (140)	3.1 (5.2)	105 (110)	30 (28)
2	69	M	12	164/65	157/86	141 (141)	3.2 (3.9)	98 (104)	35 (30)
3	63	M	11	178/96	130/95	141 (144)	2.9 (4.0)	100 (107)	28 (26)
4	43	F	8	180/104	124/82	140 (137)	3.0 (4.1)	98 (105)	31 (25)
5	39	F	5	184/132	128/80	141 (140)	3.9 (3.7)	102 (106)	29 (28)
6	76	M	9	174/100	116/74	143 (139)	2.9 (4.7)	104 (103)	29 (23)
7	68	M	6	180/105	155/76	140 (142)	3.1 (4.2)	98 (109)	32 (28)
8	69	M	5	190/95	130/70	144 (140)	2.9 (4.1)	103 (104)	29 (21)
9	59	M	7	180/116	145/99	144 (139)	2.4 (4.3)	102 (104)	35 (30)
10	55	M	8	180/110	140/74	145 (142)	3.0 (4.6)	102 (104)	30 (30)
11	59	M	6	165/102	112/68	142 (142)	3.0 (4.8)	106 (108)	30 (30)
12	50	M	6	177/117	115/80	144 (143)	3.1 (4.5)	102 (104)	31 (27)
13	44	M	6	160/110	130/82	141 (140)	3.0 (4.3)	106 (103)	29 (29)
14	64	F	8	160/98	142/60	144 (142)	3.4 (4.7)	106 (108)	29 (25)
15	52	F	13	150/104	104/76	142 (137)	3.3 (4.4)	105 (106)	24 (25)
16	52	F	5	168/102	128/91	143 (141)	2.7 (3.6)	102 (106)	32 (32)
17	54	F	17	180/110	101/71	143 (139)	3.0 (4.4)	105 (101)	33 (30)
18	59	M	8	176/116	158/78	142 (138)	2.6 (4.6)	106 (101)	29 (27)
19	44	F	9	190/122	122/78	142 (137)	2.6 (3.6)	98 (98)	32 (26)
20	61	F	14	160/110	144/72	145 (140)	2.9 (3.7)	103 (113)	35 (29)
21	68	F	5	166/108	111/78	143 (146)	2.6 (4.6)	103 (108)	30 (26)
22	66	M	11	178/108	150/92	141 (142)	3.0 (3.8)	101 (102)	31 (26)
23	73	M	10	178/100	107/66	143 (143)	3.8 (4.8)	99 (105)	31 (24)
24	56	M	15	200/125	128/85	141 (139)	3.2 (4.6)	102 (102)	32 (26)

*Blood pressure values are the average of at least three measurements.

Pheochromocytoma

Although it accounts for less than 1% of hypertensive cases, pheochromocytoma is important to diagnose because, if undetected, it potentially is fatal; it is easily curable once detected [12]. Characteristic findings are shown in Table 5. A 24-hour urine collection for catecholamines and metanephrines may provide biochemical confirmation; in doubtful cases, plasma catecholamines also may be measured (*see* Table 6). The tumors usually can be localized by an abdominal CT scan; extra-adrenal tumors may be detected by metaiodobenzylguanidine (MIBG) scans (Fig. 8) [13]. The specificity and sensitivity of various tests and their combination is shown in Figure 9. The absence of an effect of antihypertensive and other drugs on urinary normetanephrine values is shown in Figure 10. Treatment is by adrenalectomy following α-adrenergic blockade with phenoxybenzamine.

COARCTATION OF THE AORTA

Coarctation usually is diagnosed in childhood but occasionally remains undetected until adulthood. The diagnosis can be made from the routine physical examination [14]. The most striking finding is a systolic murmur best heard over the back, between the left scapula and the spine; there also may be an aortic ejection murmur arising from a bicuspid aortic valve. The femoral pulses are weak and delayed, and the blood pressure is lower in the legs than in the arms. The coarctation itself usually is situated at the site of the ductus arteriosus, just below the origin of the left subclavian artery. The diagnosis can be confirmed by echocardiography. Treatment is by surgical correction of the stenosis, which usually is performed after the child reaches 5 years of age.

Renal Parenchymal Disease

The discovery of a small kidney in a hypertensive patient does not necessarily signify renal artery stenosis; it may occur with unilateral parenchymal disease, which is commonly attributed to pyelonephritis, although glomerulonephritis is just as likely [15]. The main renal artery is small but patent; removal of the shrunken kidney may cure the hypertension. Chronic pyelonephritis typically is bilateral, but whether it actually causes hypertension is uncertain. On the other hand, chronic glomerulonephritis, which causes more parenchymal disease than pyelonephritis, certainly can. Proteinuria is more pronounced with glomerulonephritis than with pyelonephritis.

Hypertension may be the presenting feature of adult polycystic disease. Clinically, patients with this condition also may experience abdominal pain and hematuria, and the renal or associated hepatic cysts may be palpable on physical examination. The hypertension is associated with high plasma renin activity [16].

TABLE 5 CLINICAL ASPECTS OF PHEOCHROMOCYTOMA	
Five H's*	**Rule of 10**
Hypertension	10% familial
Headache	10% bilateral (adrenal)
Hyperhidrosis	10% malignant
Hypermetabolism	10% multiple
Hyperglycemia	(extra-adrenal)
	10% occur in children

*95% will have headache, hyperhidrosis, or palpitations.

TABLE 6 URINE AND BLOOD TESTS FOR PHEOCHROMOCYTOMA	
Test	**Upper limit of normal**
Urine metanephrines	1.8 mg/24 h
Urine catecholamines	1.0 mg/24 h
Urine vanillylmandelic acid	11 mg/24 h
Plasma catecholamines (norepinephrine and epinephrine)	950 pg/mL
Plasma catecholamines (after clonidine)	500 pg/mL

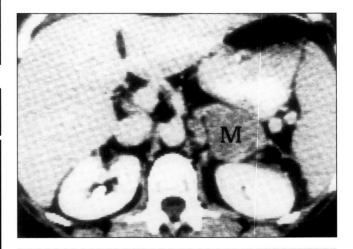

FIGURE 8 Computed tomography scan showing pheochromocytoma (*M*).

Angioplasty had little advantage over antihypertensive drug therapy in a controlled study [17] (Table 7).

Cushing's Disease

Most patients with Cushing's disease are hypertensive, although it rarely is the presenting feature [18]. The diagnosis is established by elevated plasma or urinary levels of cortisol. Treatment of the underlying condition usually cures the hypertension.

Thyroid Disorders

About 20% of hypothyroid patients have associated diastolic hypertension, which can be improved by thyroid supplementation. Systolic hypertension is characteristic of hyperthyroidism [19].

Scleroderma

In the later stages of this condition the kidneys may be affected, causing very high renin levels and severe hypertension.

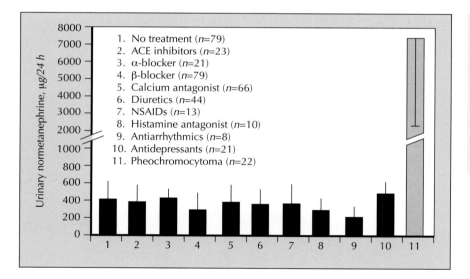

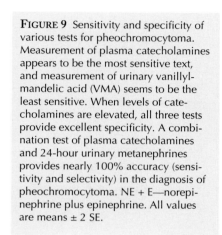

FIGURE 9 Sensitivity and specificity of various tests for pheochromocytoma. Measurement of plasma catecholamines appears to be the most sensitive text, and measurement of urinary vanillyl-mandelic acid (VMA) seems to be the least sensitive. When levels of catecholamines are elevated, all three tests provide excellent specificity. A combination test of plasma catecholamines and 24-hour urinary metanephrines provides nearly 100% accuracy (sensitivity and selectivity) in the diagnosis of pheochromocytoma. NE + E—norepinephrine plus epinephrine. All values are means ± 2 SE.

FIGURE 10 Urinary normetanephrine values in hypertensive patients on various types of drugs. Normetanephrine in urine was measured by high-pressure liquid chromatography. None of the commonly used antihypertensive agents interfered with the measurement of normetanephrine in urine. Values represent mean ± SD. ACE—angiotensin-converting enzyme; NSAID—nonsteroidal anti-inflammatory drug.

Variable	Angioplasty group, *n=56*	Drug therapy group, *n=50*	*P* value
Outcomes 3 months after randomization			
Blood pressure, *mm Hg*†			
Systolic	169±28	176±31	0.25
Diastolic	99±12	101±14	0.36
Blood pressure by automatic device, *mm Hg*			
Systolic	160±26	163±27	0.61
Diastolic	89±14	88±13	0.73
Antihypertensive drugs			
Defined daily doses, *n*	2.1±1.3	3.2±1.5	<0.001
Drugs, *n*	1.9±0.9	2.5±1.0	0.002
Serum creatinine, *mg/dL*			0.05
Median	1.2	1.3	
Range	0.7–1.9	0.6–2.6	
Creatinine clearance, *mL/min*	70±25	59±23	0.03
Abnormal renal scintigrams, *n/total n (%)*	17/47 (36)	28/40 (70)	0.002
Outcomes 12 months after randomization			
Blood pressure, *mm Hg*‡			
Systolic	160±26	163±25	0.51
Diastolic	93±13	96±10	0.25
Blood pressure by automatic device, *mm Hg*			
Systolic	152±20	162±27	0.07
Diastolic	84±10	88±13	0.13
Antihypertensive drugs			
Defined daily doses, *n*	2.5±1.7	3.1±2.3	0.10
Drugs, *n*	1.9±0.9	2.4±0.9	0.002
Serum creatinine, *mg/dL*			0.11
Median	1.2	1.2	
Range	0.6–1.9	0.6–8.2	
Creatinine clearance, *mL/min*	70±24	62±27	0.11
Abnormal renal scintigrams, *n/total n (%)*	19/53 (36)	25/44 (57)	0.04
Complications during follow-up, *n* of patients			
Occlusion of affected artery	0	8	
Rupture of affected artery	0	0	
Increase of ≥50% in serum creatinine	2	6	
Embolization of cholesterol crystals	0	2	
Groin hematoma necessitating transfusion or surgery	2	4	
Other§	2	4	

*Plus/minus values are means ±SD. To convert the values for serum creatinine to mmol/L, multiply by 88.4.

†*P*<0.001 for the comparison with systolic and diastolic pressure at randomization in the angioplasty group; *P*=0.16 for the comparison with systolic pressure at randomization; *P*=0.13 for the comparison with diastolic pressure at randomization in the drug therapy group.

‡*P*=0.001 for the comparison with systolic and diastolic blood pressure at 3 months in the angioplasty group; *P*=0.001 for the comparison with systolic pressure at 3 months; *P*=0.002 for the comparison with diastolic pressure at 3 months in the drug therapy group.

§Other complications were symptomatic hypotension at the time of angioplasty in one patient in the angioplasty group, angina pectoris in one patient, and myocardial infarction in one patient in the drug therapy group.

References and Recommended Reading

Recently published papers of particular interest have been highlighted as:

• Of interest

1. Rimmer JM, Gennari FJ: Artherosclerotic renovascular disease and progressive renal failure. *Ann Intern Med* 1993, 118:712–719.

2. Davis BA, Crook JE, Vestal RE, Oates JA: Prevalence of renovascular hypertension in patients with Grade II or IV hypertensive retinopathy. *N Engl J Med* 1979, 301:1273–1276.

3. Mann SJ, Pickering TG: Detection of renovascular hypertension: state of the art: 1992. *Ann Intern Med* 1992, 117:845–853.

4.• Derkx FHM, Schalekam P: Renal artery stenosis and hypertension. *Lancet* 1994, 334:237–239.

5. Pickering TG: Renovascular hypertension: medical evaluation and non-surgical treatment. In *Hypertension: Pathology, Diagnosis, and Management.* Edited by Laragh JH, Brenner BM. New York: Raven Press; 1990:1539–1560.

6. Müller FB, Sealey JE, Case CB, *et al.*: The captopril test for identifying renovascular disease in hypertensive patients. *Am J Med* 1986, 80:633–644.

7.• Gerber LM, Mann SJ, Muller FB, *et al.*: Response to the captopril test is dependent on the baseline renin profile. *J Hypertens* 1994, 12:173–178.

8. Mann SJ, Pickering TG, Tos TA, *et al.*: Captopril renography in the diagnosis of renal artery stenosis: accuracy and limitations. *Am J Med* 1991, 90:30–40.

9. Bravo EL: Primary aldosteronism: new approaches to diagnosis and management. *Cleve Clin J Med* 1993, 60:379–386.

10. Lifton RP, Dluhy RG, Powers M, *et al.*: A chimaeric 11 beta-hydroxylase/aldosterone synthase gene causes glucocorticoid-remediable aldosteronism and human hypertension. *Nature* 1992, 355:262–265.

11. Ghose RP, Hall PM, Bravo EL: Medical management of aldosterone-producing adenomas. *Ann Intern Med* 1999, 121:105–108.

12. Sheps SG, Jiang N-S, Klee GG, van Heerden JA: Recent developments in the diagnosis and treatment of pheochromocytoma. *Mayo Clin Proc* 1990, 65:88–95.

13. Clesham CL, Kennedy A, Lavender JP, *et al.*: Meta-iodobenzylguanidine (MIBG) scanning in the diagnosis of phaeochromocytoma. *J Hum Hypertens* 1993, 7:353–356.

14. Rocchini A: Coarctation of the aorta. In *Hypertension Primer.* Edited by Izzo JL, Black HR. Dallas: American Heart Association; 1993:107–108.

15. Brown MA, Whitworth JA: Hypertension in human renal disease. *J Hypertens* 1992, 10:701–712.

16. Chapman AB, Johnson A, Gabow PA, Schrier RW: The renin-angiotensin-aldosterone system and autosomal dominant polycystic kidney disease. *N Engl J Med* 1990, 32:1091–1096.

17. van Jaarsveld BC, Krijnen P, Pieterman H, *et al.*: The effect of balloon angioplasty on hypertension in atherosclerotic renal-artery stenosis. *N Engl J Med* 2000, 342:1007–1113.

18. Carpenter PC: Cushing's syndrome: update of diagnosis and management. *Mayo Clin Proc* 1986, 61:49–58.

19. Klein I, Ojamaa K: Thyroid diseases and hypertension. In *Hypertension Primer.* Edited by Izzo JL, Black HR. Dallas: American Heart Association; 1993:108–109.

Pheochromocytoma

Arnold L. Silva
Deping Lee

17

Key Points

- Pheochromocytoma, a rare but treatable cause of hypertension, can masquerade as a classical hypertensive or as an occult clinical mystery.

- Clinical suspicion of pheochromocytoma can be confirmed by measures of plasma or urinary normetanephrine and metanephrine or catecholamines.

- Localization of the chromaffin tumor is performed with complementary MRI and octreotide or metaiodobenzylguanidine imaging, CT scan, or positron emission tomography.

- Preoperative therapy has traditionally used α-blockers, usually phenoxybenzamine, often with the addition of β-blockade, of sufficient duration to achieve euvolemia and stable left ventricular function, but calcium channel blockers have also been shown to be a safe alternative during surgical resection.

- Operative resection requires invasive monitoring, selective anesthesia, careful dissection, appropriate control of blood pressure, colloid replacement, and autologous transfusion.

Pheochromocytoma is a rare tumor of catecholamine-secreting chromaffin cells, occurring in approximately 0.1% of patients with hypertension [1••]. The majority (> 80%) occur in the adrenal medulla with the remainder in the extra-adrenal paraganglionic system that extends from the pelvic region to the base of the skull [2]. Patients with pheochromocytoma can present with a wide variety of clinical signs and symptoms: they may present to the emergency room with a transient ischemic attack, stroke, congestive heart failure, myocardial infarction, hypercalcemia, shock, adult respiratory distress syndrome, lactic acidosis, or malignant hypertension; there is one report of seizure as an initial presentation [3]. Approximately three fourths of patients will present with the classic triad of diaphoresis, headache, or feelings of impending doom. Some, however, may only be discovered to have signs and symptoms consistent with primary hypertension or be normotensive, with only occasional episodes of elevated blood pressure [2].

Pheochromocytoma is found in 0.5% to 0.8% of autopsies. There are an estimated one to two patients with pheochromocytoma per million persons and there are between one and five patients with pheochromocytoma per thousand patients with hypertension [4•]. Investigators who conducted a 30-year surveillance of the population of Rochester, Minnesota found an average annual incidence of pheochromocytoma of 0.95 per 100,000 person-years [5]. In five of the 11 patients, pheochromocytoma was diagnosed at autopsy. Unfortunately, pheochromocytoma often remains an occult disease ending the life of the patient abruptly or gradually, but almost always prematurely. Seventy percent of patients who had an autopsy diagnosis of pheochromocytoma were undiagnosed while alive [4•]. Patients in whom symptoms were present for over 3 months (61%) had the typical symptoms of palpitations, sweating, dyspnea, and headaches. Of these, 10% had hypertension only. The pattern of symptoms was different for those patients who had them for less than 3 months—almost all had abdominal pain, vomiting, and dyspnea. In addition, one half had sweating and chest pain. The tumor occurs with equal frequency in both sexes and at any age, although it is most common in the third and fourth decades. Familial tumors are less common and manifest multiplicity, especially bilateral masses, and are often associated with medullary carcinoma of the thyroid [6]; multiple, bilateral, and extra-adrenal tumors are also more common in children [7]. These tumors occur in patients with multiple endocrine neoplasia (MEN) type II or Sipple syndrome, which is associated with medullary carcinoma of the thyroid, parathyroid adenoma, and bilateral pheochromocytoma (Table 1) [8].

Approximately 10% to 13% of pheochromocytomas are malignant [9]. Malignant forms have been shown to metastasize to lungs, liver, lymph nodes and bone, but spare the brain. The presence of distant metastasis is, unfortunately, associated with poor survival [10].

Pheochromocytoma may be associated with other neuroectodermal syndromes, such as neurofibromatosis (approximately 5% of individuals with neurofibromatosis may develop pheochromocytoma), von Hippel-Lindau disease, Sturge-Weber disease, tuberous sclerosis, and Carney's syndrome [11,12]. Pheochromocytoma may occur in association with other endocrine neoplasms, both endocrine and malignant. The cells of pheochromocytoma have similar cytochemical and ultrastructural features and a presumed common embryologic origin from the neuroectoderm, sharing amine precursor uptake and decarboxylation

[13]. Isolated tumors may arise from these tissues, or they may occur in association with other amine precursor uptake and decarboxylation cell neoplasms as part of a MEN syndrome. The screening of unselected patients with pheochromocytoma discovered 19% with von Hippel-Lindau disease and 4% with MEN type 2 (MEN-II) [13]. When family members with von Hippel-Lindau disease or MEN-II were screened for pheochromocytoma, unsuspected pheochromocytoma was found in 46% [12]. Molecular genetic testing in kindred of patients with familial pheochromocytoma allows for detection of those with RET and VHL protooncogenes to offer presymptomatic diagnosis of renal cell carcinoma [14•], medullary thyroid carcinoma [15••,16], and parathyroid adenoma [15••,16].

Pheochromocytomas arising outside the chromaffin cells of the adrenal medulla are called *functional paragangliomas* [17]. These tumors occur in the posterior mediastinum; in the sympathetic chain in the neck; in the organ of Zuckerkandl, which is ventral to the aorta at the origin of the inferior mesenteric artery; in the pelvis; and in the urinary bladder [18].

ADRENAL MEDULLARY HYPERPLASIA

Whether or not this entity exists has been a topic of controversy since it was first described more than 50 years ago [19]. The normal adrenal has a weight of 6 to 6.5 g and a medullary:cortical ratio of 1:10 (thus, a medullary weight of approximately 0.6 to 0.7 g). Some investigators have reported, however, that medullary weight has approached 1.25 to 2.0 g in patients who had hypertensive crises and

TABLE 1 PRESUMPTIVE DIAGNOSIS OF PHEOCHROMOCYTOMA			
Symptoms (in order of frequency)*	**Signs (in order of frequency)**	**Clinical syndromes**	**Familial**
Headache	Hyperhidrosis	Hypertension (character)	MEN II (Sipple's syndrome)
Palpitation or tachycardia	Paroxysmal changes in BP	Paroxysmal (50%)	Familial
Excessive perspiration	Postural hypotension	Malignant accelerated	pheochromocytoma
Anxiety, nervousness	Hypertension induced	(5%–10%)	Medullary carcinoma
Weight loss	by palpation or	Paradoxical response to:	Parathyroid adenoma
Tremor	positioning	β-blockers	MEN III
Pallor	Hypertensive retinotherapy	Imipramine, desipramine	Thickened corneal nerves
Chest or abdominal pains	Hypermetabolism	Guanethidine,	Ganglioneuromatosis
Nausea, vomiting	Neurofibromatosis	hydralazine	Marfanoid features
Malaise	Café-au-lait spots	Induction of anesthesia	Mucosal neuronomas
	Absence of hand veins	In pregnancy	von Reckinghausen's
	Axillary freckling	(1st, 3rd trimester)	neurofibramotosis
	Palpable mass (rare)	Diabetes mellitus (50%)	von Hippel–Lindau
	Acrocyanosis, shock, ARDS	Cardiomyopathy (30%)	disease
		In children	
		Multiple, bilateral, and	
		extra-adrenal tumors	

*Absence of all makes diagnoses unlikely with > 90% specificity.

ARDS—adult respiratory distress syndrome; BP— blood pressure; MEN—multiple endocrine neoplasia.

attacks similar to pheochromocytoma, but without chromaffin tumors [20,21].

Symptoms

The complaints of patients with pheochromocytoma may resemble those with primary hypertension (Table 1). Symptoms generally have two patterns, persistent or paroxysmal, which are related to a constant or pulsatile release of catecholamines [22]. Attacks occur from once every 2 months to 25 per day and last from 30 seconds to 1 week, with an average time of approximately 15 minutes. Paroxysmal attacks are rarely associated with malignancy [22].

Acute episodes with a constellation of symptoms may occur in patients with pheochromocytoma. Most commonly, these consist of sweating, palpitations, and anxiety with hypertension. Of course, most hypertensive patients with symptoms of pheochromocytoma do not have a chromaffin tumor but instead seem to have spontaneous adrenergic discharge without apparent reasons. Sometimes, the masquerade results from an identifiable cause, such as phenylpropanolamine ingestion or a Munchausen syndrome resulting from self-administration of vasoactive amines, like isoproterenol [23,24]. Kuchel, however, described patients who appear to have episodic dopamine surges that flood phenol sulfotransferase mechanisms that inactivate norepinephrine and epinephrine [25]. Some of our hypertensive patients have had excessive adrenergic tone and appeared to be "caricatures of pheochromocytoma," with surges of free norepinephrine and plasma concomitant with blood pressure elevation. The blood pressure rise in these patients responded to α- and β-receptor blockade [26].

Chromaffin tumors of the adrenal medulla commonly secrete only norepinephrine; less often, a mixture of norepinephrine and epinephrine; and rarely, epinephrine alone. Extra-adrenal pheochromocytomas secrete only norepinephrine, which is less potent than epinephrine in causing hypermetabolism and glycogenolysis. Rarely, epinephrine-like effects are seen in patients with tumors excreting only norepinephrine. The history of attacks occurring when the patient bends to one side, wears a tight girdle, or has a full bladder may help to localize or lead to the diagnosis of the tumors.

Physical Findings

Patients with pheochromocytoma often are thin from weight loss, but some remain obese (Table 1). Many have a normal physical examination. Sweating may be subtle or severe, with drenching night sweats and even dehydration. Facial or digital flushing may also occur, and the extremities may be pale. Vasospasm may be so severe that peripheral pulses are undetectable, and even gangrene may be present. Intense arterial constriction may result in falsely low brachial arterial pressure. The veins on the dorsum of the hands may not be seen because of intense vasoconstriction. Therefore, the clinician must determine whether central pulsations are present, and if they are strong, interarterial monitoring from the femoral region is indicated. Central nervous system findings are diverse and range from anxiety to frank psychosis and from transient ischemic attacks to completed strokes resulting from cerebral hemorrhage. Prior to their diagnosis, patients are frequently referred for psychiatric diagnosis and therapy.

Postural hypotension is common in pheochromocytoma, perhaps because of the reduced plasma volume [27]. The hypotension or shock that occurs after removal of a pheochromocytoma results from discontinuation of the catecholamine infusion and reexpansion of the vascular compartment. Traditionally, this complication has been minimized by the preoperative administration of oral α-blockers, such as phenoxybenzamine (POB), along with rapid expansion of the blood volume with albumin or autologous blood immediately after the tumor vessels are ligated. Nevertheless, preoperative POB administration has not been shown to reduce perioperative mortality [28]. Alternatively, preoperative calcium channel blockade has been shown to be an effective and safe antihypertensive strategy. Calcium channel blockers typically do not produce overshoot or orthostatic hypotension, making them especially useful in normotensive patients with occasional episodic rises in blood pressure [29].

ADULT RESPIRATORY DISTRESS SYNDROME

We have encountered two patients with acrocyanosis and hypertension rapidly proceeding to hypotension that was associated with marked plasma volume contraction, lactic acidosis, bilateral pulmonary infiltrates, and subsequently at autopsy or surgery, a recent hemorrhage was found in the adrenal tumor. It is exceedingly important to consider the possibility of underlying chromaffin tumor in such patients.

Myocardial Sequelae

Twenty percent to 30% of patients have specific cardiac complications of pheochromocytoma, such as left ventricular hypertrophy, catecholamine myocarditis, and dilated or obstructive cardiomyopathy [30–32]. They often exhibit the ECG abnormalities of sinus tachycardia, junctional rhythm, ventricular tachyarrhythmias, and ST-T changes of left ventricular hypertrophy and ischemia. Recovery can occur rapidly, often within 14 days of beginning therapy with α-blockade [30]. Heart rate variability measured using ambulatory 24-hour electrocardiography is reduced in patients with pheochromocytoma compared to that of patients with hypertension, and may be related in part to enhanced sympathetic as well as increased vagal tone [33].

Myocardial necrosis and fibrosis are related to the arteriolar constriction [34] and hypoxia mediated by adrenergic receptors [35] and enhanced permeability of the cell membrane to calcium [36]. There is also evidence that oxidized catecholamine products are toxic. Pheochromocytoma should be considered in patients with congestive heart failure without other obvious cause, even in normotensives. Normotensive patients may be more likely to die as a result of cardiac injury and lung edema because the diagnosis may not be suspected and the required specific α-blockade may not be given [36–38]. Thus, α-blockade must be used for a sufficient period preoperatively for repair of this cardiac dysfunction. Echocardiography can document or detect global or segmental akinesis or hypokinesis, which usually reverts over a period of days to normal after α-blocking therapy. In one series of necropsies of patients with pheochromocytoma and sudden death, five of 10 had acute myocardial infarction. Several of the young patients had far-advanced atherosclerosis, and two of our own patients in their sixth decade required coronary revascularization. One patient with pheochromocytoma, 35 years of age, sustained an acute myocardial infarction after angiography. Thus, this complication, although relatively rare, must be considered during planning for surgical correction of these tumors. In our experience, surgical excision of the pheochromocytoma in patients with stable angina, coronary artery disease, and pheochromocytoma can be performed successfully prior to eventual coronary artery bypass grafting, although there is a report of combined CABG and pheochromocytoma resection in a patient with unstable angina on maximal antianginal therapy [39]. Rarely, pheochromocytoma occurs in the intra-atrial groove or travels to the heart by extension inside the great veins.

Biochemical Assays
Urine

Urinary metanephrines remain the most reliable—as well as universally available—tests for pheochromocytoma using 24-hour values or the expression of the microgram per creatinine ratio. The sensitivity is 95/100% and the specificity 96/98%; positive and negative predictive values are, respectively, 46/47% and 100/100% for the two methods [40]. Patients should avoid stress and activities causing nonspecific elevations of catecholamines during urine collection (Table 2). We prefer to use free catecholamines for screening and use "timed urine" or express the result as *mg/h*, "per milligram of creatinine" (Table 2).

For patients with labile hypertension, urine should be collected during exacerbations, and this timed specimen can be compared with baseline. When the pattern of catecholamine excretion includes 20% or more as epinephrine, the tumor is usually found in the adrenals or in the organs of Zuckerkandl. Low levels of vanillylmandelic acid excretion do not exclude the diagnosis of pheochromocytoma. In our studies, the levels were normal in 10% to 15% of patients with known pheochromocytoma [41]. Further, false-positive results occurring in 10% to 15% can be caused by beverages high in vanillin and food such as bananas, coffee, nuts, and other fruits.

Plasma catecholamine and metanephrine

Plasma catecholamine measurements are of value in episodic crises and before and after clonidine suppression or histamine challenge. To minimize false-positive results, blood obtained 20 to 30 minutes after supine rest avoids the effect of stress and posture on catecholamine levels. The total catecholamine value in normotensive patients ranges from 100 to 500 ng/L [42]. Patients with pheochromocytoma usually have values 10 to 15 times normal. The high predictive value of a plasma catecholamine value that is greater than 2000 ng/L is offset by the low specificity when only mild-to-moderate elevations are found (Table 3). Catecholamine values of less than 2000 ng/L in various stressful states may be considered equivocal because some patients with primary hypertension have elevations ranging from 800 to 1000 g/L. Plasma catecholamine value may be normal during normotensive or asymptomatic intervals. We have encountered patients who have had normal plasma levels of norepinephrine and epinephrine, but elevated levels of normetanephrine that were greater than 500 ng/L [43,44]. Eisenhofer *et al.* [45] have described an assay of plasma normetanephrine and metanephrine that provides a more sensitive assay for supporting the theory

---

TABLE 2 EXCRETION RATES OF CATECHOLAMINES AND CATECHOLAMINE METABOLITES IN NORMAL SUBJECTS AND IN PATIENTS WITH PHEOCHROMOCYTOMA

	Normal,* μg/h	Pheochromocytoma,† μg/h
Catecholamines (free epinephrine plus norepinephrine)	2.5±0.8	10–120
Metanephrine plus normetanephrine (free plus conjugated)	16±5	30–420
Normetanephrine (free and conjugated)	10±5	30–720
Vanillylmandelic acid	240±120	500–3500

*Mean ± SD.
†Presumptive until proved otherwise.

that the methlated amines are found in the tumor. Some of these patients have had metastatic pheochromocytoma. O'Connor and Bernstein [46] demonstrated elevated chromogranin A levels in the plasma of patients with pheochromocytoma. This substance may prove helpful in the diagnosis of patients with pheochromocytoma and in excluding its diagnosis in pseudopheochromocytoma.

Clonidine Suppression Test

The clonidine suppression test has practical clinical value in patients with pseudopheochromocytoma, as described previously [47]. Because of the clinical symptoms and borderline values present in patients with pseudopheochromocytoma, the diagnosis of pheochromocytoma is considered, and frequently the elevations of the plasma catecholamines are two SD above normal. Oral clonidine, an α_2-agonist, reduces plasma norepinephrine levels in hypertensive patients consonant with its effects in lowering central and thus peripheral sympathetic tone and blood pressure [36,38]. Bravo *et al.* [48,49] applied the method of clonidine suppression of plasma norepinephrine to a population of hypertensive patients and they found no suppression in patients with pheochromocytoma, compared with a 60% to 70% reduction of plasma norepinephrine 3 hours after an oral dose of 0.3 mg of clonidine in patients without

pheochromocytoma (Fig. 1). Blood pressure was equally reduced in both groups. We do not know of any patients with pheochromocytoma in whom clonidine lowered the plasma norepinephrine level. Some of our patients have had marginally elevated plasma norepinephrine levels for many years without documentation of pheochromocytoma and have had no suppression of plasma norepinephrine level after clonidine. Thus, a positive test result, that is, suppression of norepinephrine, is strongly predictive of nonpheochromocytoma, but a negative result in the presence of marginally increased catecholamines cannot be considered presumptive evidence for the presence of a chromaffin tumor. More recent work, however, suggests that in patients with suspected pheochromocytoma, elevation of plasma normetanephrine following clonidine suppression is more reliable than using the normetanephrine level or the norepinephrine response to clonidine [45].

Pharmacologic Diagnosis

The provocative tests for diagnosis of pheochromocytoma may be dangerous. These drugs have caused hypertensive crises, cardiovascular accidents, and fatalities. The "tandem" glucagon stimulator followed by clonidine suppression test, as suggested by the NIH Group, requires a threefold increase in catecholamines after 2-mg glucagon IV then the

TABLE 3 AFTER URINARY SCREENING: DIAGNOSTIC TESTS FOR PHEOCHROMOCYTOMA
Plasma
Norepinephrine and epinephrine, supine (30–60 min)
700–1000 pg/mL (repeat, especially if urine results positive)
1000–2000 pg/mL (use clonidine suppression test; should fall to < 50%)
> 2000 pg/mL (usually diagnostic for pheochromocytoma)
Imaging
CT, 77% sensitivity overall
MRI
Scintigraphy:
131I MIBG (if CT results are negative or more than one tumor suspected)
Octreotide scan
Iodocholesterol: nonfunctional tumors in region of clips
Vena caval and regional vein sampling for catecholamine step-up
Ultrasound: pregnancy, screening, near clips
Intravenous pyelography: hypertension screening, urinary bladder
Angiography: to localize and to establish vascular connections
MIBG—metaiodobenzylguanidine.

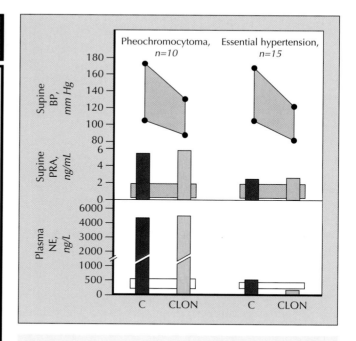

FIGURE 1 Cardiovascular and humoral responses of 10 patients with proven pheochromocytoma and 15 patients with essential hypertension who underwent the clonidine suppression test. For plasma renin activity (PRA) and plasma norepinephrine (NE), the *cross-hatched areas* indicate the mean (± 2 SD) of values obtained from healthy adult subjects of similar age. BP—blood pressure; C—control group; CLON—clonidine suppression test group. (*Adapted from* Bravo [49].)

usual response to clonidine: every one of their reported pheochromocytomas had a positive response to glucagon and no significant suppression after clonidine. If both tests were negative, no pheochromocytoma could be found. These tests should be carried out by experienced endocrinologists when indicated.

LOCALIZATION OF TUMORS

Localization of the tumor before surgery is required to decrease operative time and the incidence of cardiovascular accidents and to avert unnecessary adrenalectomy. Ninety-eight percent of pheochromocytomas are found below the diaphragm, with most sporadic cases (90%) occurring in the adrenal medulla (Fig. 2). Fifteen percent are multiple. Most of the remainder are found in the posterior mediastinum, middle ear, carotid body, and urinary bladder. Ultrasound, CT, octreotide and/or metaiodobenzylguanidine (MIBG) scintigraphy, MRI and, more recently, positron emission tomography (PET) have supplanted older methods of localization. They should be carried out by experienced radiologists using the most state-of-the-art equipment.

COMPUTED TOMOGRAPHY, MAGNETIC RESONANCE IMAGING, SCINTIGRAPHY, AND POSITRON EMISSION TOMOGRAPHY

Computed tomography correctly localized 89% of tumors, including single, intra-adrenal, bilateral adrenal, ectopic, and malignant tumors, on initial presentation in 52 patients seen over a 7-year period at the Mayo Clinic [50]. Current state-of-the-art scanners may localize as many as 95%. The Mayo Clinic study noted a localization rate of 73% for recurrent tumors; failures were attributable to small tumor size (8 mm) and artifacts resulting from surgical clips.

Scintigraphic visualization of adrenergic tissues has been made possible by the development of an analogue of guanethidine, ^{131}I-MIBG (Fig. 3) [51]. ^{131}I-MIBG is concentrated in adrenergic neurons and chromaffin tissue by uptake into norepinephrine-containing storage sites. Discrete images after 48 hours usually represent pheochromocytomas that are rich in adrenergic storage vesicles. The method delivers 0.11 total body cGy and 17.5 cGy to the normal adrenal medullas [52]. Imaging is performed 48 and 72 hours after administration of the tracer. The method is safe, reproducible, and highly specific (Fig. 4). It provides unique functional information that may be of great value when multiple tumors are expected, as in MEN [53]. False-negative results may occur in 4% to 10% of patients, often those with malignancy [54]. Medications known to inhibit norepinephrine uptake, such as labetalol and tricyclic antidepressants, should be discontinued 2 weeks before the study. Because ^{131}I-MIBG is excreted by the bladder, imaging of this region with other methods may be necessary in some patients.

Pheochromocytomas contain a high content of somatostatin receptors. Thus, the radiologic somatostatin analogue octreotide can be used to localize the primary tumor, as well as any metastases [55]. Scintigraphy with octreotide is not specific for pheochromocytoma; other neuroendocrine (*ie*, carcinoid) and some nonendocrine (*ie*, astrocytoma) tumors, granulomas (*ie*, sarcoid), and some autoimmune processes (*ie*, Graves' disease) can be visualized using this technique. However, paragangliomas may be more octreotide-positive than MIBG-positive. However, paragangliomas may be more octreotide-positive than MIBG-positive. The small size of this peptide allows for rapid clearance and low background activity. In a sample of 1000 patients, 12 of the 14 patients with pheochromocytoma were somatostatin-receptor positive. Perhaps MIBG is more useful in localization of tumors in the adrenal and renal regions because of the relatively high accumulation of ligand in the kidney. A comparison study with MIBG of patients with 17 tumors yielded the following findings: 12 tumors were pheochromocytoma or paraganglioma, octreotide scans visualized five tumors that were not found by MIBG, MIBG localized two not found by octreotide scan, and both scans localized five tumors. The authors found that 86% of scans were positive for pheochromocytoma (compared with 88% for MIBG in

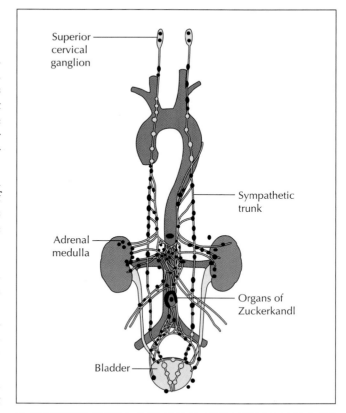

FIGURE 2 Sites of aorticosympathetic paraganglia (extramedullary chromaffin tissue) in a newborn child. Most functional paragangliomas occur below the diaphragm. (*Adapted from* Glenner and Grimbley [78].)

the literature) and that 100% of the paragangliomas were visualized with octreotide (compared with 52% for MIBG in the literature) [55].

Computed tomography can be focused on the region likely to yield a tumor. Presently, both tests are considered complementary [56]. The presence of a mass on CT does not necessarily mean a chromaffin tumor. On the other hand, some chromaffin tumors do not function or absorb MIBG [56]. If the evaluation of patients with hypertension proceeds from clinical suspicion to CT without biochemical confirmation, a small number of incidental asymptomatic adrenal masses will be uncovered, most of which will not be pheochromocytoma. Autopsy data and imaging studies suggest that finding an "incidentaloma" of the adrenal gland rarely yields a functional tumor. Of 100,000 tumors, 6500, 7000, and 35 will be pheochromocytoma, aldosteronoma, and glucocorticoid adenoma, respectively [57]. Although only 58 of 100,000 tumors will be adrenocortical carcinoma, rapid growth (or growth above 4 to 6 cm) may require excision or biopsy once pheochromocytoma is excluded [57].

Ansari *et al.* [58] have found a sensitivity of 77% and a specificity of 92% with MIBG scanning. Their accuracy rate was 96% and 90% for MIBG and CT, respectively.

Magnetic resonance imaging appears even better than CT scan for adrenal tissue characterization for both adrenal cortical adenoma and medullary pheochromocytoma and is better able to distinguish adrenal adenoma from adrenal medullary neoplasm on the basis of intensity difference. Patients with pheochromocytoma have demonstrated marked hyperintensity compared with normal liver on T2-weighted pulse sequences [59,60].

In 14 patients with malignant pheochromocytoma encompassing 40 tumor sites, three patients with more than 20 sites on MIBG scan had only one to nine sites visualized on ^{111}In-ocreotide scintigraphy; two patients had no MIBG uptake, but one of these had lung uptake with octreotide; and in nine patients with a total of 41 MIBG foci there were 33 sites of ^{111}In-ocreotide [61••]. There is some evidence that PET may also be of use for diagnostic localization of pheochromocytoma [62]. Though preliminary, this work suggests that PET may be superior to other nuclear imaging modalities including ^{131}I-MIBG. PET also offers the advantage of near immediate visualization following tracer administration as compared to MIBG, which requires a 24- to 48-hour imaging period. Further study is needed, however, to better define the role of diagnostic PET scanning in pheochromocytoma.

THERAPY

Medical Control

Advances in perioperative preparation and intraoperative patient management have had a major impact on mortality associated with pheochromocytoma surgery (Table 4). Surgical mortality was approximately 15% before 1950, and many deaths were attributable to hypovolemic shock, hypertensive hemorrhage, and anesthesia-related arrhythmias [63]. Since that time, preoperative therapy with α-blocking drugs, usually phenoxybenzamine as well as propanolol for at least 2 weeks (to allow reexpansion of blood volume), intraoperative anesthesia with improved anesthetic agents, and intraoperative or postresection

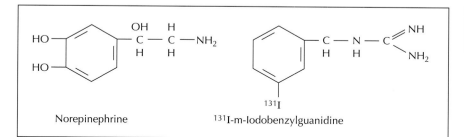

FIGURE 3 Chemical structure of metaiodobenzylguanidine.

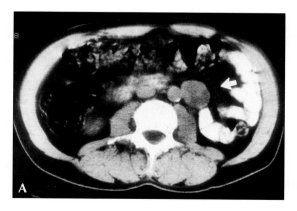
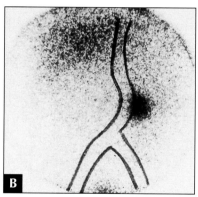

FIGURE 4 **A,** CT scan of patient with paraganglioma. Tumor is seen at tip of *arrow.* **B,** Complementary role of the metaiodobenzylguanidine scan. The functional tumor is seen adjacent to the aorta. There was a plasma norepinephrine step-up increase in the left adrenal vein as well.

volume replacement have made surgical mortality an exceptional occurrence (Table 4) [64,65]. Patients are usually prepared for surgery.

Phenoxybenzamine is a noncompetitive adrenergic blocking agent with greater selectivity for α_1 than α_2 receptors (100:1 vs 3–5:1 for phentolamine). Therapy is initiated

with one or two divided daily doses of 10 mg each. Most patients with pheochromocytoma require 20 to 40 mg/d. However, we have encountered patients who failed to respond adequately to oral phenoxybenzamine, and each has subsequently responded to intravenous phentolamine.

Prazosin hydrochloride, doxazosin mesylate, and terazosin are even more exclusive α_1-receptor blockers that have also been used with mixed success in patients with pheochromocytoma as preoperative therapy [66,67]. I do not believe that these should be relied on as the sole α-blocking agent during surgery because they only block α_1 receptors or they are "competitive" blockers [67]. The possible adverse effects of doxazosin in primary HIV patients make it less attractive as long-term monotherapy of patients with pheochromocytomas. The main role of α-blocker therapy in pheochromocytoma is to prevent vasoconstriction and to provide normalization of blood pressure. However, adverse α-agonist effects on the myocardium are also lessened, and congestive heart failure due to catecholamine myocarditis is reversed or prevented. Recent studies suggest that nonselective α-blockade with agents such as phenoxybenzamine diminish both sympathomimetic stimulation and vagal inhibition of the myocardium, as well as reduce the incidence and frequency of repetitive ventricular dysrhythmia [68]. The addition of β-receptor blockade may be indicated when tachycardia or catecholamine-induced arrhythmias are present, or when epinephrine constitutes 15% to 20% or more of total neurohormone secretion. Propranolol is added in low doses, 10 to 20 mg three to four times per day, only after α-blocking therapy has begun. Propranolol may cause paradoxical hypertension in pheochromocytoma in the absence of prior α-receptor blockade. The combined α- and β-receptor blocker labetalol has been effective in preoperative and intraoperative management [69].

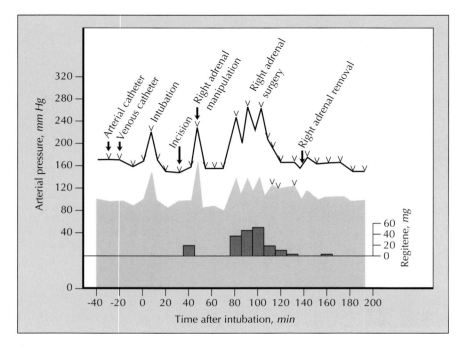

FIGURE 5 Pressor responses during operative removal of adrenal chromaffin tumor. Pressor responses were managed by bolus injections of phentolamine. Time and amount administered are indicated by *arrows* and *hatched columns*, respectively.

Calcium channel blockade, which is useful in pheochromocytoma both preoperatively and intraoperatively, reduces smooth muscle contractility and also impairs exocytosis release of norepinephrine from storage vesicles and blocks α_2 receptors. Continuous infusion of nicardipine hydrochloride during surgery has been shown to successfully suppress elevations in blood pressure during tumor excision [70]. In one case series of 113 patients with pheochromocytoma, there was no surgical mortality when calcium channel blockers were the primary antihypertensive therapy [71]. In cases of resistant hypertension, combination calcium channel and α-blockade has been shown to successfully control blood pressure.

The 5-year survival of patients with benign pheochromocytoma is approximately 96%, and that small fraction of patients (< 10%) with malignant pheochromocytoma have only a 44% survival rate [72]. Therapy for these patients with malignancies and for those who cannot tolerate surgical procedures with α- and β-blocking agents is not entirely satisfactory. For these patients, methylparatyrosine in doses of 1 to 2 g/d can reduce tumor synthesis from active sites and can normalize blood pressure for long periods—more than 15 years in some patients [73]. However, symptoms of parkinsonism, perhaps related to reduction of basal ganglia dopamine content, have been reported [74].

Phentolamine has been the traditional drug of choice for obtaining rapid control of hypertension during crisis, provocative testing, and surgery (Fig. 5). Doses of 1 to 5 mg are given as boluses, and side effects include nausea and tachycardia. Most recently, we have used esmolol hydrochloride (50–100 mg/kg/min) and/or sodium nitroprusside (1 mg/kg/min) infusion during induction and intraoperatively. At the Cleveland Clinic, conventional antihypertensives are used preoperatively with morbidity rates comparable to patients treated with α-blockers at other centers.

Chemotherapy of patients with malignant pheochromocytoma is of limited benefit. However, patients treated with cyclophosphamide, vincristine, and dacarbazine have shown regression of tumor size, reduction in catecholamine excretion, and improved quality of life, at least temporarily [75]. Systematically administered or targeted radiopharmaceuticals such as ^{131}I-labeled MIBG can be used in the therapy of metastatic pheochromocytoma. This therapy can be enhanced with consideration for tumor dosing, concomitant chemotherapy, radiosensitizers, surgical debulking, and external beam radiotherapy [76]. Whenever possible, resection of the chromaffin tumors should be accomplished as soon as the patient is adequately blocked and the cardiac function, if impaired, is returned to optimal levels. Sudden cardiac death can occur in effectively α-"blocked" patients: even those on concomitant β-blockers and ACE inhibitor therapy and without clinical evidence of dysrhythmia.

PHEOCHROMOCYTOMA IN PREGNANCY

Pregnant women with undiagnosed pheochromocytoma may die from cerebral vascular accidents, acute pulmonary edema, cardiac arrhythmias, shock, or malignancy. If pheochromocytoma is diagnosed before term, the maternal mortality is reduced to 17% or less. However, fetal mortality may remain high because of spontaneous abortion, with most deaths occurring during or just after labor. Increased catecholamine levels in maternal blood may cause fetal anoxia as a result of constriction of uterine arteries and also by heightened uterine contractions.

Maternal pheochromocytoma is extremely uncommon (only 180 patients were described in the world's literature through 1989). It is, however, often fatal (50% for the mother and 20% for the fetus) when undiagnosed (66% to 87% during pregnancy) [77]. It is then perhaps a reasonable course to perform urinary screening tests for pheochromocytoma on all pregnant patients with hypertension, and to consider diagnostic testing for those with normal blood pressure but classic signs and symptoms of pheochromocytoma. In rare cases, nausea and vomiting and epigastric distress of an occult pheochromocytoma will mimic hyperemesis gravidarum.

KEY REFERENCES

Recently published papers of outstanding interest, as identified in *References and Recommended Reading*, have been annotated.

•• Pacak K, Linehan WM, Eisenhofer G, *et al.*: Recent advances in genetics, diagnosis, localization and treatment of pheochromocytoma. *Ann Intern Med* 2001, 134:315–329.

Recent data shows high sensitivity for diagnosis of pheochromocytoma with plasma metanephrines along with improved imaging techniques, including PET.

•• Skinner MA, DeBenedetti MK, Moley JF, *et al.*: Medullary thyroid carcinoma in children with multiple endocrine neoplasia types 2A and 2B. *J Pediatr Surg* 1996, 31:177–182.

The genetic diagnosis of patients with these syndromes may allow for prophylactic surgery before the development of biochemical or clinical evidence of medullary thyroid carcinoma.

•• Tenebaum F, Lumbroso J, Schlumberger M, *et al.*: Comparison of radiolabeled ocreotide and meta-iodobenzylguanidine (MIBG) scintigraphy in malignant pheochromocytoma. *J Nucl Med* 1995, 36:1–6.

Use of octreotide to identify somatostatin receptors seems promising, especially when results from MIBG scans are negative. Moreover, octreotide images could aid in determining a treatment regimen, as well as establishing the extent of disease and prognosis.

REFERENCES AND RECOMMENDED READING

Recently published papers of particular interest have been highlighted as:

• Of interest
•• Of outstanding interest

1.•• Pacak K, Linehan WM, Eisenhofer G, *et al.*: Recent advances in genetics, diagnosis, localization and treatment of pheochromocytoma. *Ann Intern Med* 2001, 134:315–329.

2. Williams DT, Dann S, Wheeler MH: Phaeochromocytoma: views on current management. *Eur J Surg Oncol* 2003, 29:483–490. [Erratum in *Eur J Surg Oncol* 2003, 29:933.]

3. Leiba A, Bar-Dayan Y, Leker RR, *et al.*: Seizures as a presenting symptom of phaeochromocytoma in a young soldier. *J Hum Hypertens* 2003, 17:1:73–75.

4.• Platts, JK, Drew PJT, Harvey JN. Death from phaeochromocytoma: lessons from a post-mortem survey. *J Royal Coll Physicians of London* 1995, 29:299–306.

5. Beard C, Sheps SG, Kurland LT, *et al.*: Occurrence of pheochromocytoma in Rochester, Minnesota, 1950 through 1979. *Mayo Clin Proc* 1983, 58:802–804.

6. Moorehead EL Jr, Brenner MJ, Caldwell JR, *et al.*: Pheochromocytoma: a familial tumor. A study of 11 families. *Henry Ford Hosp Med J* 1965, 13:467–478.

7. Steiner AL, Goodman AD, Powers SR: Study of a kindred with phaeochromocytoma, medullary thyroid carcinoma, hyperparathyroidism and Cushing's disease: multiple endocrine neoplasia, type 2. *Medicine* 1968, 47:371–409.

8. Sipple J: The association of pheochromocytoma with carcinoma of the thyroid gland. *Am J Med* 1961, 31:163–166.

9. Manger WM, Gifford RW, JR.: *Clinical and Experimental Pheochromocytoma*. Cambridge, MA: Blackwell Science; 1996.

10. Lo CY, Lam KY, Wat MS, Lam KS: Adrenal pheochromocytoma remains a frequently overlooked diagnosis. *Am J Surg* 2000, 179:212–215.

11. Glushien A, Mansuy M, Littman D: Pheochromocytoma: It's relationship to the neurocutaneous syndromes. *Am J Med* 1953, 14:318–327.

12. Mulholland SG, Atuk NO, Walzak MP: Familial pheochromocytoma associated with cerebellar hemangioblastoma: A case history and review of the literature. *JAMA* 1969, 207:1709–1711.

13. Neumann HPH, Berger DP, Sigmund G, *et al.*: Pheochromocytomas, multiple endocrine neoplasia type 2, and Von Hippel-Lindau disease. *N Engl J Med* 1993, 329:1531–1538.

14.• Crossey PA, Eng C, Ginalska-Malinowska M, *et al.*: Molecular genetic diagnosis of von Hippel-Lindau disease in familiar phaeochromocytoma. *J Med Genet* 1995, 32:885–886.

15.•• Skinner MA, DeBenedetti MK, Moley JF, *et al.*: Medullary thyroid carcinoma in children with multiple endocrine neoplasia types 2A and 2B. *J Pediatr Surg* 1996, 31:177–182.

16. Moers AMJ, Landsaeter RM, Schaap C, *et al.*: Familial medullary thyroid carcinoma: not a distinct entity? Genotype-phenotype correlation in a large family. *Am J Med* 1996, 101:635–641.

17. Pearse AG: Common cytochemical and ultrastructural characteristics of cells producing polypeptide hormones (the APUD series) and their relevance to thyroid and ultimobranchial C cells and calcitonin. *Pro R Soc Lond [Biol]* 1968, 170:71–80.

18. Ober WB: Emil Zuckerkandl and his delightful little organ. *Pathol Annu* 1983, 18:103–119.

19. Quinan C, Berger AA: Observations on human adrenals with especial references to the relative weight of the normal medulla. *Ann Intern Med* 1993, 6:1180–1192.

20. Visser JW, Axt R: Bilateral adrenal medullary hyperplasia: A clinicopathological entity. *J Clin Pathol* 1975, 28:298–304.

21. Carney JA, Sizemore GW, Sheps SG: Adrenal medullary disease in multiple endocrine neoplasia, type 2: Pheochromocytoma and its precursors. *Am J Clin Pathol* 1976, 66:270–290.

22. Gifford R, Dvale W, Maher F, *et al.*: Clinical features, diagnosis, and treatment of pheochromocytomas. A review of 76 cases. *Mayo Clin Proc* 1964, 39:281–302.

23. Hyams JS, Leichtner AM, Breiner RG, *et al.*: Pseudopheochromocytoma and cardiac arrest associated with phenylpropanolamine. *JAMA* 1985, 253:1609–1610.

24. Lurvey A, Yusin A, DeQuattro V: Pseudopheochromocytoma after self-administered isoproterenol. *J Endocrinol Metab* 1973, 36:766–769.

25. Kuchel O: Pseudopheochromocytoma. *Hypertension* 1985, 7:151–158.

26. DeQuattro V, Campese V, Miura Y, Esler M: Sympathotonia in primary hypertension and in a caricature resembling dysautonomia. *Clin Sci* 1976, 51:435–438.

27. Waldman TA, Bradley JE: Polycythemia secondary to a pheochromocytoma with production of an erythropoiesis stimulating factor by the tumor. *Proc Soc Exp Biol Med* 1961, 108:425–427.

28. Boutros AR, Bravo EL, Zanettin G, Straffon RA: Perioperative management of 63 patients with pheochromocytoma. *Cleveland Clin J Med* 1990, 57:613–617.

29. Bravo EL: Pheochromocytoma: an approach to antihypertensive management. *Ann NY Acad Sci* 2002, 970:1–10.

30. Nanda AS, Feldman A, Liang CS: Acute reversal of pheochromocytoma-induced catecholamine cardiomyopathy. *Clin Cardiol* 1995, 18:421–423.

31. Huddle KR, Kalliatakis B, Skoularigis J: Pheochromocytoma associated with clinical and echocardiographic features simulating hypertrophic obstructive cardiomyopathy. *Chest* 1996, 109:1394–1397.

32. Scott IU, Gutterman DD: Pheochromocytoma with reversible focal cardiac dysfunction. *Am Heart J* 1995, 130:909–911.

33. Dabrowska B, Dabrowski A, Pruszczyk P, *et al.*: Heart rate variability in pheochromocytoma. *Am J Cardiol* 1995, 76:1201–1204.

34. Kline IK: Myocardial alterations associated with pheochromocytoma. *Am J Pathol* 1961, 38:539–551.

35. Simons M, Downing SE: Coronary vasoconstriction and catecholamine cardiomyopathy. *Am Heart J* 1985, 109:297–304.

36. Sardesai SH, Farrow B, Gibbons DO: Pheochromocytoma and catecholamine-induced cardiomyopathy presenting as heart failure. *Br Heart J* 1990, 63:234–237.

37. Hamada N, Akamatsu A, Joh T: A case of pheochromocytoma complicated with acute renal failure and cardiomyopathy. *Jpn J Circulation* 1993, 57:84–90.

38. Suga K, Tsukamoto K, Nishigauchi K, *et al.*: Iodine-123-MIBG imaging in pheochromocytoma with cardiomyopathy and pulmonary edema. *J Nucl Med* 1996, 37:1361–1364.

39. Seah PW, Costa R, Wolfenden H: Combined coronary artery bypass grafting and excision of adrenal pheochromocytoma. *J Thorac Cardiovasc Surg* 1995, 110:559–560.

40. Heron E, Chatellier G, Billaud E, *et al.*: The urinary metanephrine-to-creatinine ratio for the diagnosis of pheochromocytoma. *Ann Intern Med* 1996, 125:300–303.

41. Bray GA, DeQuattro V, Fisher DA, *et al.*: Catecholamines: a symposium—teaching conference. University of California, Los Angeles and Harbor General Hospital (specialty conference). *California Med* 1972, 117:32–62.

42. DeQuattro V, Chan S: Raised plasma catecholamines in some patients with primary hypertension. *Lancet* 1972, i:806–809.

43. Kobayashi R, DeQuattro V, Kolloch R, Miano L: A radioenzymatic assay for plasma normetanephrine in man and patients with pheochromocytoma. *Life Sci* 1980, 26:567–573.

44. Foti A, Adachi M, DeQuattro V: The relationships of free to conjugated metanephrine in plasma and spinal fluid of hypertensive patients. *J Clin Endocrinol Metab* 1982, 55:81–85.

45. Eisenhofer G, Goldstein DS, Walther MM, *et al.*: Biochemical diagnosis of pheochromocytoma: how to distinguish true- from false-positive results. *J Clin Endocrinol Metab* 2003, 88:2656–2666.

46. O'Connor DT, Bernstein KN: Radioimmunoassay of chromogranin A in plasma as a measure of exocytotic sympathoadrenal activity in normal subjects and patients with pheochromocytoma. *N Engl J Med* 1984, 311:764–770.

47. Goldstein DS, Levinson PD, Zimlichman R, *et al.*: Clonidine suppression testing in essential hypertension. *Ann Intern Med* 1985, 102:42–48.

48. Bravo EL, Tarazi RC, Fouad FM, *et al.*: Clonidine suppression test: a useful aid in the diagnosis of pheochromocytoma. *N Engl J Med* 1981, 305:623–626.

49. Bravo E: Clonidine-suppression test for diagnosis of pheochromocytoma. *N Engl J Med* 1982, 306:49–50.

50. Welch TJ, Sheedy PF, Heerden JA, *et al.*: Pheochromocytoma: value of computed tomography. *Radiology* 1983, 148:501–503.

51. Wieland DM, Wu J, Brown LE, *et al.*: Radiolabeled adrenergic neuron-blocking agents: adrenomedullary imaging with (131-I) iodobenzylguanidine. *J Nucl Med* 1980, 21:349–353.

52. Sisson JC, Frager MS, Valk TW, *et al.*: Scintigraphic localization of pheochromocytoma. *N Engl J Med* 1981, 305:12–17.

53. Valk TW, Frager MS, Gross MD, *et al.*: Spectrum of pheochromocytoma in multiple endocrine neoplasia: a scintigraphic portrayal using 131-I metaiodobenzylguanidine. *Ann Intern Med* 1981, 94:762–767.

54. Shapiro B, Copp JE, Sisson JE, *et al.*: Iodine-131 metaiodobenzylguanidine for the locating of suspected pheochromocytoma: experience in 400 cases. *J Nucl Med* 1985, 26:576–585.

55. Krenning EP, Kwekkeboom DJ, Bakker WH, *et al.*: Somatostatin receptor scintigraphy with [^{111}In-DPTA-D-Phe^1 and ^{123}I-Tyr^3]-octreotide: the Rotterdam experience with more than 1000 patients. *Eur J Nucl Med* 1993, 20:716–731.

56. Francis IR, Glazer GM, Shapiro B, *et al.*: Complementary roles of CT and I-MIBG scintigraphy in diagnosing pheochromocytoma. *AJR Am J Roentgenol* 1983, 141:719–725.

57. Gross MD, Shapiro B: Clinical review 50: clinically silent adrenal masses. *J Clin Endocrinol Metab* 1993, 77:885.

58. Ansari AN, Siegel ME, DeQuattro V, Gazarian LH: Imaging of medullary thyroid carcinoma and hyperfunctioning adrenal medulla using iodine-131 metaiodobenzylguanidine. *J Nucl Med* 1986, 27:1858–1860.

59. Glazer GM, Woolsey EJ, Borrello J, *et al.*: Adrenal tissue characterization using MR imaging. *Radiology* 1986, 158:73–79.

60. Fink IJ, Reinig JW, Dwyer AK, *et al.*: MR imaging of pheochromocytomas. *J Comput Assist Tomogr* 1985, 9:454–458.

61.•• Tenebaum F, Lumbroso J, Schlumberger M, *et al.*: Comparison of radiolabeled ocreotide and meta-iodobenzylguanidine (MIBG) scintigraphy in malignant pheochromocytoma. *J Nucl Med* 1995, 36:1–6.

62. Pacak K, Eisenhofer G, Carrasquillo JA, *et al.*: Diagnostic localization of pheochromocytoma: The coming age of positron emission tomography. *Ann N Y Acad Sci* 2002, 970:170–176.

63. Apgar V, Papper EM: Pheochromocytoma: anesthetic management during surgical treatment. *Arch Surg* 1951, 62:634–648.

64. Brunjes S, Johns V, Crane M: Pheochromocytoma: Postoperative shock and blood volume. *N Engl J Med* 1960, 262:393–396.

65. Deoreo GA Jr, Stewart BH, Tarazi RC, Gifford RW: Preoperative blood transfusion in the safe surgical management of pheochromocytoma. *J Urol* 1974, 111:715–721.

66. Wallace J, Gill DP: Prazosin in the diagnosis and treatment of pheochromocytoma. *JAMA* 1978, 240:2752–2753.

67. Nicholson JP, Vaughn ED, Pickering TG, *et al.*: Pheochromocytoma and prazosin. *Ann Intern Med* 1983, 99:477–479.

68. Dabrowska B, Pruszczyk P, Dabrowski A, *et al.*: Influence of alpha adrenergic blockade on ventricular arrhythmias, QTc interval and heart rate variability in phaeochromocytoma. *J Human Hypertens* 1995, 9:925–929.

69. Rosca EA, Brown JT, Tever AF, *et al.*: Treatment of pheochromocytoma and clonidine withdrawal hypertension with labetalol. *Br J Clin Pharmacol* 1976, 3:809–815.

70. Tokioka HT, Takahashi Y, Kosogabe, *et al.*: Use of nicardipine hydrochloride to control circulatory fluctuations during resection of a phaeochromocytoma. *Br J Anaesth*, 1988, 60:582–587.

71. Ulhacker JC, Goldfarb DA, Bravo EL, Novick, AC: Successful outcomes in pheochromocytoma surgery in the modern era. *J Urol* 1999, 161:3:764–767.

72. Manger WM, Gifford RW: Hypertension secondary to pheochromocytoma. *Bull N Y Acad Med* 1982, 58:139–158.

73. Sjoersdma A, Engelman K, Spector S, Undenfriend S: Inhibition of catecholamine synthesis in man with a-methyl-tyrosine, an inhibitor of tyrosine hydroxylase. *Lancet* 1965, ii:1092–1094.

74. Gitlow SE, Pertsemlidis D, Bertani LM: Management of patients with pheochromocytoma. *Am Heart J* 1971, 83:557–567.

75. Keiser HR, Goldstein DS, Wade JL, *et al.*: Treatment of malignant pheochromocytoma with combination chemotherapy. *Hypertension* 1985, 7:18–24.

76. Tristam M, Alaamr AS, Fleming JS, *et al.*: Iodine-131-metaiodobenzylguanidine dosimetry in cancer therapy: risk versus benefit. *J Nucl Med* 1996, 37:1058–1063.

77. Botchan A, Hauser R, Kupfermine M, *et al.*: Pheochromocytoma in pregnancy: case report and review of the literature. *Obstet Gyn Survey* 1995, 50:321–327.

78. Glenner G, Grimbley P: Tumors of the extra-adrenal paraganglion system. *Ann Tumor Pathol* 1974, Ser 2, fasc 9.

SELECT BIBLIOGRAPHY

Aravot DJ, Banner NR, Cantor AM, *et al.*: Location, localization and surgical treatment of cardiac pheochromocytoma. *Am J Cardiol* 1992, 69:283–285.

Ledger GA, Khosla S, Lindor NM, *et al.*: Genetic testing in the diagnosis and management of multiple endocrine neoplasia type II. *Ann Intern Med* 1995, 122:118–124.

Neumann HPH, Weistler OD: Clustering of features of von Hippel-Lindau syndrome: evidence for a complex genetic locus. *Lancet* 1991, 337:1052–1154.

Orchard T, Grant CS, van Heerden JA, Weaver A: Pheochromocytoma: continuing evolution of surgical therapy. *Surgery* 1993, 116:1153–1159.

Schulumberger C, Gicquel C, Lumbroso J, *et al.*: Malignant pheochromocytoma: clinical, biological, histologic and therapeutic data in a series of 20 patients with distant metastases. *J Endocrinol Invest* 1992, 15:631–642.

Chronic Ischemic Heart Disease

18

Tomasz Stys
Maria Stys
Peter F. Cohn

Key Points
- The pathophysiology of myocardial ischemia is related to a mismatch between coronary blood flow and myocardial oxygen requirements.
- In most patients with coronary artery disease, the angina threshold is not fixed but varies throughout the day.
- The exercise test is probably still the most important noninvasive diagnostic test.
- Patients with chronic ischemia may or may not demonstrate painful symptoms during ischemic episodes.
- Prognosis in patients with chronic ischemia relates to the severity of coronary artery disease and the degree of left ventricular dysfunction plus objective documentation of ischemia.
- Major therapeutic agents for patients with chronic ischemia are antianginal drugs (nitrates, β-blockers, calcium blockers), lipid-lowering agents, angiotensin-converting enzyme inhibitors, antiplatelet drugs (aspirin), and revascularization procedures (coronary angioplasty, coronary artery surgery).

Myocardial ischemia occurs when the coronary blood supply cannot meet the myocardial demands. This discrepancy is termed a supply–demand mismatch. Coronary blood supply is determined by the oxygen-carrying capacity and the coronary blood flow, which is regulated by numerous interacting factors. Myocardial demands are affected by changes in heart rate, contractility, and systolic wall tension; increasing heart rate is believed to be the single most important determinant of increased myocardial oxygen consumption.

In the normal heart, the coronary blood supply increases to match increasing myocardial demands. In the patient with significant coronary atherosclerotic disease, however, myocardial oxygen consumption may exceed the coronary blood supply, resulting in myocardial ischemia. Because it is at the end of the arterial blood supply, the subendocardium is the most vulnerable to ischemia.

CLINICAL PRESENTATION

The clinical presentation of myocardial ischemia resulting from coronary artery disease (CAD) ranges from asymptomatic silent ischemia to atypical angina to classic angina pectoris. Classic angina has been defined as transient precordial discomfort provoked by exertion or emotional stress and relieved by rest or nitroglycerin. The discomfort can be heaviness, pressure, or tightness in the chest. It also can radiate to the arm, neck, jaw, or back and may be provoked by exercise; cold, hot, or humid weather; heavy meals; or emotional stress. The discomfort begins gradually and reaches maximal intensity over several minutes before resolving. Classic angina eases after rest or 2 to 3

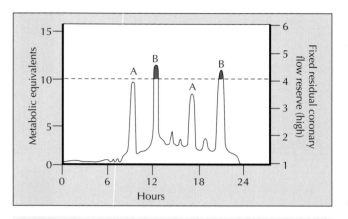

FIGURE 1 Fixed coronary artery obstructions not adequately compensated by collateral flow may reduce coronary flow reserve. In this diagram, it is reduced to only four times the resting values. The patient can exercise up to approximately 10 metabolic equivalents without having ischemia (A); however, if the patient exercises above approximately 10 metabolic equivalents, he or she will consistently develop ischemia (B). (*Adapted from* Maseri *et al.* [34].)

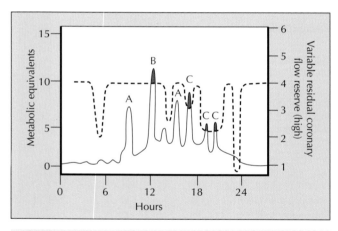

FIGURE 2 Residual coronary flow reserve may have an upper limit that is indeed fixed, but it can decrease because of mechanisms that transiently interfere with coronary blood flow. Thus, residual coronary flow reserve can vary throughout the day. Under these conditions, if the patient exercises beyond the maximal residual coronary flow reserve, the patient will always develop ischemia (B). However, the patient may also develop ischemia on other occasions after smaller degrees of exercise when residual coronary flow reserve is decreased by these functional factors (C). Occasionally, coronary flow reserve can decrease so that resting flow is impaired and ischemia occurs at rest. At other times of the day, this patient can exercise below the level of maximal residual coronary flow reserve without experiencing ischemia (A). In this case, the coronary flow reserve is fixed at approximately four times resting levels, so that the patient can exercise to approximately 10 metabolic equivalents in the absence of transient impairment of coronary flow. This level of work is compatible with most activities of daily life; hence, if the episodes of transient impairment of coronary flow reserve could be prevented, the patient would develop angina only after efforts of unusual intensity. (*Adapted from* Maseri *et al.* [34].)

minutes after nitroglycerin is taken. Most importantly, angina is *not* described as a brief, sharp, pleuritic, stabbing, localized, or migratory discomfort.

Atypical angina is a syndrome that has some similar symptoms, but lacks one or more of the criteria for classic angina. Angina equivalents are symptoms of myocardial ischemia other than angina. Exertional dyspnea is often referred to as an anginal equivalent. Others use the term to describe pain in a referred location, such as isolated exertional arm or neck discomfort not accompanied by discomfort in the chest. Variant angina is chest discomfort occurring at rest secondary to coronary vasospasm and associated with ST-segment elevation (rather than depression) on electrocardiography (ECG).

The angina threshold is the level of metabolic activity (physical or emotional) at which myocardial ischemia ensues. If this threshold is fixed, the same amount of exertion, often expressed in metabolic equivalents or as a rate–pressure product (heart rate multiplied by systolic blood pressure), provokes the patient's angina (Fig. 1). In other patients, the threshold varies throughout the day. These patients sometimes have angina at rest or with minimal exertion; at other times, they are able to exercise more vigorously (Fig. 2). Many patients have both fixed- and variable-threshold angina, which is described as mixed angina pectoris.

The clinical history may give clues to the mechanism of a patient's angina (increasing myocardial demands as seen in exertional angina and decreasing coronary blood supply in patients with angina without precipitant). This information may help to guide the physician in choosing a medication (Fig. 3).

DIAGNOSIS

The diagnosis of CAD cannot be made on physical examination; however, some findings may increase clinical suspicion of CAD. One such example is systemic hypertension. Skin xanthomas are found in patients with familial hypercholesterolemia who have an increased incidence of premature coronary artery disease. Arcus cornealis (an opaque, grayish ring at the periphery of the cornea found in young white patients) is a predictor of subsequent coronary events. The presence of carotid or femoral bruits, which is suggestive of peripheral vascular disease, increases the likelihood that the patient also has atherosclerotic heart disease. Cardiac examination may give clues to underlying organic heart disease (*eg*, if pathologic murmurs or gallops are noted) but it is by no means sensitive or specific for the diagnosis of CAD.

Noninvasive tests include exercise ECG, ambulatory ECG monitoring, nuclear imaging, and echocardiography. The exercise stress test is best used in patients who have normal findings on resting ECG. The patient exercises, commonly with either a treadmill or a stationary bicycle, and the patient's exercise duration, symptoms, blood pressure, heart rate, heart rhythm, physical examination findings, and ECG findings are analyzed. In the context of the clinical history, these parameters are evaluated to formulate a diagnostic impression.

The pretest risk (the probability of disease in the patient having the test) can be ascertained on clinical examination. Pryor and coworkers [1] concluded that the type of chest pain (typical, atypical, or nonanginal) was the most important predictor of significant coronary artery disease, followed by evidence of a prior myocardial infarction, gender, age, tobacco use, hyperlipidemia, ST-T segment changes on ECG, and a history of diabetes. Figures 4 and 5 are nomograms for estimating the likelihood of significant CAD. The post-test risk (the probability of disease in a patient with a positive test result) is assessed in light of the pretest risk and the test results (Table 1).

Exercise radionuclide ventriculography, thallium-201 stress testing, and stress echocardiography have increased the sensitivity for detecting CAD [2]. These specialized tests are commonly used in patients with abnormal baseline ECG results that make the exercise ECG findings difficult to interpret. Radionuclide and echocardiographic studies are also commonly used in patients with poor exercise capacity and those who are unable to exercise. In these circumstances, pharmacologic stress agents such as dipyridamole, dobutamine, or adenosine have been employed. The sensitivity and specificity of dipyridamole-

thallium stress testing are nearly comparable to those of exercise thallium stress testing [3]. Because of their increased cost and time of performance as well as the marginal benefit for improved detection in some patients, however, nuclear and echocardiographic stress tests are not routinely recommended as screening procedures.

In patients with chronic stable angina, the stress test has been said to provide little diagnostic information after clinical parameters are taken into account. However, the stress test can be used to monitor disease progression and the patient's response to medication. It also can assess the functional significance of a lesion detected angiographically, assess the benefits of revascularization via surgery or angioplasty, and perhaps most importantly, provide a prognostic assessment (aid in risk stratification).

Electron beam computed tomography (EBCT) is a highly sensitive technique for detection of coronary artery calcium, which is part of the development of atherosclerosis and is absent in normal vessel walls. However, its much lower specificity resulting in a high percentage of false-positive results poses a major limitation for clinical application of this method. Considering this and the method's lack of superiority to alternative noninvasive tests, EBCT is not currently recommended for diagnosis of obstructive coronary disease. The usefulness of determination of changes in calcium scores and its correlation with disease regression or progression is currently being studied [4].

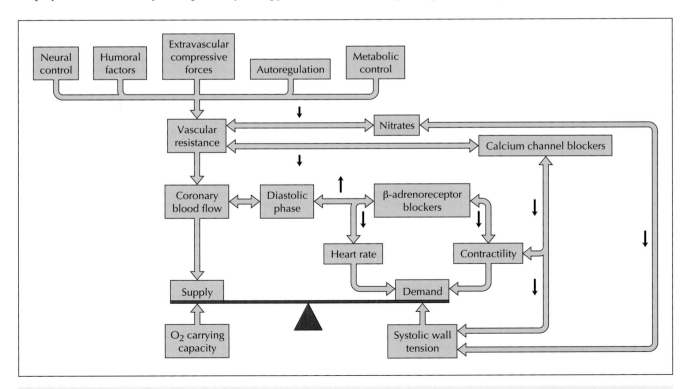

FIGURE 3 Effect of nitrates, beta-adrenoreceptor blockers, and calcium channel blockers on myocardial oxygen supply and demand. Reflex effects are not shown. (*Adapted from* Ardehali and Ports [35].)

PROGNOSIS

The prognosis in patients with chronic stable angina can be determined by the patient history, physical examination, noninvasive data, and coronary angiographic results. Some investigators believe that severe angina is consistent with a poorer outlook. Thus, the angina score, which takes into account the severity and frequency of the angina as well as the results of resting ECG, has been shown to be an independent predictor of prognosis [5]. Clinical findings suggestive of poor left ventricular function are also associated with a worse prospect.

With information obtained from the clinical examination, the clinician decides if the patient is in a low- or high-risk group. In high-risk patients (those with frequent episodes of angina and evidence of left ventricular dysfunction on clinical examination), coronary angiography with an eye toward revascularization should be performed. In low-risk patients or those in a poorly defined risk category on clinical examination, stress data have helped to delineate high- and low-risk groups. The specific criteria vary from report to report, but the conclusion remains the same: patients with poor exercise capacity and those with severe ischemia by ST response at a low workload compose a high-risk cohort (Table 2).

Radionuclide stress tests (either with ventriculography demonstrating poor resting left ventricular function or failure of the left ventricular ejection fraction to increase with exercise [6] or with perfusion imaging showing severe ischemia as evidenced by multiple reversible thallium defects), thallium uptake in the lungs, and transient postexercise left ventricular dilatation identify patients at higher risk for cardiac events [7,8]. Although left ventricular function is probably the strongest predictor of prog-

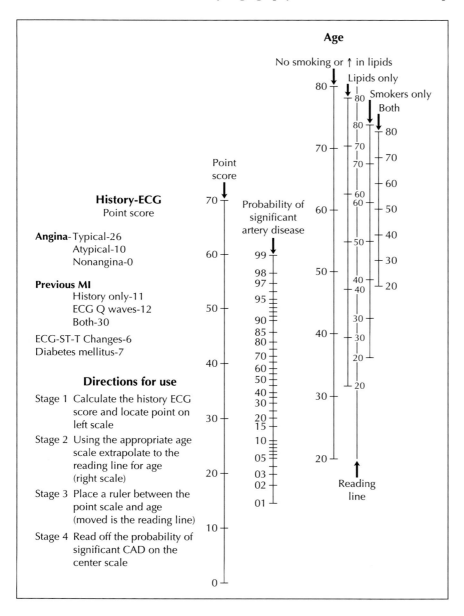

FIGURE 4 Nomogram for estimating the likelihood of significant coronary artery disease (CAD) in men. ECG—electrocardiographic; MI—myocardial infarction. (*Adapted from* Pryor *et al.* [1].)

nosis [9], the severity of the CAD has significant implications. Both the number of diseased vessels and the severity of the stenosis [9,10] correlate with survival. Left ventricular function and the severity of the CAD act synergistically in determining survival [9], and patients with left main CAD have been shown to have the worst prognosis, followed by those with severe three-vessel CAD [11].

THERAPY

The goals of therapy in managing chronic stable angina are to prolong survival, reduce the incidence of disease progression, alleviate symptoms, and improve exercise capacity. Nitrates, β-blockers, and calcium antagonists are the three classes of antianginal agents available to treat

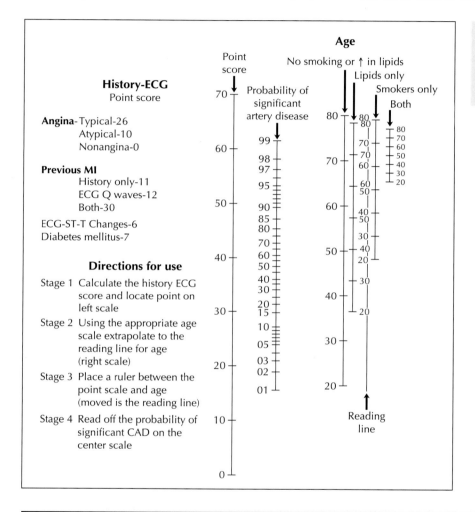

FIGURE 5 Nomogram for estimating the likelihood of significant coronary artery disease (CAD) in women. ECG—electrocardiographic; MI—myocardial infarction. (*Adapted from* Pryor *et al.* [1].)

TABLE 1 POST-TEST RISK OF OBSTRUCTIVE CORONARY DISEASE AFTER A SYMPTOM-LIMITED EXERCISE TEST*

Clinical presentation	Men, %		Women, %	
	ECG abnormal†	ECG normal‡	ECG abnormal	ECG normal
Typical angina	95	50	80	30
Probable angina	85	25	55	15
Nonspecific chest pain	40	10	10	5
Asymptomatic	30	5	5	< 1

*Patients without myocardial infarction.

†Horizontal or downsloping ST-segment depression of 1 mm or more.

‡Heart rate that is 85% or more of the age-predicted maximum.

ECG—electrocardiogram.

chronic stable angina. They can be used alone or in combination [12•,13].

Aspirin, angiotensin-converting enzyme (ACE) inhibitors, and lipid-lowering agents in the treatment of patients with chronic stable angina aim at preventing myocardial infarction (MI) and death; therefore, their major role is to improve patient survival.

Nitrates dilate coronary arteries and decrease cardiac preload. Their use is associated with reflex tachycardia, an effect that may increase myocardial demands and can be blunted by concomitant use of a β-blocker. Short-acting nitrates, which are most often administered in sublingual or buccal mucosa spray form, are often used to treat an acute episode of angina. Patients should be told to sit down when they take this type of agent, because the vasodilatation may be associated with transient hypotension and dizziness. This effect is especially prominent when there is preexistent vasodilatation, as in very hot, humid weather or after a hot shower. Most patients with chronic stable angina have a short-acting nitrate preparation prescribed for them to take on an "as-needed" basis. They also may be on a daily regimen of a longer-acting nitrate. In patients with stable exertional angina, long-acting nitrates improve exercise tolerance, increase angina threshold, and decrease ST segment depression during treadmill exercise test. At present, a multitude of preparations are available in different forms and with different half-lives. The most important aspect of long-term nitrate therapy is to ensure an adequate nitrate-free interval, which will prevent nitrate tolerance.

β-Blockers decrease heart rate and contractility and thus delay or prevent the onset of angina or the ischemic threshold. The doses of these drugs should be adjusted to reduce the heart rate to 55 to 60 bpm. In patients with more severe angina, the heart rate can be reduced to lower than 50 bpm, provided that there are no symptoms associated with bradycardia. They must be used with caution in patients who have significant bradyarrhythmias, asthma, congestive heart failure, or hypotension. They also must be used prudently in patients with diabetes mellitus and peripheral vascular disease. Because they blunt the tachycardia associated with exercise, these agents are well suited for patients with exertional or effort-induced angina. In addition, they are effective therapy for patients with angina who also have coexisting hypertension. In the absence of contraindications, β-blockers are the preferred initial therapy. The evidence for this approach is strongest in the presence of previous MI.

Calcium channel antagonists are a diverse group of agents, all of which act as vasodilators. Dilatation of the epicardial coronary arteries is the principal mechanism through which calcium channel blockers relieve vasospastic angina. Through reduction of systemic vascular resistance and reduction of blood pressure, they reduce myocardial oxygen demand. Therefore, similar to β-blockers, many calcium channel blockers can be used as antianginal and antihypertensive agents. Like β-blockers, many can be used as antianginal and antihypertensive agents. Diltiazem and verapamil can be used in patients

		Risk classification		
Study	Patients, *n*	Low	Intermediate	High
McNeer *et al.* [36]	1472	< 1 mm ST ↓ FS ≥ IV Peak HR ≥ 160 bpm		≥ 1 mm ST ↓ FS I or II
Bruce *et al.* [37] (Seattle Heart Watch)	2001	< 1 mm ST ↓ No LV dysfunction	≥ 1 mm ST ↓ No LV dysfunction	FS ≤ I Peak SBP < 130 mm Hg Cardiomegaly
Dagenais *et al.* [38]	107	≤ 2 mm ST ↓ FS ≥ IV	≤ 2 mm ST ↓ FS ≥ III	≥ 2 mm ST ↓ FS ≤ I
Schneider *et al.* [39]	80			> 1 mm ST ↓ FS I or II
Weiner *et al.* [40]	292	≤ 2 mm ST ↓ No LV dysfunction		LV dysfunction or ≥ 2 mm ST ↓ beginning in stage I
Weiner *et al.* [41] Coronary Artery Surgery Study	4083	< 1 mm ST ↓ FS ≥ III	≥ 1 mm ST ↓ FS ≥ III	≥ 1 mm ST ↓ FS ≤ I

TABLE 2 RISK STRATIFICATION BY EXERCISE TESTING

FS—final exercise stage (Bruce protocol); HR— heart rate; LV—left ventricular; SBP—systolic blood pressure; ST ↓—ST-segment depression.

with coexistent supraventricular arrhythmias, but unlike nifedipine and newer related compounds, they must be used cautiously in patients with bradyarrhythmias. Verapamil is a potent negative inotrope and is not recommended in patients with poor left ventricular systolic function. Short-acting dihydropyridine calcium antagonists have the potential to enhance the risk of adverse cardiac events and should be avoided. Long-acting calcium antagonists, including slow-release and long-acting dihydropyridines and nondihydropyridines, are effective antianginal pharmacotherapy for patients with chronic stable angina. They can be used either as initial therapy in patients in whom β-blockers are contraindicated, not tolerated, or not effective, or in combination with β-blockers [14•,15].

All three classes of antianginal drugs decrease the incidence of ischemia and improve exercise performance. These agents can be used as the sole therapy for patients stratified by noninvasive methods to a low-risk group for cardiac events or who are good candidates for revascularization. They are also often used as adjuncts to revascularization. In addition, because of its proven benefit in post–MI, unstable angina, and post–coronary bypass patients, daily aspirin use is often recommended. Aspirin has proven benefit in patients after MI, those with unstable angina, and after coronary bypass surgery. It is also effective in preventing the first heart attack in patients with stable angina as well as in asymptomatic patients. The use of aspirin in those with chronic stable angina is recommended as a strategy to decrease the risk of MI and death in this patient population [16].

The results of the Heart Outcomes Prevention Evaluation (HOPE) trial confirmed the role of ACE inhibitors in reduction of incidence of cardiovascular death, myocardial infarction, and stroke in patients who were at high risk for, or had vascular disease in the absence of heart failure. Ramipril, which was used in this study, also resulted in a very significant reduction in diabetic complications among patients with diabetes. Fewer patients were diagnosed with diabetes among those treated with ramipril during the 4-year observation period. ACE inhibitors are recommended as routine secondary prevention for patients with known CAD, particularly diabetics without severe renal disease [17,18].

The therapy directed toward improvement of survival has also expanded greatly with the use of lipid-lowering agents for this purpose. The Scandinavian Simvastatin Survival Study (4S) [19], as well as other trials, has demonstrated that treatment with 3-hydroxy-3-methylglutaryl (HMG) coenzyme reductase inhibitors significantly reduces the risk of fatal and nonfatal MI and the need for revascularization. The results of a recent large cholesterol-lowering trial, the Heart Protection Study (HPS), support the role of HMG-coenzyme reductase inhibitors in reducing morbidity and mortality not only in patients with established CAD, but also in patients with other vascular diseases, diabetes, or hypertension. The benefit of this treatment was significant among all patient subgroups, including women, the elderly, and individuals with baseline low-density lipoprotein (LDL) cholesterol of less than 100 mg/dL [20]. In general, modification of diet and exercise are less effective than statins in achieving target levels of cholesterol and LDL. Lipid-lowering pharmacotherapy is usually required in patients with chronic stable angina.

Recent prospective studies of the effect of estrogen replacement therapy on secondary prevention of coronary heart disease in women have produced disappointing results. Estrogens have been shown to exert numerous beneficial modulatory effects on the cardiovascular system, including improvement in lipid profile and endothelial function, suppression of intimal and smooth muscle cell proliferation, and numerous other beneficial effects. These observations, as well as previously reported observational clinical trials, resulted in speculations that hormone replacement therapy (HRT) should be an effective therapy in preventing CAD. The results of the Heart and Estrogen/Progestin Replacement Study (HERS) [21], as well as another recently presented trial, the Estrogen Replacement and Atherosclerosis (ERA) trial, have shown no benefit of HRT for secondary prevention of coronary heart disease in women. The Women's Health Initiative, a randomized controlled primary prevention trial of estrogen plus progestin, found that the overall health risk of this therapy exceeded its benefits [22]. At this time, the available data do not support the use of HRT in women with CAD solely for cardioprotection.

Finally, risk modification with diet counseling, antilipemic therapy, smoking cessation, and exercise programs is strongly advised. Antioxidant therapy appears to have no effect on the endpoints of cardiovascular death, cardiovascular events, stroke, or revascularization. Thus, vitamin C and E supplements or other antioxidants are not recommended for preventing or treating CAD [17]. All of these measures can be initiated by the generalist; when revascularization is indicated by refractory symptoms or markedly abnormal stress test results, referral to a specialist is appropriate.

Coronary artery bypass graft (CABG) surgery is performed to improve quality of life and prolong survival. Coronary artery bypass grafting has been shown to relieve angina more effectively than medical therapy and is effective when angina is refractory to medical therapy. The poorer the prognosis (ie, severe ischemia combined with poor left ventricular function), the greater the benefits of revascularization (albeit possibly at a higher operative risk). A meta-analysis [23] of three major randomized trials comparing initial surgery with medical management has confirmed the survival benefit achieved by surgery at 10 years after surgery for patients with three-, two-, or even one-vessel disease that included stenosis of the proximal left anterior descending (LAD) coronary artery. The survival rate of these patients was improved by surgery, whether they had normal or abnormal left ventricular function. For patients without proximal LAD stenosis, bypass surgery improved the mortality rate only for those with three-vessel disease or left main stenosis.

The role of coronary angioplasty in the treatment of chronic stable angina is evolving. A randomized trial comparing angioplasty with medical therapy in patients with single-vessel coronary artery disease reported a statistically significant improvement in exercise tolerance and anginal symptoms among the angioplasty group [24]. The angioplasty patients had a greater number of hospital days, however, as well as a higher incidence of repeated angioplasty (with its associated risks) and a higher cost than the medically treated patients. Another randomized trial, RITA (Randomised Intervention Treatment of Angina) II, comparing initial percutaneous transluminal coronary angioplasty (PTCA) with initial medical management of one-vessel CAD revealed that patients who had undergone PTCA initially had less angina; however, at 2 years after surgery, the differences between the two groups were small. The combined rates of death, MI, and nonprotocol revascularization were similar in both groups [25].

There are no PTCA versus CABG trials of patients with only chronic stable angina. A meta-analysis [26] overview of eight clinical trials compared PTCA with CABG surgery with a mean follow-up of 2.7 years. The overview showed no difference in the rate of death or nonfatal MI between the two groups. However, the angioplasty group had a statistically significant increase in subsequent revascularization procedures within the first year of follow-up. The prevalence of angina pectoris New York Heart Association class II or greater was higher in the PTCA group at 1 year, but this difference was minimized by 3 years of follow-up. The two US trials of PTCA versus CABG, the multicenter Bypass Angioplasty Revascularization Intervention (BARI) and the single-center Emory Angioplasty Surgery Trial (EAST), included both stable and unstable angina [27,28]. The results of these trials at 7 to 8 years of follow-up showed that early and late survival rates have been equivalent for both revascularization strategies. In the BARI trial, however, patients with treated diabetes had better survival rates with CABG. The latest randomized trial comparing PTCA with CABG, the European Arterial Revascularization Therapies Study (ARTS) [29], found no significant differences between the two groups with respect to mortality, stroke, or MI at 1-year follow-up. Surgery was more expensive in spite of more repeat vascularizations in the stent group.

These trials comparing initial medical treatment with initial surgery indicate that patients with left main stenosis of 50% to 70% or more and those with multivessel CAD with proximal LAD stenosis of 70% or more have a better survival rate if they have bypass surgery. Furthermore, patients with a proximal LAD lesion have a better survival rate with surgery compared with medical management, even if they have normal left ventricular function and only one-vessel disease. For these patients, PTCA may be an alternative revascularization strategy and does not appear to compromise the survival, at least for the first 7 to 8 years. Caution should be used in treating diabetic patients with PTCA, particularly in the setting of multivessel, multilesion, severe CAD.

Management of patients with angina refractory to multiple revascularization procedures or aggressive medical therapy is a real problem today. It appears to be a tribute to the success of cardiologists and cardiovascular surgeons for keeping otherwise seriously ill patients alive. For such patients, several therapies have been proposed and evaluated that either act through reduction of anginal pain by neural stimulation as in spinal cord stimulation, or through potential enhancement of myocardial perfusion (transmyocardial laser revascularization, injection of the angiogenic proteins into the heart, enhanced external counterpulsation [EECP]) [30]. Of these numerous potential future alternatives, which are still being intensively investigated, EECP deserves special interest as the only truly noninvasive procedure reporting clinical improvement in these patients. A randomized, placebo-controlled, multicenter trial evaluated the safety and efficacy of EECP. Patients (*n* = 139) with chronic stable angina, documented CAD, and a positive stress test were randomly assigned to receive EECP (35 hours of active counterpulsation) or inactive EECP over a 4- to 7-week period. EECP decreased angina frequency and time to exercise-induced ischemia [31]. Two multicenter registry studies found EECP to be generally well tolerated and efficacious, with angina symptoms improving in approximately 75% to 80% of patients [32]. Its efficacy also appears to be sustained over a long-term period after treatment [33].

REFERENCES AND RECOMMENDED READING

Recently published papers of particular interest have been highlighted as:
• Of interest

1. Pryor DB, Harrell FE Jr, Lee KL, *et al.*: Estimating the likelihood of significant coronary artery disease. *Am J Med* 1983, 75:771–780.

2. Armstrong WF, O'Donnell J, Dillon JC, *et al.*: Complementary value of two-dimensional exercise echocardiography to routine treadmill exercise testing. *Ann Intern Med* 1986, 105:829–835.

3. Francisco DA, Collins SM, Go RT, *et al.*: Tomographic thallium-201 myocardial perfusion scintigrams after maximal coronary artery vasodilation with intravenous dipyridamole: comparison of qualitative and quantitative approaches. *Circulation* 1982, 66:370–379.

4. American College of Cardiology/American Heart Association Expert Consensus document on electron-beam computed tomography for the diagnosis and prognosis of coronary artery disease. *Circulation* 2000, 102:126–140.

5. Califf RM, Mark DB, Harrell FE Jr, *et al.*: Importance of clinical measures of ischemia in the prognosis of patients with documented coronary artery disease. *J Am Coll Cardiol* 1988, 11:20–26.

6. Taliercio CP, Clements IP, Zinsmeister AR, Gibbons RJ: Prognostic value and limitations of exercise radionuclide angiography in medically treated coronary artery disease. *Mayo Clin Proc* 1988, 63:573–582.

7. Ladenheim ML, Pollock BH, Rozanski A, *et al.*: Extent and severity of myocardial reperfusion as predictors of prognosis in patients with suspected coronary artery disease. *J Am Coll Cardiol* 1986, 7:464–471.

8. Weiss AT, Berman DS, Lew AS, *et al.*: Transient ischemic dilatation of the left ventricle on stress thallium-201 scintigraphy: a marker of severe and extensive coronary artery disease. *J Am Coll Cardiol* 1987, 9:752–759.

9. Mock MB, Ringqvist I, Fisher LD, *et al.*: Survival of medically treated patients in the Coronary Artery Surgery Study (CASS) Registry. *Circulation* 1982, 66:562–568.

10. Harris PJ, Behar VS, Conley MJ, *et al.*: The prognostic significance of 50 percent stenosis in medically treated patients with coronary artery disease. *Circulation* 1980, 62:240–248.

11. Proudfit WJ, Bruschke AV, MacMillan JP, *et al.*: Fifteen year survival study of patients with obstructive coronary artery disease. *Circulation* 1983, 68:986–997.

12.• Savonito S, Ardissino D, Egstrup F, *et al.*: Combination therapy with metoprolol and nifedipine versus monotherapy in patients with stable angina pectoris. Results of the International Multi-center Angina Exercise (IMAGE) Study. *J Am Coll Cardiol* 1996, 27:311–316.

13. Dargie HJ, Ford I, Fox KM, *et al.*: Total Ischemic Burden European Trial (TIBET). Effects of ischemia and treatment with atenolol, nifedipine SR and their combination and outcome in patients with chronic stable angina *Eur Heart J* 1996, 17:104–112.

14.• Furberg CD, Psaty BM, Meyer JV: Nifedipine. Dose-related increase in mortality in patients with coronary heart disease. *Circulation* 1995, 92:1326–1331.

15. Messerli FH: Case-controlled study, meta-analysis, and bouill-abaisse: putting the calcium antagonist scare into context. *Annals of Int Med* 1995, 123:888–889.

16. Willard JE, Lange RA, Hillis LD: The use of aspirin in ischemic heart disease. *N Engl J Med* 1992, 327:175–181.

17. AHA 2002 guideline update for the management of patients with chronic stable angina—summary article: a report of the American College of Cardiology/American Heart Association Task Force on practice guidelines (Committee on the Management of Patients with Chronic Unstable Angina). *J Am Coll Cardiol* 2003, 41:159–168.

18. Yusuf S, Sleight P, Pogue J, *et al.*: Effects of an angiotensin-converting enzyme inhibitor, ramipril, on cardiovascular events in high-risk patients. The Heart Outcomes Prevention Evaluation Study Investigators. *N Engl J Med* 2000, 342:145–153.

19. MRC/BHF Heart Protection Study of cholesterol lowering with simvastatin in 20,536 high risk individuals: a randomized placebo-controlled trial. *Lancet* 2002, 360:7–22.

20. Randomized trial of cholesterol lowering in 4444 patients with coronary heart disease: the Scandinavian Simvastatin Survival Study (4S). *Lancet* 1994, 344:1383–1389.1

21. Hulley S, Grady D, Bush T, *et al.*: Randomized trial of estrogen plus progestin for secondary prevention of coronary heart disease in postmenopausal women: Heart and Estrogen/progestin Replacement Study (HERS) Research Group. *JAMA* 1998, 280:605–613.

22. Risk and benefits of estrogen plus progestin in health post-menopausal women: principal results from the Womens's Health Initiative randomized controlled trial. *JAMA* 2002, 288:321–333.

23. Yusuf S, Zucker D, Peduzzi P, *et al.*: Effect of coronary artery bypass graft surgery on survival: overview of 10-year results from randomized trials by the Coronary Artery Bypass Graft Surgery Trialists Collaboration. *Lancet* 1994, 344:563–570.

24. Parisi AF, Folland ED, Hartigan P: A comparison of angioplasty with medical therapy in the treatment of single-vessel coronary artery disease. *N Engl J Med* 1992, 326:10–16.

25. Coronary angioplasty versus medical therapy for angina: the second Randomised Intervention Treatment of Angina (RITA-2) trial: RITA-2 trial participants. *Lancet* 1997, 360:461–468.

26. Pocock SJ, Henderson RA, Rickards AF, *et al.*: Meta-analysis of randomised trials comparing coronary angioplasty with bypass surgery. *Lancet* 1995, 346:1184–1189.

27. The Bypass Angioplasty Revascularization Investigation (BARI) investigators: Comparison of bypass surgery with angioplasty in patients with multivessel disease. *N Engl J Med* 1996, 335:217–225.

28. King SB, Lembo NJ, Weintraub WS, *et al.*: A randomized trial comparing coronary angioplasty with coronary bypass surgery. Emory Angioplasty versus Surgery Trial (EAST). *N Engl J Med* 1994, 331:1044–1050.

29. Serruys PW, Unger F, Sousa JE, *et al.*, Arterial Revascularization Therapies Study Group: Comparison of coronary-artery bypass surgery and stenting for the treatment of multivessel disease. *N Engl J Med* 2001, 344:1117–1124.

30. Cohn PF: Emerging treatments for refractory angina. *ACC Curr J Rev* Jan/Feb 1999, 544–546

31. Arora RR, Chou TM, Jain D, *et al.*: The multicenter study of enhanced external counterpulsation (MUST-EECP): Effect of EECP on exercise-induced myocardial ischemia and anginal episodes. *J Am Coll Cardiol* 1999, 33:1833–1840.

32. Barness G, Feldman AM, Holmes DR Jr, *et al.*, International EECP Patient Registry Investigators, the International EECP Patient Registry (IEPR): Design, methods, baseline characteristics, and acute results. *Clin Cardiol* 2001, 24:435–442.

33. Arora RR, Chou TM, Jain D, *et al.*: The multicenter study of enhanced external counterpulsation (MUST EECP): Effect of EECP on exercise-induced myocardial ischemia and anginal episodes. *J Am Coll Cardiol* 1999, 33: 1833–1840.

34. Maseri A, Chierchia S, Kaski JC: Mixed angina pectoris. *Am J Cardiol* 1985, 56:30E–33E.

35. Ardehali A, Ports TA: Myocardial oxygen supply and demand. *Chest* 1990, 90:699–705.

36. McNeer JF, Margolis JR, Lee KL, *et al.*: The role of the exercise test in the evaluation of patients for ischemic heart disease. *Circulation* 1979, 57:64–70.

37. Bruce RA, DeRouen TA, Hammermeister KE: Noninvasive screening criteria for enhanced 4-year survival after aortocoronary bypass surgery. *Circulation* 1979, 60:638–646.

38. Dagenais GR, Rouleau JR, Christen A, Fabia J: Survival of patients with a strongly positive exercise electrogram. *Circulation* 1982, 65:452–456.

39. Schneider RM, Seaworth JF, Dohnman ML, *et al.*: Anatomic and prognostic implications of an early positive treadmill exercise test. *Am J Cardiol* 1982, 50:682–688.

40. Weiner DA, McCabe CH, Ryan TJ: Prognostic assessment of patients with coronary artery disease by exercise testing. *Am Heart J* 1983, 105:749–755.

41. Weiner DA, Ryan TJ, McCabe CH, *et al.*: The prognostic importance of a clinical profile and exercise test in medically treated patients with coronary heart disease. *J Am Coll Cardiol* 1984, 3:772–779.

SELECT BIBLIOGRAPHY

AHA 2002 guideline update for the management of patients with chronic stable angina—summary article: a report of the American College of Cardiology/American Heart Association Task Force on practice guidelines (Committee on the Management of Patients with Chronic Unstable Angina). *J Am Coll Cardiol* 2003, 41:159–168.

Detrano R, Gianrossi R, Froelicher V: The diagnostic accuracy of exercise electrocardiogram: a meta-analysis of 22 years of research. *Prog Cardiovasc Dis* 1989, 31:173–206.

Braunwald E: *Heart Disease: A Textbook of Cardiovascular Medicine*, edn 5. Philadelphia: WB Saunders; 2001.

Unstable Angina and Non–ST Elevation Myocardial Infarction

John Speer Schroeder

19

Key Points

- Unstable angina and non–ST elevation myocardial infarction are important diagnoses to establish because of a high infarction/death rate that occurs over the next few months.

- These acute coronary syndromes are caused by atherosclerosis plaque rupture with varying degrees of occlusion because of platelet thrombus at the rupture site. There is increasing evidence that underlying vascular inflammation is an important component of the acute coronary syndrome and plaque rupture.

- Diagnosis is established by a history of prolonged angina chest pain, electrocardiographic changes, and serial enzyme testing, creatine kinase, creatine kinase MB, and troponin T and I. We now recognize that any elevation of cardiac muscle–specific biomarkers reflect an acute coronary syndrome regardless of electrocardiogram and creatine kinase abnormalities.

- Therapy is directed at the platelet thrombus (aspirin, clopidogrel, unfractionated or low molecular weight heparin, glycoprotein IIb/IIIa inhibitors), prevention of coronary spasm (intravenous or topical nitroglycerin), and treatment of contributing factors such as hypertension and tachycardia with β-blockers.

- Sublingual nifedipine is contraindicated for chest pain or hypertension.

- Identification of high-risk versus low-risk patients is important for subsequent decisions regarding coronary intervention.

The syndromes of unstable angina pectoris (UAP) and non–ST elevation myocardial infarction (NSTEMI) are referred to as intermediate coronary syndromes, because they sit between predictable exertional angina on the one hand and an acute transmural ST elevation myocardial infarction (STEMI) on the other. The diagnosis is important [1,2]. These syndromes frequently precede a more serious cardiovascular event that can now be prevented with aggressive medical therapy and, in some instances, coronary interventional procedures or coronary bypass surgery.

Unstable angina has had many clinical terms through the years, including impending MI, rest angina, angina decubitus, crescendo angina, preinfarction angina, and acute coronary syndrome (ACS). A new terminology has now been agreed upon, ie, ACS divided into non–ST elevation or ST elevation. Non–ST elevation ACS may still be associated with evidence of myocardial injury tropinin I and T, albeit of lower levels. It is important for the physician to recognize the diagnosis, rapidly initiate aggressive treatment, and in most instances, obtain a cardiology consultation to assist with the patient's care.

PATHOPHYSIOLOGY

This change from an asymptomatic to an unstable state is thought to result from a rupture of an atherosclerotic plaque in the coronary artery [3,4]. As shown in Figure 1, once the plaque ruptures, exposure of the plaque contents to the bloodstream results in platelet thrombosis as part of a "repair process." Platelet aggregation releases vasoactive substances that can cause local vasoconstriction, which can further reduce the coronary lumen diameter. This complex combination of platelet thrombosis, threatening to close off the coronary artery, coronary vasospasm, and counteractive natural lytic mechanisms, attempting to lyse the platelet thrombus, combine to cause dynamic, changing degrees of coronary occlusion that lead to the unstable angina syndrome. If this process is not reversed, complete occlusion may occur, leading to a STEMI. There is increasing evidence that underlying vascular inflammation is an important component of the ACS and plaque rupture.

DIAGNOSIS

Unstable angina pectoris/NSTEMI should be suspected or included in the differential diagnosis when a patient relates a changing or crescendo pattern of chest pain consistent with myocardial ischemia. The character of the chest pain is typical for angina pectoris, (*ie*, squeezing or pressure), usually in the substernal area that may radiate into the neck, jaw, or inner aspect of either arm. Relief of the pain within 5 minutes by sublingual nitroglycerin (NTG) assists in the diagnosis. NSTEMI should be suspected when the patient has a more prolonged episode of ischemic chest pain (> 15–30 minutes) that resolves spontaneously or with subsequent therapy. Myocardial ischemia does not always present as chest pain or pressure. It may be in the epigastric area and

thought to be heartburn, gastrointestinal upset, or gastritis, or even felt in the neck, jaw, or arm. The location should not deter the physician form suspecting ACS.

Examples include the following:

1. A patient with known, stable, five-block exertional angina being treated with β-blockers and isosorbide dinitrate reports that pain suddenly began with simply walking across the room.
2. A patient calls and reports that her angina has been occurring at 3 AM the past two nights instead of just during marked exertion.
3. A patient reports that his exertional angina attacks are much more severe and may take three or four NTG tablets to relieve.
4. A woman with coronary artery disease risk factors calls at 5 AM and reports a 30-minute episode of severe substernal chest pain radiating into her left elbow.
5. A 59-year-old man who has smoked for the past 40 years comes to your office at 9 AM to get treatment for "heartburn." He relates recurring neck pain that has occurred off and on for the past 3 hours.
6. A 65-year-old man who had coronary artery bypass surgery 10 years ago reports sudden onset of "that old chest pain."
7. A patient with known hypertension reports trouble breathing and "maybe a little chest pressure" whenever she climbed three or four steps for the past week.
8. A 72-year-old woman reports two episodes of heaviness in her chest, each lasting approximately 1 hour and associated with mild diaphoresis.

These simple examples reflect the fact that UAP or NSTEMI can occur in the setting of known coronary artery disease or *de novo* disease, but the characteristics are frequently similar.

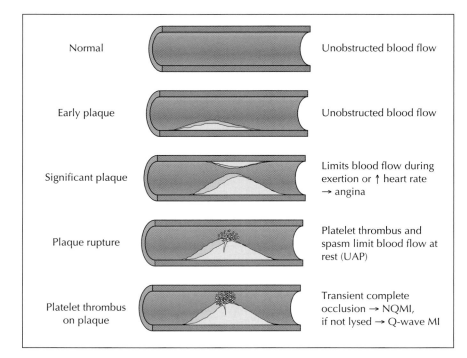

FIGURE 1 Atherosclerotic plaque in a coronary artery as it relates to clinical syndromes. NQMI—non–Q-wave myocardial infarction; MI—myocardial infarction; UAP—unstable angina pectoris.

Normal	Unobstructed blood flow
Early plaque	Unobstructed blood flow
Significant plaque	Limits blood flow during exertion or ↑ heart rate → angina
Plaque rupture	Platelet thrombus and spasm limit blood flow at rest (UAP)
Platelet thrombus on plaque	Transient complete occlusion → NQMI, if not lysed → Q-wave MI

Initial Assessment

The initial assessment of a patient presenting with symptoms that may represent UAP or NSTEMI should include a thorough history, physical examination, laboratory studies, and electrocardiography.

History

The physician should obtain a thorough patient history. Is the chest pain from myocardial ischemia? Is it typical versus atypical pain? Are there known coronary artery disease risk factors? Is there known coronary artery disease? Does NTG relieve or reduce the chest pain?

Physical examination and laboratory studies

Physical examination and laboratory studies should concentrate on whether other factors contributed to the myocardial ischemia. Is there decreased oxygen delivery (eg, anemia)? Is there increased oxygen demand, such as tachycardia secondary to new arrhythmia (eg, atrial fibrillation with rapid ventricular rate), increased heart rate, increased blood pressure, or hyperthyroidism?

Diagnostic Testing

If the patient is having acute chest pain during your interview, a trial of sublingual NTG can be helpful.

Electrocardiography

The electrocardiogram (ECG) is an essential tool in evaluating not only the cause of the patient's chest pain but also its severity. The finding of the ST-segment elevation or T-wave peaking suggests acute transmural ischemia, and the patient generally would be considered for thrombolytic therapy or acute angioplasty. If the ST elevation resolves with sublingual NTG, this suggests that coronary spasm was playing a significant role, but that the setting likely is still a ruptured, unstable atherosclerotic plaque. ST depression and abnormal T waves are consistent with myocardial ischemia, particularly if it is a change from previous ECGs or disappears with relief of chest pain after NTG. T-wave inversion suggests a recent subendocardial ischemic event that would be consistent with UAP or NSTEMI (Fig. 2). Serial ECGs are valuable in making the diagnosis of UAP or NSTEMI, because a rapidly changing pattern of ST-T waves suggests a dynamic ongoing process.

A normal ECG can be useful to rule out myocardial ischemia, but it also can be misleading. A normal ECG can be consistent with a noncardiac cause for the chest pain in approximately 10% of the patients presenting with a history consistent for unstable angina. However, a normal ECG also may reflect true posterior ischemia or be associated with a dissecting thoracic aneurysm. Exercise testing may be useful if the diagnosis at this point is still not clear. It is best to review the findings with a cardiologist before initiating exercise testing, however, because stress testing in the setting of UAP or NSTEMI may be hazardous to the patient.

Biomarkers for myocardial injury

Serial creatine kinase (CK) enzyme levels have been this standard in differentiating UAP from NSTEMI (Tables 1 and 2) in the past. Total and myocardial band creatine kinase (CK-MB) are drawn at the time of patient encounter and 8 and 24 hours after the initial patient encounter if the patient had a prolonged (> 15 minute) episode of chest pain that may have resulted in myocardial necrosis. Some patients may not have an elevated total CK, but still show evidence of NSTEMI based on an abnormal increase in the MB fraction that reflects death of myocardial tissue. Tropinin T, a regulatory protein located in the myocyte, has recently been found to be an additional monitor for adverse events in the unstable angina patient [5•,6•].

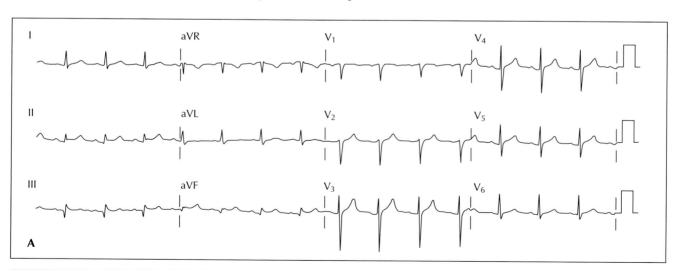

FIGURE 2 A, Twelve-lead electrocardiogram (ECG) in a patient complaining of crescendo angina chest pain. Leads qIII and AVG as well as ST-segment elevation in leads II, III, and AVF suggest an acute or recent inferior myocardial infarction.

(Continued)

Routine assessment of these cardiac-specific troponins T and I has improved the speed and accuracy of identifying myocardial necrosis and has been shown to provide prognostic value in patients with the unstable coronary syndromes. These enzyme tests have replaced CK and CK-MB in many hospitals.

We now recognize that any elevation of cardiac muscle–specific biomarkers reflects an ACS regardless of ECG and CK abnormalities. However, the decision to admit or consult a cardiologist should always be based on the history and overall patient assessment rather than an abnormal cardiac enzyme result.

TREATMENT

Initial therapy should be directed toward preventing progressive thrombus formation that could completely occlude the vessel and lead to transmural MI. Aspirin (325 mg, non–enteric coated) should be given immediately whether the initial contact is by telephone, in the office, or in the emergency room. The basis for this therapy is a 12-week study of 1266 veterans given Alka-Seltzer (Miles Inc, West Haven, CT) containing aspirin (325 mg) or placebo for 12 weeks following diagnosis of UAP [7]. The 12-week death rate was 3.3% in the placebo group and 1.6% in the aspirin group—a 51% reduction. Similar decreases occurred in fatal and nonfatal myocardial infarctions.

Nitroglycerin (usually one tablet sublingually every 5 minutes three times or until dizziness or severe headache occurs) should be used if the patient has it available and has not used it at the time of initial contact. If not available at home, this therapy should be used early during assessment of the patient in the office or the emergency department. The basis for NTG therapy includes reversal of any local coronary vasoconstriction related to the platelet thrombus as well as

causing preload and afterload reduction, resulting in lessened myocardial oxygen demand by the heart. WARNING: If the patient has taken sildenafil or other phosphodiesterase 5 inhibitors for sexual dysfunction in the past 24 hours, nitrates in all forms should not be taken because of the drug interactions, which may lead to hypotension.

A recent addition to the medical therapy at time of initial diagnosis is to give clopidogrel 300 mg followed by 75 mg per day. This recommendation is based on the CURE and PCI-CURE trials documenting further benefit over aspirin alone. Clopidogrel is an ADP inhibitor that also affects platelet aggregation at a different site on the platelet from aspirin and glycoprotein (GP) IIb/IIIa inhibitors.

In the Emergency Department

Once the initial assessment has established a probable diagnosis of UAP or NSTEMI, therapy should be directed toward treating the three ongoing processes: platelet thrombus formation, coronary vasoconstriction, and myocardial oxygen demand exceeding coronary blood supply (Table 3). Give NTG sublingually and aspirin if not previously administered. See previously mentioned sildenafil warning. Thrombolytic therapy has not been shown to be therapeutic for the UAP and NSTEMI syndromes despite the fact that early platelet thrombus formation plays a pathogenic role [8,9]. Heparin therapy has been shown to improve outcome with a further 33% decrease in risk of MI or death [10•]. Low molecular weight heparin (LMWH) has recently been shown to be more efficacious than intravenous heparin, and the LMWH enoxaparin has Food and Drug Administration approval for patients with NSTEMI [11]. It has also been shown to be more cost effective than intravenous heparin because there is less nursing care time needed for subcutaneous injections and no need for repeated laboratory tests [12].

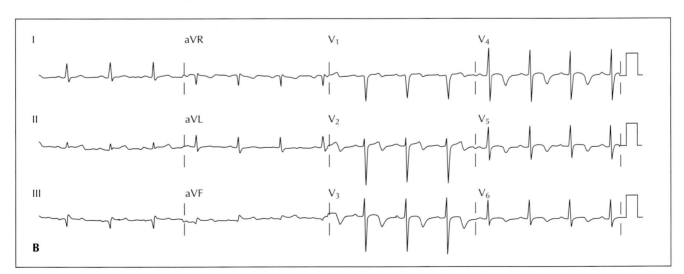

FIGURE 2 (*continued*) **B,** Twelve-lead ECG of the same patient taken 24 hours later. There is no change in the inferior leads. However, there is new T-wave inversion in anterior leads V_2 through V_6 consistent with severe anterior ischemia and/or a non–Q-wave myocardial infarction if serial creatine kinase or creatine kinase–myocardial band enzyme levels become elevated.

After initial emergency room therapy, the patient should be reassessed, and if there is continued diffuse ST-segment depression on ECG or chest pain, consider emergency coronary angiography. If there is continued ischemic chest pain, add intravenous β-blockers, increase intravenous NTG to blood pressure tolerance, and consider emergency coronary angiography. Patients who are likely to proceed to coronary angiography and angioplasty or stent placement are also candidates for a new class of therapeutic agents called GP IIb/IIIa inhibitors that decrease platelet aggregation and clotting in the intervened area of the affected coronary artery [13]. In the past, sublingual nifedipine was frequently given for ongoing chest pain or hypertension in the unstable angina patient. This is now contraindicated because of the reflex tachycardia and hypotension that may occur and because of reports of progression to acute MI or even stroke [14•]. If there is a progression to ST-segment elevation, thrombolytic therapy or acute angioplasty is indicated.

After the diagnosis of UAP is established, initiate heparin therapy. The choice of unfractionated heparin (UFH) versus LMWH should be based on whether the patient is expected to go to early interventional therapy. If early intervention is anticipated, UFH is the agent of choice. Otherwise, LMWH (enoxaparin), 1 mg/h every 12 h can be as effective with less cost and nursing care. Two trials have shown enoxaparin to be as effective or more effective than UFH. LMWH has a more predictable anticoagulant effect, does not require repeated testing with activated partial thromboplastin time (aPTT), is less likely to be initiated by activated platelets, and inhibits factor X. The ESSENCE (Efficacy and Safety of Subcutaenous Enoxaparin vs non−Q-wave Coronary Events) trial demonstrated fewer (16.6% vs 19.8%)

events (death, MI, or recurrent angina) at 14 days with enoxaparin compared with UFH. Another large-scale trial, TIMI IIB (Thrombolysis vs Myocardial Infarction) compared enoxaparin with UFH, again showing the superiority of LMWH. These results plus the simplicity of administration now provide the basis for LMWH (enoxaparin) as the agent of choice unless the patient is expected to proceed to early coronary intervention.

A new group of agents that block the final pathway for platelet formation, the GP IIb/IIIa receptors, has recently been demonstrated to provide additional benefits, particularly in high-risk patients proceeding to acute coronary intervention and stenting. Decisions regarding the initiation of this therapy in addition to heparin should be undertaken with cardiologist consultation.

Hospitalization

Generally, all patients with UAP or NSTEMI should be hospitalized for initiation of medical therapy and to monitor their course over the next 24 hours. An electrocardiographically monitored bed is useful for assessing heart rate response to therapy and to watch for ischemia-related arrhythmias.

TABLE 3 THERAPY FOR UNSTABLE ANGINA PECTORIS AND NON−ST ELEVATION MYOCARDIAL INFARCTION (NSTEMI)

1. Aspirin 325 mg
2. Sublingual nitroglycerin x 3; intravenous nitroglycerin if any residual chest pain
3. Clopidogrel 300 mg*
4. Low molecular weight heparin (enoxaparin 1 mg/kg unless serum creatine kinase > 2)
5. Intravenous beta-blocker for high blood pressure or tachycardia
6. Early cardiology consultation (or transfer)
7. Statin therapy (atorvastatin)

*Can be deferred until coronary angiography if possible coronary artery bypass graft candidate.

TABLE 1 BIOMARKERS FOR MYOCARDIAL INJURY

Creatine kinase-myocardial band total
Creatine kinase-myocardial band fraction
Troponin T
Troponin I

TABLE 2 SERUM ENZYME CHANGES IN UNSTABLE ANGINA AND NON−ST ELEVATION MYOCARDIAL INFARCTION (NSTEMI)

Time, h	CK	Unstable angina MB, %	NSTEMI CK rise CK	MB, %	NSTEMI MB rise only CK	MB, %
Normal value	< 160	< 5	< 160	< 5	< 160	< 5
0	100	3	100	3	100	3
8	120	4	260	8	160	9
24	110	3	150	7	150	7

CK—creatine kinase; MB—myocardial band.

The TIMI Risk Score has been introduced to help identify high-risk versus low-risk patients for subsequent adverse events. These include age greater than 65 years; three or more coronary artery disease risk factors; known coronary artery disease (> 50% stenosis); two or more anginal episodes in prior 24 hours; ST elevation ≥ 0.5 mm on presenting ECG; and cardiac markers. The higher the score, the more likelihood of an adverse outcome.

On the first day of hospitalization, continue daily aspirin (plain or enteric-coated). Continue LMWH until the patient is pain-free for 24 to 48 hours or the decision to proceed with angiography has been made. Add a statin and ACE inhibitor early on. The MIRACL trial demonstrated that cardiovascular events were reduced over the next 4 months when atorvastatin 80 mg was given within 96 hours of admission compared with placebo.

Cardiology Consultation

Depending on whether it is immediately available, cardiology consultation will always be necessary to assist in the initial care of the patient, particularly if myocardial ischemic chest pain is persistent. Decision points are usually based on:

• Serial ECGs and enzyme tests;
• Ongoing pain—reassessment after maximizing intravenous NTG and/or β-blocker;
• Severe pain or progressive ECGs change—urgent assessment by coronary angiography.

Subsequent Therapy

The great majority of patients with UAP or NSTEMI "cool down" on hospitalization after initial medical therapy.

Further therapeutic decisions are based on response to initial therapy and laboratory assessment. Generally, a decision will be made on whether the patient is a candidate for coronary intervention based on functional status, personal desires, and risk assessment.

Long-term medical therapy is directed toward maintaining good blood pressure control in addition to antiplatelet and antiischemic therapy. Typical regimens include the following:

1. Enteric-coated aspirin, 80 mg qd;
2. β-blocker, particularly carvedilol, which does not aggravate insulin resistance based on the COMET trial.
3. ACE inhibitor or angiotensin receptor blocker once the patient is hemodynamically stable.
4. Continued lipid lowering with a 3-hydroxy-3-methyl-glutaryl coenzyme A reductase inhibitor (statin); and
5. Hygienic measures such as low saturated fat diet, walking program, and antioxidants.

Coronary Arteriography and Intervention

Because the patient with UAP or NSTEMI is at increased risk for a major cardiovascular event over the next 12 months, assessment of the coronary anatomy is usually performed. Decisions regarding subsequent therapy are based on coronary anatomy, suitability for interventional techniques, left ventricular function, and suitability of patient for functional restoration. Figure 3 shows a tight stenosis detected by coronary angiography and treated with coronary angioplasty. Revascularization with coronary angiography is usually highly successful, with low morbidity and mortality associated with the procedure [15,16].

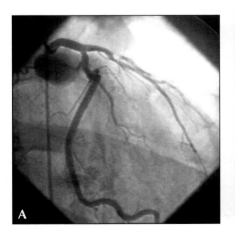 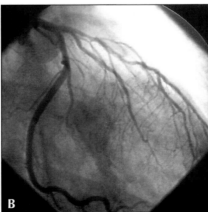

FIGURE 3 Coronary angiogram in the right anterior oblique position showing a tight proximal stenosis of the left anterior descending coronary artery before (**A**) and after (**B**) angioplasty.

REFERENCES AND RECOMMENDED READING

Recently published papers of particular interest have been highlighted as:
• Of interest

1. Braunwald E: Unstable angina. *Circulation* 1989, 80:410–414.

2. Theroux P: A pathophysiologic basis for the clinical classification and management of unstable angina. *Circulation* 1987, 75(Suppl V):V103–V109.

3. Fuster V, Badimon L, Badimon JJ, *et al.*: Mechanisms of disease: the pathogenesis of coronary artery disease and the acute coronary syndromes (first of two parts). *N Engl J Med* 1992, 326:242–250.

4. Fuster V, Badimon L, Badimon JJ, *et al.*: Mechanisms of disease: the pathogenesis of coronary artery disease and the acute coronary syndromes (second of two parts). *N Engl J Med* 1992, 326:310–318.

5.• Ohman EM, Armstrong PW, Christenson RH, *et al.*: Cardiac troponin T levels for risk stratification in acute myocardial ischemia. *N Engl J Med* 1996, 335:1333–1341.

6.• Lindahl B, Venge P, Wallentin L: Tropinin T identifies patients with unstable coronary artery disease who benefit from long-term antithrombotic protection. *J Am Coll Cardiol* 1997, 29:43–48.

7. Lewis HD Jr, Davis JW, Archibald JD, *et al.*: Protective effects of aspirin against acute myocardial infarction and death in men with unstable angina: results of a veterans cooperative study. *N Engl J Med* 1983, 309:396–403.

8. Freeman MB, Langer A, Wilson RF, *et al.*: Thrombolysis in unstable angina: randomized double-blind trial of t-PA and placebo. *Circulation* 1992, 85:150–157.

9. Ambrose JA, Hjemdahl-Monsen C, Borrico S, *et al.*: Quantitative and qualitative effects of intracoronary streptokinase in unstable angina and non–Q-wave infarction. *J Am Coll Cardiol* 1987, 9:1156–1165.

10.• Oler A, Whooley MA, Oler J, Grady D: Adding heparin to aspirin reduces the incidence of myocardial infarction and death in patients with unstable angina. *JAMA* 1996, 276:811–815.

11. Cohen M, Demers C, Gurfinkel EP, *et al.*: A comparison of low-molecular-weight heparin with unfractionated heparin for unstable coronary artery disease. *N Engl J Med* 1997, 337:447–452.

12. Mark DB, Cowper PA, Berkowitz SD, *et al.*: Economic assessment of low-molecular-weight heparin (enoxaparin) versus unfractionated heparin in acute coronary syndrome patients. Results from the ESSENCE randomized trial. *Circulation* 1998, 97:1702–1707.

13. The Platelet Receptor Inhibition in Ischemic Syndrome Management (PRISM) Study Investigators. A comparison of aspirin plus tirofiban with aspirin plus heparin for unstable angina. *N Engl J Med* 1998, 338:1498–1505.

14.• Grossman E, Messerli FH, Grodzicki T, Kowey P: Should a moratorium be placed on sublingual nifedipine capsules given for hypertensive emergencies and pseudoemergencies? *JAMA* 1996, 276:1328–1331.

15. Gibson RS, Young PM, Boden WE, *et al.*: Prognostic significance and beneficial effect of diltiazem: results from the Multicenter Diltiazem Reinfarction Study. *Am J Cardiol* 1987, 60:203–209.

16. Williams DO, Braunwald E, Thompson B, *et al.*: Results of percutaneous transluminal coronary angioplasty in unstable angina and non–Q-wave myocardial infarction. *Circulation* 1996, 94:2749–2755.

SELECT BIBLIOGRAPHY

Clinical Practice Guidelines, Unstable Angina: Diagnosis and Management AH CPR Publication #94-0602. Available from Unstable Angina Guidelines AHCPR Clearinghouse, PO Box 8547, Silver Spring, MD 20907.

Quick Reference Guide for Clinicians. AH CPR, Publication #94-0603. Available from Unstable Angina Guidelines AHCPR Clearinghouse, PO Box 8547, Silver Spring, MD 20907.

ST–Segment Elevation Myocardial Infarction

Ernst R. Schwarz
Rajiv Gupta

20

Key Points

- Myocardial infarction is defined as cardiomyocyte necrosis due to lack of oxygen supply in relationship to oxygen demand. The underlying cause in most cases is rupture of an intracoronary atherosclerotic plaque with subsequent thrombotic occlusion.

- ST elevation myocardial infarction is defined as myocardial cell necrosis with development of ST elevation on the electrocardiogram.

- The key symptom occurring with acute coronary artery occlusion is severe retrosternal chest pain, but symptoms may vary.

- Early hospitalization and intensive monitoring are required.

- Worldwide mortality of myocardial infarction is 20% to 40%; one third die within the first few hours.

- Treatment of choice is early recanalization primarily by interventional therapy if available or alternatively thrombolytic therapy, treatment of complications, and secondary prevention.

- The main prospective goal is public education, early identification, and urgent therapy.

- Future work contains the search for genetic markers for the development of acute myocardial infarction and its potential genetic modulation.

Of the cardiovascular diseases, acute myocardial infarction (MI) is the most common cause of death. The incidence of acute MI reaches 900,000 per year in the United States, and 150,000 per year in a representative state in Europe (Germany), with a mortality rate of 20% to 40%, including a 15% mortality rate before reaching the hospital. The underlying cause in most cases is atherosclerotic coronary artery disease. Acute MI can be identified by typical chest pain, electrocardiographic (ECG) changes, and subsequent characteristic elevation of cardiac enzymes.

NOMENCLATURE

The present system of classification of MI consists of ST-segment elevation myocardial infarction (STEMI) and non-ST-segment elevation myocardial infarction (NSTEMI). This classification is clinically relevant and is associated with a difference in strategy of care. STEMI mainly indicates a need for early revascularization due to a completely occluded coronary artery leading to myocardial necrosis (*eg*, transmural necrosis) whereas NSTEMI might implicate either collateralized coronary occlusion, subtotal coronary occlusion, or spontaneous reperfusion, which needs to be further risk stratified. Both conditions subsequently can result in Q-wave or non–Q-wave MI as well as in transmural or nontransmural MI.

STEMI in some, but not all, cases [1] correlates with transmural cell necrosis, whereas NSTEMI is often pathologically nontransmural or subendocardial. STEMI tends to be larger in size and has a higher in-hospital mortality.

ETIOLOGY

The underlying disease in most patients who develop MI is coronary artery disease, with atherosclerotic narrowing leading to a reduction of vessel lumen diameter and concomitant alterations of coronary blood flow. Atherosclerotic plaques are known to exist over long periods, but also may rupture suddenly for unknown reasons. Theories regarding rupture of atherosclerotic plaques include alterations of shear stress, as occurs with catecholamine or sympathetic stimulation, as well as infiltration of plaques with monocytes and release of various cytokines. The rough intimal surface attracts platelets, leading to adhesion and finally development of thrombotic occlusion of the coronary vessel. If complete coronary artery occlusion develops quickly, the patient may suffer acute chest pain as a result of myocardial ischemia. If the ischemia is severe and prolonged, MI may develop. With gradual coronary artery occlusion, the patient may be relatively asymptomatic or exhibit only exercise-induced angina. Slow coronary lumen reduction may induce the development of coronary collateral circulation, sufficient to supply oxygen to the myocardial tissue even in the setting of total occlusion. Myocardial damage is associated with elevated serum vascular endothelial growth factor (VEGF) levels. VEGF may play an important role by promoting angioneogenesis and re-endothelialization [1]. However, the development of new collaterals occurs slowly. Therefore, the management of acute coronary occlusion with MI involves shortening the time of hypoperfusion to avoid cell death.

The risk factors for development of coronary artery disease are multifactorial and include smoking, diabetes, hypertension, hyperlipoproteinemia, age, and male sex. Other risk factors include family history, hyperuricemia, lack of physical exercise, obesity, hyperhomocysteinemia, type A personality, cocaine use [2], and eventually high C-reactive protein (CRP) levels [3]. More recently, elevated fibrinogen levels were found to be associated with reduced prognosis in patients with myocardial ischemia and infarction [4]. Whether polymorphisms of different genes such as human apolipoproteins, lipoprotein lipases, serotonin receptor genes, and stromelysin genes play a role in the development of coronary artery disease and MI is currently under investigation [5–8]. The aim for primary and secondary prevention of MI is to minimize exogenous and treat endogenous risk factors.

DIAGNOSIS

The diagnosis of acute STEMI can be accurately detected by clinical symptoms, ECG findings, and enzyme analysis

[9•,10•]. However, the decision to institute revascularization therapy usually can be based on clinical findings and ECG, because laboratory confirmation of the clinical diagnosis of acute MI caused by chest pain and ST-segment elevation in ECG has been reported in 90% to 100% of cases.

Clinical Findings

Typically, patients suffer acute chest pain that is more severe and longer lasting than angina. The pain may be described as pressure, compression, constriction, squeezing, boring, or burning in the chest [2]. Prodromal symptoms such as angina pectoris during or after exercise or at rest with increasing frequency are often reported. The pain of MI characteristically radiates to the left arm, but also may involve the neck, jaw, epigastrium, right arm, or back. The chest pain is not relieved by rest or nitroglycerin administration, lasts for over 30 minutes, and is often accompanied by anxiety, apprehension, restlessness, hypotension, nausea, pallor ("pale and gray appearance"), and sweating. Between 20% and 30% of patients with acute MIs are completely asymptomatic at the onset of coronary occlusion ("silent infarcts"). In particular, in the elderly or patients with diabetes, chest pain might be less severe and other symptoms may be present, such as syncope, faintness, or dysp-

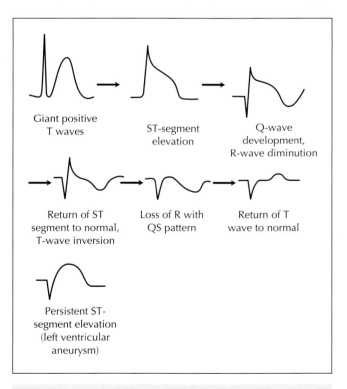

FIGURE 1 Electrocardiographic findings in myocardial infarction. Giant positive T waves are shown in hyperacute phase, followed by ST-segment elevation, then Q-wave development and R-wave diminution. Over time, the ST segment returns to normal, with loss of R wave, T-wave inversion, and sometimes T-wave pseudonormalization. There is persistent ST elevation in left ventricular aneurysm.

nea. Interestingly, only 10% to 20% of patients with acute chest pain admitted to emergency wards are diagnosed with acute MI [3], indicating similarity of symptoms due to other causes.

The acute symptoms of MI are frequently associated with stress such as anger or upsetting life events, or physical exertion [2]. Factors that increase oxygen demand or decrease oxygen supply may lead to myocardial ischemia, but the additional mechanisms that trigger plaque rupture are not fully understood.

Physical Examination

Findings on physical examination are variable. Patients may appear diaphoretic and unable to find a comfortable position. The heart rate may be rapid due to sinus tachycardia, or atrial or ventricular arrhythmia. Irregular pulse may be a result of premature atrial or ventricular beats, atrial fibrillation, heart block, or other arrhythmia. Hypotension and cool cyanotic extremities typically are present in patients with evolving cardiogenic shock or severe heart failure. Lung examination may or may not reveal rales or wheezes. Cardiac examination often demonstrates a fourth heart sound. A third heart sound and a new systolic murmur or palpable thrill may be recognized with heart failure or volume overload caused by mechanical complications such as acquired ventricular septal defect, papillary muscle rupture, or dysfunction with mitral regurgitation. Low-grade fever and pericardial friction rub may be present within the first days of MI. A single diagnostic physical sign of acute MI does not exist. Thus, the clinical appearance is variable (from the healthy-looking athlete carrying his own suitcase to the somnolent patient in cardiogenic shock). However, to detect complications of acute MI, physical examination—in particular, auscultation of the lungs and the heart—should be meticulously performed every day in all patients.

Electrocardiographic Findings

The electrocardiogram serves as the hallmark for diagnosis of acute MI because characteristic ST, T, and Q wave changes are detectable in most of the patients [4]. In the early stage of acute coronary occlusion (phase 1 or *hyperacute* phase) giant positive T waves appear with taller than normal R waves (Fig. 1). In phase 2 (*acute phase*, more commonly seen at hospital admission), ST-segment elevation is evident with a decrease in amplitude of the R wave, followed by pathologic Q wave development that lasts 0.04 seconds or more and reaches 25% of the amplitude of the R wave (pathologic Q wave, phase 3, when cell necrosis occurs over hours to days). Over time, the ST segment returns to normal with T wave inversion (terminal negative T wave); the R wave may be lost as a result of transmural necrosis and may be replaced by a QS wave (phase 4, *chronic phase*). The Q wave or QS wave persists, whereas the T wave may return to being positive. ST wave elevation may persist in cases of left ventricular dyskinesis or aneurysm. The electrocardiographic leads not representing the infarcted area may show reciprocal ST-segment alterations. A new left bundle branch block may be present and, if persistent, usually indicates large anterior wall infarction. In patients with acute chest pain who present with left bundle branch block, ST-segment elevation of 1 mm or more concordant with the QRS complex, ST-segment depression of 1 mm or more in lead V1, V2, or V3, and ST-segment elevation of 5 mm or more discordant to the QRS complex can be used for the diagnosis of acute MI [5]. In 20% of patients with acute MI, the ECG at hospital admission is normal without characteristic ST-segment changes. When possible, the current ECG tracing should be compared with previous records. Determination of myocardial infarct localization according to ECG leads is listed in Table 1.

Computerized score systems for assessment of ST-segment elevation and maximal QRS have been introduced,

TABLE 1 LOCATION OF MYOCARDIAL INFARCTION ACCORDING TO ELECTROCARDIOGRAPHIC LEADS AND INVOLVED CORONARY ARTERY

ST-segment elevation in ECG leads	Ventricular location	Probable coronary artery involved
V1 through V3	Anteroseptal	Proximal LAD, septal perforators
V2 through V4	Anteroapical	LAD, diagonal branches
I, aVL, V6	Lateral	LAD, diagonal branch, or circumflex
I, aVL	High lateral	1st diagonal branch or circumflex
I, aVL, V3 through V6	Anterolateral	Mid LAD or circumflex
I, aVL, V1 through V6	Extensive anterior	Proximal LAD
II, III, aVF	Inferior	RCA or circumflex, distal LAD
V1 through V2 (ST depression)	Posterior	Posterior descending of RCA, circumflex
II, III, aVF, V5 through V6	Posterolateral	RCA or circumflex
V1, V3R, V4R	Right ventricular	RCA

ECG—electrocardiogram; LAD—left anterior descending; RCA—right coronary artery.

which might provide a useful estimation for the extent of myocardial injury [11]. Recently, a more distinct differentiation of the coronary artery occlusion site was introduced [12••,13]: ST elevation in lead aVR, complete right bundle branch block, ST depression in lead V5 and ST elevation in V1 of greater than 2.5 mm predicts occlusion of the left anterior descending artery (LAD) proximal to the first septal perforator, whereas abnormal Q waves in V4-V6 are associated with LAD occlusion distal to the first septal perforator, and abnormal Q waves in lead aVL are associated with LAD occlusion proximal to the first diagonal branch [12••]. Furthermore, isolated ST-segment elevation in leads V7-V9 identify patients with acute posterior wall MI [14].

Laboratory Findings

After myocardial injury and cell death, cellular enzymes are released into the bloodstream. The typical time course of enzyme alterations that occur can help to determine the phase of MI [15,16]. The levels of the following enzymes can be routinely measured: creatine kinase (CK), creatine kinase isoenzyme MB (CK-MB), aspartate aminotransferase (AST), lactate dehydrogenase (LDH), and troponin T or troponin I. CK activity increases 4 to 8 hours after permanent coronary occlusion. With early spontaneous or therapeutically induced reperfusion, there is a peak in the level of CK as early as 8 hours after the onset of chest pain, with a quick recovery to normal values. In nonreperfused infarcts, the mean peak is reached at 24 hours and declines to normal within 72 hours. CK is highly sensitive for MI, but not specific, whereas CK-MB is more specific (if reaching > 10% of CK) and thus can help rule out noncardiac causes of CK elevation (eg, muscle trauma, hypothermia, diabetic ketoacidosis, rhabdomyolysis, strenuous exercise, seizures, intramuscular injection, surgery, myxedema, and cerebrovascular accident).

For clinical use, it is recommended that the CK-MB level be measured if there is CK elevation in combination with chest pain [6]. Determination of CK isoforms (MM1 to 3, MB1 and MB2) and particularly the ratio of MB2 to MB1 provide earlier information than elevation in CK-MB activity, with reliable diagnostic sensitivity [7]. Cardiac troponin T or troponin I are highly specific myofibrillar proteins and their elevation is an early marker for cardiomyocyte damage; in patients with acute MI, their levels rise as early as 3.5 hours after the onset of chest pain. Immuno-strip assays for bedside measurements provide results within 20 to 30 minutes of application of blood [17–19]. Their maximum is reached after 6 to 8 hours, and is detectable for 5 to 6 days. Even small amounts of myocardial injury without CK elevation can be specifically and sensitively detected with elevated troponin T or troponin I levels [20]. Troponin tests have presently replaced CK-MB measurements for the diagnosis of acute MI [21]. There is some evidence from small patient cohorts that monitoring of troponins provides a more than 80% sensitivity and specificity for detecting reperfusion after

therapy [22,23••] and can be used for risk stratification after MI [24]. LDH is elevated from 24 hours, peaks at days 4 to 5, and declines to normal within 10 days. It is therefore useful to measure LDH in patients with chest pain occurring days before admission. LDH has a high sensitivity but poor specificity. As long as other noncardiac causes are excluded (which might be difficult in some cases), enzyme elevation and its typical time course help to determine the age, course, and possible reoccurrence of MI. There is no general agreement regarding the required frequency of laboratory testing of cardiac biomarkers. If troponin is elevated and CK and CK-MB levels are elevated, ie, the diagnosis of MI is established by laboratory tests, there is no rationale to repeat all of these laboratory parameters, for example, once every 8 hours. Instead, further course of the MI can be followed clinically, with electrocardiography, and CK-MB estimation, eg, initially once every 8 hours for the first day and thereafter once daily until a downward trend is noted. In contrast, if chest pain is recurrent, intermittent analyses of CK-MB and troponin T are recommended for detection of reinfarction. Other enzymes, such as myosin light chains or myoglobin, are not routinely used in clinical situations to detect MI.

Imaging Techniques

Echocardiography is not required to make the diagnosis of acute MI in the setting of typical symptoms and ST-segment elevation, but may help in unclear cases. Echocardiographic examination is relatively easy to perform in the emergency ward and may be helpful for detecting regional wall motion abnormalities in patients with acute chest pain, enabling the physician to diagnose acute ischemia or evolving myocardial infarction with a sensitivity of 94% to 100% and a specificity of 84% [25]. Regional wall motion abnormalities alone cannot differentiate acute ischemia from acute infarction. The location of wall motion abnormalities provides insight into which coronary arteries are involved. Regional wall motion abnormalities favor the diagnosis of coronary artery disease, whereas global and diffuse left ventricular dysfunction favor cardiomyopathy. Global ventricular function and mechanical and hemodynamic complications such as papillary muscle rupture, septal rupture, pericardial effusion, mitral regurgitation, intraventricular thrombi, and their follow-up all can be assessed accurately by echocardiography. Stress echocardiography with low-dose dobutamine is a useful technique for differentiating dysfunctional myocardium, and viable ventricular areas from necrotic ventricular areas in the chronic phase after MI [25]. Radionuclide studies are not required in the acute phase of MI, although they may help distinguish necrotic myocardium from ischemic but viable myocardium. The potassium analogue ^{201}Tl is widely used to assess myocardial perfusion as well as to test the integrity of cell membranes to distinguish viable tissue from necrotic myocardium. ^{99m}TC isonitril (^{99m}TC sestamibi) is used for myocardial perfusion imaging and may identify myocardium at risk and residual ischemia, as well as help quantify infarct size [26–28]. However, in the acute phase, nuclear imaging is not routinely recommended, if the diagnosis is clear [29••].

TREATMENT

Acute Management

Because acute MI always represents a life-threatening event, the patient with suspected acute MI should be hospitalized immediately to minimize delay in appropriate therapy. The patient should have continuous monitoring of heart rhythm and vital signs and be observed within a coronary care or intensive care unit. An intravenous line should

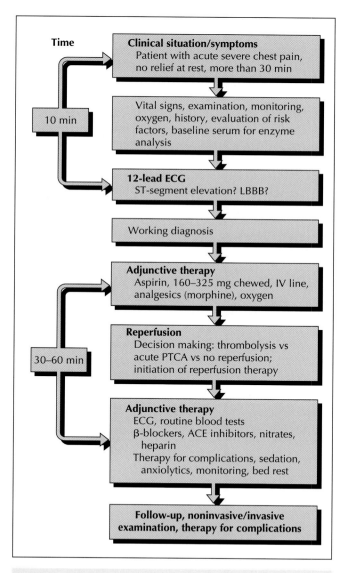

be placed. Once the patient arrives at the hospital, initial evaluation of the patient's history, coronary risk factors, physical signs, 12-lead ECG tracing, possible contraindications for reperfusion therapy, and steps for treatment should be initiated within 20 to 30 minutes ("door-to-needle time") [30,31]. In the emergency ward, the patient should immediately receive aspirin either in chewable form (in the United States) or intravenously (in Europe), oxygen by nasal prongs (blood gases may be checked, especially in patients with chronic pulmonary diseases), and sublingual, transdermal, or intravenous nitrates (unless systolic arterial pressure is less than 90 mm Hg or heart rate is less than 50 or greater than 100 beats per minute or there is presence of other contraindications for nitrate therapy such as sildenafil, vardenafil, or tadalafil intake within 24 hours). Infarct size is reduced and the frequency of non–Q-wave MIs is increased in patients using aspirin at the onset of symptoms [32,33]. In many hospitals, thrombolytic therapy can be initiated in the emergency ward. Therapy for acute MI should consist of the following six steps: 1) relief of pain, 2) relief of anxiety and restlessness, and sedation, 3) reperfusion, 4) anticoagulation, 5) therapy for complications, 6) secondary prevention (Fig. 2). For steps 1 and 2, repeated administration of opioids, ie, intravenous morphine (2 to 10 mg or more), is the treatment of choice, which can be combined with antiemetics to reduce side effects.

The patient should be monitored and have bed rest for 12 to 24 hours, ie, the patient's physical activities should be reduced for at least 12 to 24 hours because life-threatening arrhythmias, reinfarction, mechanical complications, and death occur most frequently within the first 24 hours after acute MI. Sedatives, anxiolytics, and stool softeners may be prescribed. When the patient is without pain, clear liquids can be administered prior to a heart-healthy diet with 50% of kilocalories consisting of complex carbohydrates and less than 30% of monounsaturated or unsaturated fats and including foods with high amounts of potassium, magnesium, and fibers, ie, fresh fruits, vegetables, and whole grains [29••].

Reperfusion Therapy

The main goal in the treatment of patients with acute MI is to reduce the extent of irreversible myocardial tissue damage and necrosis. Because acute thrombotic coronary occlusion is found in the majority of cases of acute STEMI [34], the acutely occluded coronary artery must be opened to reperfuse the myocardium within the shortest time interval. Early reperfusion has been convincingly shown to preserve left ventricular function and reduce morbidity and acute and long-term mortality by approximately 50%. Reopening of an acutely occluded coronary artery can be achieved, either by fibrinolytic agents, which are widely available, or by angioplasty, which requires adequate catheterization equipment and well-trained personnel. Fibrinolytic therapy should be initiated as early as possible, because overall benefit correlates inversely with time (the maximum benefit is derived if it is administered within the

FIGURE 2 In-hospital management of acute myocardial infarction. ACE—angiotensin-converting enzyme; ECG—electrocardiogram; IV—intravenous; LBBB—left bundle branch block; PTCA—percutaneous transluminal coronary angioplasty.

first 3 hours after onset of persistent chest pain, but some benefit may still be derived if administered up to at least 12 hours) [29••,35]. Even prehospital thrombolysis has been shown to be feasible and effective if an adequate infrastructure with appropriate paramedic patient selection, cardiac monitoring, and therapy for complications are available [35,36]. In the ER-TIMI trial (Early Retavase-Thrombolysis in Myocardial Infarction, 313 patients, 630 controls), prehospital administration of reteplase allowed earlier thrombolysis by a median time of 32 minutes and earlier ST-segment resolution by 30 minutes [37]. In the CAPTIM (Comparison of Angioplasty and Prehospital Thrombolysis in Acute Myocardial Infarction [840 patients]) trial, primary procedural coronary intervention (PCI) was not found to be better than prehospital thrombolysis with alteplase [38].

Thrombolytic therapy should be initiated within 60 to 90 minutes of the patient's call for medical therapy ("call-to-needle time"). Because fibrinolytic agents increase the risk of hemorrhage, including intracerebral hemorrhage, several cautions and contraindications must be considered before treatment can be initiated (Table 2). Patients with ST-segment elevation or new left bundle branch block substantially benefit from lytic therapy, with a mortality reduction of 35%. Plasminogen activators are the preferred therapeutic approach to achieve rapid thrombolysis. US Food and Drug Administration (FDA)–approved agents for intravenous application are streptokinase, anisoylated plasminogen streptokinase activator complex (APSAC, anistreplase), tissue plasminogen activator (t-PA, alteplase), and the "third-generation" thrombolytic agent recombinant plasminogen activator (rt-PA, reteplase, tenecteplase). Intracoronary application (approved for urokinase and streptokinase) is virtually obsolete. Dose regimens and characteristics of these agents are given in Table 3.

Many trials have demonstrated the efficacy of thrombolytic therapy. Most notably, the GISSI (Gruppo Italiano per lo Studio della Streptochinasi nell'Infarto Miocardico; 11,712 patients) trial in 1986 demonstrated the safety and efficacy of streptokinase if administered within 6 hours of onset of symptoms in patients with acute MI with a reduction in acute and 1-year mortality compared with that in placebo-treated controls [39,40]. Debate still exists regarding which thrombolytic agent is superior in acute MI. The TIMI-1 (Thrombolysis in Myocardial Infarction [290 patients]) study in 1987 showed a more rapid reperfusion after rt-PA compared with streptokinase (after 30 minutes and 90 minutes of initiation, 24% and 62% in rt-PA- and 8% and 31% in streptokinase-treated patients achieved TIMI flow 2 or 3, respectively) [41]. In 1990, the GISSI-2 (12,490 patients) trial demonstrated equal safety and efficacy of streptokinase and alteplase [42,43]. In 1992, ISIS-3 (Third International Study of Infarct Survival [41,299 patients] trial) revealed less reinfarction but higher rates of stroke and noncerebral bleeding as a result of t-PA administration, whereas 35-day mortality and 6-month survival were similar in those treated with t-PA, streptokinase, or APSAC [44]. The GUSTO-1 (Global Utilization of Streptokinase and Tissue Plasminogen Activator for Occluded Coronary Arteries [41,021 patients]) trial in 1993 demonstrated a lower 30-day mortality rate after the accelerated administration of t-PA plus heparin (6.3%) compared with streptokinase plus subcutaneously or intravenously administered heparin (7.2% or 7.4%, respectively) and a combination of t-PA and streptokinase plus heparin (7.0%) [45]. Moreover, an angiographic substudy in 2431 patients demonstrated that t-PA caused faster and more complete reperfusion and better regional wall motion [46]. However, there was a significant excess of hemorrhagic strokes with the use of t-PA compared with streptokinase (0.72% vs 0.54%; $P = 0.03$). The TIMI-4 trial in 1994 (382 patients) showed that front-loaded rt-PA is associated with higher rates of early reperfusion and trends toward better clinical outcome and survival compared with APSAC or a combination of both agents [47]. Results of the INJECT (International Joint Efficacy Comparison of Thrombolytics [6010 patients]) trial in 1995 compared the effects of streptokinase and the rt-PA reteplase, showing similar 35-day

TABLE 2 CONTRAINDICATIONS FOR THROMBOLYTIC THERAPY

Absolute contraindications	Relative contraindications
Major surgery or trauma or head injury within 3 weeks	Pregnancy
Active internal bleeding (except menses)	Severe hypertension
Gastrointestinal bleeding within last month	Noncompressible vascular punctures
Suspected aortic dissection	Current use of anticoagulants in therapeutic doses
Acute pericarditis	Active peptic ulcer
Known bleeding disorder	For streptokinase/anistreplase: prior exposure within 2 years or prior allergic reaction
Intracranial neoplasm	History of recent transient ischemic attacks
Hemorrhagic stroke	Hemorrhagic diabetic retinopathy, recent retinal laser therapy
Cerebrovascular accident within 6 months	Prolonged cardiopulmonary resuscitation
End-stage neoplasm	

mortality rates of 9.53% and 9.02%, and 6-month mortality rates of 12.05% and 11.02%, with similar bleeding events of 15.3% and 15.0%, respectively [48]. Additionally, the RAPID trials (Rapid-1: Reteplase Angiographic Phase II International Dose Finding Study; Rapid-2: Reteplase vs Alteplase Patency Investigation During Acute Myocardial Infarction [606 patients]) in 1995 demonstrated a more rapid and complete reperfusion following double-bolus reteplase (10 MU rt-PA bolus followed by 10 MU rt-PA after 30 min) compared with standard-dose alteplase [49]. However, the GUSTO-III trial in 2000 showed similar 1-year survival in patients with acute MI treated with alteplase versus reteplase [50•]. The InTIME-II (Intravenous nPA for Treatment of Infarcting Myocardium Early [15,078 patients]) trial in 2000 showed that lanoteplase (nPA) had similar mortality at 1 day, 30 days, 6 months, and 1 year compared with alteplase, although lanoteplase was associated with a slightly higher risk of minor and intracranial bleeding [51]. In the ASSENT-2 (Assessment of the Safety and Efficacy of a New Thrombolytic [16,949 patients]) trial, tenecteplase and alteplase had similar 30-day mortality (6.18% and 6.15%, respectively), but tenecteplase had the advantage of lower risk of bleeding and a more simple single-bolus administration [52]. The

multicenter, randomized, comparative study of recombinant versus natural streptokinase in acute MI (TERIMA) showed no differences regarding vessel patency for both drugs [53]. The third-generation agents like reteplase and tenecteplase are similar in efficacy, require a single-bolus dose, and are also easy to administer in a prehospital setting, ie, in the ambulance as it is routinely performed in some European regions with a so-called rendez-vous system (an emergency physician on board the ambulance). Although t-PA is associated with a significantly lower incidence of allergic reactions and severe hypotension compared with streptokinase, because of the higher costs of t-PA, there is still debate concerning which thrombolytic agent is the most cost-effective one in different countries. The choice of thrombolytic therapy strategy therefore depends on experience, individual risk assessment, availability, and cost-benefit analysis rather than on scientific and practical priorities, at least when choosing among streptokinase, t-PA, reteplase [54], and the newly available tenecteplase [52].

A relatively new strategy is the concomitant use of platelet glycoprotein (GP) IIb/IIIa antagonists (inhibitors of platelet aggregation) and thrombolytic agents [55–58]. Despite encouraging initial data of combination therapy

TABLE 3 COMMONLY USED THROMBOLYTIC AGENTS IN ACUTE MYOCARDIAL INFARCTION

Drug	Streptokinase	Anistreplase (APSAC)	rt-PA	Reteplase	Tenecteplase
Dose (IV)	1.5 MU in 30–60 min	30 mg in 5 min	15-mg bolus, then 0.75 mg/kg over 30 min, then 0.5 mg/kg over 60 min (max 35 mg/h); total 100 mg in 90 min	10-U bolus over 2 min; repeat 10 U bolus in 30 min	Weight-based; 30–50 mg range (max, 50 mg)
Characteristics	Produced by β-hemolytic streptococci	Complex of streptokinase and plasminogen	Recombinant single-chain alteplase	Depletion of finger, EGF, and kringle-1 from t-PA	Produced by recombinant technology using mammalian cell line
Half-life, *min*	14–20	70–120	6	13–16	20–24
Reperfusion rate, %	50–60	60–70	75–85	82–88	77–88
Antigenicity	Yes	Yes	No	Yes	Yes
Intracerebral hemorrhage, %	0.3	0.6	0.6	0.77	0.9
Additional heparin	No	No	Yes	Yes	Yes
US FDA approved	IV use	IV use	IV use	IV use	IV use
Approximate cost, US $	300	1700	2200	2200	2200

APSAC—anisoylated plasminogen-streptokinase activator complex; EGF—epidermal growth factor; IV—intravenous; rt-PA—recombinant tissue-type plasminogen activator; US FDA—US Food and Drug Administration.

with thrombolytics and GP IIb/IIIa inhibitors resulting in increased reperfusion rates in smaller trials like GUSTO-IV pilot study (528 patients) [59], TIMI-14 ([125 patients] substudy) [60], INTRO AMI (Integrilin and Low-Dose Thrombolysis in Acute Myocardial Infarction [305 patients]) study [61], and PARADIGM (Platelet Aggregation Receptor Antagonist Dose Investigation for Reperfusion Gain in Myocardial Infarction) trial [62], this did not transform into improved clinical outcomes in large randomized trials. In the GUSTO-V [16,588 patients] trial in 2001, the combination of reduced dose reteplase with 12-hour infusion of abciximab versus standard reteplase regimen was associated with similar 1-day and 30-day mortality [63•]. Although the combination therapy was associated with decrease in reinfarction, there was also an increased risk of bleeding complications. Further follow-up of these patients showed no difference in mortality at 1 year [64•]. Similarly, reduced-dose tenecteplase plus full-dose abciximab (ASSENT-3 trial [6095 patients]) or eptifibatide (Integrilin and Tenecteplase in Acute Myocardial Infarction [INTEGRITI] Phase II Angiographic Trial [189 patients]) was associated with more bleeding and was not superior to thrombolytic monotherapy [65,66•]. Currently, GP IIb/IIIa inhibitors are not being routinely used in combination with thrombolytic therapy for STEMI.

Primary percutaneous transluminal coronary Angioplasty

The updated guidelines of the American College of Cardiology/American Heart Association (ACC/AHA) for the management of patients with acute MI, published in 1999, suggested that primary percutaneous transluminal coronary angioplasty (PTCA) can serve as an alternative to thrombolysis only if performed in a timely fashion by individuals skilled in the procedure and supported by experienced personnel in high-volume centers [29••]. Indications include patients with contraindications to thrombolysis, patients at risk for bleeding, and patients with cardiogenic shock. Furthermore, early invasive strategies in patients with acute MI and nondiagnostic electrocardiogram changes are associated with lower long-term-mortality rates compared with conservative treatment [67••].

A number of studies have compared immediate angioplasty and primary intracoronary stenting to thrombolytic therapy. PAMI-1 (Primary Angioplasty in Myocardial Infarction), STAT (Stenting vs Thrombolysis In Acute Myocardial Infarction Trial [123 patients]), STOPAMI (Stent vs Thrombolysis for Occluded Coronary Arteries In Patients with Acute Myocardial Infarction [140 patients]) demonstrated a successful antegrade coronary flow in approximately 90% of patients receiving PTCA. These patients had a lower incidence of reocclusion, reinfarction, recurrent ischemia, death, coronary artery bypass grafting, and intracranial hemorrhage [68,69••,70–76], which is maintained even after a 2-year follow-up period [77•]. With the advantage of early knowledge of the coronary

anatomy and number and degree of additional stenoses, left ventricular function, and the possibility of PTCA with acute stenting, these studies suggest that PCI might be superior to thrombolytic therapy. This beneficial effect of primary coronary angioplasty versus thrombolysis was found to be maintained in elderly patients [78,79]. In the CCP (Cooperative Cardiovascular Project) involving 80,356 patients ≥65 years with acute MI, primary angioplasty was associated with a decrease in 30-day and 1-year mortality [78]. For early reperfusion and, thus, salvage of myocardial tissue and better clinical outcome, direct angioplasty should be performed with only little—if any—time delay [80••].

Primary stenting might reduce the rate of restenosis and improve survival after acute MI compared to balloon angioplasty, as suggested by PAMI and Stent-PAMI trials [81•,82] and also reduce the no-reflow and slow-reflow phenomenon with better ST segment resolution without increased costs [83,84]. In the STENTIM-2 (Stenting in Acute Myocardial Infarction [211 patients]) trial, routine stenting using Wiktor stent had less restenosis and a trend toward less clinical events and need for repeat revascularization compared with standard balloon angioplasty with provisional stenting [85]. Current practice favors stent implantation during PCI. In the first report of drug (sirolimus) eluting stents in 96 patients with STEMI, no evidence of restenosis or late luminal loss was observed at 6-month angiographic follow-up [86••]. The broader usage of drug-eluting stents has the potential to improve clinical outcomes, although randomized trials are required to confirm this prospect.

On the basis of these trials, primary percutaneous intervention is presently regarded as the reperfusion therapy of choice for STEMI. However, most trials that favored PCI may have a bias because the PCI procedures were being performed by experienced operators in high-volume centers. In real-life scenarios, patients commonly present to local hospitals that can initiate thrombolysis but lack onsite angioplasty facilities. Fewer than 25% of hospitals in the United States have PCI facilities, and these numbers are even lower around the world. Therefore, one of the main questions facing physicians working in centers without PCI facilities is whether to initiate early thrombolysis or the transfer to a PCI center. In the DANAMI-2 (DANish trial in Acute Myocardial Infarction) trial, 1572 patients were randomly assigned to PCI versus accelerated treatment with alteplase in both community hospitals (1129 patients) and primary PCI hospitals (443 patients) [87••]. Patients randomly assigned to PCI had to be transferred within 3 hours to the nearest angioplasty center (median transfer time, 67 minutes). There was a significant reduction in the composite 30-day endpoint of death, reinfarction, and disabling stroke (13.7% vs 8%; P < 0.001) in favor of PCI, the outcome driven mainly by a reduction in reinfarction rate. Similar reduction in outcome was found in PRAGUE (Primary Angioplasty in Patients Transferred from General Community Hospitals to Specialized PTCA Units

With or Without Emergency Thrombolysis [300 patients]) and PRAGUE-2 [850 patients] trials, and a nonsignificant trend toward improved outcomes was observed in the AIR PAMI (Air Primary Angioplasty in Myocardial Infarction) study [88•,89•,90].

Elective PCI traditionally has been performed in hospitals with cardiovascular surgical back-up on standby. Recently, community hospitals with cardiac catheterization facility but without an elective PCI program or onsite surgical program are beginning to offer primary PCI for STEMI. In the C-PORT (Cardiovascular Patient Outcomes Research Team) study, primary PCI (225 patients) for STEMI was performed at hospitals without on-site cardiac surgical program. No patient in the primary PCI group was sent for emergency coronary artery bypass surgery and PCI was associated with better 6-month outcomes than thrombolysis [91]. The final decision as to thrombolysis, or PCI at community hospital without surgical back-up or transfer to primary PCI center depends on a number of factors that include patient condition, anticipated transfer time, local PCI expertise, and patient and physician preference.

Procedural coronary intervention and thrombolysis have traditionally been viewed as alternative therapies. However, if used together they may combine rapidity with completeness of recanalization. The earlier disappointing results formed the basis of the classification of routine thrombolysis and PCI as a class III indication (ie, considerably harmful) in the ACC/AHA guidelines. The PACT trial (Plasminogen-activator Angioplasty Compatibility Trial) evaluated the efficacy and safety of a short-acting reduced dose fibrinolytic regimen (50 mg rt-PA) with subsequent PCI if needed. Tailored thrombolytic regimens compatible with subsequent interventions resulted in more frequent early recanalizations, associated with a better preserved left ventricular function [92•]. Also in the SPEED (Strategies for Patency Enhancement in the Emergency Department) trial, the endpoint of freedom from death, reinfarction, and urgent revascularization was 85.4% with early PCI in combination with reduced dose reteplase and abciximab versus 70.4% with non-PCI patients ($P < 0.001$) [93]. Future trials may shed further light on this promising mode of treatment.

Adjunctive Therapy

Early adjunctive therapy with thrombolysis consists of aspirin, which quickly prevents thromboxane A_2 production in platelets and prostacyclin in endothelial cells. Aspirin administration resulted in a 23% reduction in 35-day mortality rate in patients with MI; if combined with streptokinase, there was a reduction of 42% in the ISIS-2 study [94]. The ACC/AHA guidelines recommend that aspirin be administered at the time of admission to the emergency ward at a dose of 160 to 325 mg, preferably in a chewable form because of its faster absorption, followed by a daily administration indefinitely thereafter [29••,95]. In case of true aspirin allergy, dipyridamole, ticlopidine, or clopidogrel may be used.

Heparin (which forms a complex with antithrombin III, thus inactivating thrombin) is recommended with use of fibrin-specific thrombolytics such as alteplase and reteplase (70 U/kg as a bolus, followed by 15 µg/kg/h to keep the activated partial thromboplastin time [aPTT, a coagulation parameter] at 1.5 to 2.0 times control for 48 hours). Heparin also should be given for those with primary PTCA (the activated clotting time [ACT], which can be instantaneously measured in the catheter laboratory, should be 300 to 350 seconds), and in patients with large or anterior MI, known left ventricular thrombus, or previous embolic events. In patients not treated with thrombolytic therapy or with nonselected thrombolytics (streptokinase, anistreplase, urokinase), and in patients without increased risk for systemic emboli, 7500 U twice daily may be administered subcutaneously [29••]. Prolonged intravenous heparin therapy has not been shown to decrease the rate of reocclusion. Dose regimens leading to an aPTT of more than 90 seconds for hours or days are correlated with an unacceptably high risk of bleeding complications.

Currently there is a tendency to use low molecular weight heparin (LMWH) alternatively to unfractionated heparin (UFH) as adjunctive therapy in STEMI. In AMI-SK (Acute Myocardial Infarction Streptokinase [496 patients]) study, 5-day enoxaparin therapy improved ST segment resolution, patency rates at 5 to 10 days, reinfarction and the combined endpoint of death, recurrent MI or angina at 30 days [96]. In the HART II (Second Trial of Heparin and Aspirin Reperfusion Therapy [400 patients]) study, enoxaparin was as effective as UFH as adjunctive therapy with rt-PA and aspirin with a trend toward higher recanalization rates and lower reocclusion rates. There was no difference in mortality at 30 days [97]. In the ENTIRE-TIMI-23 (ENoxaparin and TNK-tPA with or without GPIIb/IIIa Inhibitor as Reperfusion strategy in ST Elevation MI- Thrombolysis In Myocardial Infarction) trial, in patients receiving full-dose tenecteplase (242 patients), the enoxaparin group showed decreased death/reinfarction rates at 30 days compared with the UFH group (4.4% vs 15.9%; $P = 0.005$) [98•]. Enoxaparin was found to reduce 90-day mortality, reinfarction, and readmission for unstable angina versus UFH and was also cost-effective in another study of 300 patients with STEMI treated with thrombolytics [99]. Although an initial pilot study on dalteparin showed improved vessel patency at 24 hours, this did not translate to an effect on mortality or reinfarction at 30 days in ASSENT Plus (Assessment of the Safety of a New Thrombolytic Plus [439 patients]) [100,101]. In the TETAMI (Treatment of Acute ST-Segment Elevation Myocardial Infarction Ineligible for Reperfusion) trial of 1224 patients ineligible for thrombolysis or PCI, of which 86.8% had STEMI, enoxaparin had a similar efficacy and safety profile to UFH [102]. More trials evaluating LMWH are currently under way, but the present data suggest that enoxaparin is as efficacious or might be even superior to UFH as adjunctive therapy to thrombolysis.

Effects of the direct antithrombin agent hirudin are similar to those of heparin. Argatroban, a small molecule direct thrombin inhibitor in combination with t-PA in patients with acute MI, might represent an alternative therapy to heparin with enhanced reperfusion rates [103]. Recombinant hirudin (lepirudin) in combination with streptokinase showed better ST segment resolution but did not significantly improve blood flow in the infarct-related artery [104]. Bivalirudin in combination with streptokinase had no effect on mortality at 30 days and was associated with an increase in mild and moderate bleeding [105]. Efegatran as an adjunct to streptokinase or t-PA was associated with a trend toward worse clinical outcomes [106,107]. Ximelagatran was found to decrease the primary endpoint of all-cause death, nonfatal MI, and severe recurrent ischemia in patients with both STEMI and non-STEMI compared with placebo [108]. Presently, thrombin inhibitors have a role as adjunctive therapy in patients who develop an allergic reaction or thrombocytopenia with heparin administration.

Studies have focused on other targets such as factor X and heparin cofactor II in the treatment of STEMI. Use of pentasaccharide, a synthetic factor Xa inhibitor, as an adjunct to alteplase had an efficacy and safety profile similar to UFH and was associated with a nonspecific trend toward lesser reocclusion rates and revascularization [109]. However, vasoflux, a LMWH derivative that inhibits activation of factor X by factor IXa and also enhances thrombin inactivation by heparin cofactor II, was not found to be efficacious and was associated with an increased risk of bleeding [110].

As mentioned earlier, the use of platelet GP IIb/IIIa inhibitors combined with rescue and primary angioplasty or thrombolysis represents a cornerstone for future therapy for patients with acute MI [111•]. The GRAPE (Glycoprotein Receptor Antagonist Patency Evaluation) study demonstrated a relatively high vessel patency rate after abciximab (without thrombolysis) administration in patients with acute MI before angioplasty [112••]. The RESTORE (Randomized Efficacy Study of Tirofiban for Outcomes and Restenosis) trial investigated the effects of tirofiban, a highly selective short-acting inhibitor of fibrinogen binding to platelet GP IIb/IIIa in patients with unstable angina or acute MI undergoing angioplasty. The RESTORE trial results found a reduction of early cardiac events related to thrombotic vessel closure compared with placebo [113]. Similarly, in the RAPPORT trial (ReoPro in Acute myocardial infarction and Primary PTCA Organization and Randomized Trial), pretreatment with abciximab before coronary angioplasty in patients with acute MI showed beneficial effects [114]. The EPISTENT (Evaluation of Platelet IIb/IIIa Inhibitor for Stenting) Investigators showed that coronary stenting with abciximab compared with stenting alone or balloon angioplasty with abciximab is associated with improved survival and appears to be an economically attractive therapy by conventional standards [115•]. Similarly, eptifibatide reduced the composite rates of death or MI in patients with percutaneous coronary inter-

ventions and those managed conservatively [116•]. Furthermore, abciximab remains clinically efficacious when re-administered as an adjunct to percutaneous coronary intervention. However, concomitant heparin administration has to be monitored carefully and warfarin therapy should be avoided. Vigilant surveillance for thrombocytopenia should be done [117]. In the ISAR-2 trial (Intracoronary Stenting and Antithrombotic Regimen-2), abciximab exerted beneficial effects in patients undergoing stenting after acute MI by reducing the 30-day rate of major adverse cardiac events. During 1-year follow-up, there was no additional benefit from a reduction in target lesion revascularization, and abciximab did not reduce angiographic restenosis [118••]. The PARADIGM (Platelet Aggregation Receptor Antagonist Dose Investigation for Reperfusion Gain in Myocardial Infarction) trial demonstrated improved patency rates in patients treated with lamifiban in conjunction with rt-PA or streptokinase [62], but the incidence of bleeding complications was also increased. In the ADMIRAL (Abciximab Before Direct Angioplasty and Stenting in MI Regarding Acute and Long-term Follow-up [300 patients]) trial, administration of abciximab before primary PCI resulted in a significant reduction of composite outcome of death, reinfarction, and urgent target vessel revascularization at 30 days (6% in the abciximab arm vs 14.6% with placebo; $P = 0.01$) and 6 months (7.4% in abciximab arm vs 15.9% in placebo arm; $P = 0.02$). The reduction in the endpoint was driven solely by a reduction in urgent target vessel revascularization [119•]. In the CADILLAC (Controlled Abciximab and Device Investigation to Lower Late Angioplasty Complications) trial, 2082 patients were randomly assigned to balloon angioplasty alone, balloon angioplasty with abciximab, stenting alone, and stenting with abciximab. Abciximab, given at the time of PCI, reduced the rate of ischemic target vessel revascularization after both stenting and balloon angioplasty and had no effect on TIMI flow rate, restenosis, or late cardiac events [120••]. This relative lack of benefit compared with the ADMIRAL trial may be related to a later administration of abciximab. Early administration of tirofiban in TIGER-PA (Tirofiban Given In the Emergency Room before Primary Angioplasty [100 patients]) was associated with improved initial angiographic results but had no effect on composite of death, reinfarction, and rehospitalization [121]. Thus overall in the setting of primary PCI, the use of GP IIb/IIIa inhibitors leads to reductions in urgent target vessel revascularization without an effect on death or reinfarction. Whether potent long-term antiplatelet therapy with oral GP IIb/IIIa antagonists will further improve outcome is unknown. SYMPHONY (Sibrafiban versus aspirin to Yield Maximum Protection from ischemic Heart events post-acute cOroNarY syndromes) was a randomized, double-blind, aspirin-controlled trial with two concentration regimens of sibrafiban, an oral peptidomimetic GP IIb/IIIa antagonist, for long-term treatment of patients after an acute coronary syndrome. Sibrafiban showed no additional benefits for secondary prevention of major ischemic events after an acute coronary syndrome but was associated with more (dose-related) bleeding complications [122,123•].

Interestingly, adjunctive adenosine with thrombolysis resulted in a 33% infarct size reduction as it has recently been demonstrated in the AMISTAD (Acute Myocardial Infarction Study of Adenosine) trial [124]. β-adrenergic blockers are known to reduce myocardial oxygen consumption, as well as acute and long-term mortality and morbidity, and should be administered intravenously as early as possible (on day 1 within 12 hours) followed by oral therapy if contraindications are excluded [125]. Furthermore, β-blockers may reduce infarct size and the incidence of ventricular fibrillation and reinfarction [126]. In the CAPRICORN (Carvedilol Post-Infarct Survival Control in LV Dysfunction [1959 patients]) trial, carvedilol in addition to ACE inhibitors and standard therapy reduced mortality and reinfarction in post-MI patients with an ejection fraction of 40% or less after a mean follow-up of 1.3 years [127•].

Mortality after MI has also been shown to be reduced in several trials comparing the use of ACE inhibitors with placebo. In the SAVE (Survival and Ventricular Enlargement) trial (n = 2231), long-term captopril therapy in patients with asymptomatic left ventricular dysfunction after acute MI was associated with a reduction in mortality and morbidity [128]. Several studies [129,130••,131,132••,133,134] confirmed the reduction of mortality as a result of ACE inhibitor administration compared with placebo, which was augmented with early administration. However, in the CONSENSUS II trial, whereas enalapril did not improve survival during a 180-day follow-up after acute MI [135], a recent meta-analysis [136••] demonstrated a reduction of sudden cardiac death in patients with ACE inhibitor therapy after acute MI. The OPTIMAAL trial (Optimal Therapy in Myocardial Infarction with the Angiotensin II Antagonist Losartan) compared losartan with captopril in 5477 patients with acute MI and evidence of heart failure or left ventricular dysfunction [137•]. The captopril group had decreased cardiovascular mortality compared to the losartan group (13.3% vs 15.3%, P = 0.03) although losartan was better tolerated. A similar decrease in mortality in post-MI patients with left ventricular dysfunction was shown with trandolapril [138]. According to the ACC/AHA guidelines, ACE inhibitors should be initiated on day 1 within hours of hospitalization in patients with evolving acute MI with ST-segment elevation or left bundle brunch block and continued indefinitely in case of impaired left ventricular function (the lower the ejection fraction, the greater the benefit).

Aldosterone blockade is useful in the treatment of heart failure or left ventricular dysfunction after acute MI. EPHESUS (Eplerenone Post-Acute Myocardial Infarction Heart Failure Efficacy and Survival Study) is a recently published trial of 6632 patients with acute MI and LV dysfunction (ejection fraction ≤ 40%) or heart failure randomly assigned to eplerenone (mean dose, 43 mg/d) or placebo within 3 to 14 days [139•]. After a mean follow-up of 16 months, eplerenone decreased the overall mortality compared to placebo (14.4% vs 16.7%, RR 0.85, P = 0.008) and cardiovascular mortality or hospitalization for cardiovascular event (26.7% vs 30.0%, RR 0.87, P = 0.02). The reduction in cardiovascular mortality was largely due to a 21% reduction in the rate of sudden death from cardiac causes.

The use of intravenous nitroglycerin is recommended during the first 48 hours and beyond this time frame in patients with recurrent angina, large infarction, and pulmonary congestion. Calcium antagonists, mainly short-acting nifedipine, may be harmful and should be avoided in patients with acute MI. If β-blockers are ineffective, verapamil or diltiazem may be used in patients with ischemia or tachycardia in the absence of left ventricular dysfunction or atrioventricular (AV) block [29••]. Administration of an ATP-sensitive potassium channel opener such as nicorandil adjunctive to primary angioplasty improved regional contractile function and reduced cardiac events after acute MI [140•] and might represent a promising future cardioprotective treatment strategy. Activation of Na^+/H^+ exchange and subsequent calcium overload in cardiac myocytes appear to play an important role in myocardial tissue injury after ischemia and reperfusion. In a multicenter, randomized, placebo-controlled clinical trial, cariporide (HOE 642) showed benefits to prevent reperfusion injury in patients with acute anterior MI treated with direct angioplasty [141].

The role of magnesium in the management has been controversial because a reduction in mortality has been reported in some studies (24% in the LIMIT-2 trial) [142-146]. However, the ISIS-4 trial could not demonstrate beneficial effects of magnesium treatment in patients with acute MI [129]. MAGIC (Magnesium in Coronaries) was a randomized, double-blind, placebo-controlled, multicenter trial involving intravenous magnesium administration within 6 hours of symptoms to 6213 high-risk patients with STEMI. No difference in 30-day mortality was observed [147]. In the ACC/AHA guidelines, magnesium administration is recommended only to correct documented magnesium deficits, especially in patients receiving diuretics, in the case of torsades de pointes with a prolonged QT interval, and in high-risk patients not receiving reperfusion therapy [29••].

Intensive insulin-glucose administration (≥24 h) during acute MI reduced long-term mortality in diabetic patients [148] and might be considered in this cohort. There is yet no role of RhuMAB (recombinant monoclonal antibody to CD18 subunit of $β_2$ integrin adhesion receptor) or Hu23F2G (antibody to CD11/CD18 integrin receptor) in improving coronary blood flow or reducing infarct size or clinical outcomes [149,150].

COMPLICATIONS OF ACUTE MYOCARDIAL INFARCTION

Arrhythmia

The incidence of arrhythmia may be as high as 100% in patients with acute MI, and it manifests predominantly as premature ventricular beats. The most serious and life-threatening arrhythmias are ventricular fibrillation and sustained polymorphic ventricular tachycardia requiring early electrical defibrillation (200 J), which is repeated if unsuc-

cessful (≥360 J). Patients with hemodynamically stable monomorphic ventricular tachycardia not associated with angina or acute heart failure may be treated with the antiarrhythmic agents lidocaine (1–1.5 mg/kg as a bolus followed

TABLE 4 MECHANICAL COMPLICATIONS OF ACUTE MYOCARDIAL INFARCTION

Complications	Management
Severe left ventricular dysfunction, left-sided heart failure *Diagnosis:* low output syndrome; tachycardia, dyspnea, orthopnea, pulmonary congestion, cyanotic limbs, oliguria, cardiac index > 2.5 L/min/m²; auscultation, chest radiography, two-dimensional echocardiography, invasive hemodynamics.	Invasive hemodynamic monitoring (Swan-Ganz catheter, intra-arterial pressure monitoring). If wedge pressure is high and blood pressure stable: diuretics (furosemide), vasodilators (nitrates, reduction of pre- and afterload), ACE inhibitors (afterload reduction); if wedge pressure is high and blood pressure low (hemodynamically unstable): dobutamine, dopamine; consider phosphodiesterase inhibitors, nesiritide, reperfusion, acute coronary angiography and PTCA, intra-aortic balloon pump
Right-sided heart failure/dysfunction due to right ventricular infarction/ischemia *Diagnosis:* prominent jugular veins, distention on inspiration, elevated venous pressure, clear lung fields, tachycardia associated with inferior myocardial infarction, echocardiography, increased right atrial pressure	Invasive hemodynamic monitoring, volume loading, maintenance of AV synchrony; avoid nitrates and diuretics; inotropic support (dobutamine); consider arterial vasodilators (sodium nitroprusside), ACE inhibitors, intra-aortic balloon pump, reperfusion, acute PTCA, emergency CABG
Cardiogenic shock *Diagnosis:* tachycardia, low pressure (cardiac index < 1.8 L/min/m²), dyspnea, tachypnea, cyanosis, shock, low urine output	Invasive hemodynamic monitoring, positive inotropic agents (dobutamine, dopamine, norepinephrine), reperfusion, acute PTCA or emergency CABG; anesthesia, artificial ventilation, intra-aortic balloon pump
Ventricular septal defect, papillary muscle rupture, acute mitral regurgitation *Diagnosis:* heart failure (dyspnea, orthopnea, tachycardia), systolic murmur, chest radiography, echocardiography, Doppler	Hemodynamic monitoring, afterload reduction, intra-aortic balloon pump, surgery
Cardiac rupture, pericardial effusion, and tamponade *Diagnosis:* low output, elevated venous pressure, tachycardia, dyspnea, shock, electrical-mechanical dissociation, echocardiography	Emergency pericardiocentesis, emergency surgery
Pericarditis, Dressler syndrome (late pericarditis) *Diagnosis:* pleuritic chest pain, pericardial friction rub	Aspirin, analgesics, follow-up echocardiography; avoid steroids and NSAIDs, if possible
Infarct extension *Diagnosis:* reappearance of CK-MB enzyme activity, chest pain, new ECG changes, left ventricular dysfunction, cardiogenic shock	Angiography and acute recanalization, revascularization, or reperfusion therapy; antiischemic medication (nitrates), anticoagulation; if possible, β-blockers, ACE inhibitor
Infarct expansion and left ventricular remodeling *Diagnosis:* echocardiography (thinning and dilation of infarct and left ventricle)	Afterload reduction, treatment of heart failure, anticoagulation, ACE inhibitors
Postinfarction angina, reinfarction *Diagnosis:* chest pain, ECG changes, heart failure, CK re-elevation if reinfarction	Nitrates, β-blockers, anticoagulation, reperfusion, early angiography and PTCA or CABG
Left ventricular aneurysm and mural thrombus *Diagnosis:* embolic events, echocardiography, ventriculography	Anticoagulation: acutely heparin and chronically warfarin recommended for 3–6 mo; consider surgical resection of aneurysm

ACE—angiotension-converting enzyme; AV—atrioventricular; CABG—coronary artery bypass grafting; CK-MB—creatine kinase myocardial band; ECG—electrocardiography; NSAIDs—nonsteroidal anti-inflammatory drugs; PTCA—percutaneous transluminal coronary angioplasty.

Cardiology for the Primary Care Physician

by 2–4 mg/min intravenously), procainamide, amiodarone, or synchronized electrical cardioversion. In the GUSTO-I and GUSTO-IIb trials, lidocaine was associated with a higher incidence of arrhythmias outside the United States. But in the United States, a lower likelihood of ventricular fibrillation and no increase in asystole, AV block, or mortality rates was reported [151]. Therefore, prophylactic use of antiarrhythmic agents (except β-receptor blockers) is not recommended [152••]. For bradyarrhythmia and heart block, either intravenous atropine or temporary transvenous (or, in some cases, transcutaneous) pacing is recommended. Indications for pacing are symptomatic bradycardia (<50 bpm) with symptoms of hypotension not responding to atropine, asystole, bilateral bundle branch block, newly developed or indeterminate bifascial block with first-degree AV block, second-degree symptomatic or Mobitz type II AV block, advanced (complete) AV block, and incessant ventricular tachycardia, which requires atrial or ventricular overdrive pacing [29••]. Atrial fibrillation is often transient and may be associated with heart failure, atrial ischemia, or pericarditis. The TRACE study (TRAndolapril Cardiac Evaluation) reported that the presence of atrial fibrillation or flutter after MI was associated with increased in-hospital mortality and 5-year mortality [153]. Patients with atrial fibrillation should be treated by either electrical cardioversion in patients with hemodynamic instability or ischemia or by rapid digitalization, β-blockade in patients without contraindications, diltiazem or verapamil, and heparin to avoid embolic events.

Hemodynamic and Mechanical Complications

Congestive heart failure may result from systolic contractile dysfunction due to large necrotic areas or to postischemic contractile wall motion abnormalities (stunned myocardium). Mechanical complications that worsen cardiac function include myocardial infarct expansion and aneurysm formation, ruptured ventricle, ventricular septal defect, papillary muscle dysfunction, and rupture (Table 4). The primary symptom is dyspnea, caused by pulmonary congestion and tachycardia. Therapy for congestive heart failure should be initiated with diuretics (furosemide, 20 mg intravenously, which may be repeated), nitrates, and oxygen, followed by positive inotropic agents (dobutamine, 2 to 20 μg/kg/min; dopamine 2 to 10 μg/kg/min intravenously). In case of severe ventricular dysfunction or cardiogenic shock, a Swan-Ganz pulmonary artery catheter for measurements of cardiac output, pulmonary artery capillary wedge pressure pulmonary and systemic resistances, and intra-aortic balloon counterpulsation should be considered. The therapeutic approaches to cardiogenic shock (with a high mortality rate), papillary muscle rupture with mitral regurgitation, cardiac rupture, postinfarction pericarditis, and other complications are summarized in Table 4.

Postinfarct Evaluation and Secondary Prevention

Coronary angiography and subsequent revascularization, either by PTCA or bypass grafting, ultimately should be performed in patients with recurrent angina or evidence of large areas of reversible ischemia on stress testing, and might be considered selectively in all survivors of acute MI. Before interventional therapy is initiated, recurrent angina should be treated with intravenous nitroglycerin, aspirin, heparin, analgesics, and β-blockers. In all patients following myocardial infarction without contraindications, long-term treatment with aspirin and β-adrenergic blockers is recommended [32,33,154] (Table 5). In the STAMI trial (Study of Ticlopidine vs. Aspirin In Myocardial Infarction) on

TABLE 5 LONG-TERM THERAPY AND SECONDARY PREVENTION AFTER MYOCARDIAL INFARCTION	
Treatment	**Comments**
Drug therapy	
Aspirin	In all patients without contraindications
β-Blockers	In all patients without contraindications
ACE inhibitors	In patients with left ventricular dysfunction
Dietary therapy	
Low saturated fats and cholesterol	Weight reduction and exercise in overweight patients
Lipid-lowering drugs	If LDL cholesterol > 100 mg/dL, HDL cholesterol < 35 mg/dL, triglycerides > 400 mg/dL
Rehabilitation	Risk factor evaluation, education, return to work (if feasible), self-control,
Physical	knowledge of limitations
Psychologic	
Socioeconomic	
Lifestyle changes	
Physical activity/exercising	
Smoking cessation	
ACE—angiotensin-converting enzyme; HDL—high-density lipoprotein; LDL—low-density lipoprotein.	

1470 survivors of acute MI treated with thrombolytics, ticlopidine was as efficacious as aspirin at 6 months follow-up [155]. ACE inhibitors should be a part of secondary prevention in patients with left ventricular dysfunction [156]. Calcium antagonists are not routinely recommended after infarction but may be selectively prescribed in patients with specific indications such as hypertension or angina in the presence of preserved left ventricular function [157•]. The prognosis after acute myocardial infarction is related to four main factors:

1. Extent of left ventricular dysfunction, including degree of left ventricular dilation
2. Presence of residual ischemia
3. Degree of electrical instability of the myocardium
4. Progression of coronary atherosclerosis

A risk stratification should be evaluated in each patient. The simple PREDICT risk score seems to be a powerful prognosticator of 6-year mortality after hospitalization [158]. Noninvasive evaluation of low-risk patients includes submaximal or symptom-limited stress ECG at 4 to 6 days

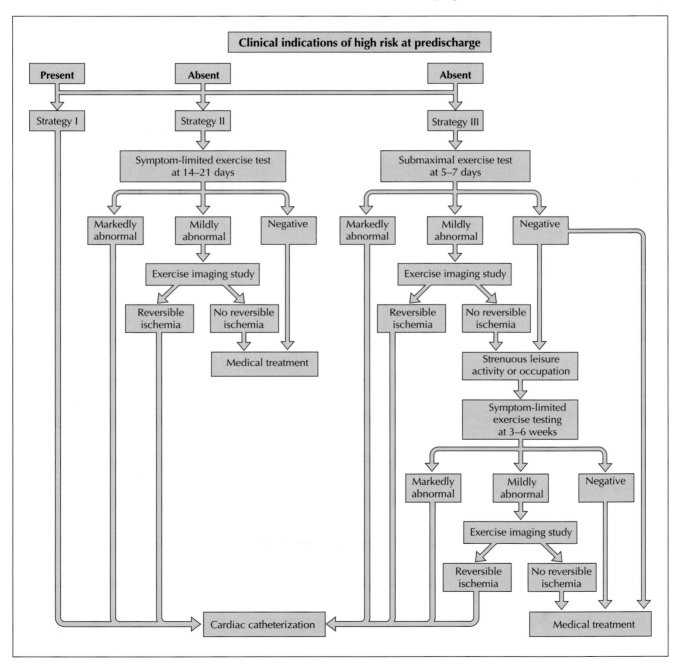

FIGURE 3 Strategies for exercise test evaluation at hospital discharge after myocardial infarction. (*Adapted from* Ryan *et al.* [164].)

or 10 to 14 days, respectively. For prognostic assessment, after mobilization, *ie*, after 1 week, submaximal exercise testing should be performed to assess potential exercise-induced angina or left ventricular dysfunction and functional capacity [159,160]. Stress ECG should be repeated early after hospital discharge and after 4 to 6 weeks. Perfusion imaging with vasodilators (dipyridamole or adenosine) or dobutamine echocardiography should be performed in patients with recurrent ischemic symptoms who are unable to exercise. Patients with evidence of reversible ischemia should be considered for coronary angiography. Knowledge of cardiac function and the coronary artery status is essential for a decision of early or delayed revascularization procedures. The postinfarction strategies for exercise testing are presented in Figure 3. Patients should be educated about risk factor modification, *ie*, cessation of smoking, necessity of physical exercise, and effective lifestyle intervention. Diet recommendations from the AHA consist of low saturated fat and cholesterol for all patients following acute MI.

Several studies like the Scandinavian Simvastatin Survival Study (4S) showed a reduction in mortality with the use of blood cholesterol-lowering agents in patients with MI [161]. Data from the CARE trial demonstrated that patients with average plasma cholesterol levels, *ie*, cholesterol below 240 mg/dL and low-density lipoprotein (LDL) cholesterol levels between 115 and 174 mg/dL, receiving pravastatin, 40 mg/d, had a reduction in risk for fatal coronary events or recurrent MI of 24% when compared with placebo-treated patients [162••]. According to the ACC/AHA guidelines, lipid-lowering drugs are recommended in patients after MI if LDL cholesterol levels are greater than 125 mg/dL (or > 100 mg/dL despite diet), triglyceride levels are greater than 400 mg/dL, and high-density lipoprotein (HDL) cholesterol levels are less than 35 mg/dL despite dietary therapy. However, according to results from the CARE trial, additional lipid-lowering drug therapy may be considered even in patients with lower (average) cholesterol levels. Social and professional rehabilitation with prescriptive exercise training and patient education is encouraged [29,163,164].

KEY REFERENCES

Recently published papers of outstanding interest, as identified in *References and Recommended Reading*, have been annotated.

•• Ryan TJ, Antman EM, Brooks NH, *et al.*: 1999 update: ACC/AHA guidelines for the management of patients with acute myocardial infarction: a report of the American College of Cardiology/American Heart Association Task Force on Practice Guidelines (Committee on management of acute myocardial infarction). *J Am Coll Cardiol* 1999, 34:890–911.

This report of the American College of Cardiology/American Heart Association Task Force on practice guidelines for the management of patients with acute myocardial infarction is a revision of the original guidelines from 1990. This update is based on current knowledge from clinical trials and contains 787 references.

•• Stone GW, Grines CL, Browne KF, *et al.*: Predictors of in-hospital and 6-month outcome after acute myocardial infarction in the reperfusion era: the primary angioplasty in myocardial infarction (PAMI) trial. *J Am Coll Cardiol* 1995, 25:370–377.

The 6-month follow-up of the comparison of primary coronary angioplasty with intravenous tissue plasminogen activator (t-PA) in patients with acute myocardial infarction demonstrated that advanced age, prior heart failure, and treatment with t-PA versus angioplasty were independently associated with increased in-hospital mortality, supporting the concept of primary angioplasty in patients with acute myocardial infarction.

•• Andersen HR, Nielsen TT, Rasmussen K, *et al.*: A comparison of coronary angioplasty with fibrinolytic therapy in acute myocardial infarction. *N Engl J Med* 2003, 349:733–742.

Patients with ST-segment elevation myocardial infarction (STEMI) presenting to community hospitals and procedural cardiac intervention (PCI) centers were randomly assigned to thrombolysis or PCI. Those at the community centers randomly assigned to PCI had to be transferred to PCI centers within 3 hours. There was a significant reduction in the composite 30-day endpoint of death, reinfarction, and disabling stroke (13.7% vs 8%; *P* < 0.001) in favor of PCI, the outcome driven mainly by a reduction in reinfarction rate. This supports the concept that primary PCI is better than thrombolysis if transfer for PCI can be done within 3 hours.

•• Latini R, Maggioni AP, Flather M, *et al.*: ACE-inhibitor use in patients with myocardial infarction: summary of evidence from clinical trials. *Circulation* 1995, 92:3132–3137.

This meeting report summarizes the data from clinical trials on angiotensin-converting enzyme (ACE) inhibition in patients with myocardial infarction and provides statements for the use of ACE inhibitors.

•• Ambrosioni E, Borghi C, Magnani B: The effect of the angiotensin-converting-enzyme inhibitor zofenopril on mortality and morbidity after anterior myocardial infarction: the Survival of Myocardial Infarction: Long-Term Evaluation (SMILE) Study Investigators. *N Engl J Med* 1995, 332:80–85.

Patients with acute myocardial infarction not receiving reperfusion therapy were randomly assigned to either zofenopril or placebo, starting 24 hours after the onset of myocardial infarction. Six-week treatment with the angiotensin-converting enzyme inhibitor zofenopril reduced mortality and the risk of severe heart failure at 6 weeks and 1 year.

•• The Task Force on the Management of Acute Myocardial Infarction of the European Society of Cardiology: Acute myocardial infarction: pre-hospital and in-hospital management. *Eur Heart J* 1996, 17:43–63.

The guidelines are provided by the European Society of Cardiology for the management and therapy for patients with acute myocardial infarction, as extrapolated from the results of clinical trials.

•• Sacks FM, Pfeffer MA, Moye, LA, *et al.*: Effect of pravastatin on coronary events after myocardial infarction in patients with average cholesterol levels. *N Engl J Med* 1996, 335:1001–1009.

This double-blind trial, which was conducted over a period of 5 years, showed that cholesterol-lowering therapy with pravastatin in patients with myocardial infarction but normal cholesterol levels (below 240 mg/dL) resulted in a significant reduction in fatal coronary events, myocardial infarction, and stroke as well as a reduction in coronary angioplasty and bypass grafting.

•• Francesco S, Pedro AL, Chi-Hang L, *et al.*: Sirolimus-eluting stent implantation in ST-elevation acute myocardial infarction: a clinical and angiographic study. *Circulation* 2003, 108:1927–1929.

This is the first report of sirolimus-eluting stents in ST segment elevation myocardial infarction (STEMI) as part of RESEARCH registry. Ninety-six patients with STEMI were treated with sirolimus-eluting stents; angiographic follow-up at 6 months showed no evidence of restenosis or late luminal loss.

•• Stone GW, Grines CL, Cox DA, *et al.*: Comparison of angioplasty with stenting, with or without abciximab, in acute myocardial infarction. *N Engl J Med.* 2002, 346:957–966.

This large randomized multicenter trial showed that abciximab tharapy during primary procedural cardiac intervention for acute myocardial infarction improved 30-day event-free survival, the outcome driven mainly by reduction of ischemic target vessel revascularization.

REFERENCES AND RECOMMENDED READING

Recently published papers of particular interest have been highlighted as:
• Of interest
•• Of outstanding interest

1. Hojo Y, Ikeda U, Zhu Y, *et al.*: Expression of vascular endothelial growth factor in patients with acute myocardial infarction. *J Am Coll Cardiol* 2000, 35:968–973.

2. Mittleman MA, Mintzer D, Maclure M, *et al.*: Triggering of myocardial infarction by cocaine. *Circulation* 1999, 99:2737–2741.

3. Lagrand WK, Visser CA, Hermens WT, *et al.*: C-reactive protein as a cardiovascular risk factor: more than an epiphenomenon? *Circulation* 1999, 100:96–102.

4. Abrignani MG, Novo G, Di Girolamo A, *et al.*: Increased plasma levels of fibrinogen in acute and chronic ischemic coronary syndromes. *Cardiologia* 1999, 44:1047–1052.

5. de Padua Mansur A, Annicchino-Bizzacchi J, Favarato D, *et al.*: Angiotensin-converting enzyme and apolipoprotein B polymorphisms in coronary artery disease. *Am J Cardiol* 2000, 85:1089–1093.

6. Gambino R, Scaglione L, Alemanno N, *et al.*: Human lipoprotein lipase HindIII polymorphism in young patients with myocardial infarction. *Metabolism* 1999, 48:1157–1161.

7. Yamada S, Akita H, Kanazawa K, *et al.*: T102C polymorphism of the serotonin (5-HT) 2A receptor gene in patients with non-fatal acute myocardial infarction. *Atherosclerosis* 2000, 150:143–148.

8. Terashima M, Akita H, Kanazawa K, *et al.*: Stromelysin promotor 5a/6a polymorphism is associated with acute myocardial infarction. *Circulation* 1999, 99:2717–2719.

9.• Parker AB, Waller BF, Gering LE: Usefulness of the 12-lead electrocardiogram in detection of myocardial infarction: electrocardiographic-anatomic correlations. *Clin Cardiol* 1996, 19:55.

10.• Sgarbossa EB, Pinski A, Barbagelata DA, *et al.*: Electrocardiographic diagnosis of evolving acute myocardial infarction in the presence of left bundle-branch block. *N Engl J Med* 1996, 334:481–487.

11. Porela P, Luotolahti M, Helenius H, *et al.*: Automated electrocardiographic scores to estimate myocardial injury size during the course of acute myocardial infarction. *Am J Cardiol* 1999, 83:949–952.

12.•• Engelen DJ, Gorgels AP, Cheriex EC, *et al.*: Value of the electrocardiogram in localizing the occlusion site in the left anterior descending coronary artery in acute anterior myocardial infarction. *J Am Coll Cardiol* 1999, 34:389–385.

13. Tsuka Y, Sugiura T, Hatadaa K, *et al.*: Clinical characteristics of ST-segment elevation in lead V6 in patients with Q-wave acute inferior wall myocardial infarction. *Coron Artery Dis* 1999, 10:465–469.

14. Matetzky S, Freimark D, Feinberg MS, *et al.*: Acute myocardial infarction with isolated ST-segment elevation in posterior chest leads V7-9: "hidden" ST-segment elevations revealing acute posterior infarction. *J Am Coll Cardiol* 1999, 34:748–753.

15. Puelo PR, Meyer D, Walthen C, *et al.*: Use of rapid assay of subforms of creatine kinase MB to diagnose or rule out acute myocardial infarction. *N Engl J Med* 1994, 331:561–566.

16. Roberts R, Kleinman NS: Earlier diagnosis and treatment of acute myocardial infarction necessitates the need for a 'new diagnostic mind-set'. *Circulation* 1994, 89:872–881.

17. Katus HA, Rempiss A, Neumann FJ, *et al.*: Diagnostic efficiency of troponin T measurements in acute myocardial infarction. *Circulation* 1991, 83:902–912.

18. Müller-Bardoff M, Freitag H, Scheffold T, *et al.*: Development and characterization of a rapid assay for bedside determinations of cardiac troponin T. *Circulation* 1995, 92:2869–2875.

19. Larue C, Calzolari C, Bertinchant JP, *et al.*: Cardiac-specific immunoenzymometric assay of troponin I in the early phase of acute myocardial infarction. *Clinical Chemistry* 1993, 39:972–979.

20. Seino Y, Tomita Y, Takano T, *et al.*: Early identification of cardiac events with serum Troponin T in patients with unstable angina. *Lancet* 1993, 342:1236–1237.

21. Falahati A, Sharkey SW, Christensen D, *et al.*: Implementation of serum cardiac troponin I as marker for detection of acute myocardial infarction. *Am Heart J* 1999, 137:332–337.

22. Apple FS: Biochemical markers of thrombolytic success. IFCC Committee on Standardization of Markers of Cardiac Damage. *Scand J Clin Lab Invest* 1999, 230(suppl.):60–66.

23.•• Tanasijevic MJ, Cannon CP, Antman EM, *et al.*: Myoglobin, creatine-kinase-MB and cardiac troponin-I 60 minute ratios predict infarct related artery patency after thrombolysis for acute myocardial infarction: results from the Thrombolysis in Myocardial Infarction study (TIMI) 10 B. *J Am Coll Cardiol* 1999, 34:739–747.

24. Ohman EM, Armstrong PW, White HD, *et al.*: Risk stratification with a point of care cardiac troponin T test in acute myocardial infarction: GUSTO III Investigators: global use of strategies to open occluded coronary arteries. *Am J Cardiol* 1999, 84:1281–1286.

25. Pierard LA, DeLandsheere CM, Berthe C, *et al.*: Identification of viable myocardium during dobutamine infusion in patients with myocardial infarction after thrombolytic therapy. *J Am Coll Cardiol* 1990, 15:1021–1031.

26. Miller GL, Herman SD, Heller GV, *et al.*: Relation between perfusion defects on stress technetium-99m sestamibi SPECT scintigraphy and the location of a subsequent acute myocardial infarction. *Am J Cardiol* 1996, 78:26–30.

27. Marcassa C, Galli M, Temporelli PL, *et al.*: Technetium-99m sestamibi tomographic evaluation of residual ischemia after anterior myocardial infarction. *J Am Coll Cardiol* 1995, 25:590–596.

28. Gibbons RJ, Miller TD, Christian TF: Infarct size measurement by single photon emission computed tomographic imaging with (99m)Tc-sestamibi: a measure of the efficacy of therapy in acute myocardial infarction. *Circulation* 2000, 101:101–108.

29.•• Ryan TJ, Antman EM, Brooks NH, *et al.*: 1999 update: ACC/AHA guidelines for the management of patients with acute myocardial infarction: a report of the American College of Cardiology/American Heart Association Task Force on Practice Guidelines (Committee on management of acute myocardial infarction). *J Am Coll Cardiol* 1999, 34:890–911.

30. Rotstein Z, Mandelzweig L, Lavi B, *et al.*: Does the coronary care unit improve prognosis of patients with acute myocardial infarction? A thrombolytic era study. *Eur Heart J* 1999, 20:813–818.

31. Somauroo JD, McCarten P, Appleton B, *et al.*: Effectiveness of a "thrombolytic nurse" in shortening delay to thrombolysis in acute myocardial infarction. *J R Coll Physicians Lond* 1999, 33:46–50.

32. Abdelnoor M, Landmark K: Infarct size is reduced and the frequency of non-Q-wave myocardial infarctions is increased in patients using aspirin at the onset of symptoms. *Cardiology* 1999, 91:119–126.

33. Mukamal KJ, Mittleman MA, Maclure M, et al.: Recent aspirin use is associated with smaller myocardial infarct size and lower likelihood of Q-wave infarction. *Am Heart J* 1999, 137:1120–1128.

34. De Wood MA, Spores J, Notske RN, et al.: Prevalence of total coronary artery occlusion during the early hours of transmural myocardial infarction. *N Engl J Med* 1980, 303:897.

35. Weaver WD, Cerqueira M, Hallstrom AP, et al.: Prehospital-initiated versus hospital-initiated thrombolytic therapy: the myocardial infarction triage and intervention trial. *JAMA* 1993, 270:1211–1216.

36. Weaver WD, Eisenberg MS, Martin JS, et al.: Myocardial infarction triage and intervention project-phase I: patient characteristics and feasibility of prehospital initiation of thrombolytic therapy. *J Am Coll Cardiol* 1990, 15:925–931.

37. Morrow DA, Antman EM, Sayah A et al.: Evaluation of the time saved by prehospital initiation of reteplase for ST-elevation myocardial infarction: results of The Early Retavase-Thrombolysis in Myocardial Infarction (ER-TIMI) 19 trial. *J Am Coll Cardiol.* 2002, 40:71-77.

38. Bonnefoy E, Lapostolle F, Leizorovicz A, et al.: Comparison of Angioplasty and Prehospital Thrombolysis in Acute Myocardial Infarction study group: Primary angioplasty versus prehospital fibrinolysis in acute myocardial infarction: a randomised study. *Lancet* 2002, 360: 825-829.

39. GISSI (Gruppo Italiano per lo Studio della Streptochinasi nell'Infarto miocardico): Effectiveness of intravenous thrombolytic treatment in acute myocardial infarction. *Lancet* 1986, I:397–401.

40. GISSI (Gruppo Italiano per lo Studio della Streptochinasi nell'Infarto miocardico): Long-term effects of intravenous thrombolysis in acute myocardial infarction: final report of the GISSI study. *Lancet* 1987, II:871–874.

41. Chesbero JH, Knatterud G, Roberts R, et al.: Thrombolysis in myocardial infarction (TIMI) trial, phase I: a comparison between intravenous tissue plasminogen activator and intravenous streptokinase. Clinical findings through hospital discharge. *Circulation* 1987, 76:142–154.

42. GISSI (Gruppo Italiano per lo Studio della Streptochinasi nell'Infarto miocardico): GISSI-2: A factorial randomized trial of alteplase versus streptokinase and heparin versus no heparin among 12,490 patients with acute myocardial infarction. *Lancet* 1990, 336:65–71.

43. GISSI (Gruppo Italiano per lo Studio della Streptochinasi nell'Infarto miocardico), The International Study Group: In-hospital mortality and clinical course of 20,891 patients with suspected acute myocardial infarction randomized between alteplase and streptokinase with or without heparin. *Lancet* 1990, 336:71–75.

44. ISIS-3 Collaborative Group: ISIS-3: a randomized comparison of streptokinase versus tissue plasminogen activator versus anistreplase and of aspirin plus heparin versus aspirin alone among 41,299 cases of suspected acute myocardial infarction. *Lancet* 1992, 339:753–770.

45. The GUSTO Investigators: An international randomized trial comparing four thrombolytic strategies for acute myocardial infarction. GUSTO-1 (Global utilization of streptokinase and tissue plasminogen activator for occluded coronary arteries). *N Engl J Med* 1993, 329:673–682.

46. The GUSTO Angiographic Investigators: The effects of tissue plasminogen activator, streptokinase, or both on coronary-artery patency, ventricular function, and survival after acute myocardial infarction. *N Engl J Med* 1993, 329:1615–1622.

47. Cannon CP, McCabe CH, Diver DJ, et al.: Comparison of front-loaded recombinant tissue-type plasminogen activator, anistreplase and combination thrombolytic therapy for acute myocardial infarction: results of the Thrombolysis in Myocardial Infarction (TIMI) 4 trial. *J Am Coll Cardiol* 1994, 24:1602–1610.

48. International Joint Efficacy Comparison of Thrombolytics: Randomized, double-blind comparison of reteplase double-bolus administration with streptokinase in acute myocardial infarction (INJECT): trial to investigate equivalence. *Lancet* 1995, 346:329–336.

49. Smalling RW, Bode C, Kalbfleisch J, et al.: More rapid, complete, and stable coronary thrombolysis with bolus administration of reteplase compared with alteplase infusion in acute myocardial infarction. *Circulation* 1995, 91:2725–2732.

50.· Topol EJ, Ohman EM, Armstrong PW, et al.: Survival outcomes 1 year after reperfusion therapy with either alteplase or reteplase for acute myocardial infarction: results from the Global Utilization of Streptokinase and t-PA for Occluded Coronary Arteries (GUSTO) III Trial. *Circulation* 2000, 102:1761–1765.

51. The InTIME-II investigators: Intravenous NPA for the treatment of infarcting myocardium early; InTIME-II, a double-blind comparison of single-bolus lanoteplase vs accelerated alteplase for the treatment of patients with acute myocardial infarction. *Eur Heart J* 2000, 21:2005–2013.

52. Assent-2 Investigators: Single-bolus tenecteplase compared with front-loaded alteplase in acute myocardial infarction: the ASSENT-2 double-blind randomised trial. Assessment of the Safety and Efficacy of a New Thrombolytic Investigators. *Lancet* 1999, 354:716–722.

53. Multicenter, randomized, comparative study of recombinant vs. natural streptokinases in acute myocardial infarct (TERIMA): the TERIMA group investigators: thrombolysis with recombinant streptokinase in acute myocardial infarct. *Thromb Haemost* 1999, 82:1605–1609.

54. Wooster MB, Luzier AB: Reteplase: a new thrombolytic for the treatment of acute myocardial infarction. *Ann Pharmacother* 1999, 33:318–324.

55. Lincoff AM, Califf RM, Topol EJ: Platelet glycoprotein IIb/IIIa receptor blockade in coronary artery disease. *J Am Coll Cardiol* 2000, 35:1103–1115.

56. Califf RM: Combination therapy for acute myocardial infarction: fibrinolytic therapy and glycoprotein IIb/IIIa inhibition. *Am Heart J* 2000, 139:S33–S37.

57. Salame M, Verheye S, More R, et al.: GPIIbIIIa inhibitors as adjunctive therapy in acute myocardial infarction. *Int J Cardiol* 1999, 69:231–236.

58. Hudson MP, Greenbaum AB, Harrington RA, Ohman EM: Use of glycoprotein IIb/IIIa inhibition plus fibrinolysis in acute myocardial infarction. *J Thromb Thrombolysis* 1999, 7:241–245.

59. Speed Group: Trial of abciximab with and without low-dose reteplase for acute myocardial infarction. Strategies for Patency Enhancement in the Emergency Department (SPEED) Group. *Circulation* 2000,101:2788–2794.

60. de Lemos JA, Antman EM, Gibson CM, et al.: Abciximab improves both epicardial flow and myocardial reperfusion in ST-elevation myocardial infarction. Observations from the TIMI 14 trial. *Circulation.* 2000,101:239–243.

61. Brener SJ, Zeymer U, Adgey AA, *et al.*: Eptifibatide and low-dose tissue plasminogen activator in acute myocardial infarction: the integrilin and low-dose thrombolysis in acute myocardial infarction (INTRO AMI) trial. *J Am Coll Cardiol*. 2002, 39:377–386.

62. The PARADIGM Investigators: Combining thrombolysis with platelet glycoprotein IIbIIIa inhibitor lamifiban: results of the platelet aggregation receptor antagonist dose investigation and reperfusion gain in myocardial infarction (PARADIGM) trial. *J Am Coll Cardiol* 1998, 32:2003–2010.

63.• Topol EJ; GUSTO V Investigators: Reperfusion therapy for acute myocardial infarction with fibrinolytic therapy or combination reduced fibrinolytic therapy and platelet glycoprotein IIb/IIIa inhibition: the GUSTO V randomised trial. *Lancet* 2001, 357:1905–1914.

64.• Lincoff AM, Califf RM, Van de Werf F *et al.*: Mortality at 1 year with combination platelet glycoprotein IIb/IIIa inhibition and reduced-dose fibrinolytic therapy vs conventional fibrinolytic therapy for acute myocardial infarction: GUSTO V randomized trial. *JAMA* 2002, 288: 2130–2135.

65. Giugliano RP, Roe MT, Harrington RA, *et al.*: INTEGRITI Investigators: Combination reperfusion therapy with eptifibatide and reduced-dose tenecteplase for ST-elevation myocardial infarction: results of the integrilin and tenecteplase in acute myocardial infarction (INTEGRITI) Phase II Angiographic Trial. *J Am Coll Cardiol* 2003, 41:1251–1260.

66.• Assessment of the Safety and Efficacy of a New Thrombolytic Regimen (ASSENT)-3 Investigators: Efficacy and safety of tenecteplase in combination with enoxaparin, abciximab, or unfractionated heparin: the ASSENT-3 randomised trial in acute myocardial infarction. *Lancet* 2001, 358:605–613.

67.•• Scull GS, Martin JS, Weaver WD, Every NR: Early angiography versus conservative treatment in patients with non-ST elevation acute myocardial infarction: MITI Investigators: Myocardial Infarction Triage and Intervention. *J Am Coll Cardiol* 2000, 15:895–902.

68. Grines CL, Browne KF, Marco J, *et al.*: A comparison of immediate angioplasty with thrombolytic therapy for acute myocardial infarction. *N Engl J Med* 1993, 328:673–679.

69.•• Stone GW, Grines CL, Browne KF, *et al.*: Predictors of in-hospital and 6-month outcome after acute myocardial infarction in the reperfusion era: the primary angioplasty in myocardial infarction (PAMI) trial. *J Am Coll Cardiol* 1995, 25:370–377.

70. Gibbons AJ, Holmes DR, Reeder GS, *et al.*: Immediate angioplasty compared with the administration of a thrombolytic agent followed by conservative treatment for myocardial infarction. *N Engl J Med* 1993, 328:685–691.

71. Zijlstra F, de Boer MJ, Hoorntje JCA, *et al.*: A comparison of immediate coronary angioplasty with intravenous streptokinase in acute myocardial infarction. *N Engl J Med* 1993, 328:680–684.

72. Kastrati A, Pache J, Dirschinger J, *et al.*: Primary intracoronary stenting in myocardial infarction: long term clinical and angiographic follow-up and risk factor analysis. *Am Heart J* 2000, 139:208–216.

73. Antoniucci D, Valenti R, Santoro GM, *et al.*: Primary coronary infarct artery stenting in acute myocardial infarction. *Am J Cardiol* 1999, 84:505–510.

74. de Boer MJ, Hoorntje JCA, Ottervanger JP, *et al.*: Immediate coronary angioplasty versus intravenous streptokinase in acute myocardial infarction: left ventricular ejection fraction, hospital mortality and reinfarction. *J Am Coll Cardiol* 1994, 23:1004–1008.

75. Le May MR, Labiraz M, Davies RF, *et al.*: Stenting versus thrombolysis in acute myocardial infarction trial (STAT). *J Am Coll Cardiol*. 2001 37: 985–991.

76. Schomig A, Kastrati A, Dirschinger J, *et al.*: Coronary stenting plus platelet glycoprotein IIb/IIIa blockade compared with tissue plasminogen activator in acute myocardial infarction. Stent versus Thrombolysis for Occluded Coronary Arteries in Patients with Acute Myocardial Infarction Study Investigators. *N Engl J Med* 2000, 343:385–391.

77.• Nunn CM, O'Neill WW, Rothbaum D, *et al.*: Long-term outcome after primary angioplasty in myocardial infarction (PAMI-I) trial. *J Am Coll Cardiol* 1999, 33:640–646.

78. Berger AK, Schulman KA, Gersh BJ, *et al.*: Primary coronary angioplasty vs thrombolysis for the management of acute myocardial infarction in elderly patients. *JAMA* 1999, 282:341–348.

79. de Boer MJ, Ottervanger JP, van't Hof AW, *et al.*: Reperfusion therapy in elderly patients with acute myocardial infarction: a randomized comparison of primary angioplasty and thrombolytic therapy. *J Am Coll Cardiol* 2002, 39:1723–1728.

80.•• Berger PB, Ellis SG, Holmes DR Jr, *et al.*: Relationship between delay in performing direct coronary angioplasty and early clinical outcome in patients with acute myocardial infarction: results from the global use of strategies to open occluded arteries in acute coronary syndromes (GUSTO-IIb) trial. *Circulation* 1999, 100:14–20.

81.• Stone GW, Brodie BR, Griffin JJ, *et al.*: Clinical and angiographic follow-up after primary stenting in acute myocardial infarction: the Primary Angioplasty in Myocardial Infarction (PAMI) stent pilot trial. *Circulation* 1999, 99:1548–1554.

82. Grines CL, Cox DA, Stone GW, *et al.*: Coronary angioplasty with or without stent implantation for acute myocardial infarction: Stent Primary Angioplasty in Myocardial Infarction Study Group. *N Engl J Med* 1999, 341:1949–1956.

83. Loubeyre C, Morice M-C, Lefevre T *et al.*: A randomized comparison of direct stenting with conventional stent implantation in selected patients with acute myocardial infarction. *J Am Coll Cardiol* 2002, 39:15–21.

84. Suryapranata H, Ottervanger JP, Nibbering E, *et al.*: Long-term outcome and cost-effectiveness of stenting vs. balloon angioplasty for acute myocardial Infarction. *Heart* 2001, 85:667–671.

85. Maillard L, Hamon M, Khalife K, *et al.*: A comparison of systematic stenting and conventional balloon angioplasty during primary percutaneous transluminal coronary angioplasty for acute myocardial infarction. *J Am Coll Cardiol* 2000, 35:1729–1736

86.•• Francesco S, Pedro AL, Chi-Hang L *et al.*: Sirolimus-eluting stent implantation in ST-elevation acute myocardial infarction: A clinical and angiographic study. *Circulation* 2003, 108:1927–1929.

87.•• Andersen HR, Nielsen TT, Rasmussen K, *et al.*: A comparison of coronary angioplasty with fibrinolytic therapy in acute myocardial infarction. *N Engl J Med*. 2003, 349:733–742.

88.• Widimsky P, Groch L, Zelizko M, *et al.*: Multicentre randomized trial comparing transport to primary angioplasty vs immediate thrombolysis vs combined strategy for patients with acute myocardial infarction presenting to a community hospital without a catheterization laboratory. The PRAGUE study. *Eur Heart J* 2000, 21:823–831.

89.• Widimsky P, Budesinsky T, Vorac D, *et al.*: Long distance transport for primary angioplasty vs immediate thrombolysis in acute myocardial infarction: final results of the randomized national multicentre trial—PRAGUE-2. *Eur Heart J* 2003, 24:94–104.

90. Grines CL, Westerhausen DR Jr, Grines LL, *et al.*: A randomized trial of transfer for primary angioplasty versus on-site thrombolysis in patients with high-risk myocardial infarction: the Air Primary Angioplasty in Myocardial Infarction study. *J Am Coll Cardiol* 2002, 39:1713–1719.

91. Aversano T, Aversano LT, Passamani E, *et al.*: Atlantic Cardiovascular Patient Outcomes Research Team (C-PORT): thrombolytic therapy vs primary percutaneous coronary intervention for myocardial infarction in patients presenting to hospitals without on-site cardiac surgery: a randomized controlled trial. *JAMA* 2002, 287:1943–1951.

92.• Ross AM, Coyne KS, Reiner JS, *et al.*: A randomized trial comparing primary angioplasty with a strategy of short-acting thrombolysis and immediate planned rescue angioplasty in acute myocardial infarction: the PACT trial: PACT investigators: Plasminogen-activator Angioplasty Compatibility Trial. *J Am Coll Cardiol* 1999, 34:1954–1962.

93. Herrmann HC, Moliterno DJ, Ohman EM, *et al.*: Facilitation of early percutaneous coronary intervention after reteplase with or without abciximab in acute myocardial infarction: results from the SPEED (GUSTO-4 Pilot) Trial. *J Am Coll Cardiol* 2000, 36:1489–1496.

94. ISIS-2 Collaborative Group: Randomized trial of intravenous streptokinase, oral aspirin, both, or neither among 17,187 cases of suspected acute myocardial infarction: ISIS-2. *Lancet* 1988, II:349–360.

95. Fuster V, Dyken ML, Vokonas PS, *et al.*: Aspirin as a therapeutic agent in cardiovascular disease. *Circulation* 1993, 87:659–675.

96. Simoons M, Krzeminska-Pakula M, Alonso A, *et al.*: Improved reperfusion and clinical outcome with enoxaparin as an adjunct to streptokinase thrombolysis in acute myocardial infarction. The AMI-SK study. *Eur Heart J* 2002, 23:1282–1290.

97. Ross AM, Molhoek P, Lundergan C, *et al.*: Randomized comparison of enoxaparin, a low-molecular-weight heparin, with unfractionated heparin adjunctive to recombinant tissue plasminogen activator thrombolysis and aspirin: second trial of Heparin and Aspirin Reperfusion Therapy (HART II). *Circulation* 2001, 104:648–652.

98.• Antman EM, Louwerenburg HW, Baars HF, *et al.*: Enoxaparin as adjunctive antithrombin therapy for ST-elevation myocardial infarction: results of the ENTIRE-Thrombolysis in Myocardial Infarction (TIMI) 23 Trial. *Circulation.* 2002,105:1642–1649.

99. Baird SH, Menown IB, Mcbride SJ, *et al.*: Randomized comparison of enoxaparin with unfractionated heparin following fibrinolytic therapy for acute myocardial infarction. *Eur Heart J* 2002, 23:627–632.

100. Frostfeldt G, Ahlberg G, Gustafsson G, *et al.*: Low molecular weight heparin (dalteparin) as adjuvant treatment to thrombolysis in acute myocardial infarction: a pilot study: biochemical markers in acute coronary syndromes (BIOMACS II). *J Am Coll Cardiol* 1999, 33:627–633.

101. Wallentin L, Bergstrand L, Dellborg M, *et al.*: Low molecular weight heparin (dalteparin) compared to unfractionated heparin as an adjunct to rt-PA (alteplase) for improvement of coronary artery patency in acute myocardial infarction-the ASSENT Plus study. *Eur Heart J* 2003, 24:897–908.

102. Cohen M, Gensini GF, Maritz F, *et al.*: The safety and efficacy of subcutaneous enoxaparin versus intravenous unfractionated heparin and tirofiban versus placebo in the treatment of acute ST-segment elevation myocardial infarction patients ineligible for reperfusion (TETAMI): a randomized trial. *J Am Coll Cardiol.* 2003, 42:1348–1356.

103. Jang IK, Brown DF, Giugliano RP, *et al.*: A multicenter, randomized study of argatroban versus heparin as adjunct to tissue plasminogen activator (TPA) in acute myocardial infarction: myocardial infarction with novastan and TPA (MINT) study. *J Am Coll Cardiol* 1999, 33:1879–1885.

104. Neuhaus KL, Molhoek GP, Zeymer U, *et al.*: Recombinant hirudin (lepirudin) for the improvement of thrombolysis with streptokinase in patients with acute myocardial infarction: results of the HIT-4 trial. *J Am Coll Cardiol* 1999, 34:966–973.

105. White H: Hirulog and Early Reperfusion or Occlusion (HERO)-2 Trial Investigators: Thrombin-specific anticoagulation with bivalirudin versus heparin in patients receiving fibrinolytic therapy for acute myocardial infarction: the HERO-2 randomised trial. *Lancet* 2001, 358:1855–1863.

106. Fung AY, Lorch G, Cambier PA, *et al.*: Efegatran sulfate as an adjunct to streptokinase versus heparin as an adjunct to tissue plasminogen activator in patients with acute myocardial infarction. ESCALAT Investigators. *Am Heart J.* 1999, 138:696–704.

107. PRIME Investigators: Multicenter, dose-ranging study of efegatran sulfate versus heparin with thrombolysis for acute myocardial infarction: The Promotion of Reperfusion in Myocardial Infarction Evolution (PRIME) trial. *Am Heart J.* 2002, 143:95–105.

108. Wallentin L, Wilcox RG, Weaver WD, *et al.*: Oral ximelagatran for secondary prophylaxis after myocardial infarction: the ESTEEM randomised controlled trial. *Lancet* 2003, 362:789–797.

109. Coussement PK, Bassand JP, Convens C, *et al.*: A synthetic factor-Xa inhibitor (ORG31540/SR9017A) as an adjunct to fibrinolysis in acute myocardial infarction. The PENTALYSE study. *Eur Heart J* 2001, 22:1716–1724.

110. Peters RJ, Spickler W, Theroux P, *et al.*: Randomized comparison of a novel anticoagulant, vasoflux, and heparin as adjunctive therapy to streptokinase for acute myocardial infarction: results of the VITAL study (Vasoflux International Trial for Acute Myocardial Infarction Lysis). *Am Heart J.* 2001, 142:237–243.

111.• Lincoff AM, Califf RM, Moliterno DJ, *et al.*: Complementary clinical benefit of coronary-artery stenting and blockade of platelet glycoprotein IIb/IIIa receptors: Evaluation of Platelet IIb/IIIa inhibition in Stenting Investigators. *N Engl J Med* 1999, 341:319–327.

112.•• van den Merkhof LF, Zijlstra F, Olsson H, *et al.*: Abciximab in the treatment of acute myocardial infarction eligible for primary percutaneous transluminal coronary angioplasty: results of the Glycoprotein Receptor Antagonist Patency Evaluation (GRAPE) pilot study. *J Am Coll Cardiol* 1999, 33:1528–1532.

113. The RESTORE Investigators: Effects of platelet glycoprotein IIb/IIIa blockade with tirofiban on adverse cardiac events in patients with unstable angina or acute myocardial infarction undergoing coronary angioplasty. *Circulation* 1997, 96:1445–1453.

114. On behalf of the ReoPro and Primary PTCA Organisation and Randomized Trial (RAPPORT) Investigators, Brener SJ, Barr LA, Burchenal JEB *et al.*: Randomized, placebo controlled trial of platelet glycoprotein IIb/IIIa blockade with primary angioplasty for acute myocardial infarction. *Circulation* 1998, 98:734–741.

115.• Topol EJ, Mark DB, Lincoff AM, *et al.*: Outcomes at 1 year and economic implications of platelet glycoprotein IIb/IIIa blockade in patients undergoing coronary stenting: results from a multicentre randomised trial. EPISTENT Investigators. Evaluation of Platelet IIb/IIIa Inhibitor for stenting. *Lancet* 1999, 354:2019–2024.

116.• Kleiman NS, Lincoff AM, Flaker GC, *et al.*: Early percutaneous coronary intervention, platelet inhibition with eptifibatide, and clinical outcomes in patients with acute coronary syndromes. PURSUIT investigators. *Circulation* 2000, 101:751–757.

117. Madan M, Kereiakes DJ, Hermiller JB, *et al.*: Efficacy of abciximab readministration in coronary intervention. *Am J Cardiol* 2000, 85:435–440.

118.•• Neumann FJ, Kastrati A, Schmitt C, *et al.*: Effect of glycoprotein IIb/IIIa receptor blockade with abciximab on clinical and angiographic restenosis rate after the placement of coronary stents following acute myocardial infarction. *J Am Coll Cardiol* 2000, 35:915–921.

119.• Montalescot G, Barragan P, Wittenberg O, *et al.*: Platelet glycoprotein IIb/IIIa inhibition with coronary stenting for acute myocardial infarction. *N Engl J Med* 2001, 344:1895–1903.

120.•• Stone GW, Grines CL, Cox DA, *et al.*: Comparison of angioplasty with stenting, with or without abciximab, in acute myocardial infarction. *N Engl J Med* 2002, 346:957–966.

121. Lee DP, Herity NA, Hiatt BL, *et al.*: Adjunctive platelet glycoprotein IIb/IIIa receptor inhibition with tirofiban before primary angioplasty improves angiographic outcomes: results of the Tirofiban Given in the Emergency Room before Primary Angioplasty (TIGER-PA) pilot trial. *Circulation* 2003, 107:1497–1501.

122. Newby LK: Long-term oral platelet glycoprotein IIb/IIIa receptor antagonism with sibrafiban after acute coronary syndromes: study design of the sibrafiban versus aspirin to yield maximum protection from ischemic heart events post-acute coronary syndromes (SYMPHONY) trial: SYMPHONY steering committee. *Am Heart J* 1999, 138:210–218.

123.• Comparison of sibrafiban with aspirin for prevention of cardiovascular events after acute coronary syndromes: a randomised trial. The SYMPHONY Investigators. Sibrafiban versus Aspirin to Yield Maximum Protection from Ischemic Heart Events Post-acute Coronary Syndromes. *Lancet* 2000, 355:337–345.

124. Mahaffey KW, Puma JA, Barbagelata NA, *et al.*: Adenosine as an adjunct to thrombolytic therapy for acute myocardial infarction: results of a multicenter, randomized placebo-controlled trial: the Acute Myocardial Infarction STudy of ADenosine (AMISTAD) trial. *J Am Coll Cardiol* 1999, 34:1711–1720.

125. First International Study of Infarct Survival Collaborative Group: Randomised trial of intravenous atenolol among 16,027 cases of suspected acute myocardial infarction: ISIS-1. *Lancet* 1986, 2:57–66.

126. Yusuf S, Peto R, Lewis J, *et al.*: Beta blockade during and after myocardial infarction: an overview of the randomized trials. *Prog Cardiovasc Dis* 1985, 27:335–371.

127.• Dargie HJ: Effect of carvedilol on outcome after myocardial infarction in patients with left-ventricular dysfunction: the CAPRICORN randomised trial. *Lancet* 2001, 357:1385–1390.

128. Pfeffer MA, Braunwald E, Moyé LA, *et al.*: Effect of captopril on mortality and morbidity in patients with left ventricular dysfunction after myocardial infarction. Results of the Survival and Ventricular Enlargement trial. *N Engl J Med* 1992, 327:669–677.

129. ISIS-4 (Fourth International Study of Infarct Survival) Collaborative Group: ISIS-4: a randomised factorial trial assessing early oral captopril, oral mononitrate, and intravenous magnesium sulphate in 58,050 patients with suspected acute myocardial infarction. *Lancet* 1995, 345:669–685.

130.•• Latini R, Maggioni AP, Flather M, *et al.*: ACE-inhibitor use in patients with myocardial infarction: summary of evidence from clinical trials. *Circulation* 1995, 92:3132–3137.

131. GISSI (Gruppo Italiano per lo Studio della Sopravvivenza nell'Infarto miocardico). GISSI-3: effects of lisinopril and transdermal glyceryl trinitrate singly and together on 6-week mortality and ventricular function after acute myocardial infarction. *Lancet* 1994, 343:1115–1122.

132.•• Ambrosioni E, Borghi C, Magnani B: The effect of the angiotensin-converting-enzyme inhibitor zofenopril on mortality and morbidity after anterior myocardial infarction: the Survival of Myocardial Infarction: Long-Term Evaluation (SMILE) Study Investigators. *N Engl J Med* 1995, 332:80–85.

133. The AIRE Study Investigators: Effect of ramipril on mortality and morbidity of survivors of acute myocardial infarction with clinical evidence of heart failure. *Lancet* 1993, 342:821–828.

134. Kober L, Torp-Pedersen C, Clarsen JE, *et al.*: A clinical trial of the angiotensin-converting enzyme inhibitor trandolapril in patients with left ventricular dysfunction after myocardial infarction. *N Engl J Med* 1995, 333:1670–1676.

135. Swedberg K, Held P, Kjekhus J, *et al.*: Effects of the early administration of enalapril on mortality in patients with acute myocardial infarction: results of the Cooperative New Scandinavian Enalapril Survival Study II (CONSENSUS -II). *N Engl J Med* 1992, 327:678–684.

136.•• Domanski MJ, Exner DV, Borkowf CB, *et al.*: Effect of angiotensin converting enzyme inhibition on sudden cardiac death in patients following acute myocardial infarction: a meta-analysis of randomized clinical trials. *J Am Coll Cardiol* 1999, 33:598–604.

137.• Duckstein K, Kjekshus J; OPTIMAAL Steering Committee of the OPTIMAAL Study Group: Effects of losartan and captopril on mortality and morbidity in high-risk patients after acute myocardial infarction: the OPTIMAAL randomised trial. Optimal Trial in Myocardial Infarction with Angiotensin II Antagonist Losartan. *Lancet* 2002, 360:752–760.

138. Torp-Pedersen C, Kober L.: Effect of ACE inhibitor trandolapril on life expectancy of patients with reduced left-ventricular function after acute myocardial infarction. TRACE Study Group. Trandolapril Cardiac Evaluation. *Lancet* 1999, 354:9–12.

139.• Pitt B, Remme W, Zannad F, *et al.*: Eplerenone, a selective aldosterone blocker, in patients with left ventricular dysfunction after myocardial infarction. *N Engl J Med* 2003, 348:1309–1321.

140.• Ito H, Taniyama Y, Iwakura K, *et al.*: Intravenous nicorandil can preserve microvascular integrity and myocardial viability in patients with reperfused anterior wall myocardial infarction. *J Am Coll Cardiol* 1999, 33:654–660.

141. Buerke M, Rupprecht HJ, vom Dahl J, *et al.*: Sodium-hydrogen exchange inhibition: novel strategy to prevent myocardial injury following ischemia and reperfusion. *Am J Cardiol* 1999(suppl G), 83:19–22.

142. Woods KL, Fletcher S: Long-term outcome after intravenous magnesium sulphate in suspected acute myocardial infarction: the second Leicester Intravenous Magnesium Intervention Trial (LIMIT-2). *Lancet* 1994, 343:816–819.

143. Gyamlani G, Parikh C, Kulkarni AG: Benefits of magnesium in acute myocardial infarction: timing is crucial. *Am Heart J* 2000, 139:37–41.

144. The MAGIC Steering Committee: Rationale and design of the magnesium in coronaries (MAGIC) study: a clinical trial to reevaluate the efficacy of early administration of magnesium in acute myocardial infarction. *Am Heart J* 2000, 139:10–14.

145. Parikka H, Toivonen L, Naukkarinen V, *et al.*: Decreases by magnesium of QT dispersion and ventricular arrhythmias in patients with acute myocardial infarction. *Eur Heart J* 1999, 20:111–120.

146. Raghu C, Peddeswara Rao P, Seshagiri Rao D: Protective effect of intravenous magnesium in acute myocardial infarction following thrombolytic therapy. *Int J Cardiol* 1999, 71:209–215.

147. The Magnesium in Coronaries (MAGIC) Trial Investigators: Early administration of intravenous magnesium to high-risk patients with acute myocardial infarction in the Magnesium in Coronaries (MAGIC) Trial: a randomised controlled trial. *Lancet* 2002, 360:1189–1196.

148. Malmberg K, Norhammar A, Wedel H, Ryden L: Glycometabolic state at admission: important risk marker of mortality in conventionally treated patients with diabetes mellitus and acute myocardial infarction: long-term results from the Diabetes and Insulin-Glucose Infusion in Acute Myocardial Infarction (DIGAMI) study. *Circulation* 1999, 99:2626–2632.

149. Baran KW, Nguyen M, McKendall GR, *et al.*: Double-blind, randomized trial of an anti-CD18 antibody in conjunction with recombinant tissue plasminogen activator for acute myocardial infarction: limitation of myocardial infarction following thrombolysis in acute myocardial infarction (LIMIT AMI) study. *Circulation* 2001,104:2778–2783.

150. Faxon DP, Gibbons RJ, Chronos NA, *et al.*: The effect of blockade of the CD11/CD18 integrin receptor on infarct size in patients with acute myocardial infarction treated with direct angioplasty: the results of the HALT-MI study. *J Am Coll Cardiol* 2002, 40:1199–1204.

151. Alexander JH, Granger CB, Sadowski Z, *et al.*: Prophylactic lidocaine use in acute myocardial infarction: incidence and outcomes from two international trials. The GUSTO-I and GUSTO-IIb Investigators. *Am Heart J* 1999, 137:799–805.

152.•• The Task Force on the Management of Acute Myocardial Infarction of the European Society of Cardiology: Acute myocardial infarction: pre-hospital and in-hospital management. *Eur Heart J* 1996, 17:43–63.

153. Pedersen OD, Bagger H, Kober L, Torp-Pedersen C: The occurrence and prognostic significance of atrial fibrillation/-flutter following acute myocardial infarction. TRACE Study group. TRAndolapril Cardiac Evaluation. *Eur Heart J* 1999, 20:748–754.

154. Goldstein RE, Andrews M, Hall WJ, *et al.*: Marked reduction in long-term cardiac deaths with aspirin after a coronary event: Multicenter Myocardial Ischemia Research Group. *J Am Coll Cardiol* 1996, 28:326–330.

155. Scrutinio D, Cimminiello C, Marubini E, *et al.*: Ticlopidine versus aspirin after myocardial infarction (STAMI) trial. *J Am Coll Cardiol.* 2001, 37:1259–1265.

156. Psaty BM, Heckbert SR, Koepsell TD, *et al.*: The risk of myocardial infarction associated with antihypertensive drug therapies. *JAMA* 1995, 274:620–625.

157.• Senior R, Basu S, Kinsey C, *et al.*: Carvedilol prevents remodeling in patients with left ventricular dysfunction after acute myocardial infarction. *Am Heart J* 1999, 137:646–652.

158. Jacobs DR Jr, Kroenke C, Crow R, *et al.*: Predict: a simple risk score for clinical severity and long-term prognosis after hospitalization for acute myocardial infarction or unstable angina: the Minnesota heart survey. *Circulation* 1999, 100:599–607.

159. Senaratne MPJ, Smith G, Gulamhusein SS: Feasibility and safety of early exercise testing using the BRUCE protocol after acute myocardial infarction. *J Am Coll Cardiol* 2000, 35:1212–1220.

160. Nakano A, Lee JD, Shimizu H, *et al.*: Reciprocal ST-segment depression associated with exercise-induced ST-segment elevation indicates residual viability after myocardial infarction. *J Am Coll Cardiol* 1999, 33:620–626.

161. The Scandinavian Simvastatin Survival Study Group: Randomized trial of cholesterol lowering in 4444 patients with coronary heart disease: the Scandinavian Simvastatin Survival Study (4S). *Lancet* 1994, 344:1383–1389.

162.•• Sacks FM, Pfeffer MA, Moye, LA, *et al.*: Effect of pravastatin on coronary events after myocardial infarction in patients with average cholesterol levels. *N Engl J Med* 1996, 335:1001–1009.

163. American Heart Association: Cardiac rehabilitation programs: a statement for healthcare professionals from the American Heart Association. *Circulation* 1994, 90:1602–1610.

164. Ryan TJ, Anderson JL, Antman EM, *et al.*: ACC/AHA guidelines for the management of patients with acute myocardial infarction. A report of the American College of Cardiology/American Heart Association Task Force on Practice Guidelines (Committee on management of acute myocardial infarction). *J Am Coll Cardiol* 1996, 28:1328–1428.

Mitral Stenosis and Regurgitation

21

Sidney C. Smith, Jr.
Park W. Willis IV

> ### *Key Points*
> - Advanced diagnostic techniques such as color flow Doppler echocardiography, and new therapeutic approaches, such as balloon mitral valvuloplasty, left ventricular unloading therapy, and direct mitral valve repair, offer improved care for patients with mitral valve disease.
> - Rheumatic heart disease remains the major cause of mitral stenosis, and outbreaks of rheumatic fever continue to occur in the United States.
> - An echocardiographic scoring system identifies patients most likely to benefit from balloon mitral valvuloplasty.
> - Physicians should make patients with mitral valve disease familiar with the new American Heart Association guidelines for prevention of infective endocarditis.
> - Resting ejection fraction remains preserved late in the course of mitral regurgitation, and exercise radionuclide ejection fractions may assist in selecting patients who are candidates for mitral valve surgery.

Over the past 20 years our understanding of the pathophysiology of mitral valve disease has increased substantially. Advanced echocardiographic methods have expanded our diagnostic capability. New therapeutic approaches such as balloon mitral valvuloplasty, left ventricular unloading therapy, and direct mitral valve repair have improved the treatment and prognosis for patients with mitral valve disease. This chapter details current trends in the diagnosis and therapy of mitral stenosis and regurgitation from the standpoint of the clinician.

MITRAL STENOSIS

Etiology and Pathophysiology

Most cases of mitral stenosis are caused by rheumatic heart disease (Table 1) [1•]. Less frequently, severe mitral annular calcification, malignant carcinoid, or rheumatoid arthritis may be the underlying cause. The clinical presentation and physical findings of left atrial myxoma can mimic rheumatic mitral stenosis. Congenital forms of mitral stenosis are rare and usually present in childhood, associated with other congenital lesions. Two thirds of patients with rheumatic mitral stenosis are female.

Because of the strong association of rheumatic heart disease with mitral stenosis, the practicing physician should be familiar with current diagnostic criteria for acute rheumatic fever. The American Heart Association has published updated Jones criteria for the diagnosis of acute rheumatic fever (Table 2) [2]. These changes emphasize the importance of establishing the initial attack of rheumatic fever and expand on the available tools to diagnose streptococcal pharyngitis with clarification of available antibody tests. Echocardiographic abnormalities without accompanying auscultatory findings are considered insufficient to be the sole criteria for valvulitis in acute rheumatic fever.

Patients with mitral valve stenosis often have no definite history of rheumatic fever in childhood or as a young adult and are usually asymptomatic until the third or fourth decade. Multiple episodes of rheumatic fever during childhood may result in an accelerated disease course causing the patient to present with mitral stenosis at an earlier age. This is especially common in patients living in underdeveloped areas and temperate zones where the disease often presents during adolescence. In general, approximately 10 years will elapse between an episode of acute rheumatic fever and the first appearance of the murmur of mitral stenosis.

The rheumatic process, presumably through an autoimmune mechanism, results in fibrosis and scarring, especially at the margins of the mitral valve leaflets. This results in fusion of the valve leaflets and shortening and thickening of the chordae tendineae. The result is progressive narrowing of the mitral valve orifice with increasing left atrial and pulmonary venous pressures. Left atrial enlargement and progressive calcification of the mitral valve follow as this process progresses. The normal valve area of 4 to 6 cm^2 is reduced to less than 2 cm^2. Severe hemodynamic changes occur at valve areas less than 1 cm^2.

Clinical Presentation

The most common presenting symptom of mitral stenosis is exertional dyspnea secondary to pulmonary venous hypertension. The majority of patients with mitral stenosis are women and symptoms often appear initially during the second trimester of pregnancy, when blood volume and cardiac output peak. Patients frequently experience orthopnea, paroxysmal nocturnal dyspnea, and progressive fatigue and weakness. Pulmonary hypertension may be associated with chest pain and hemoptysis. Approximately 50% of patients with mitral stenosis are older than 30 years and may have significant coronary artery disease. Therefore, it is important to consider multiple causes for chest pain. Hoarseness (Ortner's syndrome) may occur because of

compression of the left recurrent laryngeal nerve between the enlarged pulmonary artery, aorta, and ligamentum arteriosum. Unfortunately, systemic embolism may be the first symptom of mitral stenosis, especially in association with the development of atrial fibrillation. Although infective endocarditis is uncommon, it can complicate the clinical course of mitral stenosis [3].

The classic physical finding of mitral stenosis is a loud first heart sound (S_1) associated with a low-pitched diastolic rumble best heard at the apex, with the bell of the stethoscope, in the left lateral decubitus position. Positional variation in the intensity of the diastolic rumble may indicate that left atrial myxoma is present. A high-pitched opening snap (OS) may be heard just after the second heart sound (S_2). The S_2-OS interval narrows as the severity of mitral stenosis increases. When pulmonary hypertension develops, the amplitude of the pulmonic component of S_2 increases and a right ventricular heave may be detected. Pulmonary rales, jugular venous distention, hepatic enlargement, and peripheral edema may be present, representing generalized findings for congestive heart failure. With severe pulmonary hypertension, pulmonary regurgitation may be present (Graham Steell murmur), which should be distinguished from aortic regurgitation. Atrial fibrillation is often present as mitral stenosis progresses in severity, and characteristic ruddy cheeks (mitral facies) may be noted.

Laboratory Findings

Echocardiography is the most valuable clinical test in the management of mitral stenosis. It is useful in gauging the severity of mitral stenosis, distinguishing left atrial myxomas, and identifying coexisting atrial septal defects, thrombi, and valvular vegetations (Fig. 1). In addition,

---

TABLE 1 MITRAL STENOSIS

Etiology
Rheumatic heart disease (most common)
Congenital
Mitral annular calcification
Malignant carcinoid
Rheumatoid arthritis
Exclude
Left atrial tumor (usually myxoma)
Cor triatriatum
Associated atrial septal defect

TABLE 2 GUIDELINES FOR DIAGNOSIS OF RHEUMATIC FEVER (JONES CRITERIA, UPDATED 1992)

Major manifestations
Carditis
Polyarthritis
Chorea
Erythema marginatum
Subcutaneous nodules

Minor manifestations
Arthralgia
Fever
Elevated erythrocyte sedimentation rate
Elevated C-reactive protein
Prolonged PR interval
Evidence of antecedent group A streptococcal infection
Positive throat culture or rapid streptococcal antigen test
Elevated or increasing streptococcal antibody titer

Note: When supported by evidence of antecedent group A streptococcal infection, two major or one major and two minor manifestations indicate a high probability of rheumatic fever.

associated valvular lesions such as mitral regurgitation, aortic stenosis or regurgitation, and pulmonary and tricuspid valvular disease, which are also associated with rheumatic heart disease, may be identified. Color flow Doppler echocardiography is useful in assessing the extent of associated mitral regurgitation. Transesophageal echocardiography may help to detect left atrial thrombi (Fig. 2).

Recently, a scoring system based on the results of echocardiography has been devised to assist in identifying patients who may best benefit from balloon mitral valvuloplasty. The scoring system grades from 0 to 4+ the following four echocardiographic factors: valvular rigidity, valvular calcification, valvular thickening, and the amount of subvalvular disease; a score of 4+ represents a severely abnormal finding. Thus, a valve with severe rigidity, extensive calcification, severe thickening, and substantial subvalvular thickening would receive a score of 4 for each category, resulting in a total score of 16. Patients with mitral valve scores of 8 or less generally have the best results from balloon mitral valvuloplasty.

The electrocardiogram is useful in identifying left atrial enlargement with terminal negative P waves in V_1 and the presence of right ventricular hypertrophy pattern with increased R wave in V_1 and a rightward axis. Both of these findings reflect increasing severity of mitral stenosis. It is important to identify the presence of atrial fibrillation, because these patients will require anticoagulation therapy.

Chest radiography may be useful in identifying left atrial enlargement with elevation of the left mainstem bronchus, pulmonary venous hypertension, and the presence of mitral calcification. In general, and especially during pregnancy, the echocardiogram provides more precise and clinically valuable information for the management of patients with mitral stenosis than other noninvasive tests.

Other adjuncts to the echocardiogram in the diagnosis and management of patients with mitral stenosis include exercise testing and cardiac catheterization. Exercise testing either in association with cardiac catheterization or separately is sometimes valuable in developing management strategies for those patients with mitral stenosis of borderline severity. Cardiac catheterization before surgical intervention for mitral stenosis is generally required to identify coronary artery disease in older patients and to assess the severity of mitral stenosis using hemodynamic parameters [4]. Many patients will be identified as candidates for balloon mitral valvuloplasty and undergo cardiac catheterization for this reason.

Management

Medical therapy for mitral stenosis includes 1) antibiotic prophylaxis for infective endocarditis and recurrent rheumatic fever; 2) management of pulmonary venous hypertension and right heart failure; 3) control of atrial fibrillation; and 4) anticoagulation for prevention of thromboembolism.

The American Heart Association guidelines for antibiotic prophylaxis for infective endocarditis at the time of dental and surgical procedures should be carefully reviewed with the patient (Table 3) [5]. Wallet-sized summary cards are available from the American Heart Association to assist the patient in this regard. The guidelines for duration of long-term antibiotic therapy using 1.2 million units benzathine penicillin G monthly as prophylaxis against recurrent rheumatic fever are not well established. Generally, continuation to age 40 or later is advisable if the patient is in an occupation such as teaching, where frequent exposure to younger children with streptococcal infection may occur.

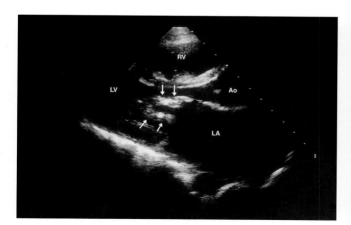

FIGURE 1 Mitral stenosis. Mid-diastolic frame from a transthoracic two-dimensional echocardiogram, in the parasternal long-axis plane, showing a thickened mitral valve with limited leaflet excursion and left atrial enlargement. Note that leaflet calcification and marked subvalvular thickening (*arrows*) would predict a suboptimal outcome after balloon dilatation. Ao—aorta; LA—left atrium; LV—left ventricle; RV—right ventricle.

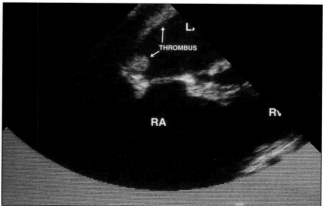

FIGURE 2 Mitral stenosis. Late diastolic frame from an intraoperative transesophageal echocardiogram, in the short-axis plane, showing left atrial mural thrombus. The finding of left atrial thrombus in a patient with mitral stenosis is a contraindication to balloon valvuloplasty. LA—left atrium; LV—left ventricle; RA—right atrium; RV—right ventricle.

Diuretic therapy is useful in managing the symptoms of pulmonary venous congestion and right heart failure; however, vigorous diuresis in the presence of significant mitral stenosis may markedly decrease cardiac output.

It is important to control the heart rate when atrial fibrillation occurs, because rapid ventricular response may increase pulmonary congestion due to shortened diastolic filling time. Thus, prompt therapy should be instituted with digoxin to control ventricular response when atrial fibrillation develops. Digoxin is not helpful in treating patients with mitral stenosis who remain in normal sinus rhythm without atrial fibrillation. β-blockers or calcium channel antagonists may be added to digoxin therapy when the ventricular rate remains poorly controlled. In patients who require prompt control of ventricular rate because of hemodynamic deterioration, intravenous diltiazem or esmolol will provide a more rapid reduction in the ventricular response than digoxin. Anticoagulation therapy should be initiated promptly when atrial fibrillation or a documented thromboembolic event has occurred. Once the ventricular rate is controlled and the patient has completed 3 weeks of anticoagulation therapy, elective pharmacologic or electrical cardioversion may be attempted.

When to Refer

Because the natural history of mitral stenosis is related to symptomatic status, the patient should be evaluated for mechanical intervention such as balloon valvuloplasty, open commissurotomy, or valve replacement as the symptoms progress beyond New York Heart Association (NYHA) class II. In patients with NYHA class II symptoms, valve area is usually less than 1.0 cm²/m² body surface area. Balloon valvuloplasty provides an acceptable alternative to open commissurotomy, with the best results occurring in patients with pliable leaflets, minimal calcification, mild leaflet thickening, and mild subvalvular fibrosis as demonstrated on echocardiography [6,7]. In patients in whom such findings are absent, mitral valve replacement or open commissurotomy should be considered [8]. Because anticoagulation with coumadin is required after valve replacement, valvuloplasty or commissurotomy are the procedures of choice for women of child-bearing age. Findings of significant mitral regurgitation or a heavily calcified valve argue for mitral valve replacement. Bioprostheses in the mitral position can carry a significant risk for embolic events in the absence of anticoagulation, particularly if atrial fibrillation of left atrial dilatation is present.

Because the number of procedures performed and the operating physician's experience have a significant impact on the outcome for both surgical and cardiac interventional procedures, physicians and patients should base the final decision regarding the choice of mechanical procedure on the results at their local institution. Published mortality rates for mitral valve replacement or open commissurotomy are generally 1% to 4%, whereas the reported mortality for balloon mitral valvuloplasty has ranged from 0% to 4%. Approximately 35% of patients undergoing balloon mitral valvuloplasty will be left with a small residual atrial septal defect which, in the majority of cases, will decrease in size or close. Ten percent of patients undergoing balloon mitral valvuloplasty will develop restenosis after 1 to 2 years. At present, balloon mitral valvuloplasty appears to be the treatment of choice for carefully selected patients with mitral

---

TABLE 3 ANTIBIOTIC PROPHYLAXIS FOR PREVENTION OF ENDOCARDITIS

Regimens for dental, oral, or upper respiratory tract procedures

Amoxicillin 3 g PO 1 h before procedure, then 1.5 g PO 6 h after initial dose

*Erythromycin ethylsuccinate 800 mg or erythromycin stearate 1 g PO 2 h before procedure, then one half the dose 6 h after initial dose

*Clindamycin 300 mg PO 1 h before procedure and 150 mg 6 h after initial dose

Regimens for genitourinary and gastrointestinal procedures

Ampicillin 2 g IV (or IM) plus gentamicin 1.5 mg/kg IV (or IM) (not to exceed 80 mg) 30 minutes before procedure, followed by amoxicillin 1.5 g PO 6 h after the initial dose. Alternatively repeat parenteral regimen may be repeated once 8 hours after initial dose

*Vancomycin 1 g IV over 1 h plus gentamicin 1.5 mg/kg IV (or IM) (not to exceed 80 mg) 1 h before procedure. May be repeated once 8 hours after initial dose

†Amoxicillin 3 g PO 1 h before procedure; then 1.5 g PO 6 hours after initial dose

*For patients allergic to amoxicillin, ampicillin, and/or penicillin.
†Alternate oral regimen for low-risk patients.
IM—intramuscularly; IV—intravenously; PO—orally.

TABLE 4 MITRAL REGURGITATION: ETIOLOGY

Acute
Ruptured chordae tendineae
Papillary muscle rupture
Endocarditis
Trauma
Prosthetic valve dysfunction

Chronic
Rheumatic heart disease
Papillary muscle dysfunction
Severe left ventricular dilatation
Endocarditis
Mitral valve prolapse
Associated with hypertrophic obstructive cardiomyopathy
Congenital abnormalities
Marfan's syndrome
Prosthetic valve dysfunction

stenosis [9], yielding an 84% 4-year survival rate in the largest multicenter registry [10]. In patients with previous surgical commissurotomies, balloon mitral valve surgery may be performed with good immediate results and continued improvement in nearly half the patients at 8 years [11].

MITRAL REGURGITATION
Etiology and Pathophysiology

Mitral regurgitation may result from a disorder of any of the components of the mitral valve, which include the annulus, anterior and posterior leaflets, chordae tendineae, and papillary muscles [12] (Table 4). Mitral regurgitation may also be caused by mitral valve prolapse. Mitral regurgitation due to involvement of the leaflets is common secondary to rheumatic heart disease and occurs more often in men than in women. With acute rheumatic fever, severe mitral regurgitation is more likely to involve the anterior leaflet, whereas chordal rupture, either primary or myxomatous in etiology, and papillary muscle ischemia generally involve the posterior leaflet. Endocarditis and Marfan's syndrome are important causes of mitral regurgitation. Degenerative annular calcification, more common in women, may also result in mitral regurgitation. Annular dilatation secondary to cardiomyopathy is an increasingly frequent cause of mitral regurgitation; varying degrees of mitral regurgitation are found in up to 30% of patients undergoing coronary artery bypass surgery [11]. Finally, prosthetic mitral valve dysfunction is becoming a more frequent cause of clinically encountered mitral regurgitation.

Mitral regurgitation results in significant backflow during systole from the left ventricle into the left atrium. The result is chronic progressive enlargement of both chambers to accommodate the regurgitant volume, which may be four to five times the forward flow when severe. Because regurgitant flow occurs at relatively low impedance into the left atrium, the left ventricular ejection fraction may be preserved late into the course of mitral regurgitation. The ejection fraction in mitral regurgitation may not serve as an accurate index of left ventricular function, and thus may lead to an erroneously favorable estimate of myocardial performance.

The sudden increase in left atrial volume and pressure associated with acute mitral regurgitation may result in severe pulmonary congestion, often in the presence of preserved left ventricular ejection fraction. Atrial fibrillation may cause significant hemodynamic compromise when it occurs in the course of either acute or chronic mitral regurgitation.

Clinical Presentation

Patients with chronic mitral regurgitation may enjoy a relatively asymptomatic course for 20 to 30 years, but finally present with symptoms of progressive weakness and fatigue. Orthopnea and systemic embolism are uncommon presenting symptoms in mitral regurgitation [1•]. In

contrast with mitral stenosis, the S_1 sound in mitral regurgitation is usually diminished. The S_2 may be widely split and an apical third heart sound (S_3) may be present. With left ventricular enlargement, the apical impulse becomes diffuse and is displaced laterally. The most prominent finding in mitral regurgitation is a holosystolic murmur beginning with S_1 and extending into the aortic component of S_2. The murmur radiates from the apex to the axilla, but may be heard at the left external edge and at the aortic area when there is marked posterior leaflet prolapse. With marked anterior leaflet prolapse, the murmur may be directed to the posterior wall of the left atrium and may be more prominent over the spine. There is little correlation between the intensity of the murmur and the severity of mitral regurgitation. The murmur may be increased in intensity by isometric exercise, which serves to distinguish it from that of aortic stenosis and hypertrophic obstructive cardiomyopathy. The location of the murmur distinguishes it from the murmur of a ventricular septal defect, which is loudest along the left sternal border and is often associated with parasternal thrill. With pulmonary hypertension, the pulmonic component of S_2 is increased and the systolic murmur of tricuspid regurgitation may be present along the left sternal border.

Laboratory Findings

As with mitral stenosis, color flow Doppler echocardiography has contributed greatly to the management of patients with mitral regurgitation (Fig. 3). It usually aids in establishing the diagnosis and helps to quantify the severity of mitral regurgitation, thereby assisting with patient management. With acute mitral regurgitation, left ventricular and left atrial chamber size may be normal. The left ventricular ejection fraction is usually preserved unless the regurgitation occurs in the setting of acute myocardial infarction, in

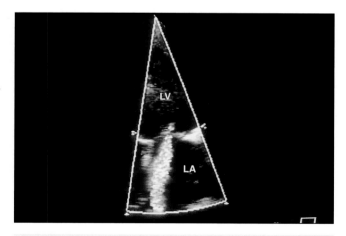

FIGURE 3 Mitral regurgitation. Late systolic frame from a transthoracic color flow Doppler study, in the apical four-chamber plane, showing turbulent flow in the left atrium caused by a high velocity jet of mitral regurgitation. LA—left atrium; LV—left ventricle. (*See* Color Plate.)

which case regional wall motion abnormalities and impaired ejection fraction may occur. Echocardiography may be particularly valuable in confirming the presence of flail mitral leaflet or endocarditis. In chronic mitral regurgitation, both left ventricular and left atrial chamber sizes are increased. Assessment of left ventricular wall stress and systolic volume may be more valuable in predicting the patient's suitability for valve replacement than the ejection fraction. Left ventricular dimensions can be followed serially in association with the regurgitant mitral jet volume to assess the results of unloading therapy. Transesophageal echocardiography is especially valuable in assessing patients undergoing mitral valve surgery as possible candidates for direct reconstructive repair rather than mitral replacement.

No electrocardiographic abnormalities are diagnostic for mitral regurgitation. Progressive left ventricular hypertrophy and left atrial enlargement are observed as the mitral regurgitation worsens. Atrial fibrillation generally occurs late in the course of mitral regurgitation. In patients with suspected acute mitral regurgitation, the electrocardiogram results may be normal, except for sinus tachycardia and evidence of acute infarction or ischemia, if that is the underlying etiology.

The chest radiograph generally demonstrates left ventricular and left atrial enlargement as chronic mitral regurgitation increases in severity. Pulmonary venous congestion may be seen as the clinical course worsens. In patients with acute mitral regurgitation, pulmonary venous hypertension may be the only finding, while left atrial and left ventricular size are normal.

Cardiac catheterization is useful in evaluating older patients with mitral regurgitation to rule out coronary artery disease, before proceeding with mitral valve surgery. In much younger patients with isolated mitral regurgitation, sufficient data may be obtained from echocardiography such that cardiac catheterization is usually unnecessary. In those with acute mitral regurgitation, marked elevation of pulmonary capillary wedge pressure may be noted with prominent regurgitant V waves. As previously mentioned, it is not unusual to find normal or above-normal ejection fractions in patients with acute regurgitation unless myocardial infarction with papillary muscle rupture is the cause, in which case regional wall-motion abnormalities usually are present. Angiographic assessment of mitral regurgitation is the most reliable system for grading mild and severe degrees of mitral regurgitation. However, angiography may not be accurate in assessing moderate regurgitation due to variation in techniques of angiographic injection or left ventricular loading conditions. This makes decisions regarding surgery more difficult when moderate regurgitation is noted; other factors previously mentioned should be carefully considered.

The V wave amplitude may also be misleading as a guide to severity of mitral regurgitation and should not be used as a reference for surgical decisions.

In patients with moderate mitral regurgitation in whom resting left ventricular ejection fraction appears preserved, exercise radionuclide ejection fractions may help to assess possible candidacy for mitral valve surgery. The inability to elevate ejection fraction with exercise may signal left ventricular dysfunction and a need for surgical intervention.

Management

Patients with acute severe mitral regurgitation should be stabilized with diuretics and afterload reduction. Nitroprusside, which acts as an arteriolar and venous dilator, should be instituted promptly and titrated to optimize systemic vascular resistance, forward cardiac output, and pulmonary capillary wedge pressures. Digoxin and inotropic agents generally are not useful, because ventricular function is usually preserved with acute mitral regurgitation.

Patients with chronic mitral regurgitation who are asymptomatic should be given antibiotic prophylaxis for infective endocarditis as outlined in the discussion for patients with mitral stenosis [5]. The incidence of embolic events is lower than that for mitral stenosis, but anticoagulation should be initiated for those patients in atrial fibrillation and patients with previous embolic events. Patients with minimal or no symptoms should receive follow-up echocardiography on a yearly basis to assess left ventricular size and function unless the mitral regurgitation is mild and ventricular dimensions are normal, in which case follow-up at longer intervals is indicated. Follow-up echo studies may not be required in patients with mild mitral regurgitation. Patients who develop symptoms should be considered for therapy with vasodilators, especially the angiotensin-converting enzyme (ACE) inhibitors and diuretics. Patients who are unable to tolerate ACE inhibitors may benefit from taking an angiotensin-receptor-blocking agent. Digoxin should be instituted for atrial fibrillation to control ventricular rate and in patients with progressive left ventricular dysfunction who are not candidates for mitral valve replacement. Symptomatic patients with left ventricular dysfunction and mitral regurgitation who are not candidates for mitral valve surgery should be considered for combined diuretic, ACE inhibitor, and digoxin therapy.

Intra-aortic balloon counterpulsation is indicated when severe hemodynamic instability is present. Surgical therapy with mitral valve replacement or repair is pursued promptly when patients cannot be stabilized hemodynamically. In cases of endocarditis, if patients can be stabilized, antibiotic therapy is started before proceeding with mitral valve replacement for acute mitral regurgitation.

When to Refer

Surgery for mitral regurgitation has evolved over the past 10 years such that reconstructive repair is performed as frequently as mitral valve replacement. The advantages of repair include lower operative mortality; preservation of the annular-chordal-papillary muscle continuity, which maintains left ventricular function; elimination of thromboembolic risk, thus obviating the need for anticoagulation; and a lower risk of late failure than might be encountered with the bioprostheses. Transesophageal echocardiography is necessary preoperatively to assess candidates for reconstructive surgery, and intraoperative Doppler color flow mapping is extremely useful in assessing the adequacy of reconstruction.

Both bioprosthetic and mechanical valves have an embolic risk and require anticoagulation in the mitral position, although the risk of emboli with a bioprosthetic valve is lower when normal sinus rhythm is present. Bioprosthetic valves generally calcify and become dysfunctional after 7 to 10 years; thus, mechanical valve replacement is preferred if reconstructive surgery is not feasible. When mitral valve replacement is performed with a prosthetic valve, every effort should be made to preserve the native valve apparatus. Ablation of the mitral valve apparatus at the time of mitral valve replacement has been shown to result in a 25% decrease in left ventricular function. The operative mortality in active centers for isolated mitral valve replacement ranges from 2% to 7% in patients with NYHA class II or III symptoms undergoing elective valve replacement and 1% to 4% for similar patients undergoing reconstructive surgery. Mortality is higher for patients with NYHA class IV symptoms as well as patients undergoing surgery for acute mitral regurgitation or those with concomitant coronary bypass surgery. Because of the improved outcome when surgery is performed earlier, surgery is recommended for most patients with isolated severe mitral regurgitation who remain symptomatic NYHA class II in association with medical therapy and have elevated end-systolic volumes of greater than 50 mL/m². End-systolic volume should be monitored carefully in asymptomatic patients with severe mitral regurgitation and ejection fractions between 55 and 70. Surgical intervention should be performed in these patients as left ventricular function deteriorates. Specifically, elective mitral valve surgery should be considered in this group of patients before ejection fraction is less than 0.50 and the end-systolic volume index greater than 50 mL/m². For patients who require mitral valve surgery, the use of computer-enhanced telemanipulation systems or robotic technology holds promise for improved outcomes with reduced morbidity and improved recovery times [13].

REFERENCES AND RECOMMENDED READING

Recently published paper of particular interest have been highlighted as:

• Of interest

1.• Braunwald E: Valvular heart disease. In *Heart Disease*, edn 5. Philadelphia: WB Saunders; 1997:1007–1035.

2. Dajani AS, Ayoub E, Bierman FZ, *et al.*: Guidelines for the diagnosis of rheumatic fever: Jones Criteria, updated 1992. *Circulation* 1993, 87:302–307.

3. McHenry MM: Systemic arterial embolism in patients with mitral stenosis and minimal dyspnea. *Am J Cardiol* 1966, 18:169–174.

4. Reis R, Roberts W: Amounts of coronary arterial narrowing by atherosclerotic plaques in clinically isolated mitral valve stenosis: analysis of 76 necropsy patients older than 30 years. *Am J Cardiol* 1986, 57:1119.

5. Dajani AS, Bisno AL, Chung KJ, *et al.*: Prevention of bacterial endocarditis. *Circulation* 1991, 83:1174–1178.

6. Wilkins GY, Weyman AE, Abascal VM, *et al.*: Percutaneous balloon dilatation of the mitral valve: an analysis of echocardiographic variables related to outcome and the mechanism of dilatation. *Br Heart J* 1988, 60:299–308.

7. Abascal VM, Wilkins GT, O'Shea JP, *et al.*: Prediction of successful outcome in 130 patients undergoing percutaneous balloon mitral valvotomy. *Circulation* 1990, 82:448–456.

8. Cosgrove DM, Stewart WJ: Mitral valvuloplasty. *Curr Prob Cardiol* 1989, 14:359–415.

9. Kirklin JW: Percutaneous balloon versus surgical closed commissurotomy for mitral stenosis. *Circulation* 1991, 83:1450–1451.

10. Dean LS, Mickel M, Bonan R, *et al.*: Four year follow-up of patients undergoing percutaneous balloon mitral commissurotomy. *J Am Coll Cardiol* 1996, 28:1452–1457.

11. Iung B, Garbarz E, Michaud P, *et al.*: Percutaneous mitral commissurotomy for restenosis after surgical commissurotomy. *J Am Coll Cardiol* 2000, 35:1295–1302

12. Olson LJ, Subramanian R, Ackerman DM: Surgical pathology of the mitral valve: a study of 712 cases spanning 21 years. *Mayo Clin Proc* 1987, 62:22.

13. Kypson AP, Nifong LW, Chitwood WR, Jr.: Robotic mitral valve surgery. *Surg Clin North Am* 2003, 83:1387–1403.

SELECT BIBLIOGRAPHY

Crawford MD, Souchek J, Oprian CA, *et al.*: Determinants of survival and left ventricular performance after mitral valve replacement. *Circulation* 1990, 81:1173–1181.

Fenster MS, Feldman MD: Mitral regurgitation: an overview. *Curr Probl Cardiol* 1995, 20:195–280.

Lee EM, Shapiro LM, Wells FC: Importance of subvalvular preservation and early operation in mitral valve surgery. *Circulation* 1996, 94:2117–2123.

Reyes VP, Rasju BS, Wynne J, *et al.*: Percutaneous balloon valvuloplasty compared with open surgical commissurotomy for mitral stenosis. *N Engl J Med* 1994, 331:961–967.

22

Mitral Valve Prolapse

Joseph S. Alpert
Richard B. Devereux

Key Points

- Mitral valve prolapse is usually a primary, dominantly inherited condition with more consistent gene expression in women than in men or children.

- Diagnosis is by midsystolic click/late systolic murmur; echocardiography confirms and documents severity.

- True mitral valve prolapse syndrome is characterized by low body weight and blood pressure, minor skeletal abnormalities, orthostatic hypotension, palpitations, and mitral regurgitation of variable degree.

- Complications are progressive mitral regurgitation, infective endocarditis, and possible risk of arrhythmic sudden death and orthostatic syncope.

- Risk factors for complications include older age, male gender, mitral regurgitant murmur, and possibly greater weight and higher blood pressure.

- Presence and severity of mitral regurgitation govern frequency and intensiveness of follow-up.

Mitral valve prolapse (MVP) is the most common abnormality of the heart in industrialized nations, affecting 3% to 4% of adults. By definition, MVP reflects abnormal systolic displacement of the mitral valve leaflets superiorly and posteriorly from the left ventricle into the left atrium. That may occur because the mitral leaflets, anulus, and chordae tendineae are enlarged in relation to left ventricular size (Fig. 1) or because they are abnormally distensible.

Although MVP has been reported to have many causes, most cases occur as a primary condition. Primary MVP is passed from affected mothers and fathers to children of both genders in a pattern indicative of autosomal dominant inheritance [1,2]. Familial MVP has an age of onset between 10 and 16 years, is more consistently expressed in women than men, and may become undetectable after middle age in mildly affected women [2]. As a result of the gender difference in the expression of primary MVP, nearly two thirds of adults with this condition are women. A small percentage of cases occur secondarily to other inheritable connective tissue diseases such as Marfan syndrome or Ehlers-Danlos syndrome. Mitral valve prolapse also may be produced by conditions, including anorexia nervosa or atrial septal defect, that make the left ventricle abnormally small.

DIAGNOSIS

In clinical practice, MVP is most commonly first recognized by auscultation. Typical auscultatory features are a midsystolic click and late systolic murmur, which is separated from the first heart sound by a silent interval but continues until the second heart sound. These sounds are best heard by listening over the left ventricular impulse and medial to it, with the patient in the supine, left decubitus, and sitting positions. Because systolic clicks may have other causes

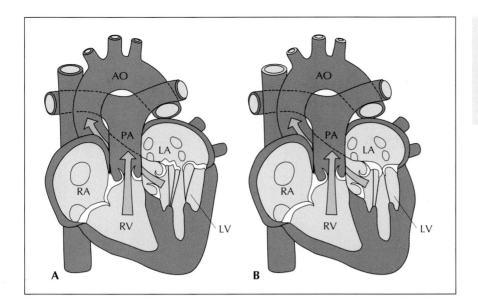

FIGURE 1 Diagram showing enlargement of mitral leaflets, annulus, and chordae **A**, in patients with mitral valve prolapse compared with **B**, findings in healthy individuals. AO—aorta; LA—left atrium; LV—left ventricle; PA—pulmonary artery; RA—right atrium; RV—right ventricle.

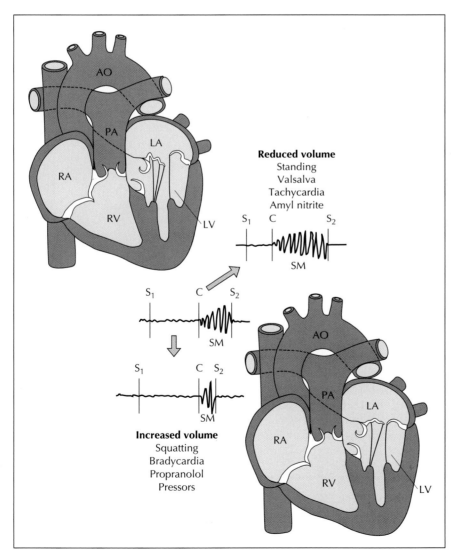

Reduced volume
Standing
Valsalva
Tachycardia
Amyl nitrite

Increased volume
Squatting
Bradycardia
Propranolol
Pressors

FIGURE 2 Effect of maneuvers that change left ventricular (LV) volume on the timing of the click (C) and murmur (SM) of mitral valve prolapse. The onset of the murmur and time of occurrence of the click move closer to the first heart sound (S_1) when LV volume is reduced and farther from it when LV volume is increased. AO—aorta; LA—left atrium; PA—pulmonary artery; RA—right atrium; RV—right ventricle; S_2—second heart sound. (*Adapted from Devereux et al.* [24].)

and mitral annular calcification may produce a late systolic murmur in older persons, it is important to perform physical maneuvers during auscultation that take advantage of the key role of valvular-ventricular disproportion in producing the manifestations of MVP [2].

As illustrated in Figure 2, maneuvers that reduce left ventricular chamber size will cause the click and onset of the murmur to move closer to the first heart sound, whereas the loudness of the click and murmur are affected by changes in blood pressure independent of changes in timing. Figure 3 shows how standard maneuvers during physical examination affect the click and murmur. It is especially important to time the onset after the first sound and continuation until the second sound of the late systolic murmur, as miscategorization caused by normal blood flow in thin-chested individuals or aortic sclerosis in older patients is a common cause of false-positive diagnoses of MVP (Fig. 4). When both a midsystolic click and late systolic murmur are present and respond appropriately to these maneuvers, the diagnosis of MVP can be made confidently by physical examination.

Late-systolic buckling of mitral leaflets on M-mode echocardiographic tracings occurs simultaneously with the midsystolic click and onset of the late systolic murmur (Fig. 5).

An accurate diagnosis can be made on M-mode recordings when continuous mitral leaflet interfaces "turn around" and move at least 2 mm posterior to the valve's C-D line in late systole (Fig. 6) [2,3]. Holosystolic posterior motion of mitral leaflets on M-mode recordings is no longer used to diagnose MVP because it may be produced artifactually by errors in ultrasound beam angulation.

Two-dimensional (2-D) and Doppler echocardiography is the mainstay of diagnosis of MVP and assessment of its severity. The condition can be accurately diagnosed by 2-D echocardiography when one or both mitral leaflets are seen to protrude or "billow" into the left atrium in systole in the parasternal or apical long-axis view (Figs. 6 and 7) [2,4]. It is important *not* to diagnose MVP based on apparent protrusion of the mitral leaflets into the left atrium that is seen only in the apical, four-chamber, 2-D view; this is a common normal consequence of the "saddle" shape of the mitral anulus (Fig. 8) [4]. Although conventional and color-

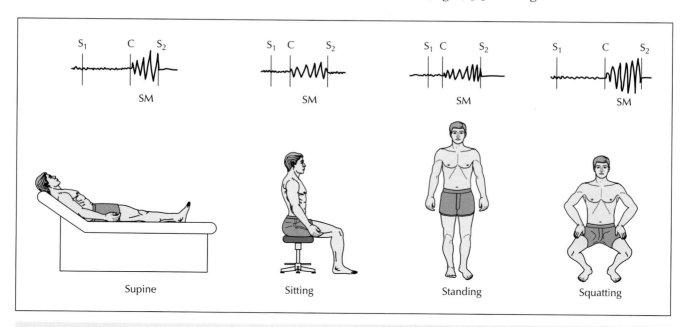

Supine   Sitting   Standing   Squatting

FIGURE 3 Effect of maneuvers during physical examination that change left ventricular chamber volume on the timing of the click (C) and murmur (SM) of mitral valve prolapse. (*Adapted from Devereux et al.* [24].)

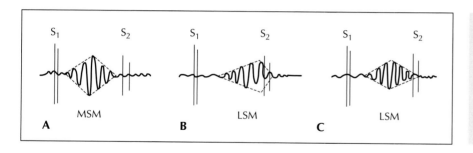

FIGURE 4 Timing of a midsystolic murmur (MSM, **A**), which begins after the first heart sound (S_1) and ends before the second heart sound (S_2); and of late systolic murmurs (LSM, **B** and **C**), which begin after S_1 but continue to or through S_2. Note that both types of murmur may have a crescendo-decrescendo configuration.

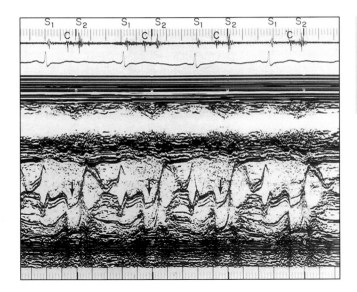

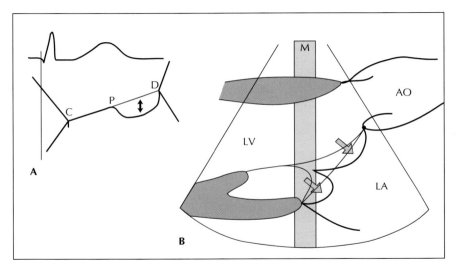

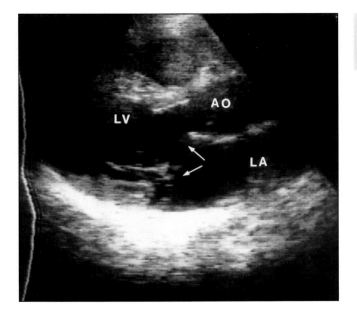

FIGURE 5 M-mode echocardiographic recording of the mitral valve demonstrating late systolic prolapse (*arrows*) and simultaneous phonocardiogram showing a midsystolic click (C) and late systolic murmur. AML—anterior mitral leaflet; IVS—interventricular septum; PML—posterior mitral leaflet; PW—posterior wall; S_1—first heart sound; S_2—second heart sound.

FIGURE 6 **A**, M-mode and **B**, two-dimensional echocardiographic diagnostic criteria of mitral valve prolapse. The condition is diagnosed when there is at least 2 mm of posterior displacement of continuous mitral leaflet interfaces behind the valve's C-D line in late systole on high-quality M-mode recordings (Figure 5) or protrusion of one or both mitral leaflets across the line connecting the hinging points of the mitral leaflets in two-dimensional long-axis views (Figure 7). AO—aorta; LA—left atrium; LV—left ventricle; M—course of M-mode beam. (*Adapted from* Devereux *et al.* [2].)

FIGURE 7 Two-dimensional echocardiogram in parasternal long-axis view showing late-systolic billowing of both mitral leaflets (*arrows*) into the left atrium (LA). AO—aorta; LV—left ventricle.

flow Doppler echocardiography are not useful in diagnosing MVP, because there are many etiologies of the mitral regurgitation, they are of great value in grading the severity of regurgitation, which is in turn the most important factor in determining the risk for major complications of MVP.

Two-dimensional echocardiography is especially useful for identifying mitral valve abnormalities associated with more severe forms of MVP. These include enlargement of the mitral leaflets and anulus [5] and prominent leaflet thickening [6], both of which are associated with severe mitral regurgitation. Billowing of one mitral leaflet segment that is so prominent it loses apposition with the appropriate segment of the other mitral leaflet is an anatomic cause of severe mitral regurgitation that can be readily visualized on 2-D echocardiography (Fig. 9) [7].

CLINICAL FEATURES

The typical auscultatory features of MVP are useful in making a diagnosis, but these features may vary considerably from one careful examination to another. Conse-

quently, up to one-fifth of patients with clinically recognized MVP confirmed by echocardiography and one-third of unselected persons with this condition may have "silent" MVP on a single examination (Table 1) [8]. As a result, it is important to examine a patient several times to determine whether a murmur is intermittently present.

Extracardiac features of primary MVP have been shown in both family studies (Table 1) and clinical series. These include a tendency to have low body weight and low blood pressure [9], which may constitute the "selective advantage" that accounts for the high population prevalence of this inherited condition. Also, thoracic bony abnormalities (including pectus excavatum, mild scoliosis, and a straight thoracic spine) occur several times more commonly among adults with MVP than among members of the general population.

A variety of symptoms were associated with the condition often enough in initial clinical reports to suggest a distinct MVP syndrome that included chest pain, dyspnea, palpitations, anxiety, and panic attacks. Carefully controlled studies have found little or no evidence,

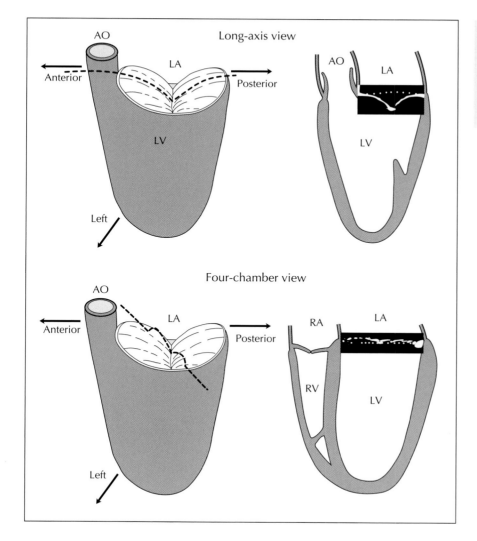

FIGURE 8 Production of artifactual mitral valve prolapse in the apical four-chamber view resulting from the saddle shape of the mitral anulus. AO—aorta; LA—left atrium; LV—left ventricle; RA—right atrium; RV—right ventricle. (*Adapted from* Levine *et al.* [5].)

however, that these symptoms—with the exception of palpitations—are truly linked to MVP (Table 2). The erroneous conclusion of previous studies appears to have resulted from selection bias, which causes more sympto-matic patients to seek experts who perform clinical studies, and from a true tendency of women to report more of these symptoms than men regardless of whether they have MVP (Table 3).

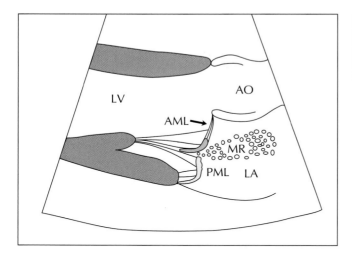

FIGURE 9 Severe posterior mitral leaflet (PML) prolapse into the left atrium (LA) producing loss of coaptation with the anterior mitral leaflet (AML) and allowing severe mitral regurgitation (MR). AO—aorta; LV—left ventricle.

TABLE 1 PREVALENCE OF AUSCULTATORY FEATURES AND EXTRACARDIAC MANIFESTATIONS OF MITRAL VALVE PROLAPSE IN INDEX CASES AND AFFECTED FAMILY MEMBERS

	First-degree relatives with MVP, n=81 (%)	First-degree relatives and spouses without MVP, n=232 (%)
Midsystolic click only	27 (33)*	7 (3)
Late systolic murmur only	14 (17)†	8 (4)
Click and late systolic murmur	13 (16)*	1 (< 1)
Holosystolic murmur only	1 (1)*	0 (0)
Thoracic bony abnormalities	33 (41)*	34 (15)*
Body weight < 90% of ideal	26 (32)*	29 (13)*
Systolic blood pressure < 120 mm Hg	43 (53)*	65 (28)*

*$P < 0.01$;
†$P < 0.001$.
MVP—mitral valve prolapse.

TABLE 2 PREVALENCE OF SYMPTOMS IN ADULT FAMILY MEMBERS WITH AND WITHOUT MITRAL VALVE PROLAPSE

	First-degree adult relatives with MVP, n=81 (%)	First-degree adult relatives and spouses without MVP, n=232 (%)
Palpitations	32 (40)	53 (23)
Atypical chest pain	14 (17)	37 (16)
Dyspnea	5 (6)	21 (9)
Panic attacks	6 (7)	11 (5)
Trait anxiety score > 50	5 (6)	14 (6)
Inferior lead electrocardiogram repolarization abnormalities	9 (11)	23 (10)

MVP—mitral valve prolapse.

Another set of symptoms that appears to be truly associated with MVP in controlled studies is syncope or presyncope caused by orthostatic hypotension [10]. The mechanism of this phenomenon is uncertain, but it may relate to the low resting blood pressure found in some patients with MVP.

COMPLICATIONS

In general, MVP is a benign condition, and most patients will never have an important complication. A minority of affected persons develop severe mitral regurgitation, infective endocarditis, neurologic events, or sudden death [11]. Because of the high prevalence of MVP, however, an appreciable number of adults have these complications (Table 4)

[3]. In our long-term experience, the rate of complications in relatively unselected patients with MVP is 1% per year or even less [12].

Severe mitral regurgitation is the most common major complication of MVP; conversely, MVP is now the most common valvular cause of severe mitral regurgitation in industrialized nations. Severe mitral regurgitation in a patient with MVP can be suspected on physical examination by a holosystolic or nearly holosystolic mitral regurgitant murmur associated with an audible third heart sound and leftward displacement of an enlarged, dynamic, left ventricular impulse (Fig. 10). Objective confirmation of this complication can be obtained by demonstrating a large mitral regurgitant jet by pulsed or color-flow Doppler

TABLE 3 RELATIONSHIP OF GENDER TO CLINICAL FEATURES OF MITRAL VALVE PROLAPSE

	Women, n=216 (%)	Men, n=185 (%)	P
Nonanginal chest pain	63 (29)	24 (13)	< 0.001
Dyspnea	50 (23)	15 (8)	< 0.001
Panic attacks	29 (13)	4 (2)	< 0.001
High trait anxiety	23 (11)	6 (3)	< 0.01
Inferior lead ST-T abnormalities	44 (20)	12 (6)	< 0.001

TABLE 4 ANNUAL OCCURRENCE IN THE UNITED STATES OF COMPLICATIONS ASSOCIATED WITH MITRAL VALVE PROLAPSE

Complication	Patients per year, n	Patients with mitral valve prolapse, n	Annual events attributable to mitral valve prolapse, n
Mitral valve surgery	16,000	25	4000
Infective endocarditis	9000	13	1150
Sudden death*	400,000	1	4000

*Figures for sudden death are less stable than for other complications, because they are based on a single study.

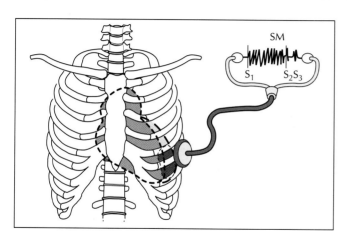

FIGURE 10 Schematic diagram of a nearly holosystolic mitral regurgitant murmur with a third heart sound (S_3) and leftward displacement of an enlarged left ventricular impulse, which is felt to the left of the midclavicular line in the fifth and sixth intercostal spaces, instead of being smaller than a quarter in diameter and being limited to one interspace in normal persons. S_1—first heart sound; S_2—second heart sound; SM—systolic murmur.

echocardiography (Fig. 11). Imaging echocardiography usually reveals left ventricular and left atrial enlargement, and it also demonstrates a spectrum of morphologic valvular abnormalities, including leaflet and annular enlargement, distortion and thickening of leaflet segments, and redundancy or rupture of chordae tendineae.

The likelihood of developing severe mitral regurgitation increases with age and is greater for men than for women with MVP [12–14]. By the age of 75 years, approximately 1.5% to 2.0% of women with MVP and 5.5% of affected men will develop regurgitation of sufficient severity to require surgical valve repair or replacement. Initially, mild regurgitation may become severe during prolonged follow-up of these patients [15]. In addition to the irreversible risk factors of age and gender, some evidence exists that high blood pressure or increased body weight may promote the progression of regurgitation [14]. Severe mitral regurgitation in association with ruptured chordae and a flail mitral valve leaflet is associated with significant morbidity and mortality [16]. Such patients should be strongly considered for mitral valve surgery.

As a complication, infective endocarditis is only one fourth as common as severe regurgitation requiring mitral valve surgery in patients with MVP (Table 4), implying a cumulative risk of less than 1% by age 75. The risk of endocarditis is increased about threefold in men compared with women, in persons older than 45 years of age compared with younger persons, and in patients with a mitral regurgitant murmur (Table 5) [17]. Whether mitral leaflet thickening or other specific morphologic abnormalities increase the risk of endocarditis independent of their role in causing mitral regurgitation has not yet been established. About one third of endocarditis cases are of dental origin, which is similar to the experience with other predisposing valvular lesions.

Neurologic ischemic events have been suggested to occur more commonly in individuals with MVP, but this association has recently been questioned [18].

Sudden death is the most feared, least understood, and perhaps the rarest major complication of MVP. An increased risk of sudden death is well established in patients with severe mitral regurgitation, but this appears to relate to the degree of regurgitation rather than MVP [19]. Instances of sudden death in patients without known severe mitral regurgitation are often associated with severe valvular deformity but also increased heart weight, suggesting that unrecognized regurgitation or some other hemodynamic overload may have been present [20,21]. To date, neither specific arrhythmias nor other electrocardiographic features such as repolarization abnormalities have been documented to identify the patient with MVP who is at increased risk of sudden death. Patients with ruptured chordae and a flail mitral valve leaflet have an increased risk of sudden death [22].

MANAGEMENT

The proper starting point of management for most patients with MVP is reassurance by the patient's primary physician that they have a condition that is generally benign and may even be marginally beneficial if they have inherited the common tendency to low body weight and low blood pressure. For a person with only a midsystolic click and no mitral regurgitant murmur on several examinations, and no evidence of mitral regurgitation by Doppler echocardiography if it is performed, no clear evidence exists that peridental endocarditis prophylaxis or other specific medication is needed. It is reasonable to reevaluate such patients at 5-year intervals.

The presence and severity of mitral regurgitation are the best indicators of the need for active treatment and more frequent follow-up (Table 6) [3]. This may be assessed

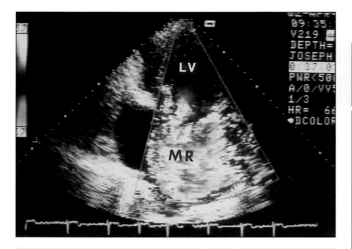

FIGURE 11 Severe mitral regurgitation (MR) demonstrated by color flow Doppler echocardiography. The multicolored MR jet fills almost the entire left atrium, which is nearly 10 cm in diameter. LV—left ventricle. (*See* Color Plate.)

TABLE 5 RELATIVE RISK OF INFECTIVE ENDOCARDITIS IN PERSONS WITH MITRAL VALVE PROLAPSE BY GENDER, AGE, AND HISTORY OF MURMUR

	Total, *n*	Male	> 45 y, *n*	History of murmur, *n*
Cases	21	13	13	15*
Controls	102	36	31	41

	Male vs. female	≥ 45 y vs. < 45 y	Present vs. absent
Odds ratio	2.98	3.72	3.72
P	0.023	0.006	0.009
95% CI	1.35, 7.86	1.40, 9.88	1.33, 10.38

*History of a murmur before development of endocarditis.
CI—confidence interval.

directly by Doppler echocardiography or indirectly by auscultation. Persons with intermittent or persistent mitral murmurs and mild regurgitation need oral antibiotic prophylaxis [23], treatment of mild hypertension, and reevaluation and echocardiography every 2 to 3 years. A person with severe regurgitation requires antibiotic prophylaxis with amoxicillin in the absence of penicillin allergy and annual reevaluation by a cardiologist or experienced internist with Doppler echocardiography and perhaps other tests (24-hour electrocardiography or exercise test) depending on the clinical circumstances. It is also logical, although not yet proven beneficial, to avoid overweight and lower even borderline elevated arterial pressure by antihypertensive drugs in patients with MVP and moderate or severe mitral regurgitation.

Patients with other manifestations of MVP may need other forms of specific management. When distressing palpitation is from frequent, single premature ventricular contractions or self-terminating paroxysms of supraventricular tachycardia at rates that do not cause hemodynamic embarrassment, treatment with a long-acting β-adrenoreceptor blocker or digoxin may give symptomatic relief. Sustained, re-entrant, supraventricular tachycardias can often be successfully eradicated by radiofrequency ablation in the electrophysiology laboratory. Rate-control with β-blockers, digoxin, or both, and anticoagulation with sodium

warfarin to prevent stroke is needed if sustained atrial fibrillation develops, usually with hemodynamically important mitral regurgitation or after mitral valve surgery. Patients with MVP and orthostatic hypotension may benefit from stopping low-salt diets, adding sodium chloride in tablet form, or if the above are not successful, taking fluorine 0.05 to 0.10 mg/d to induce expansion of the blood volume.

ACKNOWLEDGMENT

The author thanks Virginia Burns for her assistance in preparing this manuscript.

REFERENCES AND RECOMMENDED READING

1. Devereux RB, Brown WT, Kramer-Fox R, *et al.*: Inheritance of mitral valve prolapse: effect of age and sex on gene expression. *Ann Intern Med* 1982, 97:826–832.

2. Devereux RB, Kramer-Fox R, Shear MK, *et al.*: Diagnosis and classification of severity of mitral valve prolapse: methodologic, biologic and prognostic considerations. *Am Heart J* 1987, 113:1265–1280.

3. Disse S, Abergel E, Berrebi A, *et al.*: Mapping of a first locus for autosomal dominant myxomatous mitral-valve prolapse to chromosome 16p11.2-p12.1. *Am J Hum Genet* 1999, 65:1242–51.

4. Devereux RB, Kramer-Fox R, Kligfield P: Mitral valve prolapse: etiology, clinical manifestations and management. *Ann Intern Med* 1989, 111:305–317.

5. Levine RA, Triulzi MO, Harrigan P, *et al.*: The relationship of mitral annular shape to the diagnosis of mitral valve prolapse. *Circulation* 1987, 75:756–767.

6. Pini R, Devereux RB, Greppi B, *et al.*: Comparison of mitral valve dimension and motion in mitral valve prolapse with severe mitral regurgitation to uncomplicated mitral valve prolapse and to mitral regurgitation without mitral valve prolapse. *Am J Cardiol* 1988, 62:257–263.

7. Grayburn PA, Berk MR, Spain MG, *et al.*: Relation of echocardiographic morphology of the mitral apparatus to mitral regurgitation in mitral valve prolapse: assessment by Doppler color flow imaging. *Am Heart J* 1990, 119:1095–1102.

8. Devereux RB, Kramer-Fox R, Brown WT, *et al.*: Relation between clinical features of the "mitral prolapse syndrome" and echocardiographically documented mitral valve prolapse. *J Am Coll Cardiol* 1986, 8:763–772.

9. Devereux RB, Brown WT, Lutas EM, *et al.*: Association of mitral valve prolapse with low body-weight and low blood pressure. *Lancet* 1982, ii:792–795.

10. Weissman NJ, Shear MK, Kramer-Fox R, Devereux RB: Contrasting patterns of autonomic dysfunction in patients with mitral valve prolapse and panic attacks. *Am J Med* 1987, 82:880–888.

11. Freed LA, Benjamin EJ, Levy D, *et al.*: Mitral valve prolapse in the general population. The benign nature of echocardiographic features in the Framingham Heart Study. *J Am Coll Cardiol* 2002, 40:1298-1304.

12. Zuppiroli A, Rinaldi M, Kramer-Fox R, *et al.*: Natural history of mitral valve prolapse. *Am J Cardiol* 1995,75:1028-1032.

13. Devereux RB, Hawkins I, Kramer-Fox R, *et al.*: Complications of mitral valve prolapse: disproportionate occurrence in men and older patients. *Am J Med* 1986, 81:751–758.

TABLE 6 MATCHING RISK AND MANAGEMENT IN MITRAL VALVE PROLAPSE

Low risk

Subjects without mitral regurgitant murmurs or Doppler regurgitation, especially women younger than 45 years.

Management: reassurance; no clear need for antibiotics; reevaluation and echocardiography at moderate intervals (5 years).

Moderate risk

Subjects with intermittent or persistent mitral murmurs and mild Doppler regurgitation.

Management: antibiotic prophylaxis with amoxicillin or erythromycin; treat even mild established hypertension; reevaluation and echocardiography more frequently (2 to 3 years).

High risk

Subjects with moderate or severe mitral regurgitation.

Management: antibiotic prophylaxis with amoxicillin (unless allergic); optimize afterload (arterial pressure); reevaluate with Doppler echocardiography and other tests if needed annually.

Consider valve repair or replacement for exertional dyspnea or decline of left ventricular function into low-normal range.

14. Singh RG, Cappucci R, Kramer-Fox R, *et al.*: Severe mitral regurgitation due to mitral valve prolapse: Risk factors for development, progression and need for mitral valve surgery. *Am J Cardiol* 2000; 85:193–198.

15. Kolibash AJ Jr, Kilman JW, Bush CA, *et al.*: Evidence for progression from mild to severe mitral regurgitation in mitral valve prolapse. *Am J Cardiol* 1986, 58:762–767.

16. Ling LH, Enriquez-Sarano M, Seward JB, *et al.*: Clinical outcome of mitral regurgitation due to flail leaflet. *N Engl J Med* 1996, 335:1417-1423.

17. MacMahon SW, Roberts JK, Kramer-Fox R, *et al.*: Mitral valve prolapse and infective endocarditis. *Am Heart J* 1987, 113:1291–1298.

18. Orencia AJ, Petty GW, Khanderia BK, *et al.*: Risk of stroke in a population-based cohort study. *Stroke* 1995, 26:7-13.

19. Kligfield P, Hochreiter C, Niles N, *et al.*: Relation of sudden death in pure mitral regurgitation with and without mitral valve prolapse, to repetitive ventricular arrhythmias and right and left ventricular ejection fraction. *Am J Cardiol* 1987, 60:397–399.

20. Farb A, Tang AL, Atkinson JB, *et al.*: Comparison of cardiac findings in patients with mitral valve prolapse who die suddenly to those who have congestive heart failure from mitral regurgitation and to those with fatal noncardiac conditions. *Am J Cardiol* 1992, 70:234–239.

21. Morales AR, Remanelli R, Boncek RJ, *et al.*: Myxoid heart disease: an assessment of extraordinary cardiac pathology in severe mitral valve prolapse. *Hum Pathol* 1992, 23:129–137.

22. Grigioni F, Enriquez-Sarano M, Ling LH, *et al.*: Sudden death in mitral regurgiation due to fail leaflet. *J Am Coll Cardiol* 1999, 34:2078-2085.

23. Devereux RB, Frary CJ, Kramer-Fox R, *et al.*: Cost-effectiveness of infective endocarditis prophylaxis for mitral valve prolapse with our without a regurgitant murmur. *Am J Cardiol* 1994, 74:1024–1029.

24. Devereux RB, Perloff JK, Reichek N, *et al.*: Mitral valve prolapse. *Circulation* 1976, 54:3–14.

SELECT BIBLIOGRAPHY

Barlow JE, Pocock WA, Marchand P, *et al.*: The significance of late systolic murmurs. *Am Heart J* 1963, 66:443–452.

Leatham A, Brigden W: Mild mitral regurgitation and the mitral prolapse fiasco. *Am Heart J* 1980, 99:659–664.

Nishimura RA, McGoon MD, Shub C, *et al.*: Echocardiographically documented mitral-valve prolapse: long-term follow-up of 237 patients. *N Engl J Med* 1985, 313:1305–1309.

Wooley CF, Boudoulas H, eds.: *Mitral Valve Prolapse and the Mitral Valve Prolapse Syndrome.* Mt. Kisco, NY: Futura; 1988.

Aortic Stenosis and Regurgitation

Michael A. Fifer

23

Key Points

- Aortic stenosis and, less often, aortic regurgitation may cause angina in the absence of coronary artery disease.

- Sudden death is rare among truly asymptomatic patients with aortic stenosis or regurgitation.

- The "classic" physical examination findings of aortic regurgitation may be absent when regurgitation develops acutely.

- Doppler echo examination for aortic regurgitation is so sensitive that many false-positive findings occur.

- Aortic valve replacement for aortic stenosis is generally reserved for symptomatic patients, whereas surgery for aortic regurgitation may be indicated for low or decreasing left ventricular ejection fraction, even for patients without symptoms.

The clinical manifestations of aortic valve disease are heart failure, angina, syncope, and death. Aortic stenosis is particularly prevalent in the elderly population [1]. It has been increasingly appreciated that aortic regurgitation may result from diseases of the aorta rather than of the aortic valve per se [2]. Clinical recognition of aortic valve disease is critical because properly timed valve replacement may dramatically improve symptoms and prolong life.

AORTIC STENOSIS

Etiology and Pathophysiology

There are three causes of valvular aortic stenosis in adults [3]; these causes are illustrated, along with a normal valve, in Figure 1. The prevalence of congenitally bicuspid aortic valves is approximately 1% to 2%, with a male preponderance. Stenosis resulting from fibrosis, calcification, and stiffening of a bicuspid valve is the usual cause of isolated aortic stenosis in patients younger than 60 years. Less commonly, bicuspid aortic valves cause aortic regurgitation. A substantial fraction of bicuspid valves cause no hemodynamic abnormality throughout life [4]. Rheumatic aortic stenosis is characterized by thickening of the valve cusps, fusion of the commissures, and calcification. Usually, the central orifice is relatively fixed, so that some degree of regurgitation is present as well. The majority of patients with rheumatic aortic valve disease also have clinically evident mitral valve disease. Senile calcific aortic stenosis is the most common type occurring in patients older than 70 years of age, and results from progressive scarring, calcification, and stiffening of the valve without fusion of the commissures. The presence of atherosclerosis risk factors such as dyslipidemia may accelerate the progression of aortic stenosis [5].

The consequences of aortic stenosis for systole are a gradient across the aortic valve, high intraventricular pressure, a compensatory increase in ventricular wall thickness and, for a minority of patients, a decrease in ejection fraction (systolic dysfunction). The consequences of aortic stenosis for diastole are diminished distensibility of the ventricle (diastolic dysfunction) caused by the increase in wall thickness, enhanced importance of the atrial kick for ventricular filling, and the potential for sudden decompensation if the atrial kick is lost, as with atrial fibrillation.

Evaluation

Symptoms of left-sided heart failure resulting from aortic stenosis may be caused by systolic or diastolic dysfunction, or both. Whereas resting myocardial blood flow is increased, the capacity to augment flow at times of stress is correspondingly diminished, which may lead to angina or subendocardial infarction (even with no coronary artery disease); rest angina generally indicates concomitant coronary artery disease. Lightheadedness and syncope typically occur during or immediately after exertion and may result from an exercise-induced decrease in systemic vascular resistance without a proportionate increase in cardiac output or from bradyarrhythmias caused by extension of aortic valve calcification into the conduction system. Clinically apparent embolization from the aortic valve and endo-

carditis are both rare [6]. Aortic stenosis may be associated with gastrointestinal bleeding originating from angiodysplasia, usually of the ascending colon [7] and with acquired von Willebrand syndrome [8].

Hypertension may coexist with severe aortic stenosis. The pulse pressure is usually normal but may be wide, especially in older patients [9,10]. The carotid upstroke is usually weak and delayed but may be normal or nearly so in patients with hypertension and in elderly patients with atherosclerotic, noncompliant arteries. In low-output states, the carotid volume is diminished, so that it is difficult to judge the rate of increase of the upstroke. A thrill is often felt over the carotid arteries, in the suprasternal notch, or in the second right intercostal space.

The left ventricular impulse is forceful and sustained; it is displaced leftward and downward when the ejection fraction is low. The second heart sound (S_2) is single or narrowly or paradoxically split; normal splitting suggests that severe aortic stenosis is not present. A fourth heart sound (S_4) is common and reflects left ventricular diastolic dysfunction. A third heart sound (S_3) is less common and indicates systolic dysfunction [11]. An ejection click is caused by checking of the upward movement of a domed aortic valve and is best heard after the first heard sound (S_1) at the lower left sternal border or apex in the young patient with a mobile valve. It is rare in adults older than 30 years, who have calcified, immobile valves. The crescendo-decrescendo (diamond-shaped) systolic murmur of aortic stenosis is typically described as harsh, rough, or grunting. It is usually best heard in the second right intercostal space and may radiate widely to the neck, left sternal border, and apex. In elderly patients, it is often heard best at the apex, so that mitral regurgitation is erroneously suspected. The intensity of the murmur does not correlate with the severity of stenosis; it may be soft with severe stenosis and low cardiac output. A prolonged crescendo phase with a late peak suggests significant stenosis. The murmur of aortic stenosis must be distinguished from that of other cardiac lesions (Table 1). A diastolic murmur of aortic insufficiency is useful in establishing valvular aortic stenosis as opposed to hypertrophic cardiomyopathy as the cause of a systolic murmur.

The cardinal finding on the electrocardiogram (Fig. 2) is left ventricular hypertrophy, often with a "strain" pattern: ST-segment depression and T-wave inversion, usually in leads I, aV_L, and V_{4-6}. The absence of hypertrophy by electrocardiographic criteria, however, does not exclude hemodynamically significant stenosis. Other, more variable findings are left atrial abnormality, left axis deviation, and left bundle branch block. The chest roentgenogram may show calcification in the region of the aortic valve, although the technique is insensitive; on the other hand, no calcification of the valve seen by fluoroscopy in a patient older than 40 years virtually excludes severe aortic stenosis [9]. Poststenotic dilation of the ascending aorta is often seen. A "left ventricular configuration" (*ie*, rounding of the left ventricular border and apex), indicates left ventricular

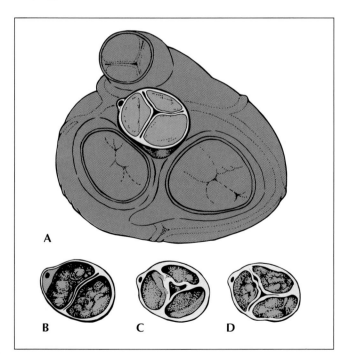

FIGURE 1 Schematic drawings showing a normal aortic valve (**A**); a calcified bicuspid valve with calcific deposits on the cusps (**B**); a rheumatic valve with commissural fusion (**C**); and a calcific tricuspid "senile" valve with calcific deposits on the cusps without commissural fusion (**D**). (*Adapted from* Sutton and Fox [30].)

hypertrophy, whereas left ventricular enlargement suggests systolic dysfunction.

There is considerable variation among physicians in the use of exercise testing to evaluate aortic stenosis. Because of the possibility of inducing angina, severe dyspnea, hypotension, or syncope, some have considered severe aortic stenosis to be a contraindication to exercise testing. Others have suggested that exercise testing is useful to establish safe levels of physical activity in asymptomatic patients with aortic stenosis. Exercise may produce ST-segment and T-wave abnormalities and even thallium defects in the absence of coronary artery disease.

Echocardiography (Fig. 3) is the mainstay of the noninvasive evaluation of aortic stenosis. The valve is seen to be thick-

TABLE 1 DIFFERENTIAL DIAGNOSIS OF AORTIC STENOSIS

	Aortic stenosis	Hypertrophic cardiomyopathy	Mitral regurgitation
Carotid upstroke	Delayed	Brisk or bisferiens, or both	Brisk
S_2	Single	Split	Split
Ejection click	Sometimes present	Absent	Absent
Murmur location	Right upper sternal border, left sternal border, apex, carotids	Left lower sternal border, apex	Apex, axilla, left sternal border
Murmur during Valsalva maneuver	Softer	Louder	Louder
Murmur of aortic regurgitation	Common	Rare	Unusual
Aortic valve calcification on chest roentgenography	Usual	Absent	Absent
Dilation of ascending aorta on chest roentgenography	Usual	Absent	Absent

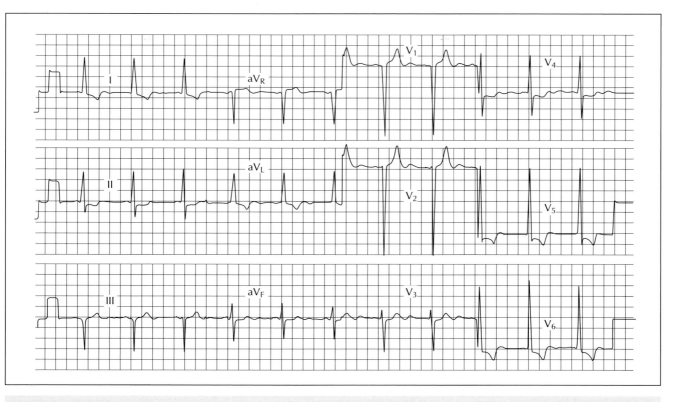

FIGURE 2 Electrocardiogram of a 77-year-old woman with senile calcific aortic stenosis reveals left ventricular hypertrophy, with a "strain" pattern (ST-segment depression and T-wave inversion) in leads I, aV_L, and V_{4-6}.

ened and calcified, and leaflet excursion is reduced. In younger patients, the valve leaflets may be mobile, but tethering of their tips results in "doming" of the valve. In some patients, the valve is bicuspid, although this finding is often obscured by thickening and calcification. The echocardiogram is more sensitive than the electrocardiogram for detecting left ventricular hypertrophy. Left ventricular ejection fraction may be calculated from a technically adequate echocardiogram. The echocardiogram is also useful for distinguishing between valvular aortic stenosis and other causes of outflow gradients, such as hypertrophic cardiomyopathy.

The noninvasive assessment of the severity of aortic stenosis has been revolutionized by Doppler echocardiogra-phy. The peak and mean aortic valve gradients are calculated from the simplified Bernoulli equation as $4v^2$, for which v is the velocity of blood flow across the valve in m/sec. The gradient may be underestimated if the Doppler beam is not aligned correctly to measure the maximum blood flow velocity. It should be recognized that the peak gradient measured by Doppler differs from (and is greater than) the peak-to-peak gradient measured during cardiac catheterization; the mean gradient may be measured by either technique and is the most useful. Doppler echocardiography may also be used to estimate aortic valve area. A technically optimal echocardiogram in a young patient who does not have risk factors for coronary artery disease may

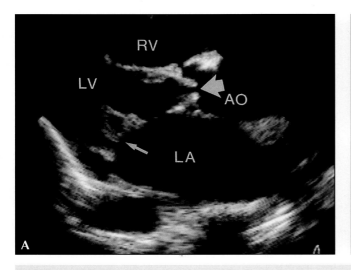
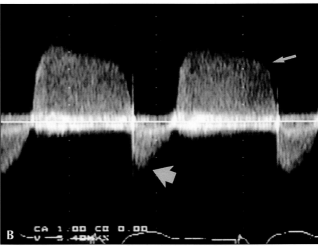

FIGURE 3 Two-dimensional echocardiogram (A) and Doppler velocity tracing (B) in a 70-year-old woman with rheumatic heart disease. The two-dimensional long-axis view in A shows the right ventricle (RV), left atrium (LA), left ventricle (LV), and aorta (AO). Two of the aortic valve leaflets (*thick arrow*) are thickened and have restricted openings. The mitral valve (*thin arrow*) is thickened and stenotic. The Doppler tracing in B, recorded from the left ventricular outflow tract, shows a peak velocity of 2.9 m/s and mean velocity of 2.1 m/s (*thick arrow*), corresponding to peak and mean gradients of 33 and 18 mm Hg, respectively. The Doppler signal in the opposite direction (*thin arrow*) demonstrates aortic regurgitation. (*Courtesy of* Michael H. Picard, MD.)

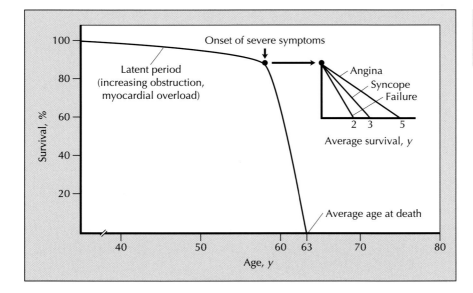

FIGURE 4 The natural history of aortic stenosis. (*Adapted from* Ross and Braunwald [31].)

preclude the need for cardiac catheterization before aortic valve replacement. Aortic valve area may also be estimated by electron beam CT or MRI.

Management

Although patients with aortic stenosis may be asymptomatic for many years, the prognosis for symptomatic patients with significant stenosis is poor, with death usually occurring within 5 years of symptom onset [12–14]. Symptoms of heart failure are the most ominous, followed by syncope and then angina (Fig. 4). Although sudden death may occur, it is almost always preceded by other symptoms in adults with aortic stenosis; the risk of sudden death in truly asymptomatic patients is low [12,15].

Patients with aortic stenosis should be questioned closely at 3- to 6-month intervals for the occurrence of angina, lightheadedness, syncope, or symptoms of heart failure and instructed to contact the physician if symptoms appear between visits. Although careful physical examination may distinguish aortic stenosis from other conditions and indicate its severity, the work-up usually includes echocardiography for confirmation. Once the presence of severe aortic stenosis is established, repeat echocardiography is generally not necessary because the indication for surgery is usually the appearance of symptoms (see the following paragraphs). The management of aortic stenosis is diagrammed in Figure 5.

Endocarditis prophylaxis should be administered according to the guidelines of the American Heart Association; this recommendation also applies to patients with bicuspid aortic valves without significant stenosis or regurgitation. Current studies are testing the hypothesis that treatment with statins will slow the progression of aortic stenosis. Asymptomatic patients with hemodynamically significant stenosis should be prohibited from occupations and sports that require heavy exertion. Most patients with asymptomatic aortic stenosis tolerate noncardiac surgery without complications [16]. Digoxin should be used for rapid supraventricular tachyarrhythmias. If nitrates are needed for concomitant coronary artery disease, they must be used cautiously for fear of inducing hypotension. Drugs with negative inotropic effects, such as β-blockers and calcium channel blockers, should be avoided. Treatment with digoxin and the careful use of diuretics may be indicated to stabilize a patient with heart failure before valve replacement. Vasodilators are relatively contraindicated. Cardiogenic shock caused by aortic stenosis should be managed with dobutamine for inotropic support, intra-aortic balloon counterpulsation if necessary, and urgent mechanical relief of aortic stenosis.

When to Refer

The patient should be referred to a cardiologist for consideration of cardiac catheterization if cardiac symptoms are present and there is clinical or echocardiographic evidence of at least moderately severe aortic stenosis. In patients with cardiac symptoms and only mild aortic stenosis, cardiology consultation may be helpful for diagnosing concomitant cardiac conditions, such as coronary artery disease or excessive left ventricular hypertrophy. Cardiology referral should also be considered, even in the absence of symptoms, if aortic stenosis is severe, so that the cardiologist may participate in the decision regarding the timing of surgery.

Until recently, the peak-to-peak and mean aortic valve gradients were generally measured at cardiac catheterization. Valve area is calculated from the mean gradient and cardiac output by means of the Gorlin equation. The normal aortic valve area is 3 to 4 cm^2; as a rule, symptoms do not occur until the valve area decreases to less than 1.0 cm^2. Surgery for aortic stenosis is generally indicated for symptomatic patients with a mean gradient of 40 mm Hg or greater and an aortic valve area of 0.8 cm^2 or less. Patients with low cardiac output, low gradient, and low calculated valve area present a thorny management problem that is beyond the scope of this chapter [17]. If it is necessary to assess the severity of coexisting aortic regurgitation, supravalvular aortography is performed. Because much information may be obtained from a technically optimal echocardiogram, the

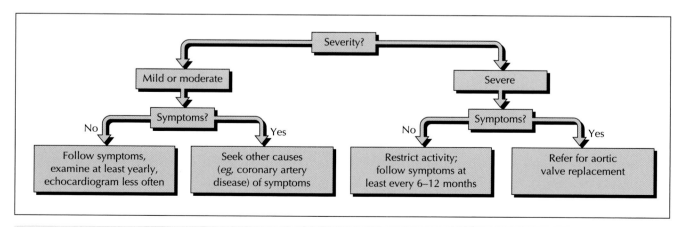

FIGURE 5 Management of aortic stenosis.

principal indication for cardiac catheterization in adults is to assess the severity of coexisting coronary artery disease by coronary arteriography; this approach is generally deemed necessary in patients older than 40 years and in younger patients with risk factors for atherosclerosis. If the presence of severe aortic stenosis is evident from clinical and noninvasive evaluation, then cardiac catheterization may be limited to coronary arteriography.

Aortic valve replacement is indicated for patients with even mildly symptomatic severe aortic stenosis if they have no major concomitant noncardiac conditions. Coronary bypass grafting is a generally accepted, if unproven, adjunct to valve replacement in patients with coronary artery disease. Advanced age is not in itself a contraindication to surgery because otherwise healthy octogenarians undergo valve replacement with acceptable mortality and morbidity

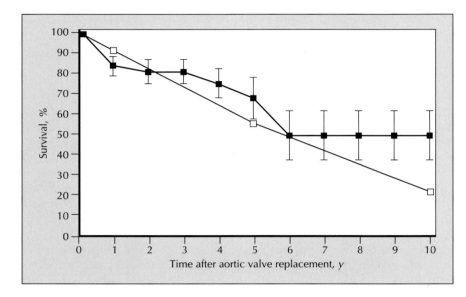

FIGURE 6 Actuarial survival curve for octogenarians undergoing aortic valve replacement for aortic stenosis (*closed squares*). For comparison, actuarial survival curve for unselected 80-year-old persons (*open squares*) from US census data is also shown. (*Adapted from* Levinson *et al.* [18].)

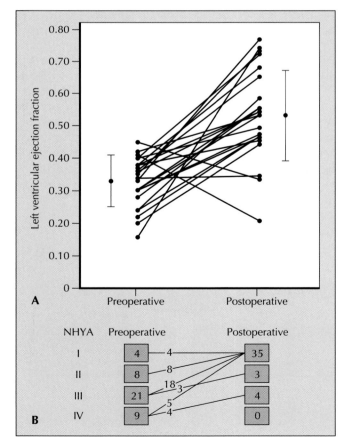

FIGURE 7 Change in New York Heart Association (NYHA) class (**A**) and left ventricular ejection fraction (**B**) after aortic valve replacement for aortic stenosis in patients with low preoperative ejection fraction and no significant associated cardiac abnormalities. (*Adapted from* Rediker *et al.* [19].)

Cardiology for the Primary Care Physician

(Fig. 6) [18]. Similarly, even severe left ventricular systolic dysfunction is not a contraindication to valve replacement if the depression of ejection fraction is caused by severe aortic stenosis and not by another condition, such as coronary artery disease, because clinical outcome is almost invariably good and the ejection fraction improves postoperatively in such cases (Fig. 7) [19]. Surgery is sometimes advocated for asymptomatic patients with aortic stenosis if 1) they are young and have very vigorous lifestyles; 2) they have a markedly abnormal response to exercise during formal testing; 3) they have progressive cardiac enlargement or depression of left ventricular ejection fraction; or 4) they have left heart filling pressures that are markedly elevated at rest or with exercise. These indications for valve replacement are not established [20].

Whereas mechanical valves require lifelong anticoagulation therapy with warfarin, bioprosthetic valves degenerate more quickly than mechanical valves, especially in younger patients. For these reasons, young and middle-aged patients usually receive mechanical valves, whereas elderly patients and patients with contraindications to anticoagulation usually receive bioprosthetic valves.

In patients with absolute contraindications to aortic valve replacement (eg, metastatic cancer or severe emphysema), percutaneous balloon aortic valvuloplasty may be offered as palliative therapy. Although this technique may provide lasting benefit for young patients with congenital aortic stenosis, it provides only temporary relief for adults with calcific aortic stenosis; restenosis of the valve within 1 year is the rule. Percutaneous aortic valvuloplasty may also have a role as a "bridge" to valve replacement in moribund patients with severe aortic stenosis. A catheterization laboratory procedure for placement of an aortic valve prosthesis without surgery has recently been introduced and is being evaluated.

AORTIC REGURGITATION

Etiology and Pathogenesis

Aortic regurgitation may result from diseases causing deformity of the valve leaflets or, alternatively, from diseases causing dilation or distortion of the aortic root, with resultant failure of the leaflets to coapt. This distinction is vital because the causes of aortic regurgitation associated with the two mechanisms differ substantially (Table 2) [2,21]. Like rheumatic aortic stenosis, rheumatic aortic regurgitation is usually accompanied by clinically important rheumatic mitral stenosis or regurgitation, or both. The manifestations of chronic and acute aortic regurgitation are disparate (Table 3) [22]. With chronic aortic regurgitation, there is a gradual and marked increase in left ventricular end-diastolic volume. Left ventricular distensibility is increased, such that there is only a modest increase in end-diastolic pressure. Total left ventricular stroke volume increases, forward stroke volume (total stroke volume minus the volume regurgitated across the aortic valve back into the ventricle) is maintained, ejection fraction is initially normal, and heart rate does not increase markedly. Aortic systolic pressure is high, diastolic pressure is low, and pulse pressure is wide. With long-standing volume overload of the ventricle, there is an eventual loss of myocardial contractility, with consequent increase in end-systolic volume and decrease in ejection fraction. The loss of myocardial contractility may be irreversible. In acute aortic regurgitation (as caused by endocarditis or aortic dissection), regurgitation into an unprepared left ventricle results in a marked increase in end-diastolic pressure, which is transmitted backward to the left atrium and pulmonary circulation, resulting in pulmonary congestion. Total left ventricular stroke volume increases minimally, forward stroke volume falls, and there is compensatory tachycardia in an attempt to maintain cardiac output. Prominent widening of the pulse pressure (and the corresponding physical signs of chronic aortic regurgitation; see the following paragraphs) is absent. The manifestations of aortic regurgitation described in the following paragraphs are of the chronic form unless otherwise noted.

Evaluation

Patients with chronic aortic regurgitation may have no symptoms until left ventricular contractile dysfunction and marked cardiomegaly are apparent. The most common symptoms are those of left-side heart failure: dyspnea on exertion, orthopnea, paroxysmal nocturnal dyspnea, and fatigue. Angina is much less common than that in aortic stenosis but may be caused by increased myocardial oxygen demand associated with hypertrophy in the face of a

TABLE 2 CAUSES OF AORTIC REGURGITATION	
Conditions causing deformity of aortic valve leaflets	**Conditions causing dilation or dissection of aortic root**
Congenitally bicuspid valve	Idiopathic (annuloaortic ectasia)
Rheumatic fever	Aortic dissection
Endocarditis	Chronic, severe hypertension
Trauma	Inflammatory diseases (eg, ankylosing spondylitis)
Myxomatous ("floppy") valve with prolapse	Connective tissue diseases (eg, Marfan syndrome)
Inflammatory diseases (eg, systemic lupus erythematosus)	Syphilitic aortitis
Radiation	Nonspecific aortitis

decreased supply associated with low perfusion (aortic diastolic) pressure. Syncope is rare. Prominent neck pulsations may be noted by the patient, and the high stroke volume may be experienced as uncomfortable palpitations, especially when the patient lies down. Patients with acute aortic regurgitation may have severe dyspnea, weakness, hypotension, and cardiovascular collapse.

In cases of severe chronic aortic regurgitation, the aortic diastolic pressure is usually 60 mm Hg or less. The pulse pressure (which should be measured by the physician) is wide, with muffled sounds continuing to a pressure as low as 0 mm Hg; in such cases, the aortic diastolic pressure correlates best with the onset of muffled (phase IV) Korotkoff sounds. The wide pulse pressure manifests as various peripheral signs, such as Corrigan's pulse (rapid rise and collapse), Quincke's pulse (flushing and blanching of the capillary bed in the fingertips, seen by transmitting a light through the fingers), Duroziez's sign (systolic and diastolic murmurs over a femoral artery lightly compressed by the stethoscope), and "pistol shot" systolic sounds over the femoral artery. The peripheral arterial pulsation may be bisferiens.

The left ventricular impulse is displaced downward and leftward. An S_3 may indicate left ventricular systolic dysfunction [23] or merely left ventricular dilation [11]. A systolic murmur is usually present and reflects the increased total stroke volume traversing the left ventricular outflow tract. A relatively soft, high-pitched, blowing decrescendo diastolic murmur is best heard with the diaphragm of the stethoscope in held expiration with the patient sitting up and leaning forward. It is typically heard at the mid or lower left sternal border in primary valve disease; auscultation predominantly at the right upper sternal border suggests root disease. The length and intensity [24] of the murmur correlate with the severity of regurgitation, except in acute aortic regurgitation. Aortic regurgitation may cause a mid and late diastolic rumble at the apex (Austin-Flint murmur), which is distinguished from the murmur of mitral stenosis by the absence of an opening snap and of a loud S_1. In acute aortic regurgitation, there is tachycardia, peripheral vasoconstriction, normal pulse pressure without the peripheral signs of chronic aortic regurgitation, a normal left ventricular impulse, and a short, relatively soft diastolic murmur.

The electrocardiogram shows left ventricular hypertrophy in most patients with chronic aortic regurgitation but not in patients with acute aortic regurgitation. ST-segment and T-wave abnormalities, left atrial abnormality, left axis deviation, or left bundle branch block may be present. Chest roentgenogram shows left ventricular enlargement. The ascending aorta is dilated, markedly so if root disease is the cause of regurgitation. Acute aortic regurgitation produces a roentgenogram characterized by pulmonary edema with normal heart size.

The echocardiogram (Figs. 3 and 8) images both the valve leaflets and the aortic root and is the most useful test, invasive or noninvasive, for determining the cause of regurgitation. Valve abnormalities that may be detected include thickening of cusps, prolapsed or flail leaflets, and vegetations. Transthoracic and, in particular, transesophageal echocardiography are useful for detecting proximal aortic dissection. The echocardiogram may be used for serially assessing left ventricular size and systolic function, which are critical for determining the timing of aortic valve replacement in asymptomatic or minimally symptomatic patients. Doppler echocardiography is so

TABLE 3 CHRONIC VERSUS ACUTE AORTIC REGURGITATION

	Chronic	Acute
Symptoms	Often none; exertional dyspnea, orthopnea, paroxysmal nocturnal dyspnea	Dyspnea, often severe and at rest; weakness
Appearance	Often normal	Dyspneic, pale, diaphoretic
Heart rate	Normal	Fast
Pulse pressure	Wide	Normal or slightly widened
Peripheral signs of aortic regurgitation	Present	Absent
Left ventricular impulse	Heaving, displaced laterally and inferiorly	Normal
Murmur	Long	Short
Left ventricular hypertrophy on electrocardiogram	Present	Absent
Cardiomegaly on chest roentgenography	Present	Absent
Pulmonary congestion on chest roentgenography	Absent	Present
Pulmonary capillary wedge pressure	Normal or mildly elevated	Markedly elevated

sensitive for detecting valvular regurgitation that it generates "false positives"; a useful rule is that if aortic regurgitation is not discernible by careful cardiac auscultation (see the preceding paragraphs), then it is not responsible for symptoms. Doppler echocardiography is moderately useful for grading the severity of regurgitation. Radionuclide ventriculography provides the ratio of stroke volume ejected by the left ventricle to that ejected by the right ventricle, a useful estimate of the severity of aortic regurgitation in the absence of shunts or other regurgitant lesions. Failure of the ejection fraction to increase during exercise has been proposed as a test of left ventricular reserve in patients with aortic regurgitation, but the validity of this criterion for determining the timing of aortic valve surgery has not been established [25].

Management

Like patients with aortic stenosis, patients with aortic regurgitation may be asymptomatic for many years. Sudden death may occur, but it is rare in asymptomatic patients [12,26]. Although low left ventricular ejection fraction in aortic stenosis is usually reversed with relief of afterload excess by valve replacement, low ejection fraction in aortic regurgitation often reflects irreversible loss of myocardial contractility.

The work-up of aortic regurgitation includes carefully questioning the patient for symptoms of heart failure, inquiring into the cause of regurgitation, and meticulously assessing left ventricular systolic function. When indicated on clinical grounds or by echocardiography, the erythrocyte sedimentation rate for inflammatory disease, serology for syphilis, and blood cultures for endocarditis should be obtained. The patient should be evaluated clinically every 3 to 6 months, and left ventricular systolic function should be assessed by echocardiography or radionuclide ventriculography (one or the other should be performed consistently, rather than switching from one to the other) every 6 to 12 months. The management of chronic aortic regurgitation is shown schematically in Figure 9.

Patients with asymptomatic but severe aortic regurgitation should avoid heavy exertion, including competitive sports. Systolic hypertension should be treated, usually with an angiotensin-converting enzyme inhibitor. Long-term therapy with vasodilators (hydralazine, 3 mg/kg/d [27], or enalapril, 20 mg bid [28]) reduces left ventricular volume. It has been reported that treatment with nifedipine, 20 mg bid, delays the need for aortic valve replacement [29]. Endocarditis prophylaxis is necessary. Digoxin, diuretics, and vasodilators are indicated for symptomatic patients with contraindications to cardiac surgery or in preparation for surgery. Drug therapy for acute aortic regurgitation includes diuretics, oral and intravenous vasodilators (in particular, afterload reduction with drugs such as nitroprusside), and, as indicated, inotropic support (usually with dobutamine). Urgent or emergency aortic valve surgery, even with active endocarditis, may be life-saving. Intraaortic balloon counterpulsation is not useful because inflation of the balloon in diastole worsens regurgitation across the aortic valve.

When to Refer

Patients should be referred to a cardiologist if they have symptoms or signs of heart failure and aortic regurgitation is evident on physical examination. Asymptomatic patients

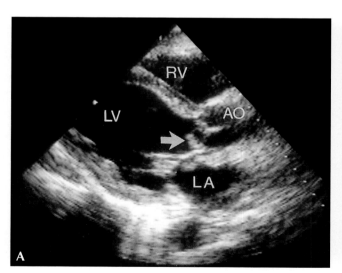

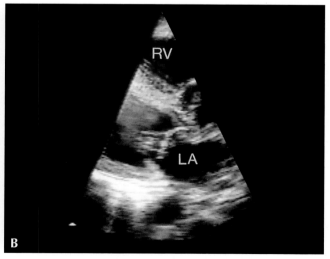

FIGURE 8 Two-dimensional echocardiogram without (A) and with (B) a superimposed color Doppler signal from a 49-year-old man with severe aortic regurgitation and an aortic root abscess. The right ventricle (RV), left atrium (LA), left ventricle (LV), and aorta (AO) are shown. The left ventricle is dilated. One aortic valve leaflet visualized in end-diastolic frame is in the normal position in the aorta, but the other (arrow) has prolapsed into the left ventricular outflow tract. The thickened area between the aorta and the left atrium is the abscess. The light blue color Doppler signal depicts the jet of regurgitation through the aortic valve into the left ventricle. (See Color Plate.) (Courtesy of Michael H. Picard, MD.)

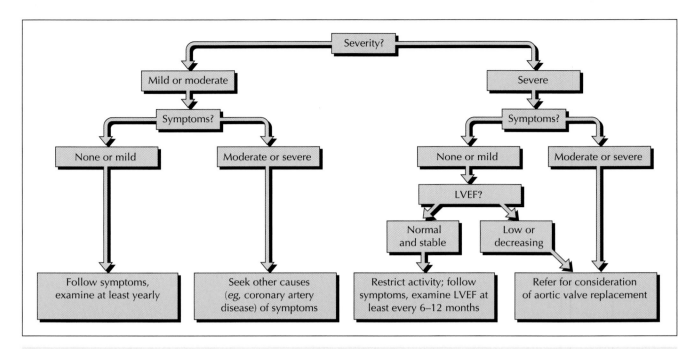

FIGURE 9 Management of aortic regurgitation. Serial left ventricular ejection fraction (LVEF) determinations for an individual
patient should be obtained consistently from either echocardiography or radionuclide ventriculography.

with aortic regurgitation should be promptly referred if left
ventricular ejection fraction is low or in the low-normal
range or if serial noninvasive studies indicate that it is
decreasing over time.

The definitive test for grading aortic regurgitation is
supravalvular aortography performed as part of cardiac
catheterization. The regurgitant fraction, derived from a
comparison of total (angiographic) and forward (eg, ther-
modilution) left ventricular stroke volume, is fraught with
error and is a less useful index of the severity of regurgitation. Right-side heart catheterization, left ventriculography, and—for patients older than 40 years or for younger
patients with atherosclerosis risk factors—coronary arteriography are also performed.

If there is no noncardiac contraindication, surgery is
performed if aortic regurgitation is severe and symptoms
are more than minimal. Surgery should be strongly considered for asymptomatic or minimally symptomatic patients
if left ventricular ejection fraction is mildly or moderately
impaired, if there is a decline in left ventricular ejection
fraction within the normal range, if there is very marked
left ventricular dilation [26], or if there is marked dilation
of the ascending aorta. Patients with severe depression of
ejection fraction may not benefit from valve surgery.

The usual operation for valve disease is aortic valve
replacement, although a minority of patients are successfully treated with valve repair. The considerations regarding
type of valve prosthesis are similar to those for surgery for
aortic stenosis. Patients with root disease require aortic
repair, usually accompanied by valve replacement, often
with a composite graft.

REFERENCES AND RECOMMENDED READING

1. Lindroos M, Kupari M, Heikkila J: Prevalence of aortic valve abnormalities in the elderly: an echocardiographic study of a random population sample. *J Am Coll Cardiol* 1993, 21:1220–1225.

2. Olson LT, Subramanian R, Edwards WD: Surgical pathology of pure aortic insuffficiency: a study of 225 cases. *Mayo Clin Proc* 1984, 59:835–841.

3. Subramanian R, Olson LJ, Edwards WD: Surgical pathology of pure aortic stenosis: a study of 374 cases. *Mayo Clin Proc* 1984, 59:683–690.

4. Fenoglio JJ, McAllister HA, DeCastro CM, *et al.*: Congenital bicuspid aortic valve after age 20. *Am J Cardiol* 1977, 39:164–169.

5. Chan K: Is aortic stenosis a preventable disease? *J Am Coll Cardiol* 2003, 42:593-599.

6. Selzer A: Changing aspects of the natural history of valvular aortic stenosis. *N Engl J Med* 1987, 317:91–98.

7. King RM, Pluth JR, Giuliani ER: The association of unexplained gastrointestinal bleeding with calcific aortic stenosis. *Ann Thorac Surg* 1987, 44:514–516.

8. Vincentelli A, Susen S, Le Tourneau T, *et al.*: Acquired von Willebrand syndrome in aortic stenosis. *N Engl J Med* 2003, 349:343-349.

9. Levinson GE: Aortic stenosis. In *Valvular Heart Disease*, edn 2. Edited by Dalen JE, Alpert JS. Boston: Little, Brown and Company; 1987:197–282.

10. Lombard JT, Selzer A: Valvular aortic stenosis: a clinical and hemodynamic profile of patients. *Ann Intern Med* 1987, 106:292–298.

11. Folland ED, Kriegel BJ, Henderson WG, *et al.*: Implications of third heart sounds in patients with valvular heart disease. *N Engl J Med* 1992, 327:458–462.

12. Turina J, Hess O, Sepulci F, Krayenbuehl HP: Spontaneous course of aortic valve disease. *Eur Heart J* 1987, 8:471–483.

13. Horstkotte D, Loogen F: The natural history of aortic valve stenosis. *Eur Heart J* 1988, 9(suppl E):57–64.

14. Aronow WS, Ahn C, Kronzon I, Nanna M: Prognosis of congestive heart failure in patients aged ≥ 62 years with unoperated severe valvular aortic stenosis. *Am J Cardiol* 1993, 72:846–848.

15. Pellikka PA, Nishimura RA, Bailey KR, Tajik AJ: The natural history of adults with asymptomatic, hemodynamically significant aortic stenosis. *J Am Coll Cardiol* 1990, 15:1012–1017.

16. Torscher LC, Shub C, Rettke SR, Brown DL: Risk of patients with severe aortic stenosis undergoing noncardiac surgery. *Am J Cardiol* 1998, 81:448–452.

17. Carabello BA: Advances in the hemodynamic assessment of stenotic cardiac valves. *J Am Coll Cardiol* 1987, 10:912–919.

18. Levinson JR, Akins CW, Buckley MJ, *et al.*: Octogenarians with aortic stenosis: outcome following aortic valve replacement. *Circulation* 1989, 80(suppl I):I-49–I-56.

19. Rediker DE, Boucher CA, Block PC, *et al.*: Degree of reversibility of left ventricular systolic dysfunction after aortic valve replacement for isolated aortic stenosis. *Am J Cardiol* 1987, 60:112–118.

20. Braunwald E: On the natural history of severe aortic stenosis. *J Am Coll Cardiol* 1990, 15:1018–1020.

21. Guiney TE, Davies MJ, Leech GJ, Leatham A: The aetiology and course of isolated severe aortic regurgitation: a clinical, pathological, and echocardiographic study. *Br Heart J* 1987, 58:358–368.

22. Morganroth JM, Perloff JK, Zeldis SM, Dunkman WB: Acute severe aortic regurgitation: pathophysiology, clinical recognition, and management. *Ann Intern Med* 1977, 87:223–232.

23. Abdulla AM, Frank MJ, Erdin RAJ, Canedo MI: Clinical significance and hemodynamic correlates of the third heart sound gallop in aortic regurgitation: a guide to optimal timing of cardiac catheterization. *Circulation* 1981, 64:464–471.

24. Desjardins VA, Enriquez-Sarano M, Tajik AJ, *et al.*: Intensity of murmurs correlates with severity of valvular regurgitation. *Am J Med* 1996, 100:149–156.

25. ACC/AHA guidelines for the management of patients with valvular heart disease [review]. *J Am Coll Cardiol* 1998, 32:1486-1588.

26. Bonow RO, Lakatos E, Maron BJ, *et al.*: Serial long-term assessment of the natural history of asymptomatic patients with chronic aortic regurgitation and normal left ventricular systolic function. *Circulation* 1991, 84:1625–1635.

27. Greenberg B, Massie B, Bristow JD, *et al.*: Long-term vasodilator therapy of chronic aortic insufficiency: a randomized double-blinded, placebo-controlled clinical trial. *Circulation* 1988, 78:92–103.

28. Lin M, Chiang H, Lin S, *et al.*: Vasodilator therapy in chronic asymptomatic aortic regurgitation: enalapril versus hydralazine therapy. *J Am Coll Cardiol* 1994, 24:1046–1053.

29. Scognamiglio R, Rahimtoola SH, Fasoli G, *et al.*: Nifedipine in asymptomatic patients with severe aortic regurgitation and normal left ventricular function. *N Engl J Med* 1994, 331:689–694.

30. Sutton GC, Fox KM: *A Color Atlas of Heart Disease: Pathological, Clinical and Investigatory Aspects.* London: Current Medical Literature; 1990:136–137.

31. Ross J Jr, Braunwald E: Aortic stenosis. *Circulation* 1968, 37(suppl V):V-61–V-67.

SELECT BIBLIOGRAPHY

Bonow RO, Carabello B, de Leon AC Jr, *et al.*: ACC/AHA guidelines for the management of patients with valvular heart disease: a report of the American College of Cardiology/American Heart Association Task Force on practice guidelines (committee on management of patients with valvular heart disease). *J Am Coll Cardiol* 1998, 32:1486–1582.

Braunwald E: Valvular heart disease. In *Heart Disease*, edn 5. Edited by Braunwald E. Philadelphia: WB Saunders Co.; 1997:1035–1053.

Rahimtoola SH: Perspective on valvular heart disease: an update. *J Am Coll Cardiol* 1989, 14:1–23.

Waller BF, Howard J, Fess S: Pathology of aortic valve stenosis and pure aortic regurgitation: a clinical morphologic assessment—Parts I and II. *Clin Cardiol* 1994, 17:85–92, 150–156.

Tricuspid and Pulmonic Valve Disease

William R. Pitts
L. David Hillis

24

Key Points

- Congenital anomalies of the tricuspid and pulmonic valves constitute 10% to 15% of all congenital heart disease.

- Pulmonic stenosis is the most common congenital right-sided valvular abnormality and is effectively treated by balloon valvuloplasty.

- Pulmonic regurgitation usually results from pulmonary arterial hypertension, and its prognosis is largely determined by the underlying disease process.

- Tricuspid stenosis is nearly always caused by rheumatic disease and is never seen without concomitant mitral or aortic involvement.

- Tricuspid regurgitation (TR) usually results from right ventricular dilatation; patients with TR present with right-sided heart failure.

The tricuspid and pulmonic valves are often overlooked during evaluation of suspected cardiac disease. This is particularly true in the United States, where the incidence of rheumatic valvular disease has declined and other disease processes involving the right-sided valves (*eg*, infective endocarditis in intravenous drug abusers) have increased in frequency.

TRICUSPID VALVE DISEASE

Congenital

Congenital anomalies of the tricuspid valve account for only 1% to 3% of congenital heart disease. Only tricuspid atresia and Ebstein's anomaly are of clinical importance, and almost all patients with the former are diagnosed and surgically corrected in infancy or early childhood.

In Ebstein's anomaly, the septal and inferior tricuspid valve leaflets are displaced away from the tricuspid annulus into the right ventricle. The anterior leaflet retains its normal attachment to the atrioventricular groove and is typically large and redundant. The displacement of the valve apparatus divides the right ventricle into 1) an inlet portion, which is functionally part of the right atrium (the so-called *atrialized* portion) and 2) a distal, functionally small right ventricular chamber. Associated anomalies include an interatrial communication (atrial septal defect or patent foramen ovale) in 75% of cases, ventricular septal defect, pulmonary stenosis or atresia, and mitral valve prolapse [1]. In addition, as many as 25% of patients with Ebstein's anomaly have ventricular preexcitation, most commonly via a right-sided accessory atrioventricular pathway [2].

Most patients with Ebstein's anomaly survive to adulthood, and an occasional patient lives into the seventh or eighth decade. Early (fetal or neonatal) presentation usually is associated with other cardiac abnormalities and portends a poor prognosis [3]. Most patients are asymptomatic until the third or fourth decade, when dyspnea, fatigue, or cyanosis appear insidiously. In 15% to 20% of cases, sudden death caused by tachydysrhythmias may be the presenting manifestation. The onset of right heart failure portends a poor prognosis and is the most common cause of death.

On physical examination, the arterial and jugular venous pulses are usually normal. The first heart sound (S_1) is usually loud and widely split, as is the second heart sound (S_2); multiple systolic clicks as well as right-sided gallops may be heard. A murmur of tricuspid regurgitation is almost invariably present at the left lower sternal border and characteristically becomes louder with inspiration [4].

The electrocardiogram (ECG) usually reveals sinus rhythm, although supraventricular arrhythmias may be seen. Tall P waves, a prolonged PR interval, and complete or incomplete right bundle branch block are common (Fig. 1). Chest radiography usually demonstrates globular cardiomegaly and evidence of an enlarged right atrium. Echocardiography is extremely valuable in identifying the anatomic relationship between the tricuspid valve and right heart chambers as well as in assessing right ventricular function, tricuspid regurgitation, and intracardiac shunting [5]. Finally, the diagnosis of Ebstein's anomaly may be made at catheterization by recording a simultaneous intracardiac pressure and electrogram with a single catheter. When this catheter is withdrawn from the right ventricle to the right atrium, a right ventricular electrical potential continues to be recorded after the pressure contour has changed to a right atrial waveform. Right ventricular angiography is usually diagnostic. In most subjects with Ebstein's anomaly, transthoracic echocardiography provides all the information that is needed, and, as a result, catheterization is unnecessary.

Management of the patient with Ebstein's anomaly is based on the severity of disease. An acyanotic patient with minimal symptoms is managed conservatively, whereas the patient with class III or IV heart failure, a cardiothoracic ratio of 0.65 or greater, severe cyanosis, or paradoxic embolization may benefit from surgical repair [6,7]. Valve repair is preferable to valve replacement because it is associated with lower mortality rates and fewer long-term compli-

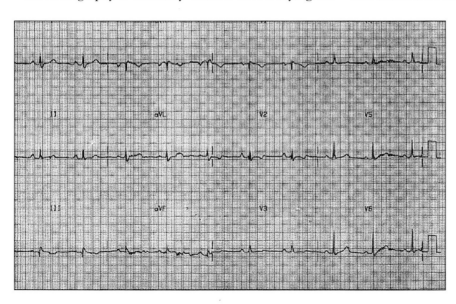

FIGURE 1 Electrocardiogram from a patient with Ebstein's anomaly demonstrating a prolonged PR interval, peaked P waves, and an incomplete right bundle branch block.

TABLE 1 CAUSES OF FUNCTIONAL OR ANATOMIC TRICUSPID STENOSIS
Tricuspid valve vegetations
Tumor (myxoma, leiomyoma, metastatic melanoma)
Thrombus (ball valve)
Carcinoid syndrome
Löffler's endocarditis
Postsurgical (following tricuspid annuloplasty)
Constrictive pericarditis
Methysergide

TABLE 2 SYMPTOMS OF TRICUSPID STENOSIS
Easy fatigability (because of reduced cardiac output)
Right upper quadrant abdominal discomfort (because of hepatic congestion)
Anorexia, nausea, vomiting, and eructation (because of passive congestion of the gastrointestinal tract)
Syncope/near syncope
Periodic cyanosis (because of right-to-left intracardiac shunting through a patent foramen ovale)
Vague retrosternal chest discomfort

cations [8]. If valve replacement is necessary, a bioprosthesis is preferable to a mechanical prosthesis [9]. Refractory tachydysrhythmias may be treated at the time of surgery.

Acquired
Tricuspid stenosis

Tricuspid stenosis (TS) is uncommon and results almost exclusively from rheumatic scarring; other causes of functional and anatomic TS are listed in Table 1. Isolated rheumatic TS in the absence of concomitant mitral involvement, aortic involvement, or both is rare.

Patients with TS usually have symptoms related to their predominant left-sided valvular abnormality. Indeed, the absence of pulmonary congestion in a patient with severe mitral stenosis should raise the suspicion of concomitant TS. Symptoms that are primarily related to TS result from peripheral venous congestion or a reduced cardiac output (Table 2).

On physical examination, the patient with TS has jugular venous dist ntion with prominent A waves and hepato- jugular reflux. Hepatomegaly with presystolic pulsation, ascites, peripheral edema, and pleural effusions are common. The auscultatory findings are usually dominated by concomitant left-sided valvular disease. S_1 is increased in intensity, as is the pulmonic component of S_2 (if pulmonary hypertension is present). The murmur of TS may be confused with that of mitral stenosis, but careful auscultation can usually distinguish them (Table 3).

Both the diastolic murmur and the opening snap of TS are augmented by maneuvers that increase flow across the tricuspid valve (*eg*, inspiration).

The ECG of the patient with TS usually shows right atrial enlargement. The PR interval is often slightly prolonged, and ECG evidence of concomitant mitral stenosis is often present. Atrial dysrhythmias are usually indicative of coexistent mitral valve disease. On chest radiography, the patient has right atrial enlargement with rightward displacement of the right lower cardiac contour. Echocardiography and Doppler ultrasound provide a qualitative assessment of the severity of TS [10]. At catheterization, right atrial and ventricular pressures are recorded simultaneously (Fig. 2). A mean diastolic gradient across the tricuspid valve of 2 to 3 mm Hg is suggestive of TS. Provocative maneuvers during catheterization (*eg*, deep inspiration, exercise, volume infusion) may magnify a small resting pressure gradient.

The patient with isolated TS may be asymptomatic for years. Once symptoms develop, sodium restriction and diuretics are effective in relieving peripheral venous congestion. Once medically refractory symptoms develop, surgical correction via open commissurotomy or valve replacement should be recommended. If valve replacement is required, a bioprosthesis is preferable because of its proven durability in the tricuspid position and the increased risk of a thromboembolic complication with a mechanical prosthesis in this position [11,12].

	Mitral stenosis	Tricuspid stenosis
Location	Apex	Left lower sternal border
Quality	Rumbling	Rumbling
Intensity	Louder	Softer
Pitch	Lower	Higher
Timing	Mid-diastole	Mid-diastole
Duration	Longer	Shorter
Opening snap	Earlier	Later and increases with inspiration

TABLE 3 COMPARISON OF AUSCULTATORY FEATURES IN MITRAL AND TRICUSPID STENOSIS

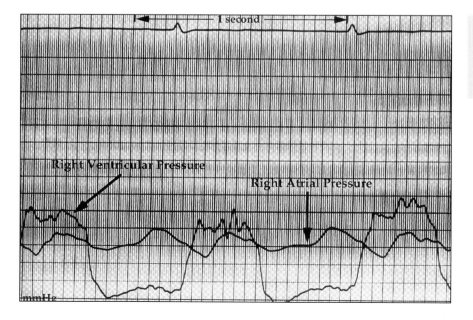

FIGURE 2 Simultaneous right atrial and ventricular pressure tracings in a patient with tricuspid stenosis. There is a gradient of 11 mm Hg across the tricuspid valve during diastole.

Tricuspid regurgitation

Tricuspid regurgitation (TR) may be functional or organic. Functional TR is far more common than organic TR and results from dilatation of the right ventricular and tricuspid anulus. Right ventricular dilatation, in turn, may result from pulmonary hypertension of any cause, right ventricular outflow obstruction (valvar, supravalvar, or infundibular), right ventricular infarction, or dilated cardiomyopathy. Organic TR may result from a variety of disease processes (Table 4). Recently, TR caused by infective endocarditis has appeared with increasing frequency, most commonly in intravenous drug abusers. The causative organism is usually *Staphylococcus aureus*. Fortunately, most of these patients respond to medical therapy and have a better prognosis than those with left-sided endocarditis. Organic TR is generally well tolerated in the absence of elevated right ventricular systolic pressure; indeed, the surgical procedure of choice in the patient with right-sided endocarditis refractory to medical therapy is tricuspid or pulmonic valve excision *without* immediate valve replacement [13].

Symptoms of TR are similar to those of tricuspid stenosis. On physical examination, the patient usually has distended neck veins with prominent V waves, hepatomegaly that may be pulsatile, ascites, and peripheral edema. Cardiac examination may reveal a prominent right ventricular impulse. On auscultation, S_1 is typically diminished, and the pulmonic component of S_2 may be prominent in the presence of pulmonary hypertension. A holosystolic murmur is present at the left lower sternal border and characteristically increases in intensity with inspiration (Carvallo sign). In addition, a right ventricular gallop (S_3) and a diastolic rumble ("relative" tricuspid stenosis) may be audible.

Common ECG features include right axis deviation, right atrial enlargement, and right ventricular hypertrophy. Chest radiography reveals right atrial and right ventricular enlargement. Two-dimensional echocardiography with Doppler color flow mapping is useful for detecting TR and estimating right ventricular peak systolic pressure. Recent studies have shown a good correlation between proximal regurgitant jet size (measured with transthoracic color flow mapping) and regurgitant fraction in subjects with tricuspid regurgitation [14]. At catheterization, right atrial and right ventricular diastolic pressures are elevated. A right ventricular systolic pressure greater than 60 mm Hg suggests a functional etiology of TR, whereas a systolic pressure less than 40 mm Hg implies organic valvular disease. Although right ventricular angiography will demonstrate regurgitation of radiographic contrast material into the right atrium, quantitation of TR by this method is imprecise.

Treatment of functional TR is directed at the underlying disease process. In the absence of pulmonary hypertension, TR usually does not require surgical treatment; when surgical therapy is necessary, tricuspid annuloplasty with (Carpentier) or without (De Vega) a prosthetic ring may be performed [15]. When valve replacement is indicated, a bioprosthesis is preferred. If surgery is not feasible, medical therapy with sodium restriction, digoxin, and diuretics should be employed.

PULMONIC VALVE DISEASE

Congenital

Valvular pulmonic stenosis (PS) is almost always congenital and is present in about 7% of patients with congenital heart disease. Acquired PS is exceedingly rare but may result from rheumatic scarring, infective endocarditis, trauma, malignant carcinoid syndrome, cardiac tumors, or an aneurysm of a sinus of Valsalva [16].

The patient with PS is frequently asymptomatic. He or she eventually may note exertional dyspnea, fatigue, syncope, or chest pain; peripheral edema and other evidence of peripheral venous congestion may develop if right ventricular failure occurs. If the foramen ovale is patent, intermittent or continuous right-to-left intracardiac shunting with resultant clubbing or cyanosis may occur.

On physical examination, the patient may have evidence of right ventricular failure (peripheral edema, hepatomegaly, jugular venous distention), right ventricular lift at the left sternal border, and a systolic thrill over the pulmonic area (second left intercostal space). On auscultation, S_1 is normal, and S_2 is widely split but moves with respiration. The pulmonic component is soft and markedly delayed. A harsh, crescendo–decrescendo systolic murmur is loudest over the pulmonic area, but is audible along the left sternal border. An ejection click that softens or even disappears with inspiration may be heard at the pulmonic area.

The ECG may reveal right axis deviation, right ventricular hypertrophy, right atrial enlargement, and

---

TABLE 4 CAUSES OF ORGANIC TRICUSPID REGURGITATION

Rheumatic
Infective endocarditis
Ebstein's anomaly
Right ventricular papillary muscle dysfunction
Myxomatous degeneration
Carcinoid syndrome
Trauma
Tricuspid valve prolapse
Connective tissue disorders (rheumatoid arthritis, systemic lupus erythematosus, Marfan syndrome)
Right atrial myxoma
Methysergide
Endomyocardial fibrosis
Thyrotoxicosis

---

complete or incomplete right bundle branch block (Fig. 3). Chest radiography demonstrates diminished pulmonary vascular markings and a markedly dilated main pulmonary artery. Cardiomegaly may be present. Two-dimensional echocardiography with Doppler ultrasound is useful to visualize the pulmonic valve, to assess the severity of stenosis, and to identify coexisting anomalies [17]. Cardiac catheterization demonstrates a pressure gradient during systole between the right ventricle and pulmonary artery. The severity of PS is quantitated according to the right ventricular peak systolic pressure (Table 5).

Many adults with mild or moderate PS are asymptomatic and require no treatment. Survival among such patients is excellent, with 94% alive 20 years after diagnosis [18]. When undergoing elective dental or surgical procedures, they should receive antibiotic prophylaxis against infective endocarditis. In contrast, patients with severe valvular stenosis should have the stenosis relieved, because only 40% of such patients do not require intervention within 10 years of diagnosis [18]. Surgical valvotomy, balloon valvuloplasty, or (rarely) valve replacement is warranted for the indications outlined in Table 6. Balloon valvuloplasty is currently the procedure of choice for relief of valvular PS; its results are excellent and comparable to surgical valvotomy [19,20].

Acquired

Similar to TR, acquired pulmonic regurgitation (PR) may be functional or organic. Functional PR usually results from pulmonary arterial hypertension, regardless of etiology. Rarely, it occurs with idiopathic dilatation of the pulmonary artery [21]. Organic PR is relatively rare; it may occur with infective endocarditis, rheumatic scarring, chest trauma, carcinoid syndrome, syphilis, or following balloon valvuloplasty or surgical valvotomy.

The patient with functional PR presents with symptoms induced by the underlying disease. Organic PR in the absence of pulmonary hypertension may be well tolerated for many years. When severe and long standing, it may cause symptoms and signs of right ventricular failure.

Cardiac examination may reveal a palpable pulsation over the pulmonic area. On auscultation, S_2 is widely split, with an accentuated pulmonic component. A blowing, decrescendo diastolic murmur is audible in the second and third left intercostal spaces and increases in intensity with inspiration. A systolic ejection murmur caused by increased flow across the pulmonic valve is frequently heard. If right ventricular dilatation and decompensation have occurred, a right-sided S_3 and holosystolic murmur of TR may be present.

The ECG demonstrates right axis deviation, right ventricular hypertrophy, and possibly right bundle branch

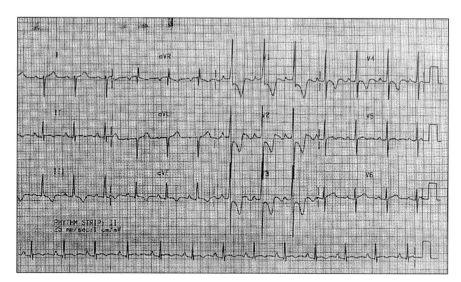

FIGURE 3 Electrocardiogram from a patient with congenital pulmonic stenosis showing right axis deviation, right atrial enlargement, and right ventricular hypertrophy with strain.

TABLE 5 GRADING OF VALVULAR PULMONIC STENOSIS	
Right ventricular peak-systolic pressure, *mm Hg**	Grade
30–49	Mild
50–99	Moderate
≥100	Severe

*As determined at cardiac catheterization.

TABLE 6 INDICATIONS FOR BALLOON PULMONIC VALVULOPLASTY OR SURGICAL TREATMENT
Symptoms attributable to the stenosis
Intermittent or continuous cyanosis
Right ventricular peak systolic pressure >100 mm Hg, even without symptoms

block. Chest radiography shows right ventricular enlargement and dilatation of the pulmonary artery. Echocardiography may reveal right ventricular dilatation, paradoxic motion of the interventricular septum during systole, and occasionally diastolic fluttering of the tricuspid valve. As with TR, a small amount of PR is seen in most normal subjects (93%) with Doppler color flow mapping. At catheterization, right ventricular systolic and diastolic pressures are similar to pulmonary arterial pressures provided that PS is not present. With pulmonary angiography, there is reflux of contrast material into the right ventricle.

The prognosis of a patient with functional PR is determined by the underlying disease process, and therapeutic measures should be tailored accordingly. Organic PR is usually benign. In the occasional patient in whom severe PR causes right ventricular failure despite medical therapy, surgical intervention is warranted.

REFERENCES AND RECOMMENDED READING

1. Giuliani ER, Fuster V, Brandenberg RO, Mair DD: Ebstein's anomaly: the clinical features and natural history of Ebstein's anomaly of the tricuspid valve. *Mayo Clin Proc* 1979, 54:163–173.

2. Smith WM, Gallagher JJ, Kerr CR, *et al.*: The electrophysiologic basis and management of symptomatic and recurrent tachycardia in patients with Ebstein's anomaly of the tricuspid valve. *Am J Cardiol* 1982, 49:1223–1234.

3. Celemajer DS, Bull C, Till JA, *et al.*: Ebstein's anomaly: presentation and outcome from fetus to adult. *J Am Coll Cardiol* 1994, 23:170–176.

4. Brickner ME, Hillis LD, Lange RA: Congenital heart disease in adults. *N Engl J Med* 2000, 342:334–342.

5. Shiina A, Seward JB, Tajik AJ, *et al.*: Two-dimensional echocardiographic-surgical correlation in Ebstein's anomaly: preoperative determination of patients requiring tricuspid valve plication vs. replacement. *Circulation* 1983, 68:534–544.

6. Driscoll DJ, Mottram CD, Danielson GK: Spectrum of exercise intolerance in 45 patients with Ebstein's anomaly and observations on exercise tolerance in 11 patients after surgical repair. *J Am Coll Cardiol* 1988, 11:831–836.

7. Mair DD: Ebstein's anomaly: natural history and management. *J Am Coll Cardiol* 1992, 19:1047–1048.

8. Vargas FJ, Mengo G, Granja MA, *et al.*: Tricuspid annuloplasty and ventricular plication for Ebstein's malformation. *Ann Thorac Surg* 1998, 65:1755–1777.

9. Kiziltan HT, Theodoro DA, Warnes CA, *et al.*: Late results of bioprosthetic tricuspid valve replacement in Ebstein's anomaly. *Ann Thorac Surg* 1998, 66:1538–1545.

10. Pearlman AS: Role of echocardiography in the diagnosis and evaluation of severity of mitral and tricuspid stenosis. *Circulation* 1991, 84(suppl 1):193–197.

11. Guerra F, Bortolotti U, Thiene G, *et al.*: Long-term performance of the Hancock bioprosthesis in the tricuspid position. A review of 45 patients with 14-year follow-up. *J Thorac Cardiovasc Surg* 1990, 99:838–845.

12. Kobayashi Y, Nagata S, Ohmori F, *et al.*: Serial doppler echocardiographic evaluation of bioprosthetic valves in the tricuspid position. *J Am Coll Cardiol* 1996, 27:1693–1697.

13. Arbulu A, Holmes RJ, Asfaw I: Tricuspid valvulectomy without replacement. Twenty years' experience. *J Thorac Cardiovasc Surg* 1991, 102:917–922.

14. Rivera JM, Vandervoort P, Mele D, *et al.*: Value of proximal regurgitant jet size in tricuspid regurgitation. *Am Heart J* 1996, 131:742–747

15. McGrath LB, Gonzalez-Lavin L, Bailey BM, *et al.*: Tricuspid valve operations in 530 patients. Twenty-five year assessment of early and late phase events. *J Thorac Cardiovasc Surg* 1990, 99:124–133.

16. Waller BF, Howard J, Fess S: Pathology of pulmonic valve stenosis and pure regurgitation. *Clin Cardiol* 1995, 18:45–50.

17. Richards KL: Assessment of aortic and pulmonic stenosis by echocardiography. *Circulation* 1991, 84(suppl 1):182–187.

18. Hayes CJ, Gersony WM, Driscoll DJ, *et al.*: Second natural history study of congenital heart defects: results of treatment of patients with pulmonary valvar stenosis. *Circulation* 1993, 87(suppl I):28–37.

19. Rao PS: Transcatheter treatment of pulmonary outflow tract obstruction: a review. *Prog Cardiovasc Dis* 1992, 35:119–158.

20. Chen CR, Cheng TO, Huang T, *et al.*: Percutaneous balloon valvuloplasty for pulmonic stenosis in adolescents and adults. *N Engl J Med* 1996, 335:21–25.

21. Ansari A: Isolated pulmonary valvular regurgitation: current perspectives. *Prog Cardiovasc Dis* 1991, 33:329–344.

SELECT BIBLIOGRAPHY

Braunwald E: Valvular Heart Disease. In *Heart Disease. A Textbook of Cardiovascular Medicine*, edn 5. Edited by Braunwald E. Philadelphia: WB Saunders; 1994:1054–1060.

Bonow RO, Carabello B, DeLeon AC Jr, *et al.*: ACC/AHA guidelines for the management of patients with valvular heart disease. *J Am Coll Cardiol* 1998, 32:1468–1588.

Hypertrophic Cardiomyopathy

Ranjan Dahiya
Gregg M. Yamada

25

Key Points

- Familial hypertrophic cardiomyopathy (HCM) is an autosomal dominant disorder linked to mutations in proteins that comprise the cardiac sarcomere.

- In obstructive HCM, systolic anterior motion of the mitral valve leaflet creates a subaortic pressure gradient.

- Echocardiography is the most useful study in the diagnosis of HCM, providing both anatomic and physiologic information.

- Sudden death is the most devastating consequence of HCM, and is associated with high risk features such as syncope, prior cardiac arrest, family history of sudden death, and nonsustained ventricular tachycardia on Holter monitoring.

- Medical therapy, including β-blockers, calcium channel blockers, and antiarrhythmic agents, is the initial treatment for most patients with HCM.

- Surgical therapy or alcohol septal ablation should be considered for patients refractory to medical therapy.

The most characteristic morphologic feature of hypertrophic cardiomyopathy (HCM) is left ventricular hypertrophy. Hypertrophy of the nondilated left ventricle results in abnormal diastolic function and can produce a dynamic subaortic pressure gradient. The pattern of left ventricular hypertrophy is typically asymmetrical, primarily involving the anterior and basal septum; however, other segments may be selectively involved.

ETIOLOGY

Hypertrophic cardiomyopathy occurs in less than 0.2% of the population, and approximately 45% of these cases are sporadic [1]. Familial HCM is inherited in an autosomal dominant fashion and results from mutations in proteins that comprise the cardiac sarcomere [2••]. Phenotypic expression of HCM varies within families due to the interplay of both modifier genes and enviromental factors [3,4].

PATHOPHYSIOLOGY

Hypertrophic cardiomyopathy may be either obstructive or nonobstructive depending on the presence or absence of a dynamic subaortic pressure gradient (Fig. 1). In the majority of patients with left ventricular outflow tract obstruction, systolic anterior motion of the mitral valve leaflet is the mechanism of mechanical outflow obstruction. Hypertrophy of the ventricular septum results in narrowing of the left ventricular outflow tract. Consequently, during ventricular systole, blood is expelled at a higher velocity, creating a Venturi effect near the anterior mitral leaflet. The mitral leaflet is drawn into contact with the ventricular septum, creating a subaortic gradient and resulting in ventricular outflow obstruction (Fig. 2). The severity of the pressure gradient may vary at rest, during exercise, or after pharmacologic therapy. A much less common mechanisim of left ventricular outflow obstruction occurs when there is muscular apposition of the ventricular myocardium [2••].

Nonobstructive HCM is characterized by left ventricular hypertrophy in the absence of a resting pressure gradient. Diastolic dysfunction, due to decreased compliance and incomplete relaxation of the hypertrophied ventricle, leads to impaired early diastolic filling and increased left ventricular end-diastolic pressure (LVEDP). Myocardial ischemia may result from increased myocardial oxygen demand in the absence of coronary artery disease (Fig. 3).

CLINICAL MANIFESTATIONS

The clinical presentation of HCM is variable. Many patients are asymptomatic. The most common symptoms include dyspnea (diastolic dysfunction), exertional angina (myocardial ischemia), fatigue, near syncope, and syncope (decreased cardiac output or arrhythmias). The morphologic and functional severity of the cardiomyopathy is not necessarily correlated with the severity of the clinical symptoms. Patients with minimal hypertrophy may have severe complaints, whereas those with marked hypertrophy may be relatively asymptomatic.

The cardiac examination is abnormal in patients with significant subaortic pressure gradients. The characteristic systolic murmur of HCM is harsh in character, with a crescendo–decrescendo pattern. The murmur is heard best between the left sternal border and the cardiac apex and often radiates to the axilla. In patients with prominent gradients, the murmur tends to be holosystolic at the cardiac apex because of accompanying mitral regurgitation. Abrupt standing and Valsalva maneuver accentuate the murmur of HCM, whereas squatting and isometric handgrip diminish it. The apical impulse is displaced laterally, and a systolic thrill is often palpable. Additionally, forceful atrial contraction combined with interrupted systolic flow due to left ventricular outflow obstruction may generate a triple apical impulse (Fig. 4).

DIAGNOSIS

Echocardiography is the most useful study in the diagnosis of HCM, providing morphologic and functional information (Fig. 5). The most characteristic finding is asymmetrical septal hypertrophy, which contributes to the narrowing of the left ventricular outflow tract. Variable degrees of mitral regurgitation are present in patients with outflow gradients. Diastolic dysfunction occurs in most patients with HCM, even in the absence of a ventricular outflow gradient, but the presence of diastolic dysfunction does not always correlate with clinical symptoms [5].

The most characteristic electrocardiographic features include nonspecific ST segment and T wave changes, left ventricular hypertrophy, abnormal Q waves in the anterolateral and inferior leads (pseudoinfarction pattern), and left atrial enlargement. Large amplitude (> 10 mm), inverted T waves in the left precordial leads may identify patients with apical HCM, but the clinical significance of these T-wave inversions is uncertain [6].

The chest radiograph often is unrevealing. The left ventricle may be prominent, but the cardiac silhouette usually is not enlarged. The left atrium and atrial appendage may be prominent secondary to increased pressure and associated mitral regurgitation.

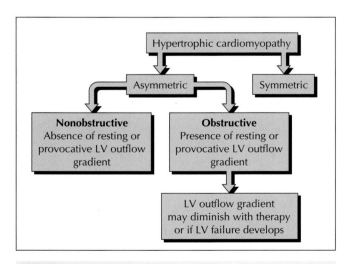

FIGURE 1 Classification of hypertrophic cardiomyopathy (HCM). LV—left ventricular.

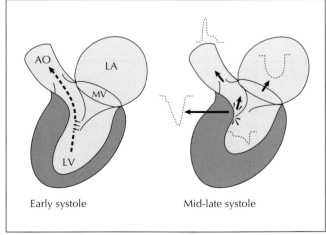

FIGURE 2 Mechanism of systolic anterior motion of the mitral leaflet in obstructive hypertrophic cardiomyopathy. AO—aorta; LA—left atrium; LV—left ventricle; MV—mitral valve. (*Adapted from* Wigle [30].)

Cardiac catheterization is performed if surgery is contemplated or if the diagnosis remains uncertain despite noninvasive assessment. Typically, a left ventricular outflow gradient is detected, and LVEDP is increased. Variable degrees of atherosclerosis may be present.

Risk stratification for sudden cardiac death is an important component in the work-up of HCM and should be performed in conjunction with a comanaging cardiologist. Risk stratification relies less on electrophysiologic testing than in the past. Instead, risk factors for sudden death such as syncope, previous cardiac arrest, abnormal exercise blood pressure, nonsustained ventricular tachycardia on Holter monitor, or family history of sudden cardiac death are used to determine whether an implantable defibrillator (ICD) should be implanted. ICD therapy is superior to antiarrhythmic therapy in high-risk groups, providing nearly absolute protection against life-threatening arrhythmias [7••].

COURSE AND PROGNOSIS

The clinical course is variable. It is not known why some patients remain clinically stable for years and only mildly symptomatic, whereas others deteriorate more rapidly [8]. Sudden death is the most devastating sequela of HCM, with an annual mortality rate of 2% to 3% in patients younger than 30 years of age [9]. Much of the published literature, however, has originated from tertiary care centers and may overestimate the actual mortality rate in the general population because of selection bias [10].

Left ventricular outflow obstruction, with a corresponding gradient greater than 30 mm Hg, has been shown to be a strong independent predictor of disease progression in hypertrophic cardiomyopathy. The severity of the gradient, however, does not appear to correlate with disease progression [11]. Nonsustained ventricular tachycardia on Holter monitoring is associated with an 8% annual mortality rate [12]. However, ventricular tachycardia is poorly predictive of sudden death in the absence of presyncope, or syncope [13]. Although ventricular arrhythmias are the most common cause of sudden death, acute hemodynamic derangements (both physiologic and pharmacologic) that augment the outflow gradient and diminish diastolic filling also may play a role.

Patients with mild hypertrophy without resting outflow gradients, or nonobstructive HCM, have a more favorable prognosis [14]. The prognosis in patients older than 60 years is similar to that in younger patients and appears related to cardiac function [15]. Patients with asymptomatic HCM also should be restricted from competitive athletics; however, noncompetitive athletics are not contraindicated (*eg*, walking, bicycling).

Decreased LV cavity size	HCM	MR, AS
Valsalva, standing, exercise, tachycardia, hypovolemia, inhalation of amyl nitrite	↑	↓
Increased LV cavity size		
Squatting, passive elevation of patient's legs, isometric handgrip, administration of phenylephrine	↓	No change or slight ↑

FIGURE 4 Response of murmurs of hypertrophic cardiomyopathy (HCM), aortic stenosis (AS), and mitral regurgitations (MR) to various maneuvers. LV—left ventricular.

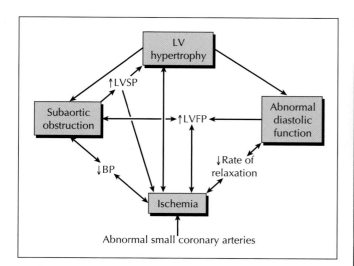

FIGURE 3 Pathophysiologic interrelationships of left ventricular (LV) hypertrophy, subaortic obstruction, diastolic dysfunction, and myocardial ischemia in hypertrophic cardiomyopathy. BP—blood pressure; LVFP—left ventricular filling pressure; LVSP—left ventricular systolic pressure. (*Adapted from* Maron *et al.* [31].)

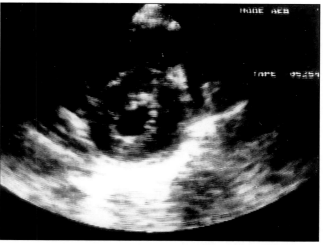

FIGURE 5 Echocardiogram of hypertrophic cardiomyopathy as seen in the short-axis view. (*Courtesy of* Linda A. Pape, MD.)

Ventricular tachycardia and ventricular fibrillation are the principal mechanisms of sudden cardiac death in young patients with HCM. ICDs may be effective in aborting sudden death episodes in high-risk patients [16].

Both medical and nonmedical treatment options decrease the left ventricular outflow gradient. The four treatment options presently available for patients with symptomatic HCM with documented outflow gradients are medical therapy, surgical myectomy, dual chamber pacing, and transcatheter septal ablation.

Medical Therapy

The most commonly used drugs, all with proven efficacy in alleviating symptoms, are β-blockers, calcium channel blockers, and antiarrhythmic agents.

β-blockers are effective in alleviating angina, dyspnea, and other symptoms of HCM. Overall clinical improvement, however, may be seen in only one third to one half of all patients treated. Mechanisms of action include a decrease in myocardial oxygen consumption (negative inotropy), increased diastolic filling time (decreased heart rate), and inhibition of sympathetic stimulation during exercise. The effect of β-blockers on the incidence of sudden death has not been determined conclusively.

Verapamil is the most frequently used calcium channel blocker for the treatment of HCM. It alleviates symptoms and improves exercise function in approximately two thirds of patients who have failed β-blocker therapy [17]. A more recent report has corroborated symptomatic improvement observed in patients with HCM taking verapamil, but found no increase in exercise capacity [18]. Mechanisms of action include a decrease in the systolic left ventricular outflow gradient through negative inotropic effects and an improvement in diastolic function. Verapamil should be used with great caution in patients with severe left ventricular outflow gradients and elevated left ventricular end-diastolic pressures [19]. The effect of verapamil on sudden death remains undetermined. Only limited information is available on the use of other calcium channel blockers in the treatment of HCM.

Disopyramide is a type IA antiarrhythmic agent with negative inotropic properties that effectively relieves symptoms of HCM and improves exercise capacity [20]. Although disopyramide is potentially effective in treating supraventricular and ventricular arrhythmias in patients with HCM, a clear survival benefit remains to be proved [21].

Medical therapy with negative inotropes, including β-blockers, calcium channel blockers, and antiarrhythmic agents, are widely used. These negative inotropes are thought to decrease the acceleration of blood leaving the left ventricle, which subsequently delays mitral leaflet ventricular septal contact, thereby decreasing the obstructive pressure gradient [22].

Nonmedical Therapy

Patients who remain or become symptomatic after conservative medical management have the options of surgical septal myectomy, alcohol ablation, or dual chamber pacing.

Septal myectomy

Patients refractory to medical therapy are considered for ventricular septal myotomy–myectomy with possible mitral valve replacement following cardiac catheterization. Cardiovascular surgery to remove portions of the left ventricular septum is effective at reducing symptoms in the majority of patients with HCM. The operative mortality rate is approximately 5%, and a majority of patients report long-term symptomatic improvement. The beneficial effects of this procedure are preserved in excess of 20 years [23••,24••,25].

Transcatheter alcohol septal ablation

Alcohol septal ablation has increasingly become an alternative to surgery when medical therapy alone is no longer effective. Absolute alcohol in small quantities is injected into the arteries supplying the myocardial septum. This produces an infarction in the hypertrophied tissue thereby reducing septal mass and alleviating outflow obstruction. Potential complications include complete heart block or inadvertent myocardial infarction in locations other than the hypertrophied septum. One study comparing surgical myectomy with alcohol septal ablation found both techniques comparable in reducing outflow gradients [26]. Alcohol septal ablation is now more commonly performed than surgical myectomy [27]. However, according to the American College of Cardiology & the European Society of Cardiology expert consensus panel, surgical myectomy is still considered the gold standard [2••]. Alcohol septal ablation should be confined to those patients who fail medical therapy and are not good operative candidates.

Dual chamber pacemaker implantation

Dual chamber pacing is an additional method for decreasing left ventricular outflow tract obstruction. Pacing-induced contraction of the right ventricle causes an inward motion of the interventricular septum in systole. This results in increased left ventricular outflow diameter and a lessened gradient. Initial observational reports have not been replicated in randomized trials, and the effectiveness of dual chamber pacing remains inconsistent [28,29].

WHEN TO REFER

Patients with HCM should be comanaged with a cardiology consultant. These patients require close follow-up for development and monitoring of symptoms. In addition, patients with HCM should receive subacute bacterial endocarditis prophylaxis.

REFERENCES AND RECOMMENDED READING

Recently published papers of particular interest have been highlighted as:

•• Of outstanding interest

1. Maron BJ, Bonow RO, Cannon RO, *et al.*: Hypertrophic cardiomyopathy: interrelations of clinical manifestations, pathophysiology, and therapy. *N Engl J Med* 1987, 316:780–789.

2.•• Maron and McKenna *et al*: ACC/ESC Expert Consensus Document on Hypertrophic Cardiomyopathy. *J Am Coll Cardiol* 2003, 42: 1687–1713.

3. Osterop AP, Kofflard MJ, Sandkuijl LA, *et al.* AT1 receptor A/C1166 polymorphism contributes to cardiac hypertrophy in subjects with hypertrophic cardiomyopathy. *Hypertension* 1998, 32:825–830.

4. Lechin M, Quinones MA, Omran A, *et al.* Angiotensin-I converting enzyme genotypes and left ventricular hypertrophy in patients with hypertrophic cardiomyopathy. *Circulation* 1995, 92:1808–1812.

5. Nihoyannopoulos P, Karatasakis G, Frenneaux M, *et al.*: Diastolic function in hypertrophic cardiomyopathy: relation to exercise capacity. *J Am Coll Cardiol* 1992, 19:536–540.

6. Alfonso F, Nihoyannopoulos P, Stewart J, *et al.*: Clinical significance of giant negative T waves in hypertrophic cardiomyopathy. *J Am Coll Cardiol* 1990, 15:965–971.

7.•• Maron BJ, Shen W-K, Link MS, *et al.*: Efficacy of implantable cardioverter-defibrillators for the prevention of sudden death in patients with hypertrophic cardiomyopathy. *N Engl J Med* 2000, 342:365–373.

8. McKenna WJ: The natural history of hypertrophic cardiomyopathy. *Cardiovasc Clin* 1988, 19:135–142.

9. McKenna WJ, England D, Doi YL, *et al.*: Arrhythmia in hypertrophic cardiomyopathy. I: Influence on prognosis. *Br Heart J* 1981, 46:168–172.

10. Spirito P, Chiarella F, Carratino L, *et al.*: Clinical course and prognosis of hypertrophic cardiomyopathy in an outpatient population. *N Engl J Med* 1989, 320:749–755.

11. Maron MS, Olivotto I, Betocchi S, *et al.*: Effect of left ventricular outflow tract obstruction on clinical outcome in hypertrophic cardiomyopathy. *N Engl J Med* 2003, 348:295–303.

12. Maron BJ, Savage DD, Wolfson JK, Epstein SE: Prognostic significance of 24 hour ambulatory electrocardiographic monitoring in patients with hypertrophic cardiomyopathy: a prospective study. *Am J Cardiol* 1981, 48:252–257.

13. Fananapazir L, Chang AC, Epstein SE, McAreavey D: Prognostic determinants in hypertrophic cardiomyopathy: prospective evaluation of a therapeutic strategy based on clinical, Holter, hemodynamic and electrophysiological findings. *Circulation* 1992, 86:730–740.

14. Aron LA, Hertzeanu L, Enrique FZ, *et al.*: Prognosis of nonobstructive hypertrophic cardiomyopathy. *Am J Cardiol* 1991, 67:215–216.

15. Pelliccia F, Cianfrocca C, Romeo F, Reale A: Natural history of hypertrophic cardiomyopathy in the elderly. *Cardiology* 1991, 78:329–333.

16. Maron BJ, Shen WK, Link MS, *et al.*: Efficacy of implantable cardioverter-defibrillators for the prevention of sudden death in patients with hypertrophic cardiomyopathy. *N Engl J Med* 2000, 342:365–373.

17. Rosing DR, Idanpaan-Heikkila U, Maron BJ, *et al.*: Use of calcium-channel blocking drugs in hypertrophic cardiomyopathy. *Am J Cardiol* 1985, 55 (Suppl):185B–195B.

18. Gilligan DM, Chan WL, Joshi J, *et al.*: A double-blind, placebo-controlled crossover trial of nadolol and verapamil in mild and moderately symptomatic hypertrophic cardiomyopathy. *J Am Coll Cardiol* 1993, 21:1627–1629.

19. Epstein S, Rosing D: Verapamil: Its potential for serious complications in patients with hypertrophic cardiomyopathy. *Circulation* 1981, 64:437–439.

20. Hartmann A, Kuhn J, Hopf R, *et al.*: Effect of propranolol and disopyramide on left ventricular function at rest and during exercise in hypertrophic cardiomyopathy. *Cardiology* 1992, 80:81–88.

21. Blanchard DG, Ross J: Hypertrophic cardiomyopathy: prognosis with medical or surgical therapy. *Clin Cardiol* 1991, 14:11–19.

22. Sherrid MV, Pearle G, Gunsburg DZ: Mechanism of benefit of negative inotropes in obstructive hypertrophic cardiomyopathy. *Circulation* 1998, 97:41–47.

23.•• McCully RB, Nishimura RA, Tajik AJ, *et al.*: Extent of clinical improvement after surgical treatment of hypertrophic obstructive cardiomyopathy. *Circulation* 1996, 94:467–471.

24.•• Schulte HD, Borisov K, Gams E, *et al.*: Management of symptomatic hypertrophic obstructive cardiomyopathy–long-term results after surgical therapy. *Thorac Cardiovasc Surg* 1999, 47:213–218.

25. McIntosh CL, Maron BL: Current operative treatment of obstructive hypertrophic cardiomyopathy. *Circulation* 1988, 78:487–494.

26. Nagueh SF, Ommen SR, Lakkis NM, *et al.*: Comparison of ethanol septal reduction therapy with surgical myectomy for the treatment of hypertrophic obstructive cardiomyopathy. *J Am Coll Cardiol* 2001; 38:1701–1706.

27. Maron BJ. Role of alcohol septal ablation in treatment of obstructive hypertrophic cardiomyopathy. *Lancet* 2000;355:425–426.

28. Maron BJ, Nishimura RA, McKenna WJ, *et al.*: Assessment of permanent dual-chamber pacing as a treatment for drug-refractory symptomatic patients with obstructive hypertrophic cardiomyopathy: a randomized, double-blind, crossover study (M-PATHY). *Circulation* 1999, 99:2927–2933.

29. Nishimura RA, Trusty JM, Hayes DL, *et al.*: Dual-chamber pacing for hypertrophic cardiomyopathy: a randomized, double-blind, crossover trial. *J Am Coll Cardiol* 1997;29:435–441.

30. Wigle ED: Hypertrophic cardiomyopathy: a 1987 viewpoint [editorial]. *Circulation* 1987, 73:311–322.

31. Maron BJ, Bonow RO, Cannon RO, *et al.*: Hypertrophic cardiomyopathy: interrelations of clinical manifestations, pathophysiology, and therapy. *N Engl J Med* 1987, 316:844–852.

Congestive Cardiomyopathy
Mohammad Asif

26

> ## Key Points
> - Document borderline heart disease by imaging for size and function.
> - B-type natriuretic peptide can be used as a diagnostic tool.
> - Low ejection fraction without symptoms can benefit from treatment.
> - Angiotensin converting enzyme inhibitors improve mortality.
> - Digoxin improves symptoms but not mortality.
> - The diuretic dosage should be carefully adjusted according to patient's circulatory status.
> - An angiotensin receptor blocker can be added to the regimen of heart failure treatment.
> - A selective subset of patients may respond to the use of β-blockers.
> - Heart transplantation should be considered in refractory cases.

INTRODUCTION

The incidence of heart failure (HF) is growing at an epidemic proportion. Currently, 5 million Americans suffer from HF at an incidence rate of 550,000 new cases diagnosed each year. This costs our health care system $22.2 billion in health care expenditures per year [1]. HF is also associated with substantial morbidity; it is the most frequent cause of hospitalization in the elderly with 990,000 hospitalizations per year [1].

CLINICAL PRESENTATION

Congestive cardiomyopathy is usually associated with impaired systolic function of the ventricle. In some patients, diastolic function may be the predominant abnormality and require a different therapeutic approach. More often, however, this alteration is combined with systolic dysfunction. Symptoms usually develop gradually after an asymptomatic period with cardiac dysfunction. There are three cardinal symptoms, any of which may predominate: fatigue (caused by low cardiac output), dyspnea (Table 1) [2], and weight gain (often with venous and hepatic congestion). Some patients have noncongestive symptoms including palpitations, chest pains, fainting spells, and lightheadedness. Orthopnea, paroxysmal nocturnal dyspnea, chronic cough, abdominal distention, right upper quadrant pain, or nausea also may be present. Occasionally, the first symptom to occur is secondary to an embolic event.

CAUSES OF CONGESTIVE CARDIOMYOPATHY

Consideration of the etiologic factor that may precipitate or play a role in the development of the diffuse myocardial disease is crucial to preventing or ameliorating the process (Table 2). More frequent causes include hypertension, alcohol consumption, age, viral infection, and drug toxicity.

Hypertension is a leading cause of heart failure resulting from both systolic and diastolic dysfunction, even without significant coronary atherosclerosis. Early symptoms are often caused by diastolic dysfunction of the left ventricle [3]. Many patients with hypertension have evidence of abnormal left ventricular relaxation and filling, even without left ventricular hypertrophy [4].

Alcoholism is one of the most common, identifiable causes of cardiomyopathy. Over time, excessive alcohol consumption can lead to heart muscle disease without evident malnutrition. Although no specific cardiovascular markers exist, plasma tests used in the diagnosis of liver injury and urinary ethanol levels may be helpful. Progression of heart disease may be delayed or even reversed in patients who abstain from alcohol.

The normal aging process may be associated with a decline of ventricular diastolic function, whereas ventricular systolic function is unaltered at rest. Elderly persons are more prone to develop diastolic HF if they also have hypertension. The prevalence of systolic hypertension attributable to increased arterial stiffness is high among the elderly.

Presentation of patients with heart muscle disease caused by a viral infection is quite varied. Patients may have a distinct viral syndrome with severe cardiovascular compromise that may be fatal or may spontaneously resolve. Acute fulminating myocarditis is usually associated with left ventricular dysfunction, which may progress to dilated cardiomyopathy.

Doxorubicin and other anthracycline antitumor agents are causes of dose-related and irreversible toxic cardiomyopathy. Evidence also supports the concept that a specific diabetic cardiomyopathy without accelerated coronary atherosclerosis or hypertension increases the incidence of heart failure, more so in females than males [5]. Finally, morbid obesity may cause circulatory congestion associated with increased blood volume and arterial pressure as well as eccentric hypertrophy.

FUNCTIONAL ABNORMALITIES

During the early stages of the disease, stroke volume is maintained despite decreased ejection fraction by increased end-diastolic volume. Increased ventricular wall stress stimulates myocyte hypertrophy, which may normalize wall stress. With further reductions of the ejection fraction,

---

TABLE 1 MECHANISMS OF DYSPNEA IN HEART FAILURE

Decreased pulmonary function
   Decreased compliance
   Increased airway resistance
Increased ventilatory drive
   Hypoxemia—↑ PCW
   V/Q mismatching—↑ PCW
   ↑ CO_2 production—↓ CO-lactic acidosis
Respiratory muscle dysfunction
   Decreased strength
   Decreased endurance
   Ischemia

CO—cardiac output; PCW—mean pulmonary capillary wedge pressure; V/Q—ventilation/perfusion.

TABLE 2 ETIOLOGIES OF CONGESTIVE CARDIOMYOPATHY

Frequent incidence
Hypertension
Ethyl alcohol abuse
Viral infection
Age
Idiopathic

Less frequent incidence
Metabolic
   Nutritional–obesity, thiamine
   Endocrinologic–diabetes mellitus, myxedema
   Uremia
   Amyloid
   Electrolyte imbalance
Infectious
   Bacterial
   Mycobacterial
   Parasitic
   Spirochetal
   Rickettsial
   Fungal
Immune
   Transplantation rejection
   Autoimmune disease (collagen diseases)
   Peripartum
Toxic
   Chemotherapeutic agents
   Catecholamines
   Cocaine
   Cobalt
Familial
   Myotonia dystrophica
   Progressive muscular dystrophy
   Neuromyopathic
Hypersensitivity
   Methyldopa
   Penicillin
   Sulfonamides
   Tetracycline
   Phenylbutazone

ventricular volume and stress increase and stroke volume decreases (Table 3) [6]. Increased heart rate may sustain normal cardiac output. Fluid retention, which is initially adaptive, may further increase ventricular volume, leading to pulmonary and systemic venous congestion. Multiple neurohumoral mechanisms, including the release of circulating norepinephrine and stimulation of the renin-angiotensin system, are activated. Peripheral circulation undergoes local changes in response to heart failure: fractional distribution of blood flow to the kidneys, limbs, and splanchnic beds decreases, whereas blood flow to the heart and brain is preserved [7,8]. The diminished exercise capacity of limb muscles in patients with HF may be due in part to chronically diminished nutritive perfusion [9,10••]. Renal hypoperfusion and altered intrarenal hemodynamics may contribute to sodium and water retention [11,12••]. Atrial natriuretic factor partly counteracts the undesirable fluid retention promoted by vasopressin. During the advanced stage, these neurohumoral mechanisms override serum osmolarity homeostasis, causing a decrease in serum sodium levels and resistance to medical therapy.

Up to 40% of symptomatic patients have diastolic HF. The mechanisms responsible for diastolic dysfunction (Fig. 1) despite normal systolic function are decreased compliance (increased stiffness) and impaired ventricular relaxation [13,14]. Hence, the left ventricle is unable to fill adequately at normal diastolic pressures (Table 4). Reduced left ventricular filling volume leads to decreased stroke volume and symptoms of low cardiac output, whereas increased filling pressure leads to pulmonary congestion.

Physical Examination

Physical signs vary according to when a patient is seen during the natural history of congestive cardiomyopathy.

TABLE 3 SYSTOLIC VS. DIASTOLIC DYSFUNCTION IN HEART FAILURE		
Parameters	**Systolic**	**Diastolic**
History		
Coronary heart disease	++++	+
Hypertension	++	++++
Diabetes	+++	+
Valvular heart disease	++++	–
Paroxysmal dyspnea	++	+++
Physical examination		
Cardiomegaly	+++	+
Soft heart sounds	++++	+
S_3 gallop	+++	+
S_4 gallop	+	+++
Hypertension	++	++++
Mitral regurgitation	+++	+
Rales	++	++
Edema	+++	+
Jugular venous distention	+++	+
Parameters	**Systolic**	**Diastolic**
Chest roentgenogram		
Cardiomegaly	+++	+
Pulmonary congestion	+++	+++
Electrocardiogram		
Low voltage	+++	–
Left ventricular hypertrophy	++	++++
Q waves	++	+
Echocardiogram		
Low ejection fraction	++++	–
Left ventricular dilation	++	–
Left ventricular hypertrophy	++	++++

Plus signs suggestive of dysfunction (the number reflects relative weight); minus signs not very suggestive.

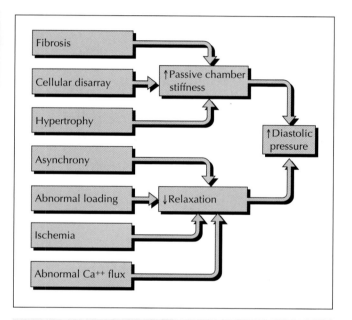

FIGURE 1 Factors responsible for diastolic dysfunction and increased left ventricular diastolic pressure (*Adapted from* Gaasch and Izzi [13].)

TABLE 4 PARAMETERS OF LEFT VENTRICULAR DIASTOLIC FILLING MEASURED BY DOPPLER ECHOCARDIOGRAPHY	
Peak E	79 ± 26 cm/sec
Peak A	48 ± 22 cm/sec
E/A	1.7 ± 0.6
E Deceleration time	184 ± 24 msec
E Deceleration rate	5.6 ± 2.7 m/sec
Isovolumetric relaxation time	74 ± 26 msec
Peak pulmonary venous AR wave	19 ± 4 cm/sec

Commonly, the patient has tachypnea, tachycardia, and usually sinus but occasionally atrial fibrillation. Systolic blood pressure may be normal, high, or low. Pulse pressure is narrow, reflecting a diminished stroke volume; there may be pulsus alternans. Jugular veins are frequently distended with a prominent V wave, a sign of tricuspid regurgitation. The liver may be enlarged and pulsatile, and ascites and peripheral edema may be present. The apical impulse is usually displaced laterally and inferiorly. The most prominent and useful finding on auscultation is a loud third heart sound, best heard with the bell of the stethoscope placed lightly over the cardiac apex with the patient in the left lateral position. During diastolic HF, however, a fourth heart sound is most common (Table 4). Systolic murmurs of functional mitral and tricuspid regurgitation may be present. Patients may have physical signs of congested lungs and pleural effusion if seen before treatment.

Laboratory Evaluation

B-type natriuretic protein

B-type natriuretic protein (BNP) is a cardiac neurohormone specifically secreted from the cardiac ventricles as a response to ventricular volume expansion and pressure overload. Currently, BNP elevation > 100 is considered diagnostic for detecting HF in symptomatic patients presenting with signs and symptoms suggesting HF. Several studies examining the utility of BNP as a possible screening marker to help detect asymptomatic early HF have yielded mixed results (Fig. 2) [15–18]. Three small studies have suggested that natriuretic peptides can be used as a guide to follow a patient's response to therapy [19–21]. BNP levels have been shown to predict future cardiac events (Table 5) [22].

Chest radiography reveals varying degrees of cardiomegaly and pulmonary venous congestion, ranging from pulmonary venous redistribution to frank pulmonary edema in the acutely ill patient. Kerley's B lines and peribronchial cuffing as signs of interstitial edema are common during the acute phase.

Electrocardiography (ECG) commonly reveals sinus tachycardia with nonspecific ST-T wave changes and an intraventricular conduction defect (IVCD). Other ECG abnormalities are shown in Figure 3 [23]. Holter monitoring shows a high incidence of

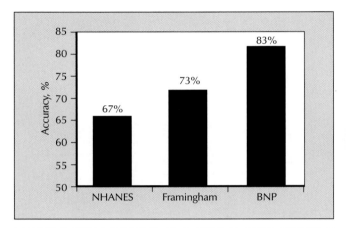

FIGURE 2. The utility of B-type natriuretic peptide (BNP) as a possible screening marker to help detect asymptomatic early heart failure. NHANES—National Health and Nutrition Examination Survey.

	Endpoint	
BNP	**Yes**	**No**
Increase	15 (52%)	14 (48%)
Decrease	7 (16%)	36 (84%)

TABLE 5 B-TYPE NATRIURETIC PEPTIDE (BNP) AND PREDICTION OF CLINICAL EVENTS*

*72 patients with class II–IV heart failure. Followed serial BNP levels and 30-day events (endpoint). Decreasing BNP levels = decrease events.

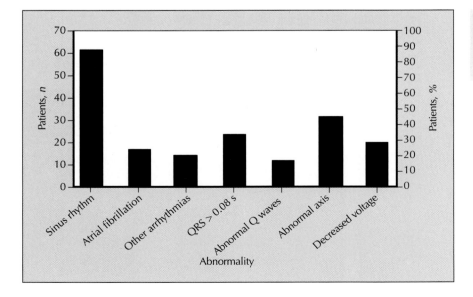

FIGURE 3 Electrocardiographic findings in a series of 74 patients with congestive cardiomyopathy. (*Adapted from* Kristinsson [23].)

ventricular extrasystoles, which are frequently complex. More than 70% of patients have multiformed ventricular extrasystole or ventricular couplets, and 30% to 70% have episodic nonsustained (≥ 3 beats in series and < 30 seconds) or sustained (> 30 seconds) ventricular tachycardia [24•]. Less common, but by no means infrequent, are atrial extrasystole and supraventricular tachycardia. There is no consensus that complex or frequent ventricular arrhythmias predict sudden (presumably arrhythmic) death, but they do appear to predict total mortality. At least one annual baseline 24-hour Holter recording with repeat monitoring is recommended. Unfortunately, an unremarkable Holter recording (≤ 1000 ventricular extrasystole per 24 hours) does not exclude the possibility of future sudden death.

Electrophysiologic studies may be helpful for patients with repeated runs of sustained monomorphic tachycardia or arrhythmia-induced syncope or near-syncope who have reliably induced ventricular tachycardia. In these patients, electrophysiologic study can be used to select the optimal antiarrhythmic drugs [7]. If these antiarrhythmic drugs fail to suppress the arrhythmia, the patient should have an automatic cardioverter/defibrillator device implanted.

The echocardiographic features of congestive cardiomyopathy are characteristic (Figs. 4 and 5; Table 6). Echocardiography is very useful for excluding heart failure secondary to a primary valvular disease. It is sometimes difficult to distinguish between this cardiomyopathy and ischemic left ventricular failure, because segmental wall-motion abnormalities characteristic of ischemic disease are also observed in cardiomyopathy. Radionuclide ventriculo-

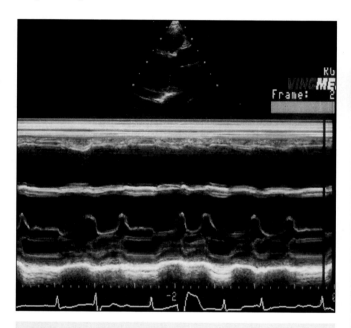

FIGURE 4 M-mode echocardiogram of a patient with congestive cardiomyopathy. The left ventricular (LV) and right ventricular (RV) cavities are dilated, and systolic motion of the interventricular septum and the LV posterior wall is decreased. Note the increased E–to–septal point separation. LV cavity in diastole = 60 mm; RV cavity in diastole = 35 mm.

TABLE 6 ECHOCARDIOGRAPHIC FINDINGS IN DILATED CARDIOMYOPATHY

M-mode

Increased diastolic dimensions of left ventricular and possibly right ventricular cavity

Decreased left ventricular fractional shortening

Decreased mitral valve opening in diastole

Increased E–to–septal point separation

Increased left atrial size

Pericardial effusion

Two-dimensional

Four-chamber dilation

Decreased ejection fraction

Possible mural thrombus (any chamber)

Pericardial effusion

Doppler studies (including color Doppler)

Demonstrate tricuspid and mitral regurgitation

Estimate pulmonary hypertension

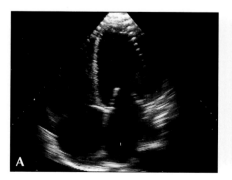
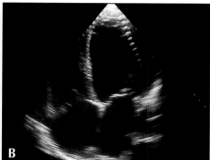
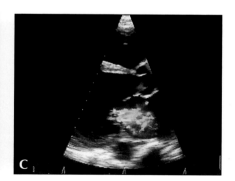

FIGURE 5 Four-chamber view in diastole (A), and systole (B) of a patient with congestive cardiomyopathy. Note the dilation of all four chambers of the heart. In a color Doppler study (C) the parasternal long-axis view shows functional mitral regurgitation.

TABLE 7 HEMODYNAMIC PARAMETERS IN CONGESTIVE CARDIOMYOPATHY

Systolic failure

Right-side heart catheterization
  Increased systemic and pulmonary vascular resistance
  Increased right ventricular end-diastolic pressure
  Increased mean pulmonary artery pressure
  Increased pulmonary capillary wedge pressure (reflects left ventricular filling pressure)
  Decreased cardiac index
Left-side heart catheterization
  Increased left ventricular end-diastolic pressure
  Increased left ventricular systolic and diastolic volume
  Decreased ejection fraction

Diastolic failure

Right-side heart catheterization
  Increased right ventricular end-diastolic pressure
  Increased mean pulmonary artery pressure
  Increased pulmonary capillary wedge pressure
  Decreased cardiac index
Left-side heart catheterization
  Increased left ventricular end-diastolic pressure
  Normal left ventricular systolic volume
  Normal left ventricular diastolic volume
  Normal ejection fraction

graphy is usually not needed unless the echocardiographic study is inadequate.

Cardiac catheterization is not routinely done unless a question exists of ischemic heart disease. Parameters obtained from right- and left-side heart catheterization are listed in Table 7. Endomyocardial biopsy is not useful except when a diagnosis of myocarditis or infiltrative disease is considered.

TABLE 8 NEW YORK HEART ASSOCIATION FUNCTIONAL CLASSIFICATION

Class I
No limitation during ordinary physical activity. Does not cause undue fatigue, dyspnea, or palpitation.

Class II
Slight limitation of physical activity. Ordinary physical activity results in fatigue, palpitation, dyspnea, or angina.

Class III
Marked limitation of physical activity. Although patients are comfortable at rest, less than ordinary activity will lead to symptoms.

Class IV
Inability to carry on any physical activity without discomfort. Symptoms of congestive failure are present even at rest; with any physical activity, discomfort is increased.

TABLE 9 DIFFERENTIAL CHARACTERISTICS OF THE CARDIOMYOPATHIES

Anatomic feature	Dilated	Hypertrophic	Restrictive
Dilated ventricular cavities	+	–	–
Dilated atrial cavities	+	+	±
Hypertrophied left ventricular walls	±	+	±
Asymmetric septal hypertrophy	–	±	–
Increased heart weight	+	+	+
Abnormally thickened intramural arteries	–	+	±
Intracardiac thrombus	+	–	±
Thickened anterior mitral valve leaflet	–	+	±
Myocardial fiber disarray	–	+	–
Functional			
Systolic function	D	I	N
Diastolic function	N or abnormal	Abnormal	Abnormal
Dynamic left ventricular outflow gradient	–	±	–
Systolic anterior motion of the mitral valve	–	±	–
"Square root sign" in ventricular pressure tracings	–	–	+

D—decreased; I—increased; N—normal.

Assessment of Functional Status

Severity of heart failure is estimated by clinical and radiographic examination, measures of ventricular performance (ejection fraction and serial hemodynamic parameters measured with right heart catheterization), and exercise capacity. All these methods have limitations when used independently. In practice, the most frequently used methods are clinical, radiographic, and echocardiographic.

Patients are often classified according to the New York Heart Association (NYHA) scheme (Table 8). This classification is relatively subjective, however, and only assesses functional capacity and the degree of disability. It is not a measure of the severity of left ventricular dysfunction.

Differential Diagnosis

The differential diagnosis includes all causes of congestive heart failure. Organic valvular or congenital heart disease usually can be readily differentiated; principal differential causes include coronary artery disease with ischemic left ventricular failure, restrictive cardiomyopathy, hypertrophic cardiomyopathy, pulmonary disease, rheumatic heart disease, and effusoconstrictive pericardial disease (Table 9). Heart muscle disease secondary to specific etiologies must be recognized early to enhance the potential for reversibility.

In coronary heart disease, there often is a history of angina or myocardial infarction. Electrocardiograms can show evidence of previous myocardial infarction but may be misleading, because Q waves are present in some patients

TABLE 10 PRECIPITATING FACTORS IN CHRONIC HEART FAILURE	
Precipitant	**Patients,** *n*
Lack of compliance	64
With diet	22
With drugs	6
With both (diet and drugs)	37
Uncontrolled hypertension	44
Cardiac arrhythmias	29
Atrial fibrillation	
Atrial flutter	7
Multifocal atrial tachycardia	1
Ventricular tachycardia	1
Environmental factors	19
Adequate therapy	17
Pulmonary infection	12
Emotional stress	7
Administration of inappropriate medications	
Fluid overload	4
Myocardial infarction	6
Endocrine disorders (thyrotoxicosis)	1

with congestive cardiomyopathy and normal coronary arteries on coronary angiography.

Clinical Course and Prognosis

The clinical course of congestive cardiomyopathy is usually steadily downhill over a period of 3 to 6 years, during which time progressive deterioration in exercise tolerance occurs and the heart size increases. (Data collected from the Framingham Heart Study between the years 1948 to 1988 indicate that the median survival was 3.2 years for males and 5.4 years for females.) Patients become increasingly refractory to diuretics, leading to escalating dose requirements and, in turn, progressive electrolyte imbalance and a further increase in plasma catecholamine levels. A sudden, symptomatic deterioration should alert the clinician to look for exacerbating factors (Table 10). The most useful means of following the clinical course of the disease is a careful history and physical examination, including body-weight measurements. Serial chest radiographs, echocardiographs, or both to evaluate increasing heart size are helpful.

The single most powerful prognostic factor is ejection fraction, and in patients with ejection fractions under 20%, the 1-year mortality rate is more than 50% (Table 10). Male gender has also been shown to be associated with a high mortality rate. Adequate total body magnesium stores serve as an important prognostic indicator because of an amelioration of arrhythmia, digitalis toxicity, and hemodynamic abnormalities [25]. When the NYHA class is integrated with maximal oxygen consumption during exercise, the mortality rate is 20% per year in patients in class III with a VO$_2$max of 10 to 15 mL/kg/min and rises to 60% in patients in class IV or VO$_2$max of less than 10 mL/kg/min [26••]. The distance walked in 6 minutes predicted both morbidity and mortality in the SOLVD trial [27]. Percent of predicted VO$_2$max achieved provides important information that can be used to stratify risk in the ambulating patient with heart failure with ischemic or dilated etiology that exceeds that provided by measurement of VO$_2$max have an excellent short-term prognosis when treated medically and heart transplant can be deferred [28•]. Half of all deaths from severe congestive cardiomyopathy occur suddenly, associated with a tachy- or bradyarrhythmia. Less common (but important) in patients who are subjectively well with less severe ventricular dysfunction is sudden death from a major thromboembolic event.

The treatment of HF consists of nonpharmacologic and pharmacologic management. Nonpharmacologic management consists of restrictions of salt intake to 2 to 3 g/d, regular exercise as symptoms permit, and treating a correctible cause of ischemia by revascularization and valvular disease (Fig. 6). Factors that contribute to the survivability of patients with congestive heart failure (CHF) are outlined in Table 11; associated causes of sudden death are addressed in Table 12.

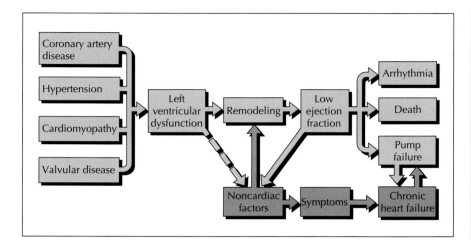

FIGURE 6 Management of congestive heart failure. The treatment of heart failure involves counteracting two related but largely independent processes. Left ventricular dysfunction, regardless of cause (coronary artery disease, cardiomyopathy, hypertension, or valvular disease), develops through ventricular remodeling that results in a dilated chamber with a low ejection fraction, leading to episodes of arrhythmia, progressive pump failure, and premature death. Noncardiac factors (neurohormonal stimulation, endothelial dysfunction, vascoconstriction, and renal sodium retention) may or may not be stimulated by left ventricular dysfunction, vasoconstriction, and renal sodium retention) may or may not be stimulated by left ventricular dysfunction, but ultimately contribute to the same progressive process of cardiac remodeling; the noncardiac factors independently cause the dyspnea, fatigue, and edema that are characteristic of the clinical syndrome of congestive heart failure. (*Adapted from* Cohn [29].)

TABLE 11 FACTORS AFFECTING SURVIVAL IN PATIENTS WITH CONGESTIVE HEART FAILURE

Clinical
Coronary artery disease etiology
New York Heart Association class
Exercise capacity
Heart rate at rest
Systolic arterial pressure
Pulse pressure
S_3

Hemodynamic
LV ejection fraction
RV ejection fraction
LV stroke work index
LV filling pressure
Right atrial pressure
Maximal O_2 uptake
LV systolic pressure
Mean arterial pressure
Cardiac index
Systemic vascular resistance

Biochemical
Plasma norepinephrine
Plasma renin
Plasma vasopressin
Plasma atrial natriuretic peptide
Serum sodium
Serum potassium
Total potassium stores
Serum magnesium

Electrophysiologic
Frequent ventricular asystole
Complex ventricular arrhythmias
Ventricular tachycardia
Atrial fibrillation/flutter

LV—left ventricular; RV—right ventricular.

TABLE 12 CAUSES OF SUDDEN DEATH IN HEART FAILURE

Underlying cause	Rhythm observed
Acute myocardial ischemia or infraction (coronary artery disease or embolus)	VT (usually polymorphic) or VF, bradycardia, EMD
Pulmonary embolism	Bradycardia, EMD
Embolic or hemorrahgic stroke	Bradycardia, polymorphic
Drugs prolonging QT interval	Polymorphic VT
Electrolyte depletion (potassium, magnesium)	Polymorphic VT
Hyperkalemia	Bradycardia Apparent VT*
Exaggerated vagal reflexes	Sinus bradycardia Complete heart block
Primary arrhythmia	
Ventricular tachyarrhythmias	VT, VF Sinus bradycardia
Conduction system disease	Complete heart block

EMD—electromechanical dissociation; VF—ventricular fibrillation; VT—ventricular tachycardia.
*Rhythms during hyperkalemia are frequently diagnosed as ventricular tachycardia. These may also be "sinoventricular rhythms" in which the prolonged conduction causes absence of apparent atrial activity and marked widening of the QRS complex.

Pharmacologic Management
Systolic dysfunction

Various circulating neurohormonal agents have a very important role in the pathophysiology of HF, but measurement of their levels is of little value in the routine assessment and management of patients with HF [11]. Myocarditis is a rare cause of rapidly progressive HF and requires myocardial biopsy to establish the diagnosis. There is no evidence that immunosupressive therapy is beneficial [11].

Goals for the management of systolic dysfunction are as follows:

1. Short-term goal: relief of symptoms and improvement of the quality of life; drugs include diuretics, vasodilators, and digoxin.
2. Long-term goal: prolonging life by slowing, halting, or actually reversing the progressive left ventricular dysfunction.
3. Prevention of life-threatening ventricular arrhythmias and systemic emboli.
4. Ultimately, the proper selection of patients for cardiac transplantation.
5. Cardiac rehabilitation.
6. New approaches.

Diuretics in patients with fluid overload can relieve circulatory congestion and the accompanying pulmonary and peripheral edema. Thiazide diuretics administered intermittently two or three times weekly may be adequate to maintain normal intravascular volume in mild states of congestion, but the daily administration of a loop diuretic such as furosemide is necessary when the congestion is more severe or when impaired renal function reduces the response to thiazides. In more resistant cases proximal tubular diuretics such as metolozone, 2.5 mg to 5 mg daily or intermittently given 1 hour before furosemide, may be effective while monitoring serum potassium levels [12••].

Vasodilators: Data from the V-HeFT I and II trials [11] established the role of isosorbide dinitrate (ISN) and hydralazine for patients with functional class II and III HF. Although angiotensin-converting enzyme (ACE) inhibitors are the cornerstone of treatment for heart failure, ISN and hydralazine should be considered when ACE inhibitors are not tolerated because of symptomatic hypotension, azotemia, hyperkalemia, cough, rash, or angioedema. Although the target daily dose in clinical trials was 300 mg of hydralazine and 160 mg of ISN, an initial dose of 5 to 10 mg of ISN three times daily and 10 mg of hydralazine four times daily should be gradually increased toward the target level as long as tolerated. A minimal 10-hour nitrate-free period at night should be maintained to avoid nitrate tolerance.

Digoxin: Although the therapeutic efficacy of digoxin in patients with HF and normal sinus rhythm has long been controversial, recent evidence indicates that drug therapy withdrawal can adversely affect symptoms of heart failure. The most recently completed trial by the Digitalis Investigation Group (DIG) showed no significant effect of digoxin on mortality but reduction in the hospitalization rate in the DIG group as compared with the placebo group [12••]. The dose of digoxin should be calculated according to creatinine clearance, and levels should be monitored in patients with renal insufficiency.

Inotropes: The use of dobutamine and phosphodiesterase inhibitors to temporarily improve cardiac output and renal blood flow is effective in lessening symptoms and relieving refractory salt and water retention. These drugs improve quality of life and decrease hospital stays, but long-term survival benefit is unclear and warrants further evaluation [30•]. A low dose of dobutamine (2–5 μ/kg/min) or milrinone (0.375–0.75 μg/kg/min) after a loading dose of 50 μg/kg is being used in severely decompensated cases as well as in outpatients for 12 to 24 hours, or continuous outpatient therapy in patients in whom weaning is difficult as an inpatient [11].

ACE inhibitors have a favorable effect on preventing the progression of left ventricular dysfunction [12••]. Current recommendations based on the SOLVD, SAVE, GISSI-III, ISIS-IV, V-HeFT-II, and CONSENSUS trials are to use ACE inhibitors for all patients with significant reduction of left ventricular ejection fraction (LVEF%) less than 30% unless contraindicated. The starting dose may be as low as 6.25 mg or 12.25 mg of capoten three times daily or 2.5 mg of enalapril every day with a goal to gradually increase the dose to a level that has been shown to reduce mortality (*ie*, 150 mg of capoten, 20 mg of enalapril, 20 mg lisinopril, or 10 mg of quinapril). Preliminary evidence from one trial suggests that ACE inhibitors may reduce the risk of coronary ischemic events and improve the endothelial dysfunction [31]. The selective angiotensin II receptor blocker, losartan, has all the benefits of conventional ACE inhibitors with an advantage in that there is no disruption of prostaglandin and bradykinin biosynthesis [32]. Treatment with losartan provides beneficial effects on survival [33]. Losartan and enalapril increase oxygen consumption at peak exercise (peak VO_2) in patients with CHF. This effect is synergistic when the two drugs are combined [34]. One advantage of the use of ACE inhibitors to relieve symptoms is that they tend to conserve potassium by reducing the secretion of aldosterone. Consequently, hypokalemia induced by diuretics can often be prevented without the need for supplemental potassium or a potassium-sparing diuretic.

Calcium channel blockers: The results of short-term studies indicate that heart rate–lowering calcium channel blockers can provide benefits for patients with CHF [35]. Some data suggest that these calcium channel blockers may regress left ventricular dysfunction [36]. Amlodipine may produce favorable hemodynamic and neurohumoral effects in the setting of left ventricular dysfunction [37]. The antioxidant activity of amlodipine may also contribute to its potential benefit in those with nonischemic cardiomyopathy and atherosclerosis [38]. Reduction in mortality from treatment with amlodipine suggests a possible benefit in the microvasculature [39]. Amlodipine promotes kinin-mediated nitric oxide production in coronary microvessels of failing hearts. This may partly be responsible for the beneficial effect of amlodipine in the treatment of patients with heart failure [40].

β-Blockers: Several trials using metoprolol have suggested that long-term β-blockade may reduce morbidity and mortality in patients with chronic HF [25]. Carvedilol, a second generation β-blocker with vasodilator ($α_1$-blocking) and antioxidant properties revealed a 65% reduction in mortality [26••]. Further studies suggest that in addition to its favorable effects on survival, carvedilol produces important benefits in patients with moderate to severe HF treated with digoxin, diuretics, and an ACE inhibitor [27].

The Carvedilol or Metoprolol European Trial (COMET) is a comparison study of two β-blockers: carvedilol 25 mg twice daily and immediate-release (IR) metoprolol tartrate 50 mg twice daily. Patients who received carvedilol had significantly lower all-cause mortality than patients who received IR metoprolol tartrate (33.9% vs 39.5%) (Table 13).

Angiotensin receptor blockers: The most recent study of angiotensin receptor blockers (ARBs) in HF, the Candesartan in Heart Failure-Assessment of Reduction in Mortality and Morbidity (CHARM) program, was designed to answer some very specific questions to better describe the role of ARBs in HF and show where ARBs fit into a plan for managing and treating patients with HF [41].

The CHARM program comprised three independent,

multicenter, randomized trials involving 7601 HF patients (NYHA class II–IV) with an average age of 64 to 67 years. The program included three groups of patients forming three distinct, autonomous trials (Table 14). The first trial, CHARM Added, included patients with left ventricular dysfunction (LVEF < 40%) who were already taking an ACE inhibitor. The second trial, CHARM Alternative, addressed whether candesartan is a reasonable choice for patients who are ACE-inhibitor intolerant (LVEF < 40%).

A third trial, CHARM Preserved, included patients with normal systolic left ventricular function (LVEF > 40%). Patients in each trial were randomized to either candesartan (titrated to 32 mg once daily) or placebo treatment, and all patients were followed for at least 2 years.

In CHARM Alternative, patients in the candesartan group were 23% less likely to experience cardiovascular death or HF hospitalization compared with those in the placebo group (40% vs 33%).

In CHARM Added, candesartan treatment in addition to standard therapy reduced the risk of cardiovascular death or hospitalizations by 15% relative to placebo treatment (37.9% vs 42.3%).

In contrast to V-HeFT, data from CHARM Added demonstrated a significant benefit for the triple combination of an ACE inhibitor, ARB, and β-blocker.

In the CHARM Preserved trial, results showed an 11% reduction in the primary outcome with candesartan compared with placebo (22% vs 24.3%). Thus, although previous studies supported ARBs mainly as an alternative to ACE inhibitors in HF treatment, the CHARM program findings clearly support the use of candesartan as part of combination therapy or in place of ACE inhibitor therapy for the treatment of HF, irrespective of LVEF.

Anticoagulants: Because thromboembolism is a potential complication with heart failure, many physicians administer anticoagulation therapy to patients with an ejection fraction of less than 20% or with an intracardiac thrombus [11].

Antiarrhythmics: With atrial fibrillation of new onset or uncertain duration an attempt should be made to convert to normal sinus rhythm. Failure to convert should then be managed with β-blockers, or in some cases, amiodarone [28•]. Occasionally, catheter ablation or modification of the atrioventricular node with a dual-chamber pacemaker is

---

TABLE 13 BENEFITS OF BETA-BLOCKADE IN PATIENTS WITH HEART FAILURE

Reduction of heart rate and blood pressure
Reduction of arterial and ventricular arrhythmias
Inhibition of sympathetic nervous system activity
Inhibition of the renin-angiotensin-aldosterone system
Improvement of ventricular structure and function
Protection from ischemic effects

TABLE 14 CHARM PROGRAM STUDIES

Study	Patient group	Goal
CHARM Alternative (*n* = 2548)	EF < 40	To determine whether candesartan is better than placebo for treatment of systolic HF in patients who are ACE-inhibitor intolerant
CHARM Added (*n* = 2028)	EF < 40	To determine whether candesartan is effective as add-on therapy to ACE inhibitors and beta-blockers in patients with systolic HF
CHARM Preserved (*n* = 3025)	EF > 40	To determine whether candesartan is effective in preserved-LVEF HF

ACE—angiotensin-converting enzyme; EF—ejection fraction; HF—heart failure; LVEF—left ventricular ejection fraction.

Cardiology for the Primary Care Physician

attempted for atrioventricular synchrony and improvement of congestive heart failure [42••]. Antiarrhythmic drugs are not recommended for ventricular arrhythmia in dilated cardiomyopathy except for the treatment of ventricular tachycardia. Amiodarone substantially reduces cardiac death and hospitalization in nonischemic patients with CHF better than other antiarrhythmic agents [43]. Radiofrequency catheter ablation is less effective for ventricular tachycardia in patients with dilated cardiomyopathy. Implantable cardioverter defibrillator (ICD) implantation in high-risk patients without symptoms is a feasible approach that may result in benefit in some patients. A large-scale randomized trial currently under way will determine the risk/benefit ratio of this management [44].

Cardiac resynchronization therapy: Cardiac resynchronization therapy (CRT) involves the use of biventricular pacemakers that are synchronized to each patient's intrinsic sinus rhythm. One pacemaker is programmed to stimulate the right ventricle with a conventional lead; the second stimulates the left ventricle through a coronary sinus lead.

The Multicenter In Sync ICD Randomized Clinical Evaluation (MIRACLE-ICD) tested CRT in combination with an ICD device in 369 patients with moderate-to-severe HF. The study showed that CRT/ICD improved quality of life and exercise duration in patients with moderate-to-severe HF [45]. A recent large-scale clinical trial, Comparison of Medical Therapy and Pacing and Defibrilla-

tion in Chronic Heart Failure (COMPANION), compared the effect of CRT devices, with or without ICDs, to optimal pharmacologic therapy in 1520 patients with moderate-to-severe HF. CRT devices yielded significant reductions compared with optimal pharmacologic therapy in the primary outcome, combined all-cause mortality, and hospitalization, regardless of defibrillator capabilities [46]. In addition, patients who received a resynchronization pacemaker plus defibrillator had a statistically significant reduction in all-cause mortality.

Transplantation: Heart transplantation should be considered in patient with heart failure refractory to drug therapy if there are no contraindications to the procedure (Table 15). Before labeling a patient refractory to medical treatment, however, physicians should step back and re-examine the patient for possible common errors in the management of HF, including other underlying medical conditions, infection, neoplasm, inadequate doses of medicine, and the treatment of diastolic versus systolic dysfunction. Cardiac transplantation improves the survival rate to about 60% after 6 years (Fig. 7).

Cardiac rehabilitation and exercise: Intense physical activity should be discouraged, but moderate exercise to tolerance should be strongly encouraged. Regular physical exercise corrects endothelial dysfunction and improved exercise capacity in patients with CHF [47]. A moderate-intensity home-based combined walking and resistance program for

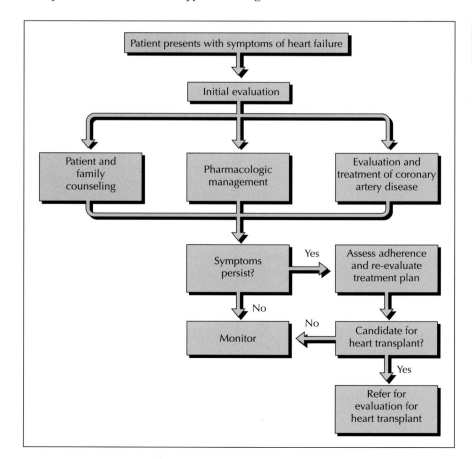

FIGURE 7 Evaluation of patient who presents with symptoms of heart failure.

patients with class II to III HF is safe and effective in reducing symptoms and improving quality of life [48]. Home-based intervention reduces out-of-hospital deaths and hospitalization in those with CHF [49] (Fig. 8).

New approaches and future treatments: Drugs that inhibit the sympathetic nervous system of the renin–angiotensin system (including ibiopamide, imidazole receptor agents, α_2 adrenergic receptor agents, neural endopeptidase inhibitors, atrial natriuretic peptide, BNP, angiotensin II receptor antagonists, modulators of sympathetic activity, growth hormone, interferon alpha-2, thymomodulin, and drugs that manipulate nitrous oxide generation, tumor necrosis factor, and calcium sensitizers) are in various stages of evolution as probable therapies for patients with HF. In the future it may be possible to stimulate the regrowth of myocardial cells or correct genetic abnormalities in patients with HF.

Nonpharmacologic approaches: Transplantation remains the definite surgical option for the failing heart. Five-year survival rates of 70% to 80% for patients receiving triple immunosuppressive agents have been reported. Surgical procedures, such as cardiomyoplasty, including that of the lastissimus dorsi patch, and the use of mechanical ventricular assist devices as a bridge, are encouraging; however, long-term benefit has yet to be determined [50•,51,52•,53,54].

Diastolic dysfunction

An ideal agent with purely neurotropic properties that selectively enhances myocardial relaxation without affecting left ventricular contractility or peripheral vasculature is not available. The goal of drug therapy in diastolic dysfunction is to reduce symptoms by lowering the elevated filling pressure without significantly reducing cardiac output. This reduction can be accomplished by the judicious use of diuretics and nitrates, avoiding dehydration and hypotension. β-blockers, ACE inhibitors, and calcium channel blockers have been proposed to improve diastolic dysfunction directly by augmenting ventricular relaxation or

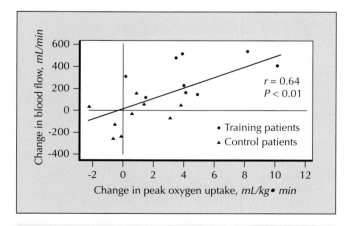

FIGURE 8 Change in peak oxygen uptake correlated with changes in endothelium-dependent peripheral blood flow.

improving compliance. Agents with pure inotropic actions are not indicated in patients with normal systolic dysfunction. Patients with diastolic dysfunction that is refractory to optimal medical/surgical management should be evaluated for heart transplantation [11].

Special Subsets of Congestive Heart Failure

Diabetes mellitus and heart failure

Type 2 diabetes mellitus substantially increases the lifetime risk of both developing and dying from HF. While this appears to be explained in part by the well-known association of diabetes witih hypertension, dyslipidemia, and coronary atherosclerosis, additional pathophysiologic mechanisms linking type 2 diabetes and HF have recently been suggested. These include the potentially adverse effects of hyperglycemia on endothelial function and redox state, effects of excess circulating glucose and fatty acids on cardiomyocyte ultrastructure, intracellular signaling and gene expression, and the possibility that diabetes may impair recruitment of the myocardial insulin-responsive glucose transport system in response to ischemia. Because many of these putative pathophysiologic mechanisms should be amenable to normalization of the diabetic metabolic milieu, strategies designed to more carefully control circulating levels of glucose and fatty acids might conceivably delay or prevent the development of HF [55].

Chronic obstructive pulmonary disease, arthritis, and heart failure

Patients with chronic obstructive pulmonary disease (COPD) may have left ventricular failure because of a coexistent cardiac disorder or right ventricular failure from pulmonary hypertension. An acute respiratory tract infection may precipitate right ventricular failure and should be treated. Alveolar hypoxia should be corrected by improving alveolar ventilation. Loop diuretics should be used cautiously. If bronchospasm is not present, β-blockers may be given to patients with COPD and left ventricular failure. ACE inhibitors should be used to treat left ventricular failure. Digitalis should not be used in patients with left ventricular failure due to COPD. Nonsteroidal anti-inflammatory drugs are contraindicated in patients with CHF. There are controversial data on the negative interaction between aspirin and ACE inhibitors in patients with CHF. Patients with arthritis and CHF needing larger doses of aspirin for pain relief may be treated with acetaminophen, tramadol, or Percoset if necessary for chronic severe pain [56].

Depression and heart failure

The prevalence rates of depression in CHF patients range from 24% to 42%. The selective serotonin reuptake inhibitors are recommended, whereas the tricyclic antidepressants are not recommended for depression in CHF patients. The combination of a selective serotonin reuptake inhibitor with cognitive-behavioral therapy is often the most effective treatment [57].

Skeletal muscle abnormalities in heart failure patients: relation to exercise capacity and therapeutic implications

Recent studies suggest that changes in the periphery, like those occurring in the skeletal muscles of patients with chronic HF, might play an important role in the origin of symptoms and exercise intolerance in this condition. Biochemical and histologic changes in the skeletal muscles of chronic HF patients relate to the degree of exercise intolerance better than hemodynamic parameters. A reduction in skeletal muscle mass represents another important determinant of exercise intolerance in chronic HF patients. The relationship between skeletal muscle changes and exercise intolerance sugests the possibility of modifying the peripheral changes in order to improve functional capacity in chronic HF patients. Recent studies have shown that the administration of ARBs can improve the properties of the skeletal muscles. Similarly, exercise training allows improvement in peak oxygen consumption, which parallels important biochemical and histologic changes in the skeletal muscles [58].

KEY REFERENCES

Recently published papers of outstanding interest, as identified in *References and Recommended Reading*, have been annotated.

•• Stelken AM, Younis LT, Jennison SH, *et al.*: Prognostic value of cardiomyopathy exercise testing using percent achieved of predicted peak oxygen uptake for patient with ischemic dilated cardiomyopathy. *J Am Cardiol* 1996, 27:345–352.

Showed that percent achieved of predicted VO_2max is a better predictor for long-term outcome, and that patients with more than 75% predicted VO_2max can be handled medically.

•• Cohn JN: The management of chronic heart failure. *N Engl J Med* 1996:490–498.

Recent review article on the management of chronic heart failure (CHF) clears up controversies in the treatment of heart failure as well as failure in the treatment of CHF.

•• Packer M, Bristow M, Cohn JN, *et al.*: Carvedilol US Heart Failure Study Group: Effect of carvedilol on morbidity and mortality in patient with chronic heart failure. *N Engl J Med* 1996, 334:1349–1355.

Carvedilol reduces the risk of death significantly as well as hospitalization for cardiovascular causes.

•• Packer M, Colucci WS, Sackner-Bernstein JD: Double blind placebo controlled study of the effects of carvedilol in patients with moderate to severe heart failure: the PRECISE trial. *Circulation* 1996, 94:2793–2799.

Indicates role of dual-chamber pacemaker in dilated or hypertophic cardiomyopathy.

REFERENCES AND RECOMMENDED READING

Recently published papers of particular interest have been highlighted as:

• Of interest

•• Of outstanding interest

1. American Heart Association: *2003 Heart and Stroke Statistical Update*. Dallas: American Heart Association; 2003.

2. Mancini DM: Pulmonary factors limiting exercise capacity in patients with heart failure. *Prog Cardiovasc Dis* 1995, 37:347–370.

3. Iriate MM, Olea JP, Sagastagoitia D, *et al.*: Congestive heart failure due to hypertensive ventricular diastolic dysfunction. *Am J Cardiol* 1995, 76:43d–47d.

4. Cuocolo A, Sax FL, Brush JE, *et al.*: Left ventricular hypertrophy and impaired diastolic filling in essential hypertension: diastolic mechanism for systolic dysfunction during exercise. *Circulation* 1990, 81:978–986.

5. Shehadeh A, Regan TJ: Cardiac consequences of diabetes mellitus. *Clin Cardiol* 1995, 18:301–305.

6. Young JB: Assessment of heart failure. In *Heart Failure: Cardiac Function and Dysfunction*. Edited by Colucci WS. Philadelphia: Current Medicine; 1995:7.1–7.20.

7. Kulick DL, Bhandari AK, Hong R, *et al.*: Effect of acute hemodynamic decompensation on electrical inducibility of ventricular arrhythmia in patient with dilated cardiomyopathy and complex non-sustained ventricular arrhythmia. *Am Heart J* 1990, 119:878–883.

8. Douban S, Brodsky M, Whong D: Significance of magnesium in CHF. *Am Heart J* 1996, 132:664–671.

9. Bittner V, Weiner DH, Yusuf H, *et al.*: Prediction of mortality and morbidity with a six minute walk test in patient with LV dysfunction. *JAMA* 1993, 270:1702–1707.

10.•• Stelken AM, Younis LT, Jennison SH, *et al.*: Prognostic value of cardiomyopathy exercise testing using percent achieved of predicted peak oxygen uptake for patient with ischemic dilated cardiomyopathy. *J Am Cardiol* 1996, 27:345–352.

11. ACC/AHA Task Force Report: Guidelines for the evaluation and management of heart failure. *Circulation* 1995, 92:2764–2784.

12.•• Cohn JN: The management of chronic heart failure. *N Engl J Med* 1996:490–498.

13. Gaasch WH, Izzi G: Clinical diagnosis and management of left ventricular diastolic dysfunction. In *Cardiac Mechanics and Function in the Normal and Diseased Heart*. Edited by Hori M, Suga H, Baan J, Yellin EL. New York: Springer-Verlag; 1989:296.

14. Vasan RS, Benjamin EJ, Levy D: Prevalence, clinical features and prognosis of diastolic heart failure. *J Am Cardiol* 1995, 26:1556–1574.

15. Luchner A, Burnett JC, Jougasaki M, *et al.*: Evaluation of brain natriuretic peptide as marker of left ventricular dysfunction and hypertrophy in the population. *J Hypertens* 2000, 18:1121–1128.

16. Smith H, Pickering RM, Struthers A, *et al.*: Biochemical diagnosis of ventricular dysfunction in elderly patients in general practice: observational study. *BMJ* 2000, 320:906–908.

17. Suzuki T, Yamaoki K, Nakajma O, *et al.*: Screening for cardiac dysfunction in asymptomatic patients by measuring B-type natriuretic peptide levels. *Jpn Heart J* 2000, 41:205–214.

18. Vasan RS, Benjamin EJ, Larson MG, *et al.*: Plasma natriuretic peptides for community screening for left ventricular hypertrophy and systolic dysfunction: the Framingham Heart Study. *JAMA* 2002, 288:1252–1259.

19. Kazanegra R, Cheng V, Garcia A, *et al.*: A rapid test for B-type natriuretic peptide correlates with falling wedge pressures in patients treated for decompensated heart failure: a pilot study. *J Cardiol Fail* 2001, 7:21–29.

20. Murdoch DR, McDonagh TA, Byrne J, *et al.*: Titration of vasodilator therapy in chronic heart failure according to plasma brain natriuretic peptide concentration: randomized comparison of the hemodynamic and neuroendocrine effects of tailored versus empirical therapy. *Am Heart J* 1999, 138:1126–1132.

21. Troughton RW, Frampton CM, Yandle TG, *et al.*: Treatment of heart failure guided by plasma aminoterminal brain natriuretic peptide (N-BNP) concentrations. *Lancet* 2000, 355:1126–1130.

22. Cheng V, Kazanagra R, Garcia A, *et al.*: A rapid bedside test for B-type peptide predicts treatment outcomes in patients admitted for decompensated heart failure: a pilot study. *J Am Coll Cardiol* 2001, 37:386–391.

23. Kristinsson A: *Diagnosis, National History, and Treatment of Congestive Cardiomyopathy.* PhD Thesis: University of London, 1969.

24.• Doval HC, Nul DR, Granceli HO, *et al.*: for The GESICA-GEMA Investigation: Nonsustained ventricular tachycardia in severe heart failure: independent marker of increased mortality of sudden death. *Circulation* 1996, 94:3198–3203.

25. Rhman MA, Daly PA, Hara K, *et al.*: Reduction in muscles sympathetic nerve activity after long term metoprolol for dialated cardiomyopathy. *Br Heart J* 1995, 74:431–436.

26.•• Packer M, Bristow M, Cohn JN, *et al.*: Carvedilol US Heart Failure Study Group: Effect of carvedilol on morbidity and mortality in patient with chronic heart failure. *N Engl J Med* 1996, 334:1349–1355.

27. Doval HC, Nul DR, *et al.*: Randomized trial of low dose amio-darone in severe congestive heart failure (GESICA). *Lancet* 1994, 344:493–498.

28.• Nishimura RA, Symanski JD, Hurrell DC, *et al.*: Dual chamber pacing for cardiomyopahty. *Mayo Clin Proc* 1996, 71:1077–1087.

29. Cohn JN: The management of congestive heart failure. *N Engl J Med* 1996, 335:490–498.

30.• Jennison SH, Dhar SC, Derfler MC: Outpatient use of continuous IV milranone in heart failure. *Congest Heart Fail* 1996, 2:15–20.

31. Yousef S, Pepine CJ, Grace C, *et al.*: Effect of cactopril on myocardial infarction and unstable angina in patient with low ejection fraction. *Lancet* 1992, 340:1173–1178.

32. Awan NA, Mason DT: Direct selective blocking of the vascular angiotensin-II receptor in therapy for hypertension and severe CHF. *Am Heart J* 1996, 131:177–185.

33. Sharma D, Buyse M, Pitt B, Rucinska EJ: Meta-analysis of observed mortality data from all-controlled, double-blind, multiple-dose studies of losartan in heart failure. Losartan Heart Failure Mortality Meta-analysis Study Group. *Am J Cardiol* 2000, 85:187–192.

34. Guazzi M, Palermo P, Pontone G, *et al.*: Synergistic efficacy of enalapril and losartan on exercise performance and oxygen consumption at peak exercise in congestive heart failure. *Am J Cardiol* 1999, 84:1038–1043.

35. Daterman KW: Intercenter variability in outcome for patients treated with direct coronary angioplasty during acute myocardial infarction. *Am Heart J* 1998, 135(suppl):310–319.

36. Bonow RO, Udelson JE: Left ventricular diastolic dysfunction as a cause of congestive heart failure. Mechanisms and management. *Ann Intern Med* 1992, 117:502–510.

37. Krombach RS, Clair MJ, Hendrick JW, *et al.*: Amlodipine therapy in cogestive heart failure: hemodynamic and neurohormonal effects at rest and after treadmill exercise. *Am J Cardiol* 1999, 84(Suppl 4A):3L-15L.

38. Mason RP, Mak IT, Trumbore MW, Mason PE: Antioxidant properties of calcium antagonists related to membrane biophysical interactions. *Am J Cardiol* 1999, 84(Suppl 4A):16L-22L.

39. Lui PP, Mak S, Stewart DJ: Potential role of the microvasculature in progression of heart failure. *Am J Cardiol* 1999, 84(Suppl 4A):23L-26L.

40. Zhang X, Kichuk MR, Mital S, *et al.*: Amlodipine promotes kinin-mediated nitric oxide production in coronary microvessels of failing human hearts. *Am J Cardiol* 1999, 84(Suppl 4A):27L-33L.

41. McMurray JV, Ostergren J, Swedberg K, *et al.*: Effects of candesartan in patients with chronic heart failure and reduced left ventricular systolic functions taking angiotensin-converting enzyme inhibitors: the CHARM Added Trial. *Lancet* 2003, 362:767–771.

42.•• Packer M, Colucci WS, Sackner-Bernstein JD: Double blind placebo controlled study of the effects of carvedilol in patients with moderate to severe heart failure: the PRECISE trial. *Circulation* 1996, 94:2793–2799.

43. Massie BM, Fisher SG, Deedwani PC, *et al.*: Effect of amio-darone on clinical status and LV function with CHF. *Circulation* 1996, 93:2128–2134.

44. Levine JH, Waller T, Hoch D, *et al.*: ICD use in patient with no symptoms and at high risk. *Am Heart J* 1996, 131:59–65.

45. Young JB, Abraham WT, Smith AL, *et al.*: Combined cardiac resynchronization and implantable cardioversion defibrillation in advanced chronic heart failure: the MIRACLE ICD Trial. *JAMA* 2003, 289:2685–2694.

46. Bristow M, Saxon L, Boehmer J, *et al.*: Cardiac resynchronization therapy reduces hospitalization and cardiac resynchronization therapy and implantable defibrillation reduces mortality in chronic HF: results of the COMPANION trial. Presented at *American College of Cardiology 52nd Annual Scientific Sessions.* March 30–April 2, 2003. Chicago, IL.

47. Hambrecht R, Fiehn E, Weigl C, *et al.*: Regular physical exercise corrects endothelial dysfunction and improves exercise capacity in patients with chronic heart faiure. *Circulation* 1998, 98:2709-2715.

48. Oka RK, DeMarco T, Haskell WL, *et al.*: Impact of a home-based walking and resistance training program on quality of life in patients with heart failure. *Am J Cardiol* 2000, 85:365-369.

49. Stewart S, Vandenbroek AJ, Pearson S, Horowitz JD: Prolonged beneficial effects of a home-based intervention on unplanned readmissions and mortality among patients with congestive heart failure. *Arch Intern Med* 1999, 159:257–261.

50.• Fazio S, Sabatini D, Capaldo B, *et al.*: A preliminary study of growth hormone in the treatment of dilated cardiomyopathy. *N Engl J Med* 1996, 334:809–814.

51. Dickstein K, Manhenke C, Aarsland T, *et al.*: Acute hemodynamic and neurohumoral effects of moxonidine in congestive heart failure secondary to ischemic or idiopathic dilated cardiomyopathy. *Am J Cardiol* 1999, 83:1638–1644.

52.• Moreira LF, Stolf NA, Braile DM, *et al.*: Dynamic cardiomy-oplasty in South America. *Ann Thorac Surg* 1996, 61:408–412.

53. Little WC, Downes TR: Clinical evaluation of left ventricular diastolic performance. *Prog Cardiovasc Dis* 1990, 32:273–290.

54. Stevenson WG, Stevenson LW, Middlekauff HR, Saxon LA: Sudden death prevention in patients with advanced ventricular dysfunction. *Circulation* 1993, 38:2953-2961.

55. Jagasia D, McNulty PH: Diabetes and heart failure. *Congest Heart Fail* 2003, 9:133-141.

56. Aronow WS: Treatment of heart failure in older persons. *Congest Heart Fail* 2003, 9:142-147.

57. Guck TP, Elsasser GN, Kavan MG, Barone EJ: Depression and congestive heart failure. *Congest Heart Fail* 2003, 9:163-169.

58. Nicoletti I, Cicoira M, Zanolla L, *et al.*: Skeletal muscle abnormalities in chronic heart failure patients: relation to exercise capacity and therapeutic implications. *Congest Heart Fail* 2003, 9:148-154.

27

Restrictive Cardiomyopathy

Jonathan E.E. Fisher
Edward A. Fisher
Martin E. Goldman

> ### Key Points
> - The hallmark of restrictive cardiomyopathy is abnormal diastolic filling of the ventricles, which are stiff because of fibrosis, hypertrophy, or secondary infiltration.
> - The classic Doppler echocardiographic finding is rapid diastolic ventricular inflow and early cessation of diastolic flow.
> - Differential diagnosis includes congenital, valvular, hypertensive, and pericardial disease (especially constrictive pericarditis).
> - Endomyocardial biopsy can differentiate restriction from constriction and other causes of heart failure.
> - Conventional treatment can temporize by relieving symptoms caused by restricted diastolic ventricular filling and subsequent passive right- and left-sided congestion.

Cardiomyopathies (diseases affecting the myocardium) are categorized as restrictive, hypertrophic, or dilated. Restrictive cardiomyopathy, the least common of these, is manifested by impaired diastolic filling of the ventricles, which are stiff because of fibrosis, hypertrophy, or secondary infiltration. Restrictive cardiomyopathies are more common in Africa, the tropics, and subtropics than in North America and Europe. The etiology of restrictive cardiomyopathy may be primary, including idiopathic, or secondary, resulting from a known cause or associated with a disease affecting other organ systems.

Right and left ventricular chamber sizes are usually normal, and systolic function may be preserved until late in the disease course. Wall thickness may be normal or increased, depending on the etiology [1]. Importantly, the diagnosis of restrictive cardiomyopathy is made in the absence of congenital, valvular, hypertensive, or pericardial disease, and it is essential to differentiate it from constrictive pericarditis as the latter may be surgically treated. Clinical presentation and hemodynamic data of the two may be very similar, but echocardiography, endomyocardial biopsy, CT, and MRI may assist in differentiating the two diseases (Table 1).

Idiopathic causes of restrictive cardiomyopathy include idiopathic restrictive cardiomyopathy, endomyocardial fibrosis, and eosinophilic myocardial disease. Common secondary causes of restrictive physiology caused by myocardial infiltration include amyloidosis (which is the most common outside the tropics), sarcoidosis, glycogen storage disease (including Fabry's disease), carcinoid, and hemochromatosis. Less frequently observed are fibroelastosis (in infants), tumors, pseudoxanthoma elasticum, and collagen vascular diseases.

CLINICAL MANIFESTATIONS

As a result of increased myocardial stiffness, intracavitary ventricular pressure increases with minimal increases in volume, causing diastolic dysfunction and systolic dysfunction. Patients may be asymptomatic, but because either ventricle may be involved, they can present with either right heart failure (jugular venous distention, peripheral edema, and ascites) or left heart failure (dyspnea, paroxysmal nocturnal dyspnea, or orthopnea). Because of the diastolic filling abnormality and limited ability to increase cardiac output, decreased exercise tolerance and fatigue are common. One third of patients with idiopathic restrictive cardiomyopathy may present with thromboembolic complications [2].

Presentation is very similar to that of constrictive pericarditis, which must be excluded. The degree of jugular venous distention correlates with the severity of disease. The most prominent jugular venous pulse is the rapid *y* descent. Jugular venous pressure may paradoxically increase with inspiration (Kussmaul's sign). Peripheral edema, ascites, and hepatomegaly are present late in the disease. A left ventricular apical impulse may be palpable in restrictive cardiomyopathy, but not with constriction. The first and second heart sounds are normal, and there is usually a third and, less commonly, a fourth heart sound. Low output late in the disease may be characterized by sinus tachycardia and weak peripheral pulses.

DIAGNOSIS

The most common and characteristic electrocardiographic (ECG) findings are low voltage (especially considering the usual increased verticular wall thickness), nonspecific ST-segment and T-wave abnormalities, left-axis deviation, and pseudo–myocardial infarction (Q waves mimicking infarction). Chest radiography often shows a normal heart size with signs of pulmonary edema, although an enlarged silhouette may be seen, often caused by atrial enlargement, especially in the presence of mitral or tricuspid regurgitation. There is no pericardial calcification.

M-mode and two-dimensional echocardiography generally confirm normal left and right ventricular size and are important in excluding hypertrophic cardiomyopathy and valvular heart disease. Both atria are often dilated, due to increased filling pressures, as are the pulmonary veins, vena cavae, and hepatic veins [3]. Unfortunately, ECG diagnosis of pericardial thickening is technique dependent (*eg*, gain) and does not correlate well with pericardial thickness of pathologic specimens [4,5]. Digitized M-mode echocardiograms analyzing instantaneous rates of change of left ventricular chamber and posterior wall dimensions have been used with some success to study left ventricular filling abnormalities and differentiate restrictive cardiomyopathy from constrictive pericarditis. The rate of maximum left ventricular posterior wall diastolic thinning is significantly slower in restrictive cardiomyopathy than in pericardial constriction [6], and the diastolic filling period and minimal dimension to peak rate of filling interval are prolonged in restrictive cardiomyopathy, but shortened in constriction [7]. Thus, ventricular filling occurs earlier and more completely in constriction than in restriction because of the latter's noncompliant myocardium.

With constriction, the abnormal pericardium impedes normal ventricular filling and elevates end-diastolic pressures, whereas with restriction, the abnormal myocardium elevates diastolic pressures. During inspiration, the right ventricle fills as its free wall bulges out; however, with constriction, this occurs at the expense of left ventricular filling. The rigid pericardial restraint inhibits diastolic expansion of the right ventricular free wall, and the pliant interventricular septum bulges into the left ventricle, limiting its filling. With expiration, the opposite occurs: the left ventricle fills as the septum bulges into the right ventricle. These respiratory variations in ventricular filling can be detected by two-dimensional and Doppler echocardiography.

Two-dimensional echocardiography can image respiratory variations in ventricular dimensions as well as the

---

TABLE 1 RESTRICTIVE CARDIOMYOPATHY VERSUS CONSTRICTIVE PERICARDITIS		
	Restrictive	**Constrictive**
Physical examination		
Kussmaul's sign	±	+
Apical impulse	+	–
Regurgitation	+	–
ECG		
Low voltage	+	+<50%
Pseudoinfarction	+	–
Atrial arrhythmias	+	–
Echo		
LV wall thickness	↑	nl
Ground glass myocardium	(amyloid)	–
Thickened pericardium	–	+
Doppler		
Respiratory variation	–	+
Hepatic vs diastolic flow	↑insp	↑exp
Hemodynamics	>5mm>	RVEDP=
LVEDP	RVEDP	LVEDP
Myocardial biopsy	abn	nl
Pericardial biopsy	nl	abn
CT/MRI		
Myocardium	abn	nl
Pericardium	nl	abn

LV—left ventricular; LVEDP—left ventricular end-diastolic pressure; RVEDP—right ventricular end-diastolic pressure; abn—abnormal; nl—normal; insp—inspiration; exp—expiration.

undulating interventricular septum characteristic of constriction. Other distinctive features of constriction include abnormal diastolic flattening of the left ventricular posterior wall and early pulmonic valve opening. Hatle et al. [8] used pulsed Doppler echocardiography to differentiate constrictive pericarditis from restrictive cardiomyopathy, demonstrating respiratory-dependent changes in inflow velocity filling patterns across the mitral and tricuspid valves in patients with constriction but not with restriction. Patients with constriction showed marked changes in left ventricular isovolumic relaxation time and early mitral and tricuspid velocities at the onset of inspiration and expiration, which were not seen in patients with restriction or in normal controls. Patients with restriction, however, were more likely to have diastolic mitral or tricuspid regurgitation, indicative of marked elevation of ventricular diastolic pressure.

Tissue Doppler imaging of mitral annular motion is a less preload-dependent means of assessing restrictive diastolic filling. With this technique, elevated left ventricular filling pressures are manifest with a severe < 8 ms and an E/E >15 [9].

Appleton et al. [10] studied 14 patients with restrictive myocardial filling using pulsed Doppler echocardiography. The most striking abnormalities of patients with restriction were the short periods (<150 ms) of mitral and tricuspid deceleration, indicative of rapid equalization of atrial to ventricular diastolic pressures and an early end to ventricular diastolic filling. In addition, deceleration time across the tricuspid valve was even shorter during inspiration than during apnea. Flow reversal across one of the atrioventricular (AV) valves in mid or late diastole (ie, diastolic mitral or tricuspid regurgitation) was seen in 11 of 14 patients because at end-diastole ventricular pressures were higher than atrial pressures. Hepatic vein flow velocities demonstrated a reversal of normal systolic (represented by x) to diastolic (represented by y) predominance. (Normally, both x and y are positive as they move toward the right atrium). In eight of 14 patients, systolic forward flow velocity intervals were less than diastolic intervals, and six had forward flow only in diastole. The inspiratory increase in venous flow reversal is a sensitive indicator of restriction of right heart filling.

Color-flow Doppler echocardiography has also been used to differentiate restriction from constriction. Mancuso et al. [11] studied six patients with restrictive cardiomyopathy and seven with constrictive pericarditis. They found moderate or severe mitral and tricuspid regurgitation in all patients with restrictive cardiomyopathy, but only trivial regurgitation in two control subjects and one patient with constriction.

Ultrasonic tissue characterization uses quantitative backscatter imaging to detect abnormal cardiac tissues and can identify the soft-tissue acoustic characteristics of the restrictive cardiomyopathies. Sound waves are attenuated and reflected differently by the denser fibrosed and infiltrated myocardium. Backscatter imaging estimates the amount of ultrasound energy reflected from the myocardium back to the transducer [12]. Backscatter varies through the cardiac cycle, with peak levels at end-diastole and lowest levels at end-systole [13]. Perez et al. [14] used the magnitude of cyclic variation of integrated backscatter to differentiate abnormal myocardium in diabetic versus normal patients. Similar application in patients with amyloid, sarcoid, and primary restriction may be useful in detecting cardiac involvement before ventricular function has been affected and when treatment of the cardiomyopathy may be possible.

Magnetic resonance imaging also has been used to diagnose restrictive cardiomyopathy. Although MRI demonstrates a thickened pericardium in constriction, suggestive findings of restriction include enlarged atrial chambers, thick ventricular walls, impaired ventricular filling (demonstrated by a prominent signal within the atria at all phases of the cardiac cycle consistent with stasis of blood secondary to elevated ventricular diastolic pressure), and normal pericardial thickness [15]. More recently, MRI flow mapping of the mitral valve has been used to assess numerous diastolic indices including early to atrial filling (E/A) ratio and E wave deceleration time. These have been validated by comparison with echocardiographic Doppler indices [16]. CT can detect the pericardial abnormalities of constriction [17].

Hemodynamic and angiographic evaluation during cardiac catheterization shows that both constriction and restriction manifest preserved systolic function, prominent and rapid decline in ventricular pressures at the onset of diastole, and a rapid increase in pressure, forming a dip and plateau suggestive of a square-root sign (Fig. 1) [18–20]. In restriction, left atrial pressure may exceed that of the right by 9 mm Hg, and left ventricular filling pressure usually exceeds that of the right by more than 5 mm Hg [19]. Also in restriction, the left ventricle is usually more involved than the right; with constriction, the abnormal pericardium constrains both ventricles equally. Thus, to differentiate restrictive from constrictive physiology in patients who have elevated end-diastolic pressures in both ventricles, a rapid intravenous infusion of saline will maximize the separation of left from right ventricular end-diastolic pressure only in restriction [21,22]. Pulmonary artery systolic pressure is usually elevated (> 45 mm Hg) with restriction and lower with constriction [23].

Coronary arteriography has been used to accentuate the pericardial thickening and lack of motion of major epicardial coronary arteries in most patients with constriction but not restriction [24]. In contrast to the major arteries, the septal perforators have an exaggerated motion in constrictive, but limited motion in restrictive cardiomyopathy [25]. Endomyocardial biopsy is the definitive method to differentiate restriction from constriction and other causes of heart failure; a specific etiology of restriction was identified in 15 of 30 patients studied with class III or IV heart failure, with 11 patients with amyloidosis [26]. Myocyte diameter, nuclear area, and severity of fibrosis can be measured on the biopsy specimen. Myocyte hypertrophy and interstitial fibrosis are frequently found in restriction as well as hypertrophic cardiomyopathy, but without the latter's myocardial disarray [27].

TREATMENT AND PROGNOSIS

Conventional treatment of restrictive cardiomyopathy is directed toward relief of symptoms caused by restricted diastolic ventricular filling and subsequent passive right- and left-sided congestion. Diuretics are used to reduce peripheral edema and ascites. Angiotensin-converting enzyme (ACE) inhibitors should be used with caution because they may reduce ventricular filling to an excessive degree, reducing cardiac output [28]. Digoxin should also be avoided because it may be arrhythmogenic, especially in patients with amyloidosis. With the onset of atrial fibrillation and loss of atrial contribution to cardiac output, decompensation often occurs. Attempts should be made to maintain sinus rhythm, and amiodarone may be helpful. If patients are at risk for thromboembolic events (atrial fibrillation and low cardiac output) they may benefit from anticoagulation. Calcium-blocking agents have been useful in treating diastolic abnormalities in patients with hypertensive or hypertrophic cardiomyopathy, but these agents also must be used with caution in patients with restriction because of their vasodilating effects. Glucocorticoid steroids and cytotoxic agents may play a role in specific causes of restrictive cardiomyopathy.

Patients with primary restrictive cardiomyopathy have a reasonably good 5-year survival rate, which may result from early diagnosis and recognition by noninvasive techniques. Of 26 Japanese patients, only two with idiopathic restriction died within 1 year, two died within 5 years, and 6 others died after 10 years [29]. Once the onset of heart failure occurs, however, mean survival decreases significantly. Mean survival has been reported to be 9 years after the onset of initial symptoms, but only 5 years following the onset of heart failure [30]. Of eight children studied (age range, 1 to 10 years), those having evidence of heart failure with systemic venous congestion and whose biopsies were consistent with idiopathic restrictive cardiomyopathy had a median survival of only 1.4 years [31].

PRIMARY CAUSES

Idiopathic Restrictive Cardiomyopathy

Idiopathic restrictive cardiomyopathy characteristically produces a modest increase in heart weight. Atria are enlarged and atrial appendage thrombi are often noted. A left atrial dimension greater than 60 mm carries a particularly poor prognosis [32]. Ventricular chamber size and wall thickness are usually normal, and systolic function may be normal. Patchy endocardial fibrosis is commonly noted. The disease is occasionally familial and may or may not be associated with distal skeletal myopathy [33–35]. There may be a genetic predisposition to this disease and, in some patients, a genetic locus associated with myopathic syndromes [36]. In children, in whom the prognosis appears to be worse than in adults, studies with very small

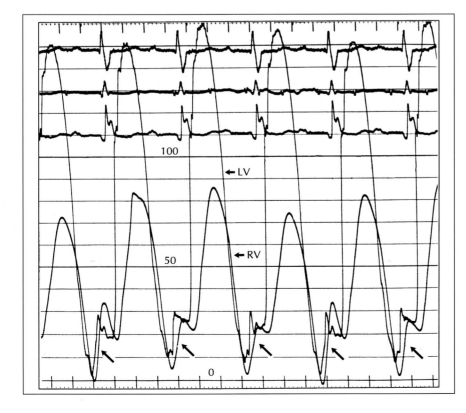

FIGURE 1 Restrictive cardiomyopathy. Hemodynamic tracings demonstrating a sharp pressure increase (*arrows*) in mid-diastole in both the left (LV) and right ventricles (RV). Note that diastolic pressures in the two ventricles are similar.

patient populations suggest that idiopathic restrictive cardiomyopathy may be more common in girls [37]. A review of the Mayo Clinic database found eight children with the disease between 1975 and 1993 [37]. Five of these patients who had pulmonary venous congestion at presentation had a median survival of only 1 year. The clinical course of idiopathic cardiomyopathy in adults is probably better [38].

Endomyocardial Fibrosis

Tropical endomyocardial fibrosis is a progressive disease that occurs most commonly in children and young adults living in Africa, particularly Uganda and Nigeria, as well as India, Brazil, and other tropical regions, where it may be endemic and cause up to 25% of deaths caused by heart disease [39,40]. Clinically, patients with endomyocardial fibrosis present with pulmonary and venous congestion. Pathologically, ventricular involvement predominates with extensive fibrous endocardial lesions of the inflow portion of the right and left ventricles and involvement of the mitral and tricuspid valves. Mural thrombi can occur in up to 41% of cases [41].

The ECG demonstrates ST-segment T-wave abnormalities, decreased voltage, and right atrial enlargement. Atrial arrhythmias are frequent. Echocardiography may demonstrate dilated atria, thickened right ventricular wall with obliteration of the apex, and increased echodensity of the myocardium. Thrombi may be seen in both ventricles. Varying degrees of tricuspid and mitral regurgitation are seen, depending on the extent of distortion of their respective annuli [42]. In contradistinction to Chagas' disease (in which an apical aneurysm forms), in endomyocardial fibrosis, the apex is involved with the fibrous process and preserved systolic ventricular function may be present.

Endomyocardial biopsy can confirm the diagnosis. Two-year mortality rate is approximately 50% [43], and medical therapy is not very successful. Surgical excision and stripping of the fibrous endothelial layer of endocardium and valve replacement have been successful, but this carries a high operative mortality (15% to 25%) [41,44]. In a recent study [45] of 83 patients who underwent endocardial decortication and AV valve repair or replacement, the actuarial 17-year survival was 55%. A transaortic approach to excision of apical fibrosis has recently been described and may offer the advantage of better visualization of the left ventricular apex then the classic transatrial approach; in addition, the risk of arrhythmia, dysfunction, bleeding and late aneurysm formation that accompany a transventricular resection may be avoided with the new approach [46].

Hypereosinophilic Syndrome

Hypereosinophilia (> 1500 eosinophils/mL) is seen as a response to parasitic infections, allergies and hypersensitivity, connective tissue diseases, neoplasias, autoimmune disorders, and cutaneous diseases. When no underlying cause is found, it is called idiopathic. The clinical diagnosis of idiopathic hypereosinophilic syndrome (IHES) connotes end-organ (heart, central nervous system, kidney, lung, gastrointestinal, and skin) dysfunction. IHES demonstrates a predilection for men (9:1), typically age 20 to 50. Cardiac involvement, occurring in approximately 50% of cases, is the most serious clinical presentation [47]. The disease may be caused by local deposition of toxic eosinophilic proteins, including cationic protein and major basic protein, which ultimately cause fibrosis (Fig. 2).

In 1936, Löffler described "fibroplastic parietal endocarditis with blood eosinophilia" in two patients with severe blood eosinophilia (70%), severe chronic congestive heart failure, and mitral regurgitation. At autopsy, there was extensive fibrous thickening of the endocardium of both ventricles with overlying thrombus in the left ventricle [48]. In 1948, Davies et al. [49] described patients with endomyocardial fibrosis in West Africa and noted that the mural endocardial fibrosis and thrombosis were mostly limited to the ventricular inflow tracts and often involved the posterior AV valves, decreasing their mobility. In 1956, Gerbaux et al. [50] suggested that endomyocardial fibrosis and Löffler's endocarditis were essentially the same disease, and indeed, autopsied hearts from patients with these disorders were found to be indistinguishable by Fauci et al. [47]. It is very possible that these disorders are the same disease simply seen at different stages of development.

The characteristic cardiac lesion of the hypereosinophilic syndrome is endocardial fibrosis and thrombus formation. Most evidence suggests that the endothelial damage initiates thrombosis. Large mural thrombi may occur in either ventricle, impairing filling and serving as a potential thromboembolic source despite preserved systolic function. The AV valves are often involved and become regurgitant. "Merlon sign" (basal hypercontractility on echocardiography) may be present and contrasts with the hypocontractile apex [51].

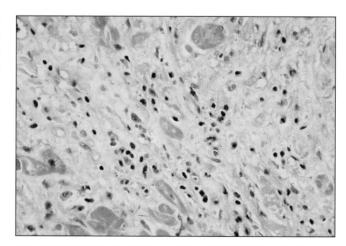

FIGURE 2 Hypereosinophilic syndrome. Endomyocardial biopsy demonstrating areas of scarring with mixed inflammatory infiltrate containing scattered eosinophils.

Magnetic resonance imaging may be helpful in establishing the diagnosis of IHES. Abnormally high signal intensity in the subendocardium in the T2-weighted sequence is suggestive of infiltration and may help direct biopsy acquisition. Cine MRI typically reveals regional hypokinesia and AV valvular regurgitation [52].

Heart failure and restrictive symptoms progress rapidly and medical treatment (*ie*, digitalis, diuretics, afterload-reducing agents, and anticoagulation) and surgical treatment may be beneficial. Glucocorticoid steroids and cytotoxic agents (hydroxyurea, interferon alfa) have improved the prognosis of patients with hypereosinophilic syndromes, which has traditionally been poor with only transient response to medical therapy [43]. After several anecdotal reports of its efficacy, Cortes *et al.* [53] studied the effects of low dose (100 mg daily) imatinib mesylate in nine patients with IHES; five patients responded within 4 weeks of therapy initiation, and four of these had a sustained complete remission. Imatinib is a selective tyrosine kinase inhibitor known to inhibit c-*abl*, *Bcr-Abl*, c-*kit* and platelet-derived growth factor receptor (PDGF) [53–55] and has shown efficacy in the treatment of Philadelphia chromosome–positive chronic myeloid leukemia [56]. Cools *et al.* [57] treated 11 IHES patients with imatinib and demonstrated sustained normalization of eosinophil counts for at least 3 months in nine patients. They also determined that many cases of IHES result from a novel fusion tyrosine kinase—FIP1L1-PDGFRa—that is the target of imatinib.

Secondary Causes

Amyloidosis

Amyloidosis is a systemic disease caused by extracellular deposition of insoluble amyloid protein fibrils that accumulate in tissues and cause pressure atrophy and dysfunction of the infiltrated organs. Cardiac involvement is the most common cause of death in primary amyloidosis [58], which is composed of an NH_2-terminal portion of an immunoglobulin light chain or fragment [59] (designated AL amyloid) originating from a monoclonal population of plasma cells, which may be derived from a malignant clone (Fig. 3). AA amyloid is found in amyloidosis secondary to various chronic inflammatory diseases such as rheumatoid arthritis, Crohn's disease, and suppurative processes such as tuberculosis, osteomyelitis, and bronchiectasis. Six types of familial amyloidosis (AF) involve amyloid-related transthyretin (prealbumin) [60]. Senile systemic amyloidosis (AS) has been found in the hearts of elderly patients at autopsy, and is usually not of clinical significance (Fig. 4) [61]. Of 153 patients with primary amyloidosis studied by Gertz and Kyle [62], 41% had cardiac involvement and 27% evidence of heart failure. These patients had the worst prognosis: median survival was 7.7 months and 5-year survival 2.4%. In contrast, the 48% of patients who presented with renal symptoms and primary nephrotic syndrome had a 5-year survival rate of 20%. Cardiac involvement is less common in secondary or familial amyloidosis [62], but cardiac deposition is common in senile amyloidosis (an autosomal dominant disease). It may contribute to diastolic dysfunction, which is commonly seen, or to significant systolic dysfunction, which is rarely seen (Fig. 4) [63]. In patients older than 60 years in the United States, isolated cardiac involvement is four times more common in blacks than whites, and 4% of blacks are heterozygous for an amyloidogenic allele of the normal serum carrier protein transthyretin (isoleucine substituted valine at position 122) [64].

Amyloid deposition between myocardial fibers may involve all cardiac chambers as well as the media of the intramural coronary arteries (Fig. 5) [65]. Patients may present with evidence of restrictive cardiomyopathy with venous congestion and congestive heart failure, arrhyth-

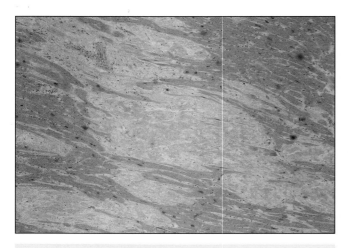

FIGURE 3 Cardiac amyloidosis. Nodular interstitial deposits of amyloid separating myocytes. This pattern is seen with amyloid light-chain amyloidosis.

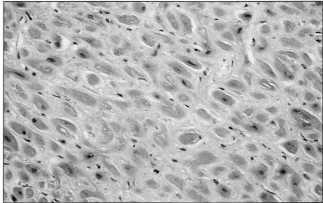

FIGURE 4 Cardiac amyloidosis. Interstitial pattern of amyloid deposition surrounding individual myocytes. This pattern is seen with senile amyloidosis.

mias, and orthostatic hypotension. Amyloid neuropathy, which occurred in 19% of the 153 patients studied by Gertz and Kyle [62] at the Mayo Clinic, may cause orthostatic hypotension. The ECG is important in the diagnosis of amyloidosis. In contrast to the thick walls observed by echocardiography, ECGs may show diffusely diminished voltage because of the replacement of normal myocardium by amyloid [65]. Left-axis deviation may also be seen. Atrial fibrillation and ventricular arrhythmias are seen, particularly in those with more severe infiltration. Ventricular conduction delays are the most common conduction abnormality, and premature ventricular beats are the most common arrhythmia.

Two-dimensional echocardiography is extremely sensitive for detecting cardiac amyloid. Assessment of patients with amyloidosis is based on M-mode and two-dimensional echocardiographic documentation of increased myocardial wall thickness, increased atrial septal thickness, increased right ventricular thickness, as well as the distinctive "ground glass" appearance of the myocardium. A total of 132 patients with biopsy-proven systemic amyloidosis were studied by Cueto-Garcia *et al.* [66] at the Mayo Clinic. The average age was 62.5 + 9.5 years, and 64% were men. A total of 58% of patients presented in congestive heart failure and 48% had M-mode fractional shortening of less than 30%, indicative of systolic dysfunction. However, left ventricular enlargement was seen in only 4% of patients. Using two-dimensional echocardiography, a granular, sparking appearance of the myocardium was seen in 47% of patients, and left atrial enlargement was seen in 61%. A totally normal echocardiogram was found in 19% of patients. Importantly, clinical congestive heart failure correlated strongly with greater wall thickness, ground glass appearance of the myocardium, and left atrial enlargement. Patients with the thickest mean ventricular wall thickness had the poorest survivor rates [66], especially mean left

ventricular wall thickness greater than 15 mm and mean right ventricular wall thickness greater than 7 mm [67]. Other echocardiographic markers of poor prognosis are right ventricular dilatation [68], and mitral E wave deceleration time of less than 150 ms [69].

The ground glass appearance of the myocardium, which has a greater impedance mismatch then normal interstitial material, may be caused by the amorphous amyloid deposition, which replaces collagen bundles in the myocardium [70]. Newer techniques of tissue characterization and quantitative ultrasonic imaging may identify the acoustic abnormalities of cardiac amyloidosis [12]. ^{201}Tl washout rate has been shown to be faster in amyloidosis and may have prognostic value [71]. MRI can confirm increased right atrial and right ventricular wall thickness, and lower signal intensity with both TE20 and TE60 in comparison to both patients with hypertrophic cardiomyopathy and healthy control subjects [72].

Although distinctive echocardiographic features are adequate evidence for the diagnosis of amyloidosis, definitive diagnosis is made by tissue biopsy. Abdominal fat aspirate is preferable to biopsy of rectal mucosa, gingiva, liver, or kidney. Transvenous endomyocardial biopsy of either ventricle confirms cardiac amyloidosis.

Clinical management of patients with amyloidosis is based on treatment of their symptoms. Diuretics are used to reduce venous congestion. Calcium blockers are relatively contraindicated because of their negative inotropic effect [73]. In addition, ACE inhibitors should be used with caution because they may significantly reduce ventricular filling and lead to decreased cardiac output. Patients may be sensitive to digitalis, which may predispose them to significant arrhythmias because of the selective binding of digoxin to amyloid fibers in the heart [65].

AL amyloid is typically treated with chemotherapy to eradicate the amyloidogenic clone and improve organ

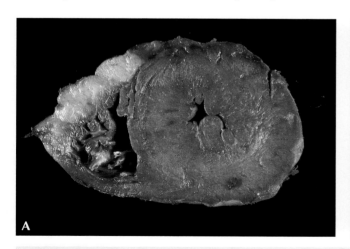
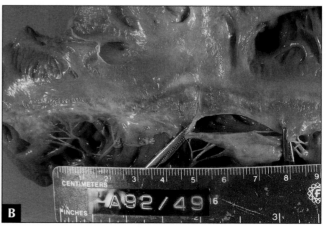

FIGURE 5 Cardiac amyloidosis. **A,** Cross-section through right and left ventricles (LV) demonstrating thickening of LV wall. The myocardium has a somewhat pale and waxy appearance.

B, Endocardial amyloid deposits of right atrium and tricuspid valve. Note the waxy appearance.

function. Melphalan and prednisone improved survival to 12.2 months compared with 8.4 months for colchicine treatment [74]. High-dose chemotherapy with autologous peripheral blood stem cell transplantation can be performed in selected patients with limited organ involvement to eradicate the plasma cell producing the amyloid protein. In a study of 25 patients, 68% were alive at 24 months [75]. Heart transplantation for patients with amyloidosis may be associated with an intermediate survival and potential recurrence in the allograft [76,77]. Dubry *et al.* [78] found that among 10 mostly AL-type amyloid-related heart transplant recipients, postoperative mortality was high (20%), and amyloid recurrence was common, occurring in six patients, between 5 and 60 months after transplant.

Reactive (AA) amyloid can be ameliorated with successful treatment of the underlying inflammatory disease process.

Familial amyloidotic polyneuropathy results from any one of over 80 described mutations of the transthyretin gene (*TTR*). Because *TTR* is synthesized only in the liver, liver transplantation (with or without concomitant heart transplantation) is often curative in this disorder [79].

Sarcoidosis

Sarcoidosis is a multisystem granulomatous disorder of unknown etiology, with an estimated prevalence of 10 to 70 cases per 100,000 [80]. The disease occurs most commonly in adults and is more common in blacks than in whites. Involvement is manifested by bilateral hilar adenopathy, pulmonary infiltrates, and typical cutaneous and ocular lesions.

Although cardiac involvement is clinically recognizable in only 5% of patients with proven sarcoidosis, pathologic evidence of myocardial granulomas is found in approximately 25% of cases. Antemortem diagnosis is made with endomyocardial biopsy, but a negative biopsy does not rule out the disease because of its patchy involvement. Noncaseating granulomas may infiltrate the myocardium, with the preponderant deposition in the left ventricular free wall and basal intraventricular septum, but also in the right ventricle, papillary muscles, and atria [80]. These granuloma eventually fibrose, and ventricular aneurysms may occur [81]. The clinical spectrum ranges from asymptomatic to arrhythmias (especially ventricular), conduction abnormalities, heart failure (right and/or left sided), or sudden death. Ventricular tachycardia may occur in 23% of patients with myocardial sarcoidosis [82].

The prognosis is much worse if myocardial involvement exists. The most common cause of death is sudden cardiac arrest, presumably on the basis of ventricular tachycardia and complete heart block. Patients also develop pulmonary fibrosis with respiratory failure and cor pulmonale [83]. Syncope may be common, either because of cardiac arrhythmias or pulmonary dysfunction.

The ECG may show repolarization abnormalities, ST-segment T-wave abnormalities, arrhythmias, varying degrees of AV block, and Q waves mimicking myocardial infarction [82]. Eighty-eight patients with systemic sarcoidosis were studied with two-dimensional echocardiography by Burstow *et al.* [84], who found that 12 (15%) had echocardiographic evidence of left ventricular systolic dysfunction (segmental wall motion abnormalities in eight and global dysfunction in four). ^{201}Tl has been used to detect myocardial perfusion defects in patients with sarcoidosis [85], and gallium scanning has also proven useful in detecting regions of myocardial involvement. However, Yamagishi *et al.* [86] studied the diagnostic accuracy of 13N-NH3/18F-FDG positron emission tomography (PET) in detecting disease activity among 17 patients with biopsy-proven cardiac sarcoid. The detection of ^{13}N-NH3 defects and/or increased ^{18}F-FDG uptake were significantly more sensitive markers for active cardiac sarcoid than ^{201}Tl defects and abnormal ^{67}Ga accumulation. Moreover, PET images were diagnostic for treatment response in seven patients after 1 month of steroid therapy.

Vignaux *et al.* [87] and Chandra *et al.* [88] demonstrated the utility of MRI in diagnosing cardiac sarcoid involvement and in accurately assessing response to therapy after 1 year; MRI findings closely correlated with clinical cardiac status.

The clinical manifestations of sarcoidosis are treated with appropriate conventional therapy, including heart failure medications, pacemaker implantation, and antiarrhythmic agents. Bajaj *et al.* [89] reported the use of an automatic implantable cardioverter defibrillator in a 31-year-old woman who had recurrent sudden cardiac death. She continued to be well at 18 months at the time of the report [89]. Because the 1-year mortality of cardiac sarcoidosis may be 60%, with many patients dying suddenly, consideration of aggressive investigation and management of the ventricular arrhythmias, including automatic intracardiac defibrillator implantation, may improve the overall mortality [83]. In addition, steroids may be beneficial in improving pulmonary and cardiac manifestations. Although heart failure is the second leading cause of death in cardiac sarcoidosis, transplantation is probably not a viable alternative because of the risk of recurrence.

Fabry's Disease

Fabry's disease (Fabry-Anderson disease or angiokeratoma corporis diffusum) is an X-linked disorder of glycosphingolipid metabolism caused by an enzyme deficiency (α-galactosidase A) leading to lipid deposition (ceramide trihexosidase) in the vasculature of various organs, precipitating myocardial, cerebral, and renal dysfunction. Accumulation of the glycosphingolipid in the lysosomes of the cardiac tissue can cause increased ventricular wall thickness, mitral valve prolapse, and ascending aortic dilatation [90]. In fact, Nakao *et al.* [91] found that among 230 consecutive male patients with left ventricular hypertrophy, seven (3%) had an atypical variant of Fabry's disease with isolated cardiac involvement. Although heterozygous females may have mild disease manifestions, hemizygous males develop symptoms early in life. Patients may present with parasthesias and typical skin lesions, which are small, erythematous, punctate, and blanching vascular lesions (angiokeratomas). Patients may develop congestive heart failure related to myocardial involvement, systemic hypertension, mitral regurgitation, or significant ventricular myocardial deposition simulating hypertrophic cardiomyopathy, as well as renal failure [92]. A case in which two sisters presenting with complete heart block and left ventricular hypertrophy (LVH) were found to have an atypical variant of Fabry's disease with isolated biopsy-proven cardiac involvement was recently described [93].

A patient with Fabry's disease who had evidence of endothelial infiltration of his coronary arteries presented with angina and myocardial ischemia and was treated with successful coronary bypass surgery [94]. Diagnosis of Fabry's disease is confirmed by a very low level of α-galactosidase activity and endomyocardial biopsy. Pieroni et al. [95] found that echocardiography tissue Doppler imaging (TDI) of the mitral valve annulus could detect preclinical cases of Fabry's disease. They found significantly lower systolic, early (Ea) and late (Aa) diastolic velocities, as well as lower Ea/Aa and higher E/Ea ratios among asymptomatic male mutation-carriers without evidence of LVH compared with healthy noncarrier control subjects. This technique may allow early screening and diagnosis before LVH develops.

The only specific therapy for Fabry's disease is recombinant human α-galactosidase A replacement therapy, which has clinically proven safety and efficacy in reducing lysosomal substrate storage. Therapy should be initiated early in all male patients with Fabry's disease and in female carriers with clinically manifest disease [96–98].

In Gaucher's disease, deficiency of the enzyme β-glucocerebrocidase results in accumulation of cerebroside in organs, including the heart, but rarely causes clinical cardiac problems or ventricular dysfunction [99]. However, Goldman et al. [90] have recently described the high incidence—30% of untreated patients and 7.4% of patients receiving enzyme replacement therapy (ERT)—of mild asymptomatic pulmonary hypertension (right ventricular systolic pressure 35 to 55 mm Hg) among 134 consecutive patients with type I Gaucher's disease screened by echocardiography. In that study, they found that several variables were associated with progression to severe pulmonary hypertension: splenectomy, poor compliance to therapy, family history of a sibling with Gaucher's and pulmonary hypertension, female gender, and an excess of the ACE I allele. ERT and vasodilators helped ameliorate cases of severe pulmonary hypertension [100]. Hurler's syndrome also causes a restrictive cardiomyopathy caused by deposition of mucopolysaccharide in the myocardial interstitium, as well as the coronary arteries and valves [101].

Carcinoid Heart Disease

Carcinoid heart disease occurs in 50% to 70% of patients with classic carcinoid syndrome and metastatic tumors [102]. Carcinoid tumor, most commonly originating in the appendix, secretes serotonin, which causes cutaneous flushing and bronchoconstriction. These tumors occur with an incidence of one to two per 100,000 per year in the United States [103]. Usually, serotonin is inactivated by the liver, but hepatic metastasis facilitates development of carcinoid heart disease. For this reason, hepatic dearterialization with chemoembolization or hepatic artery ligation is a current treatment option with variable success [104]. The right side of the heart is affected more than the left because of pulmonary inactivation of the humoral substances [105]. Grossly visible, focal, fibrous lesions can be seen on the mural endocardium of the right atrium, right ventricle, or left ventricle, and diffuse or focal thickening of the tricuspid and pulmonic valves can be seen with rare involvement of left-sided valves. Histologic examination reveals fibrous tissue devoid of elastic fibrils [106].

Two-dimensional echocardiography may reveal dilated right-sided chambers with a thickened, echodense, immobile tricuspid valve that is severely incompetent because of immobile leaflets. The pulmonic valve is also thickened and may be stenotic. Similar valve pathology has been found to occur in patients exposed to the methysergide ergotamine and most notably the anorectic agents fenfluramine and dexfenfluramine, leading the Food and Drug Administration to withdraw Fen-phen from the market [107]. Progression of carcinoid valvular heart disease correlated with clinical and biochemical markers [105,108]. Patients are treated with α-adrenergic receptors and serotonin blockers. Diuretics may be useful reducing the symptoms of severe tricuspid regurgitation. Surgical treatment of patients with carcinoid heart disease with replacement of the tricuspid and or pulmonic valve with heterografts has been successful [109]. Interferon treatment has been attempted with some success.

Hemochromatosis

Hemochromatosis results from excessive iron deposition because of increased iron absorption (primary hemochromatosis) or excessive transfusions or oral intake [110]. Two missense mutations, C282Y and H63D, in the HFE gene on the short arm of chromosome 6 are responsible for most cases of hereditary hemochromatosis (HH), although over a dozen mutations have been described [111–114]. Hemochromatosis is one of the most common genetic diseases, with a prevalence of 1:200 to 1:500 among Northern Europeans and as high as 1:100 in Ireland [115]. HH is inherited as an autosomal recessive trait leading to increased iron absorption, and clinical manifestations include skin hyperpigmentation, diabetes mellitus, cardiac impairment, arthropathy, and hypogonadism. Clinical sequelae result from deposition in the liver, pancreas, heart, and pituitary, causing fibrosis and organ failure.

Cardiac involvement is the presenting manifestation in about 15% of patients. Iron deposition is greatest in the ventricles, followed by the left and right atria [116,117]. Congestive heart failure is common and is the principal cause of death in untreated patients. The heart may be enlarged and misdiagnosed as idiopathic cardiomyopathy. The ECG may show ST-segment and T-wave abnormalities and arrhythmias, particularly supraventricular. Endomyocardial biopsy can document cardiac involvement. Patients with hemochromatosis have been successfully treated with venisection [118,119]. Chelation therapy has also been used successfully in the treatment of patients with congestive cardiomyopathy caused by iron overload [120]. The role of orthotopic liver transplantation in selected patients with hemochromatosis is currently under investigation in a multicenter trial [115].

Anthracycline Toxicity, Radiation, and Drug-Induced Fibrous Endocarditis

Anthracyclines cause a dilated cardiomyopathy, but the ensuing endomyocardial fibrosis can also result in a restrictive cardiomyopathy [121]. The diastolic dysfunction can appear years after treatment and may not be related to dose [122]. A growing body of evidence suggests that supplementation with glutamine may diminish the cardiotoxicity associated with anthracyclines [123] and there are limited data to suggest a similar protective effect of low molecular weight heparin [124]. Endomyocardial fibrosis can also be caused by drugs, including serotonin, methysergide [125], ergotamine, mercurial agents, and busulfan, and the diagnosis may require the performance of a myocardial biopsy [126]. Radiation can also cause myocardial and endocardial interstitial fibrosis and an ensuing restrictive cardiomyopathy.

CONCLUSIONS

Restrictive cardiomyopathy is the least common of the major primary cardiomyopathies; however, restriction should be suspected in patients with unexplained diastolic dysfunction. Two-dimensional and Doppler evaluation are frequently diagnostic, but endomyocardial biopsy is definitive. Unfortunately, therapeutic modalities are limited for management of most patients with restrictive heart disease. Because of the similar presentation of constrictive heart disease, however, which is surgically treatable, a full investigation of the underlying disease of a patient presenting with elevated end-diastolic pressure and suspected restrictive disease is warranted.

REFERENCES AND RECOMMENDED READING

1. Richardson P, McKenna W, Bristow M, *et al.*: Report of the 1995 World Health Organization/International Society and Federation of Cardiology Task Force on the Definition and Classification of Cardiomyopathies. *Circulation* 1996, 93:841–842.

2. Hirota Y, Shimizu G, Kita Y, *et al.*: Spectrum of restrictive cardiomyopathy: report of the national survey in Japan. *Am Heart J* 1990, 120:188–194.

3. Tam JW, Shaikh N, Sutherland E: Echocardiographic assessment of patients with hypertrophic and restrictive cardiomyopathy: imaging and echocardiography. *Curr Opin Cardiol* 2002, 17:470–477.

4. Voelkel AG, Pietro DA, Follard ED, *et al.*: Echocardiographic features of constrictive pericarditis. *Circulation* 1978, 58:871–875.

5. Plehn JF, Friedman BJ: Diastolic dysfunction in amyloid heart disease: restrictive cardiomyopathy or not. *J Am Coll Cardiol* 1989, 13:54–56.

6. Morgan JM, Raposo L, Clague JC, *et al.*: Restrictive cardiomyopathy and constrictive pericarditis: Non-invasive distinction by digitized M-mode echocardiography. *Br Heart J* 1989, 61:29–37.

7. Janos GG, Kalavathy A, Meyer RA, *et al.*: Differentiation of constrictive pericarditis and restrictive cardiomyopathy using digitized echocardiography. *J Am Coll Cardiol* 1983, 1:541–549.

8. Hatle LK, Appleton CP, Popp RL, *et al.*: Differentiation of constrictive pericarditis and restrictive cardiomyopathy by Doppler echocardiography. *Circulation* 1989, 79: 357–370.

9. Garcia MJ, Thomas JD, Klein AL: New Doppler echocardiographic applications for the study of diastolic function. *J Am Coll Cardiol* 1998, 32:865–875.

10. Appleton CP, Hatle LK, Popp RL, *et al.*: Demonstration of restrictive ventricular physiology by Doppler echocardiography. *J Am Coll Cardiol* 1988, 11:757–768.

11. Mancuso L, D'Agostino A, Pitrolo F, *et al.*: Constrictive pericarditis versus restrictive cardiomyopathy: the role of Doppler echocardiography in differential diagnosis. *Int J Cardiol* 1991, 31:319–328.

12. Skorton DJ, Miller JG, Wickline SA, *et al.*: Ultrasonic characterization of cardiovascular tissue. In *Cardiac Imaging*. Edited by Marcus ML, Schelbert HR, Skorton DJ, Wolf GL. Philadelphia: WB Saunders; 1991:886–895.

13. Vered Z, Barzilai B, Mohr GA, *et al.*: Quantitative ultrasonic tissue characterization with real-time integrated backscatter imaging in normal human subjects and in patients with dilated cardiomyopathy. *Circulation* 1987, 76:1067–1073.

14. Perez JE, McGill JB, Santiago JV, *et al.*: Abnormal myocardial acoustic properties in diabetic patients and their correlation with the severity of disease. *J Am Coll Cardiol* 1992, 19:1154–1162.

15. Sechtem U, Higgins CB, Sommerhoff BA, *et al.*: Magnetic resonance imaging of restrictive cardiomyopathy. *Am J Cardiol* 1987, 59:480–482.

16. Paelinck BP, Lamb HJ, Bax JJ, *et al.*: Assessment of diastolic function by cardiovascular magnetic resonance. *Am Heart J* 2002, 144:198–205.

17. Sutton FJ, Whitley NO, Applefeld MM, *et al.*: The role of echocardiography and computed tomography in the evaluation of constrictive pericarditis. *Am Heart J* 1985, 109:350–355.

18. Meaney E, Shabetai R, Bhargava V, *et al.*: Cardiac amyloidosis, constrictive pericarditis and restrictive cardiomyopathy. *Am J Cardiol* 1976, 38:547–556.

19. Shabetai R: Pathophysiology and differential diagnosis of restrictive cardiomyopathy. *Cardiovasc Clin* 1988, 19:123–132.

20. Benotti JR, Grossman W: Restrictive cardiomyopathy. *Ann Rev Med* 1984, 35:113–125.

21. Bush CA, Stang JM, Wooley DF, *et al.*: Occult constrictive pericardial disease: diagnosis by rapid volume expansion and correction by pericardiectomy. *Circulation* 1977, 56:924–930.

22. Pacold I, Hwang MH, Palac RT, *et al.*: The effects of rapid volume expansion on the right and left cardiac filling pressures after coronary artery bypass surgery. *Chest* 1988, 93:1144–1147.

23. Child JS, Perloff JK: The restrictive cardiomyopathies. *Cardiol Clin* 1988, 6:289–316.

24. Alexander J, Kelley MJ, Cohen LS, *et al.*: The angiographic appearance of the coronary arteries in constrictive pericarditis. *Radiology* 1979, 131:609–617.

25. Soto B, Shin MS, Arciniegas J, *et al.*: The septal arteries in the differential diagnosis of constrictive pericarditis. *Am Heart J* 1984, 108:332–336.

26. Schoenfeld MH, Supple EW, Dec GW Jr, *et al.*: Restrictive cardiomyopathy versus constrictive pericarditis: role of endomyocardial biopsy in avoiding unnecessary thoracotomy. *Circulation* 1987, 75:1012–1017.

27. Katritsis D, Wilmshurst PT, Wendon JA, *et al.*: Primary restrictive cardiomyopathy: clinical and pathologic characteristics. *J Am Coll Cardiol* 1991,18:1230–1235.

28. Bengur AR, Beekman RH, Rocchini AP, *et al.*: Acute hemodynamic effects of captopril in children with a congestive or restrictive cardiomyopathy. *Circulation* 1991, 83:523–527.

29. Hirota Y, Shimizu G, Kita Y, *et al.*: Spectrum of restrictive cardiomyopathy: report of the national survey in Japan. *Am Heart J* 1990, 120:188–194.

30. Siegel RJ, Shan PK, Fishbein MC, *et al.*: Idiopathic restrictive cardiomyopathy. *Circulation* 1984, 70:165–169.

31. Lewis AB: Clinical profile and outcome of restrictive cardiomyopathy in children. *Am Heart J* 1992, 123:1589–1593.

32. Ammash NM, Seward JB, Bailey KR, *et al.*: Clinical profile and outcome of idiopathic restrictive cardiomyopathy. *Circulation* 2000, 101:2490–2496.

33. Fitzpatrick AP, Shapiro LM, Rickards AF, Poole-Wilson PA: Familial restrictive cardiomyopathy with atrioventricular block and skeletal myopathy. *Br Heart J* 1990, 63:114–118.

34. Katritsis D, Wilmshurst PT, Wendon JA, *et al.*: Primary restrictive cardiomyopathy: clinical and pathologic characteristics. *J Am Coll Cardiol* 1991, 18:1230–1235.

35. Aroney C, Bett N, Radford D: Familial restrictive cardiomyopathy. *Aust NZ J Med* 1988,18:877–878.

36. Kushwaha SS, Fallon JT, Fuster V: Restrictive cardiomyopathy. *N Engl J Med* 1997, 336:237–242.

37. Cetta F, O'Leary PW, Seward JB, Driscoll DJ. Idiopathic restrictive cardiomyopathy in childhood: diagnostic features and clinical course. *Mayo Clin Proc* 1995, 70:634–640.

38. Benotti JR, Grossman W, Cohn PF. Clinical profile of restrictive cardiomyopathy. *Circulation* 1980, 61:1206–1212.

39. Valiathan MS, Balakrishnan KG, Kartha CC, *et al.*: A profile of endomyocardial fibrosis. *Indian J Pediatr* 1987, 54:229–236.

40. Gupta PN, Valiathan MS, Balakrishnan KG, *et al.*: Clinical course of endomyocardial fibrosis. *Br Heart J* 1989, 62:450–454.

41. Metras D, Coulibaly AQ, Quattara K: Recent trends in the surgical treatment of endomyocardial fibrosis. *J Thorac Cardiovasc Surg* 1987, 28:607–613.

42. Berensztein CS, Pineiro D, Marcotegui M, *et al.*: Usefulness of echocardiography and Doppler echocardiography in endomyocardial fibrosis. *J Am Soc Echocardiography* 2000, 13:385–392.

43. Barretto AC, da Luz PL, de Oliveira SA, *et al.*: Determinants of survival in endomyocardial fibrosis. *Circulation* 1989, 80(Suppl 1):177–182.

44. Valiathan MS, Balakrishnan, KG, Sankarkumar R, *et al.*: Surgical treatment of endomyocardial fibrosis. *Ann Thorac Surg* 1987, 43:68–73.

45. Moraes F, Lapa C, Hazin S, *et al.*: Surgery for endomyocardial fibrosis revisited. *Eur J Cardiothorac Surg* 1999:15:309–312.

46. Joshi R, Abraham S, Kumar AS: New approach for complete endocardiectomy in left ventricular endomyocardial fibrosis. *J Thorac Cardiovasc Surg* 2003, 125:40–42.

47. Fauci AS, Harley VB, Robert WC, *et al.*: The idiopathic hypereosinophilic syndrome: clinical, pathologic, and therapeutic considerations. *Ann Intern Med* 1982, 97:78–92.

48. Löffler W, *et al.*: Endocarditis parietalis fibroplastica mit bluteosinophile. Ein eigenartiges krankheitsbild. *Schweiz Med Wochenschr* 1936, 66:817–820.

49. Davies JNP, *et al.*: Endocardial fibrosis in Africans. *East Afr Med J* 1948, 25:10.

50. Gerbaux A, de Brux J, Bennaceur M, *et al.*: L'endocardite parietale fibroplastique avec eosinophile sanguine endocardite de Löffler. *Bull et Men Soc Med Hop Paris* 1956, 72:456–465.

51. Berensztein CS, Pineiro D, Marcotegui M, *et al.*: Usefulness of echocardiography and Doppler echocardiography in endomyocardial fibrosis. *J Am Soc Echocardiogr* 2000, 13:385–392.

52. Puvaneswary M, Joshua F, Ratnarajah S: Idiopathic hypereosinophilic syndrome: magnetic resonance imaging findings in endomyocardial fibrosis. *Australas Radiol* 2001, 45:524–527.

53. Cortes J, Ault P, Koller C, *et al.*: Efficacy of imatinib mesylate in the treatment of idiopathic hypereosinophilic syndrome. *Blood* 2003, 101:4714–4716.

54. Druker BJ, Tamura S, Buchdunger E, *et al.*: Effects of a selective inhibitor of the Abl tyrosine kinase on the growth of Bcr-Abl positive cells. *Nat Med* 1996, 2: 561–566.

55. Buchdunger E, Zimmermann J, Mett H, *et al.*: Inhibition of the Abl protein-tyrosine kinase in vitro and in vivo by a 2-phenylaminopyrimidine derivative. *Cancer Res* 1996, 56:100–104.

56. Kantarjian H, Sawyers C, Hochhaus A, *et al.*: Hematologic and cytogenetic responses to imatinib mesylate in chronic myelogenous leukemia. *N Engl J Med* 2002, 346:645–652.

57. Cools J, DeAngelo DJ, Gotlib J, *et al.*: A tyrosine kinase created by fusion of the PDGFRA and FIP1L1 genes as a therapeutic target of imatinib in idiopathic hypereosinophilic syndrome. *N Engl J Med* 2003, 348:1201–1214.

58. Gertz MA, Lacy MQ, Dispenzieri A: Amyloidosis: recognition, confirmation, prognosis and therapy. *Mayo Clinic Proc* 1999, 74:490–494.

59. Osserman EF, Takatsuki K, Talal N, *et al.*: The pathogenesis of "amyloidosis": studies on the role of abnormal gamma globulins and gamma globulin fragments of the Bence Jones (L-polypeptide) type in the pathogenesis of "primary" and "secondary amyloidosis," and the "amyloidosis" associated with plasma cell myeloma. *Semin Hematol* 1964, 1:3–86.

60. Varga J, Wohlgethan JR, *et al.*: The clinical and biochemical spectrum of hereditary amyloidosis. *Semin Arthritis Rheum* 1988,18:14–28.

61. Steiner I: Prvni popis "senilniho" amyloidusrdce-I. Soyka, 1876 [Eng abstr]. *Praha Cesk Patol* 1984, 20:11–13.

62. Gertz MA, Kyle RA: Primary systemic amyloidosis: a diagnostic primer. *Mayo Clin Proc* 1989, 64:1505–1519.

63. Pomerance A: Senile cardiac amyloidosis. *Br Heart J* 1965, 27:711–718.

64. Jacobson DR, Pastore RD, Yaghoubian MD, *et al.*: Variant-sequence transthyretin (isoleucine 122) in late-onset cardiac amyloidosis in black Americans. *N Engl J Med* 1997, 336:466–473.

65. Falk RH, *et al.* Cardiac amyloidosis. In *Progress in Cardiology*. Edited by Zipes DP, Rowlands, DJ. Philadelphia: Lea and Febiger; 1989:143.

66. Cueto-Garcia L, Reeder GS, Kyle RA, *et al.* Echocardiographic findings in systemic amyloidosis: spectrum of cardiac involvement and relation to survival. *J Am Coll Cardiol* 1985, 6:737–743.

67. Cueto-Garcia L., Reeder GS, Kyle RA, *et al.*: Echocardiographic findings in systemic amyloidosis: spectrum of cardiac involvement and relation to survival. *J Am Coll Cardiol* 1985, 6:737–743.

68. Patel AR, Dubrey SW, Mendes LA, *et al.:* Right ventricular dilation in primary amyloidosis: an independent predictor of survival. *Am J Cardiol* 1997, 80:486–492.

69. Klein AL, Hatle LK, Taliercio CP, *et al.*: Prognostic significance of Doppler measures of diastolic function in cardiac amyloidosis. A Doppler echocardiography study. *Circulation* 1991, 83:808–816.

70. Pinamonti B, Picano E, Ferdeghnin EM, *et al.* Quantitative texture analysis in two-dimensional echocardiography: application to the diagnosis of myocardial amyloidosis. *J Am Coll Cardiol* 1989, 14:666–671.

71. Kodama K, Hamada M, Kuwahara T *et al.*: Rest-redistribution thallium201 myocardial scintigraphic study in cardiac amyloidosis. *Int J Imaging* 1999, 15:371–378.

72. Fattori R, Rocchi G, Celletti F, *et al.*: Contribution of MRI in the differential diagnosis of cardiac amyloidosis and symmetric hypertrophic cardiomyopathy. *Am Heart J* 1998, 136:824–830.

73. Gertz MA, Falk RH, Skinner M, *et al.*: Worsening of congestive heart failure in amyloid heart disease treated by calcium channel-blocking agents. *Am J Cardiol* 1985, 55:1645.

74. Kyle RA, Greipp PR: Primary systemic amyloidosis: comparison of melphalan and prednisone versus placebo. *Blood* 1978, 52:818–827.

75. Comenzo RL, Vosburgh E, Falk RH, *et al.*: Dose intensive melphalan with blood stem cell support for treatment of Al amyloidosis: survival and responses in 25 patients. *Blood* 1998, 91:3662–3670.

76. Hosenpud JD, DeMarco T, Frazier OH, *et al.*: Progression of systemic disease and reduced long term survival in patients with cardiac amyloidosis undergoing heart transplantation: follow-up results of a multicenter survey. *Circulation* 1991, 84(suppl):338–343.

77. Dubrey SW, Burke MM, Khagani A, *et al.*: Long term results of heart transplantation in patients with amyloid heart disease. *Heart* 2001, 85:202–207.

78. Dubrey S, Simms RW, Skinner M, Falk RH: Recurrence of primary amyloidosis in a transplanted heart with four-year survival. *Am J Cardiol* 1995, 76:739–741.

79. Conraads VM, Colpaert CG, Van Hoof V, *et al.*: Systemic amyloidosis: diagnosis before treatment. *J Heart Lung Transplant*, 2002, 21:932–934.

80. Sharma ONP, *et al.*: *Sarcoidosis, Clinical Management.* Boston: Butterworth; 1978:4–7.

81. Temple-Camp CR: Sarcoid myocarditis: a report of three cases. *NZ Med J* 1989, 102:501–502.

82. Roberts WC, McAllister HA, Ferrans VJ, *et al.*: Sarcoidosis of the heart: a clinicopathologic study of 35 patients (Group I) and review of 78 previously described necropsy patients (Group II). *Am J Cardiol* 1977, 63:86.

83. Roberts WC, McAllister HA Jr, Ferrans VJ, *et al.*: Sarcoidosis of the heart. *Am J Med* 1977, 63:86–108.

84. Burstow DJ, Tajik AJ, Bailey KR, *et al.*: Two-dimensional echocardiographic findings in systemic sarcoidosis. *Am J Cardiol* 1989, 63:478–482.

85. Kinney EL, Jackson GL, Reeves WC, *et al.*: Thallium-scan myocardial defects and echocardiographic abnormalities in patients with sarcoidosis without clinical cardiac dysfunction: an analysis of 44 patients. *Am J Med* 1980, 68:497–503.

86. Yamagishi H, Shirai N, Takagi M, *et al.*: Identification of cardiac sarcoidosis with (13)N-NH(3)/(18)F-FDG PET. *J Nucl Med* 2003, 44:1030–1036.

87. Vignaux O, Dhote R, Duboc D, *et al.*: Clinical significance of myocardial magnetic resonance abnormalities in patients with sarcoidosis: a 1-year follow-up study. *Chest* 2002, 122:1895–1901.

88. Chandra M, Silverman ME, Oshinski J, Pettigrew R: Diagnosis of cardiac sarcoidosis aided by MRI. *Chest* 1996, 110:562–565.

89. Bajaj AK, Kopelman HA, Echt DS: Cardiac sarcoidosis with sudden death: treatment with the automatic implantable cardioverter defibrillator. *Am Heart J* 1988, 116:557–560.

90. Goldman ME, Cantor R, Schwartz MF, *et al.*: Echocardiographic abnormalities and disease severity in Fabry's disease. *J Am Coll Cardiol* 1986, 7:1157–1161.

91. Nakao S, Takenaka T, Maeda M, *et al.*: An atypical variant of Fabry's disease in men with left ventricular hypertrophy. *N Engl J Med* 1995, 333:288–293.

92. Cantor W, Butany J, Iwanochko M, Liu P: Restrictive cardiomyopathy secondary to Fabry's disease. *Circulation* 1998, 98:1457–1459.

93. Doi Y, Toda G, Yano K: Sisters with atypical Fabry's disease with complete atrioventricular block. *Heart* 2003, 89:e2.

94. Fisher EA, Desnick RJ, Gordon RE, *et al.*: Fabry disease: an unusual cause of severe coronary artery disease in a young man. *Ann Intern Med* 1992, 117:221–223.

95. Pieroni M, *et al.*: Early detection of Fabry cardiomyopathy by tissue Doppler imaging. *J Am Coll Cardiol* 2003, 41(6 Suppl B):415.

96. Desnick RJ, Brady R, Barranger J, *et al.*: Fabry disease, an under-recognized multisystemic disorder: expert recommendations for diagnosis, management, and enzyme replacement therapy. *Ann Intern Med* 2003, 138:338–346.

97. Schiffmann R, Kopp JB, Austin HA III, *et al.*: Enzyme replacement therapy in Fabry disease: a randomized controlled trial. *JAMA* 2001, 285:2743–2749.

98. Eng CM, Guffon N, Wilcox WR, *et al.*: Safety and efficacy of recombinant human alpha-galactosidase A–replacement therapy in Fabry's disease. *N Engl J Med* 2001, 345:9–16.

99. Smith RL, Hutchins GM, Sack GH Jr, Ridolfi RL: Unusual cardiac, renal and pulmonary involvement in Gaucher's disease: interstitial glucocerebrocidase accumulation, pulmonary hypertension and fatal bone marrow embolization. *Am J Med* 1978, 65:352–360.

100. Mistry PK, Sirrs S, Chan A, *et al.*: Pulmonary hypertension in type 1 Gaucher's disease: genetic and epigenetic determinants of phenotype and response to therapy. *Mol Genet Metab* 2002, 77:91–98.

101. Renteria VG, Ferrans VJ, Roberts WC: The heart in the Hurler syndrome: gross, histologic and ultrastructural observations in five necropsy cases. *Am J Cardiol* 1976, 38:487–501.

102. Lundin L, Hansson HE, Landelius J, *et al.*: Surgical treatment of carcinoid heart disease. *J Thorac Cardiovasc Surg* 1990, 100:552–561.

103. Moertel CG, Weiland LH, Nagorney DM, Dockerty MB: Carcinoid tumor of the appendix: treatment and prognosis. *N Engl J Med* 1987, 317:1699–1701.

104. Moller JE, Connolly HM, Rubin J, *et al.*: Factors associated with progression of carcinoid heart disease. *N Engl J Med* 2003, 348:1005–1015.

105. Millward JJ, Blake MP, Byrne MJ, *et al.*: Left heart involvement with cardiac shunt complicating carcinoid heart disease. *Aust NZ J Med* 1989, 19:716.

106. Ross EM, Roberts WC: The carcinoid syndrome: comparison of 21 necropsy subjects with carcinoid heart disease to 15 necropsy subjects without carcinoid heart disease. *Am J Med* 1985, 79:339–354.

107. Pritchett AM, Morrison JF, Edwards WD, *et al.*: Valvular heart disease in patients taking pergolide. *Mayo Clin Proc* 2002, 77:1280–1286.

108. Denney WD, Kemp WE, Anthony LB, *et al.*: Echo and biochemical evaluation of the development and progression of carcinoid heart disease. *J Am Coll Cardiol* 1998, 32:1017–1022.

109. Lundin L, Landelius J, Andren B, *et al.*: Transesophageal echocardiography improves the value of cardiac ultrasound in patients with carcinoid heart disease. *Br Heart J* 1990, 64:190–194.

110. McLaren GD, Muir WA, Kellermeyer RW, *et al.*: Iron overload disorders: natural history, pathogenesis, diagnosis and therapy. *CRC Crit Rev Clin Lab Sci* 1983,19:205–266.

111. Pietrangelo A, Camaschella C: Molecular genetics and control of iron metabolism in hemochromatosis. *Haematologica* 1998, 83:456–461.

112. Burke W, Thomson E, Khoury MJ, *et al.*: Hereditary hemochromatosis: gene discovery and its implications for population-based screening. *JAMA* 1998, 280:172–178.

113. Cazzola M: Novel genes, proteins, and inherited disorders of iron overload: iron metabolism is less boring than thought. *Haematologica* 2002, 87:115–116.

114. Camaschella C, Roetto A, De Gobbi M: Genetic haemochromatosis: genes and mutations associated with iron loading. *Best Pract Res Clin Haematol* 2002, 15:261–276.

115. Whittington CA, Kowdley KV: Haemochromatosis [review]. *Aliment Pharmacol Ther* 2002, 16:1963–1975.

116. Short EM, Winkle RA, Billingham ME, *et al.*: Myocardial involvement in idiopathic hemochromatosis: morphologic and clinical improvement following venisection. *Am J Med* 1981, 70:1275–1279.

117. Vigorita VJ, Hutchins GM: Cardiac conduction system in hemochromatosis: clinical and pathologic features of six patients. *Am J Cardiol* 1979, 44:418–423.

118. Evans J, *et al.*: Treatment of heart failure in hemochromatosis. *Br Med J* 1979, 1:1075–1078.

119. Easley RM, Schreiner BF, Yu PN, *et al.*: Reversible cardiomyopathy associated with hemochromatosis. *N Engl J Med* 1972, 287:866–867.

120. Rahko PS, Salerni R, Uretsky BF, *et al.*: Successful reversal by chelation therapy of congestive cardiomyopathy due to iron overload. *J Am Coll Cardiol* 1986 8:436–440.

121. Mortensen SA, Olsen HS, Baandup U: Chronic anthracycline cardiotoxicity: haemodynamic and histopathological manifestations suggesting a restrictive endomyocardial disease. *Br Heart J* 1986, 55:274–282.

122. Bu'Lock FA, Mott MG, Oakhill A, Martin RP: Left ventricular diastolic function after anthracycline chemotherapy in childhood: relation with systolic function, symptoms, and pathophysiology. *Br Heart J* 1995, 73:340–350.

123. Savarese DM, Savy G, Vahdat L, *et al.*: Prevention of chemotherapy and radiation toxicity with glutamine. *Cancer Treat Rev* 2003, 29:501–513.

124. Deepa PR, Varalakshmi P: Protective effect of low molecular weight heparin on oxidative injury and cellular abnormalities in adriamycin-induced cardiac and hepatic toxicity. *Chem Biol Interact* 2003, 146:201–210.

125. Mason JW, Billingham ME, Friedman JP: Methysergide-induced heart disease: a case of multivalvular and myocardial fibrosis. *Circulation* 1977, 56:889–890.

126. Billingham ME: Pharmacotoxic myocardial disease: an endomyocardial study. *Heart Vessels Suppl* 1985, 1:278–282.

28

Infectious Myocarditis

Nagib T. Chalfoun
Martin E. Goldman

Key Points
- Infectious myocarditis has an acute phase with a clinical spectrum ranging from no symptoms to severe heart failure.
- The chronic phase of illness may result from autoimmune mechanisms triggered by the initial infection without residual evidence of the inciting agent.
- Endomyocardial biopsies have limited value in most patients and should be reserved for specific subgroups.
- The value of immunosuppressive therapy has not been established.
- Therapy should be directed to the inciting infectious agent if specific therapy is available and to alleviating symptoms of heart failure and treating arrhythmias if life-threatening.

Myocarditis is an inflammation of the muscle of the heart, primarily associated with an infectious agent, although other substances may also precipitate an inflammatory response by the myocardium. Although most episodes of infectious myocarditis are clinically silent and resolve spontaneously, noninvasive technologies, such as cardiac ultrasound, enable recognition and diagnosis of even mild, asymptomatic cases. However, the other end of the spectrum of myocarditis is an acute presentation with severe heart failure. In addition, some patients may develop dilated cardiomyopathy years after their silent episode of myocarditis. Because of its varied presentation, the actual incidence of infectious myocarditis is difficult to assess. The estimated incidence of cardiac involvement in all viral infections is 5% [1]. The mean annual incidence of acute infectious myocarditis in a defined subpopulation (Finnish Military conscripts) was 0.02%, confirmed by myocardial enzyme release and serially evolving ECG changes [2]. Recent findings of elevated high-sensitivity C-reactive protein, serum amyloid A, interleukin-6, and soluble intercellular adhesion molecule type 1 (ICAM-1), markers of inflammation, have heightened interest in the possible relation of chronic or remote infection and atherosclerosis [3].

DISEASE MECHANISM

In animal models, viral myocarditis is a two-component disease with an initial phase of direct cytopathogenic myocardial damage, viral replication, minimal myocyte necrosis or cellular infiltrate. The infectious phase may last 7 to 14 days, usually followed by a complete recovery. A second phase that develops as the virus is cleared involves activation of the immune response against a myocardial or viral shared antigen, resulting in myocyte destruction and ultimately congestive failure [2]. A cellular mechanism is the principal immune response causing cardiac dysfunction. Recognition of an immunogenic epitope by antigen-specific T lymphocytes leads to macrophage and lymphocyte infiltration. T cells of the CD4 phenotype are responsible for the recognition, activation, proliferation, and differentiation of subgroups of effect, or lymphocytes. This immune response leads to a release of inflammatory cytokines, including interferon gamma, tumor necrosis factor, interleukins (ILs)-2, -3, -4, -5, -6, and -10. These cytokines lead to differentiation of B lymphocytes into antibody-secreting plasma cells and T lymphocytes into CD4 cells and cytotoxic CD8 cells. The latter attach to the target cells and lyse them by disrupting their plasma membrane and their DNA. Adhesion cell activation is essential for leukocyte activation and lymphocytic endothelial cell interaction, which precedes transendothelial migration. Monocytes are differentiated into activated macrophages, which release damaging proteases and cytokines. Cardiac dendritic cells and macrophages are in front of the inflammation, and T cells are found at a distance from the necrotic areas. Myocarditis induced by group B coxsackievirus is characterized by scattered foci of myocardial necrosis and infection of myocytes by the virus. Then the virus is undetectable in the myocardium and a mononuclear cell infiltration (macrophages, T lymphocytes, and natural killer cells) appears. In the chronic phase, macrophages and T cells are abundant, but the virus itself is not found. Cardiac dysfunction may be caused by the number of damaged and necrosed contractile myocytes, densensitization of cardiac β-adrenergic receptors, and modification of the regulatory protein Gi, uncoupling

TABLE 1 INFECTIOUS ETIOLOGIES OF MYOCARDITIS

Viral	**Bacterial**	**Metazoal**
Adenovirus	*Bacteroides fragilis*	Cysticercosis
Coxsackievirus	*Bartonella henselae*	*Echinococcus*
Cytomegalovirus	Brucellosis	Schistosomiasis
Echovirus	Clostridia	Trichinosis
Epstein-Barr virus	*Chlamydia pneumoniae*	
Hepatitis	*Chlamydia psitacci*	**Fungal**
Human immunodeficiency virus	*Chlamydia trachomatis*	Actinomycosis
Influenza	*Coxiella burnetti* (Q fever)	Aspergillosis
Mumps	Diphtheria	Blastomycosis
Mycoplasma pneumoniae	Ehrlichiosis (*Anaplasma phagocytophila*)	Candidiasis
Poliomyelitis	Endocarditis-associated myocarditis	Histoplasmosis
Rabies	*Escherichia coli*	
Retrovirus	Gonococcus	**Rickettsial**
Rubella	*Klebsiella*	Q fever
Rubeola	*Listeria*	Rocky Mountain spotted fever
Varicella	*Mycoplasma pneumoniae*	Typhus
	Meningococcus	
	Proteus	
	Pseudomonas	
	Rickettsia	
	Salmonella typhi	
	Staphylococcus	
	Streptococcus	
	Tuberculosis	
	Spirochetal	
	Leptospirosis	
	Lyme disease	
	Syphilis	
	Protozoal	
	Amebiasis	
	Chagas' disease (*Trypanosoma cruzi*)	
	Toxoplasmosis	

adrenergic receptors [4]. Sole and Liu [5] have proposed a multifactorial mechanism of myocarditis, including repetitive cycles of microvascular constriction and spasm and reperfusion, which causes dissolution of the myocardial matrix and diffuse loss of cardiac muscle mass, ultimately leading to myocardial failure.

CLINICAL PRESENTATION AND DIAGNOSIS

Myocarditis can be caused by a bacterial, fungal, parasitic, rickettsial, or spirochetal organism, but viral agents are the most common infectious etiology (Table 1). The family of enteroviruses appear to be the major pathogens responsible, with more than 50% of human cases attributable to Coxsackie B virus [6]. In the 10-year period from 1975 through 1985, the World Health Organization reported that Coxsackie B viruses carried the highest incident of cardiovascular disease (34.6 in 1000), followed by influenza B (17.4 in 1000), influenza A (11.0 in 1000), Coxsackie A (9.1 in 1000), and cytomegalovirus (CMV; eight in 1000) [7]. The spectrum of clinical manifestations of viral myocarditis ranges from a totally asymptomatic response to severe congestive heart failure or life-threatening arrhythmias. Symptoms may consist of viral prodrome, myalgia, rhinorrhea, mild fatigue, shortness of breath, palpitations, chest pain, and fever. Importantly, the symptoms of myocarditis may mimic an acute myocardial infarction, with classic ECG changes and serum markers of myocardial injury [8].

Physical examination may be normal or include sinus tachycardia and ventricular gallops and evidence of pulmonary congestion. A chest radiogram may demonstrate normal or enlarged cardiac silhouette with evidence of pulmonary congestion.

The ECG may demonstrate sinus tachycardia, ST-T wave abnormalities, Q waves, atrial abnormalities, or conduction defects. Morgera et al. [9] reviewed the ECGs of 45 consecutive patients who had a histologic diagnosis of active myocarditis. The ECG pattern was abnormal in 43 of the 45 patients. Among patients with cardiac symptoms of short duration (<1 month), normal P waves, atrioventricular (AV) block, and repolarization abnormalities were common. However, patients with a longer clinical history had atrial abnormalities (ie, left atrial enlargement and atrial fibrillation), left ventricular hypertrophy, and left bundle branch block (LBBB). Supraventricular arrhythmias were noted in 20% of patients. Complete and advanced AV block were observed in 15% of patients and were not reliable markers of myocardial damage [9]. Patients with abnormal QRS complexes had more severe left ventricular impairment and a higher frequency of hypertrophy and fibrosis. The presence of LBBB was the ECG abnormality that correlated best with the most severe left ventricular dysfunction. Patients who had right bundle branch block (RBBB) had a shorter clinical history and higher right

ventricular filling pressures. In the group of 13 patients who died, sudden death occurred in four of the nine patients who had abnormal QRS complexes [9]. Thus, the presence of an abnormal QRS or LBBB on the ECG of a patient with myocarditis implies more severe myocardial damage and a poorer prognosis.

Significant ventricular arrhythmias are another serious complication of myocarditis and may be the initial presentation. Wiles et al. [10] obtained myocardial biopsies in 33 young patients who presented with significant ventricular arrhythmias but structurally normal hearts. Fourteen (or 42%) had histologic abnormalities of the myocardium, including myocyte hypertrophy; enlarged, irregularly shaped nuclei; and increased interstitial fibrosis. Three patients (or 9%) had evidence of focal lymphocytic myocarditis with adjacent myocyte damage and necrosis.

Serologic studies, including creatine kinase and MB isoenzyme fractions, may be abnormal, indicating myocardial damage. Identification of viral particles in throat swabbing, stool or blood samples, or an increase in viral antibody titers may be useful but are not specific for the diagnosis of viral myocarditis.

With recent analysis of the genome of cardiotropic viruses, radiolabeled genetic probes can identify a viral signal in biopsy specimens even if there is no evidence of an inflammatory response. Bowles et al. [11], using a Coxsackie B viral probe, found virus-specific RNA sequences in up to 50% of patients with myocarditis or dilated cardiomyopathy (DCM) [11]. Sole and Liu [5] used the polymerase chain reaction (PCR) to rapidly duplicate and amplify specific DNA sequences for analyzing endomyocardial biopsy specimens. PCR from tracheal aspirates amplified the same viral genome as endomyocardial biopsy samples in seven patients [12]. Thus, genetic probe techniques may elucidate the complex relationship between viral infections and myocarditis.

NONINVASIVE IMAGING IN MYOCARDITIS

The gold standard for diagnosing myocarditis is endomyocardial biopsy; however, this method is invasive and has potential complications, in addition to sampling error due to the potentially focal nature of the disease [13].

Echocardiography facilitates the initial diagnosis and frequent noninvasive monitoring of the patient's clinical course [14]. The findings may be nonspecific and mimic noninfectious myocarditis, other causes of DCM, and even acute myocardial infarction [15]; therefore the echocardiographic findings must be correlated with the entire clinical picture [16].

The echocardiogram may be normal or demonstrate varying degrees of left and right ventricular dysfunction, which may be focal or global (Fig. 1). In the initial stages of the disease, the echocardiogram is usually normal or minimally abnormal as myocyte necrosis and inflammation begin in the epicardial region. As the myocarditis progresses to the endocardium, then focal or regional, right or/and left ventricular dysfunction appears. DCM with impaired systolic and diastolic dysfunction appears late in the disease [16]. Pinamonti et al. [17] found that over one third of patients can have normal systolic and diastolic function. Fifty percent of patients in this study had increased left ventricular size and decreased function. Wall motion abnormalities ranged from regional hypokinesis to akinesis, dyskinesis, or even aneurysm. The right ventricle was enlarged in 20% of patients, with decreased function in 12%. Fifteen percent of patients had a left and/or right ventricular thrombus. Some patients (20%) had restrictive physiology. Nieminen et al. [18] correlated severity of clinical myocarditis and regional abnormalities on echocardiography. In general, myocarditis more frequently involved the inferior (26%) and anterior (18%) walls, while the postero-lateral wall was involved in only 9% of cases. Mild myocarditis was associated with hyperkinesis of spared ventricular regions in 92%; this finding was absent in patients with severe myocarditis. Ten percent of patients had a pericardial effusion, which did not correlate with the severity of the disease. Some investigators have reported transient increases in left ventricular wall thickness during the acute phases of myocarditis, which could represent edema secondary to inflammation [19]. Doppler findings may include mild valvular regurgitation or diastolic dysfunction, which may precede systolic abnormalities. Echocardiographic tissue characterization and more sensitive indices of systolic and diastolic myocardial performance may detect subtle abnormalities in those with myocarditis [20]. Patients with chronic or healed myocarditis have an increased tissue Doppler index; however, this technique cannot discern between myocarditis and other causes of edema or fibrosis [16].

Radionuclide imaging may confirm biventricular involvement. An abnormal left ventricular response to exercise, by either radionuclear gated blood pool scanning (MUGA) or exercise echocardiography, may demonstrate abnormal ventricular reserve, even with normal resting function. A study by Quigley et al. [21] examining patients 6 to 8 months after their initial presentation with myocarditis showed that seven of nine patients with normal MUGA scans at rest had a decreased left ventricular ejection fraction (LVEF) with exercise [21].

Antimyosin autoantibodies are associated with deterioration of systolic and diastolic left ventricular function in patients with chronic myocarditis [22]. Monoclonal antimyosin antibodies radiolabeled with ^{111}In may reveal diffuse uptake because cellular myosin is released into the extracellular fluid caused by myocardial necrosis and cellular disruption [23]. In a study of patients with suspected myocarditis, antimyosin antibody imaging had a sensitivity of 100% and a specificity of 58% [24]. This imaging modality promises to be a sensitive screening tool when it becomes more commercially available.

[67]Ga may also demonstrate diffuse uptake but has a high sensitivity and low specificity [25]. In one study [26], ^{67}Ga had a negative predictive value of 98% and positive predictive value of 36%. The authors concluded that ^{67}Ga scintigraphic imaging is useful for screening for myocarditis and may decrease the need for repeat endomyocardial biopsies.

T_2-weighted MRI can detect early myocarditis due to edema [27]. Gagliardi et al. [28] studied 11 patients with suspected myocarditis with MRI and showed that the MRI region of interest was predictive of myocarditis on biopsy. Recently, ^{99m}Tc-MIBI myocardial perfusion imaging has been studied for use in myocarditis. Sun et al. [29] found regions of hypoperfusion with MIBI imaging in all 46 patients with a clinical diagnosis of myocarditis. The results

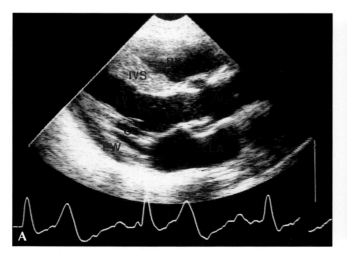
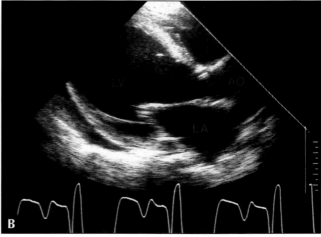

FIGURE 1 Two-dimensional echocardiogram. **A,** Long-axis view, systolic frame: normal wall thickening and cavity size. **B,** Dilated and severely hypocontractile left ventricle. A—anterior leaflet of the mitral valve; Ao—aorta; C—chordae tendonae; EFF—pericardial effusion; IVS—interventricular septum; LA—left atrium; LV—left ventricle; PW—posterior LV wall; RV—right ventricle.

were significantly correlated to ST-T segment changes, elevated cardiac enzymes, and decreased left ventricular function on echocardiography. Positron emission tomography in the diagnosis of myocarditis has not yet been defined. Larger studies are warranted to confirm the clinical utility of these new imaging modalities.

ENDOMYOCARDIAL BIOPSY

Sutton et al. [30] first described the transthoracic needle biopsy technique in human subjects in 1956. Subsequently, Sakakibra and Konno [31] reported the currently used technique: performing an endomyocardial biopsy with a fluoroscopically guided transvenous bioptome to sample the apex, free wall, and septum of the right ventricle. Usually the right internal jugular vein is the preferred biopsy entry sight, with the subclavian veins as alternatives.

In more than 4000 biopsies performed at Stanford University in the 1970s, the morbidity was less than 1% and there were no deaths [32]. Rare complications of transvenous endomyocardial biopsy include pneumothorax, ventricular or atrial arrhythmias, bradycardia, hypotension, and perforation of the right ventricular free wall and tricuspid regurgitation caused by damaged chordae tendineae [33]. Echocardiographic guidance can substantially reduce the incidence of complications as well as radiation exposure [34]. In 1000 consecutive endomyocardial biopsies performed in children, there was one death (a 2-week-old infant with DCM) and nine right ventricular perforations from the femoral venous approach (eight in children with DCM and one after transplantation) [35]. Usually more than five small tissue samples (1 to 3 mm) are required to obtain representative samples of the myocardium. Importantly, myocardial tissue more than 5 mm below the endocardial surface is not sampled by the bioptome. Because myocarditis may be a focal disease involving only 5% of the myocardium, sampling errors account for most false-negative diagnoses and may occur in up to 40% of patients [36]. A larger number of biopsy specimens have a greater diagnostic yield. Histologically defined myocarditis has been diagnosed in only 5% to 30% of patients clinically suspected to have myocarditis, in up to 41% of patients with acutely dilated cardiomyopathy, and in up to 63% of patients with chronic dilated myopathy [37–39]. In a study of 100 consecutive right ventricular endomyocardial biopsies, positive biopsy results were found in only 11% of patients clinically thought to have myocarditis [40].

Because of differing patient populations, sampling error, and conflicting criteria for defining myocarditis, the Dallas criteria were established by consensus in an effort to standardize histological criteria [41] (Table 2). This classification was based on findings of the first biopsy, defined as either myocarditis with or without fibrosis, borderline myocarditis, or no myocarditis compared with subsequent biopsies. Patients are then categorized as having ongoing or persistent myocarditis, resolving or healing myocarditis

(Fig. 2), or resolved, healed myocarditis. The classification was defined by the type, distribution, and extent of cellular infiltrate and fibrosis. Specific lymphocyte counts formerly considered critical were no longer recommended. By providing a standardized histologic terminology, the Dallas criteria have been valuable in comparing and combining treatment modalities of different institutions.

However, these morphologic criteria lack clinical correlation and are also prone to sampling error and interobserver variability. Thus, Lieberman et al. [42] introduced a clinicopathologic description of myocarditis combining clinical and histologic findings. Their four categories were fulminant myocarditis, acute, chronic active, and chronic persistent patients. The fulminant group had an acute onset of symptoms with significant left ventricular dysfunction. Their endomyocardial biopsies demonstrated foci of active myocarditis, and these patients went on to complete recovery or death. Immunosuppressive therapy was of no benefit. Patients categorized as having acute myocarditis had a distinct onset of cardiac symptoms with varying degrees of congestive heart failure. Their biopsies demonstrated active or borderline myocarditis according to the Dallas criteria, and they usually had resolution of their myocarditis. Immunosuppressive therapy was sometimes beneficial. The chronic active subset had varying degrees of left ventricular dysfunction, with biopsies demonstrating active or borderline myocarditis. They developed DCM, and immunosuppressant therapy was of no benefit. Patients with chronic persistent myocarditis had varying degrees of left ventricular dysfunction and no significant symptoms of congestive heart failure, and their biopsies also demonstrated active or

TABLE 2 DALLAS CRITERIA
Initial biopsy
Myocarditis, with or without fibrosis
Borderline
No myocarditis
Inflammation
Type: eosinophilic, giant cell, granulomatous, lymphocytic, neutrophilic, mixed
Distribution: interstitial, endocardial
Extent: mild, moderate, severe
Fibrosis
Type: pericellular, perivascular, replacement
Distribution: interstitial, endocardial
Extent: mild, moderate, severe
Subsequent biopsies
Ongoing (persistent)
Resolving (healing)
Resolved (healed)

borderline myocarditis. The classification of Lieberman *et al.* [42] is similar to that used for viral hepatitis. Although the group's subsets of patients were small, their classification attempts to integrate clinical and pathologic findings [43]. Whether this classification will be more practical than the Dallas criteria has yet to be proven.

NATURAL HISTORY AND TREATMENT OF VIRAL MYOCARDITIS

As discussed above, infectious myocarditis is most frequently caused by viruses. Myocarditis can result in one of three outcomes: 1) complete recovery; 2) continued rapid progression to heart failure, with the patient developing DCM; or 3) apparent short-term recovery followed by a latent asymptomatic period of variable duration, followed later by congestive heart failure and arrhythmias [44]. The natural history of myocarditis varies with the etiology. Many patients with viral myocarditis have little or no symptoms and have a totally benign course. In a recent study [45] of 147 patients with myocarditis by endomyocardial biopsy, 93% of those with "fulminant" myocarditis on the basis of clinical presentation (fever, rapid onset, and hemodynamic compromise) were alive at follow-up (mean, 5.6 years) without transplant compared with only 45% for patients with acute myocarditis. Those with fulminant myocarditis tend to have less significant left ventricular dilation and greater septal wall thickness, with more significant left ventricular systolic function improvement at 6 months follow-up [46]. Patients that do not show improvement in their left ventricular function in the first 6 months have a 59% mortality [47]. The incidence of viral myocarditis resulting in DCM is estimated to be 10% to 20% [5]. Cardiac autoantibodies of the organ-specific type were found in 28 of 110 (25%) patients with DCM presenting with heart failure and arrhythmias compared with only one of 160 (1%) patients with ischemic heart failure and seven

of 200 (3%) in healthy controls. At follow-up visit (14+12 months), cardiac autoantibodies were found in only 10%, with a lower anti-α myosin antibody titer than at diagnosis [48]. Thus, direct evidence of a viral infection may decrease as time elapses from the acute infection. Another study by Marti *et al.* [49] found antimyosin uptake (with ^{111}In-labeled monoclonal antimyosin antibodies), indicative of sarcolemma disruption and irreversible myocyte damage, in 16 of 19 patients (84%) with chronic idiopathic DCM. RNA viral sequences were detected in endomyocardial biopsies from four of these 16.

Treatment should be geared to managing specific clinical symptoms with the standard regimen for heart failure and arrhythmias. In the early phases of myocarditis, bed rest may be beneficial in limiting myocardial oxygen consumption and ventricular wall stress. Competitive athletic sports should be avoided for at least 6 months, until the symptoms and arrhythmias have abated and heart size and function have recovered [50]. Patients with congestive heart failure are treated with diuretics, vasodilators, angiotensin-converting enzyme inhibitors, and digitalis. Patients with myocarditis may be sensitive to digitalis during the acute stages of myocarditis. The calcium channel blocking agent verapamil, by blocking replication of certain viruses, inhibiting IL-2 messenger RNA, and preventing the microvascular spasm, improved the clinical and pathologic course of experimental murine myocarditis [51]. If a patient presents with symptomatic bradyarrhythmias or AV block, a temporary pacemaker should be inserted. Ventricular arrhythmias, if prolonged and symptomatic, may require electrophysiologic study for selection of appropriate management. Consideration of prolonged observation in a monitored setting to determine if the inflammatory process is transient may obviate the necessity to treat with potential proarrhythmic agents or even automatic implantable cardioverting devices. Nonsteroidal anti-inflammatory agents (NSAIDs) may increase myocardial damage in the

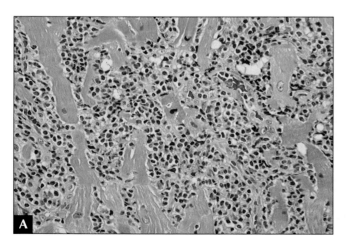

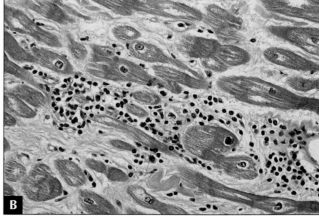

FIGURE 2 Viral myocarditis. **A,** First biopsy showing severe lymphocytic myocarditis with myocyte necrosis. **B,** Follow-up biopsy 6 months later showing resolving myocarditis with fibrosis and residual lymphocytic infiltrate.

early phase (first 2 weeks) and should be avoided [52]. Immunosuppressive therapy has been used for many years but has not been documented to be of substantial benefit.

Because of the varying criteria used and the small number of patients reported from individual centers, the National Health Institute–sponsored Myocarditis Treatment Trial was established [53]. Enrollment was initiated in 1986 and was completed in 1990. Approximately 10% of the 2200 patients screened with suspected myocarditis had positive biopsy results. The Myocarditis Treatment Trial was designed to evaluate the efficacy of immunosuppression in patients with acute myocarditis. The randomized ill patients with unexplained heart failure and a histologic diagnosis of myocarditis with an ejection fraction of less than 45% were randomized to treatment with prednisone supplemented with either cyclosporine or azathioprine or, as controls, to no immunosuppressive therapy. The primary outcome was LVEF at 28 weeks. The 10% mean improvement in LVEF in the treated group was no different from the 7% improvement in the control group. There was also no significant difference in mortality between the two groups. The mortality rate for the entire group was 20% at 1 year and 56% at 4.3 years [53].

The T-helper cell associated cytokine IL-10 was very effective in improving survival in a murine model of acute viral myocarditis [54]. Although treatment of patients with myocarditis with immune globulin has not affected mortality, it did improve LVEF in a small group of patients with postpartum cardiomyopathy [55].

At 2-year follow-up, 21 of 26 (81%) patients with idiopathic myocarditis or idiopathic DCM with an LVEF of less than 45% treated with immunotherapy consisting of interferon alfa and thymomodulin improved their LVEF compared with only eight of 12 (66%) patients given standard therapy. At 2 years, 73% of treated patients improved their functional class compared with only 25% of conventionally treated patients [56].

Both mechanical support and extracorporeal membrane oxygenation have been used with varying success in patients with acute myocarditis and hemodynamic compromise [57].

Currently, cardiac transplantation is offered to patients with end-stage cardiomyopathy. Early cardiac transplantation may be an alternative for patients with acute myocarditis with a fulminant course who do not respond to conventional therapy or a trial of immunosuppressive agents. However, O'Connell et al. [58] reported that 12 patients with acute myocarditis treated with transplantation had a 2.2-fold increase in rejection episodes and a significant decrease in 1-year survival compared with control subjects (60% vs 80% for the controls). A larger retrospective study of 26 patients with active myocarditis who underwent transplant had a higher rejection rate than patients without myocarditis, but their 5-year mortality rate was 55% compared with 63% for control patients [59].

Because of the variation in diagnostic yield from biopsies and the controversy regarding the appropriate therapeutic response, the indications for an endomyocardial biopsy for suspected myocarditis should be limited to patients with unexplained heart failure and normal coronary arteries who are having progressive deterioration in their clinical course or who present with significant ventricular ectopy. Although immunosuppressive therapy cannot be recommended routinely for patients with biopsy proven acute myocarditis, a 2-month treatment trial may be worthwhile for patients with fulminant myocarditis with rapidly progressive heart failure or life-threatening arrhythmias. Unfortunately, based on current data, one cannot predict which patients with myocarditis will respond to immunosuppressive treatment. A meta-analysis of reports on a mixed cohort of biopsied and not biopsied patients with myocarditis demonstrated that a mean of 57% of patients improved with standard therapy and restricted physical activity alone. This figure was similar to spontaneous improvement rate in biopsy positive patients in the Myocarditis Treatment Trial (53%) [60].

VIRAL MYOCARDITIS

Specific Agents

Coxsackie virus A and B, echovirus, and influenza are the most common viruses causing myocarditis, Coxsackie B being the most frequent [6–7]. Clinical manifestations such as pleurodynia, generalized myalgias, and arthralgic and upper respiratory symptoms should raise the suspicion of a viral etiology. Patients may have pleuritic or pericarditic chest pain and diffuse ST-T wave abnormalities on the ECG. Elevated antibody titers to cardiotropic viruses are reported in more than 50% of asymptomatic adults and are probably caused by silent viral infection; they are of little value in establishing the diagnosis of myocarditis [61]. However, the advent of PCR techniques to detect viruses within the myocardium has provided some new information on the etiology of disease in viral myocarditis. In a recent study by Bowles et al. [62] in 2003, 624 adults and children with clinically diagnosed myocarditis based on the Dallas criteria of borderline or definite myocarditis, and 149 with DCM by histologic verification had PCR performed for specific viruses. Thirty-eight percent of patients with myocarditis had amplification of viral genome; interestingly, adenovirus ("the common cold virus") was the most common (59%), followed by enterovirus (36%), CMV (8%), parvovirus (3%), influenza A (2%), herpes simplex virus (2%), Epstein-Barr virus (EBV) (1%), and respiratory syncytial virus (RSV) (0.5%). Eleven percent of patients had dual infection. Twenty percent of patients with DCM had detectable viruses; only adenovirus and enterovirus were detected. The adenovirus-positive patients had typically mild or borderline myocarditis by Dallas criteria, whereas enteroviruses had more acute myocarditis and inflammatory infiltrates. The latter may be the reason why adenovirus myocarditis was overlooked in the past.

Treatment is geared to specific symptoms. AV block may require temporary pacemaker implantation. Immunosuppressive therapy in the acute phase may be deleterious and their benefit in the second phase of illness is unclear. Ribavarin, gancyclovir, and acyclovir are partially beneficial for RSV pneumonitis and CMV disease in post-transplant patients, but there are currently no approved therapies for adenovirus or enterovirus infections [62].

In many patients, viral myocarditis is a benign illness and there is complete recovery without sequela. Patients who have left ventricular dysfunction may stabilize or even demonstrate spontaneous improvement in approximately 50% of patients [53, 60, 63]. In the above study by Bowles *et al.* [62], the overall mortality from myocarditis was 51% when combining all age groups; for adults, there were 38% deaths, 11% continued to have left ventricular dysfunction, and 51% improved.

HIV

Thirty-six million adults and children are living with HIV/AIDS; 5.3 million were newly infected in the year 2000 [64]. Cardiac pathology has been reported to occur in 28% to 73% of patients with AIDS [65], and can be manifested by myocarditis, DCM, endocarditis, pericardial effusion, pulmonary hypertension, malignant neoplasms, and drug-related toxicity [66]. In 1989 Levy reported that 32 of 62 patients (53%) with HIV (Table 3) had evidence of cardiac abnormalities, either by echocardiogram, ECG, or Holter monitoring [61]. Cardiomyopathy has become a significant complication of HIV-1 infection, occurring in 6.2% of 450 patients studied prospectively [67]. The Gruppo Italiano per lo Studio Cardiologico (GISCA) group [68] in 1998 collected autopsy samples from 440 AIDS patients, and found dilated cardiomyopathy in 2.7% of patients, of whom 17% had endocarditis and 41% had pericardial effusions. In addition, 40% to 52% of these patients had evidence of myocarditis. No etiologic factor was identified in 80% of these patients.

Echocardiography can detect asymptomatic pericardial effusions or biventricular dysfunction. Clinical congestive heart failure may occur in 10% to 25% of patients with AIDS [69]. Clinical characteristics associated with severe symptomatic cardiac dysfunction included low CD4 T-cell counts, myocarditis associated with nonpermissive cardiotropic virus infection on endomyocardial biopsy, and persistent elevation of anti-heart antibodies. Virus-related myocarditis and cardiac autoimmunity probably play a role in the pathogenesis of progressive cardiac injury [70].

The mechanism of myocardial involvement in patients with AIDS may be related to primary viral infection with HIV or secondary to cytomegalovirus, Coxsackie B, herpes simplex 2 or other cardiotropic viruses, other infectious agents (tuberculosis, toxoplasmosis, or *Cryptococcus neoformans*), ischemic cardiomyopathy, malnutrition, and, in intravenous drug abusers, cocaine-related damage. In the GISCA study [68], HIV-1 nucleic acid sequences were detected by in situ DNA hybridization in 35% of patients, 85% of whom had active myocarditis confirmed by histology. Coinfection with Coxsackie virus was 32%, Epstein-Barr 8%, and CMV 4%. Baroldi *et al.* [71] found evidence of cardiac lymphocytic infiltrate in 20 of 26 patients (or 77%) with AIDS; although nine of the 26 patients met the Dallas criteria for myocarditis, none of the patients had cardiac symptoms. In a study by Anderson and Virmani [72] of 71 AIDS patients, necropsy demonstrated the incidence of fungal, mycobacterial, and protozoal opportunist pathogens to be 58%, 42%, and 80%, respectively, with no evidence of direct HIV viral involvement. Kaposi's carcinoma was found in 49% of heart specimens and 52% of patients had histologic evidence of myocarditis.

Mortality secondary to progressive heart failure, lethal ventricular arrhythmias, or pericardial tamponade may be as high as 18%. Symptoms and manifestations of heart failure are treated with digoxin, diuretics, afterload reduction, and vasodilators. Treatment alternatives are limited in patients with AIDS because of their underlying immune deficiency. However, when the cardiac manifestations are disproportionate to other clinical signs of disease and treatable fungal or mycobacterial involvement is suspected, myocardial biopsy may be worthwhile to direct specific treatment. Pentamidine, which is used to treat patients with *Pneumocystis carinii* pneumonia, may precipitate ventricular arrhythmias and should be used with caution because of the frequency of clinical and subclinical cardiac involvement in AIDS.

Highly active antiretroviral therapy (HAART) has significantly improved survival rates in HIV and improved quality of life. However, HAART is not available to the majority of patients with HIV worldwide, and it is expected that HIV-associated heart failure may soon become one of the leading causes of heart failure worldwide [73]. There is no evidence to date that HAART therapy benefits HIV-associated cardiomyopathy [74]. However, the incidence of myocarditis from mycobacteria (especially nontuberculous), CMV, *Cryptococcus*, *Aspergillus*, *Candida*, *Histoplasma*, and *Coccidioides* has been decreased by HAART [75]. Myocarditis from enterovirus, EBV, and interestingly HIV-1 does not seem to have decreased in incidence [75]; the incidence of cardiac Kaposi sarcoma has been decreased by HAART, whereas no effect has been observed on cardiac lymphomas.

Table 3 Cardiac Involvement in Acquired Immunodeficiency Syndrome	
Myocarditis	**Malignant**
Viral	Kaposi's sarcoma
Opportunistic infections	Lymphoma
Autoimmune	
	Toxicity
Pericarditis	Cocaine
Autoimmune	Pentamidine
Infectious	Other drugs

It must be noted that although HAART has several benefits listed above, up to 60% of patients will develop lipodystrophy, hyperlipidemia, hyperglycemia, and/or insulin resistance [76,77]. In fact, there was a fourfold increase in myocardial infarction in patients on HAART in the Frankfurt HIV-Cohort study, compared with the pre-HAART period [78].

GIANT CELL MYOCARDITIS

Giant cell myocarditis, identified by the presence of giant cells in the myocardium, aorta, and other major arteries, is part of the spectrum of systemic giant cell arthritis (temporal arthritis). Occasionally associated with autoimmune diseases such as myasthenia gravis, lupus, and thyrotoxicosis, giant cell myocarditis has an acute course manifested by chest pain and dyspnea. Bradyrhythmias and tachyrhythmias are common. Patients with the disease may respond to corticosteroid therapy adjusted to the erythrocyte sedimentation rate [79].

BACTERIAL MYOCARDITIS

Bacterial myocarditis is uncommon, with a prevalence of 0.2%–1.5% in postmortem patients [80]. The common pathogens causing bacterial myocarditis are listed in Table 1. The most common cause is *Staphylococcus aureus*. The list is continuously expanding, most recently with the addition of *Bartonella henselae* [81], *Chlamydia pneumoniae*, and trachomatis [82]. Predisposing factors for bacterial myocarditis include bacteremia, neutropenia, myocardial infarction, osteomyelitis, and recent surgery [80].

The hallmark of bacterial myocarditis is the development of microabscesses [16]. The infection reaches the myocardium in one of three manners: 1) sepsis with myocardial seeding (most common), 2) embolism from the coronaries of valvular endocarditis, or 3) direct invasion from an adjacent focus such as valvular endocarditis, pericarditis, or pneumonia [80]. Bacteremia during a myocardial infarction can also cause abscess formation at the site of the infarcted tissue [83]. Typically, large or microabscesses are formed within the myocardium; however, there have been case reports of diffuse bacterial myocarditis without abscess formation in patients infected with meningococcus [84] and group B streptococcus [85].

Most patients present with signs of sepsis, with or without heart failure. Blood cultures are typically positive [80]. Complications of bacterial myocarditis are similar to those of viral myocarditis, and include left or right ventricular dysfunction and conduction disturbances. Some cases progress to myocardial rupture with secondary purulent pericarditis [80]. Treatment includes antibiotics targeted at the causative pathogen. Surgical drainage of the primary extracardiac focus of infection is recommended; it is unclear whether myocardial abscess drainage/removal is beneficial, because bacterial myocarditis tends to present with multiple microabscesses [80].

Some specific bacterial infections are worth noting. Diphtherial myocarditis may occur in up to 20% of patients with diphtheria infection [86]. DCM with congestive heart failure may develop rapidly and is the most common cause of death in those with diphtheria. Antitoxin therapy, erythromycin, or penicillin G and diuretics are the mainstays of treatment. Streptococcal myocarditis is one of the major manifestations of acute rheumatic fever pancarditis after a β-hemolytic streptococcal infection and may be the etiology of left ventricular dysfunction seen many years after the initial infection. Although ECG abnormalities, primarily ST-T and Q-Tc, may be frequent in those with typhoid fever (caused by *Salmonella typhi*), clinical myocarditis is rare. Bradycardia may be a harbinger of myocarditis. Treatment of patients with typhoid fever includes trimethoprim-sulfamethoxazole or ceftriaxone.

Lyme Carditis

Lyme disease is a nonfatal multiorgan disorder caused by *Borrelia burgdorferi* and may involve the heart, nervous system, skin, and muscles. The spirochete is transmitted by a tick, *Ixodes damini*, which is found in the Western states. The white-tailed deer is the dominant host for the adult tick. The initial manifestation of Lyme disease is a characteristic skin rash, erythema migrans, which occurs in 60% to 80% of cases, which may clear without therapy. Additional symptoms that develop include fever, myalgias, arthralgias, headache, lymphadenopathy, and fatigue [87]. Late persistent infection is manifested by arthritis in 40% to 50% of patients, clinical nerve palsies and meningoencephalitis in 7% to 19% of patients. Cardiac involvement may be seen 2 to 6 weeks after the tick bite in 1.6% to 10% of patients [88]. Myocarditis in particular can occur with or without pericarditis; myopericarditis occurred in 15% of patients with Lyme disease reported to the Centers for Disease Control between 1983 and 1986 [89].

The ECG may demonstrate no abnormality or mild ST-T abnormalities. The most common cardiac manifestation is varying degrees of AV block at the level of AV node. McAlister *et al.* [90] found an incidence of AV block in 87% of 52 cases of Lyme carditis that they reviewed. A review of Lyme carditis found that complete heart block was the most common form of AV block. Sixty-eight percent of the patients had a supraventricular origin to their block on electrophysiology studies, and one third showed evidence of diffuse disease in the conduction system as evidenced by simultaneously prolonged intra-atrial, atrio-His, and His-ventricular conduction [91]. The AV block usually resolves, without requiring a permanent pacemaker, within 1 to 2 weeks [90]. ^{67}Ga or ^{111}In antimyosin antibody scanning results may be positive.

Patients with Lyme carditis are usually treated with penicillin G 20 MU/d or oral ceftriaxone 2 g/d intravenously for 14 days; oral doxycycline 100 mg twice daily; or amoxicillin 500 mg, three times daily for 14 to 21 days [88]. Antibiotics are effective in treating the sequelae of Lyme disease carditis, although most of the cardiac manifestations are self-limited. A retrospective review by Sangha *et al*. [92] of patients treated for Lyme disease showed that there was no statistically significant difference in the prevalence of cardiac events compared to the general population. Whether Lyme disease can cause DCM is still debated [93].

PARASITIC MYOCARDITIS
Trypanosomiasis (Chagas' Disease)

Chagas' disease is caused by the hemoflagellate protozoan parasite *Trypanosoma cruzi* and is the leading cause of cardiac disease in South and Central America, especially in Brazil, Chile, and Argentina [94]. The clinical course of Chagas' disease is triphasic and includes an acute, indeterminate, or latent and chronic stage. The acute disease follows a parasitic infection transmitted to humans through the bite of a blood-sucking insect of the order *Hemiptera*, family Reduviidae, (the reduviid bug), which harbors the parasite in its gastrointestinal tract. At night, while the bug feeds on humans by piercing their skin, the bug may defecate, releasing trypanosomes, which may enter the skin after the affected person scratches the bite. Localized swelling of the infected area is called a chagoma. The bug may bite around the human eye, leading to a conjunctival infection and unilateral periorbital edema and swelling of the eyelid called "Romaña's sign" [94]. The acute phase of the disease is caused by trypanosomal transformation to a flagellate form in which they enter the bloodstream and infect the myocardial and muscle cells and the glia of the nervous system. Acute disease manifestations include fever, myalgias, vomiting, diarrhea, meningeal irritation, lymphadenopathy, hepatosplenomegaly, and myocarditis [95]. During this phase, parasites are seen in the cardiac fibers with a marked lymphocytic infiltrate and contraction band necrosis (Fig. 3) [96].

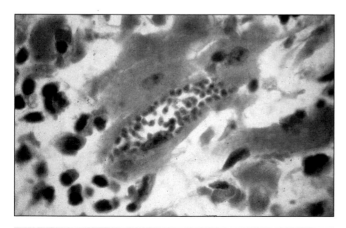

FIGURE 3 Myocarditis in acute Chagas' disease. Parasites forming a pseudocyst are seen within a cardiac myocyte. Note the surrounding inflammatory infiltrate.

An acute myocarditis may develop with prolongation of the PR interval, low QRS voltage, and heart failure. Symptoms of the acute phase resolve spontaneously within 3 to 4 months in more than 85% of infected individuals. After a latent period of clinical quiescence that may last for 10 to 50 years after the initial infection (average, 20 years), approximately 30% of patients develop chronic Chagas' disease. Cardiac manifestations of the chronic phase include congestive heart failure (most common), arrhythmias, conduction defects, thromboemboli, or sudden death [97]. Megaesophagus or megacolon may develop as well.

Diagnosis is confirmed by parasites in the myocardium (Fig. 3), the complement fixation test (Machado-Guerreiro test), and enzyme-linked immunosorbent assay. Xenodiagnosis, in which the patient suspected of having Chagas' disease is bitten by a reduviid bug sucking parasites into its intestine, may have positive results in 30% to 40% of patients with chronic Chagas' disease. In a study of 16 patients with chronic Chagas' heart disease, with histologic evidence of myocarditis, *T. cruzi* antigen was detected in 11 of 16 and in 10 of 14 regions with moderate to severe myocarditis [98]. A recent study of 91 patients with positive serology for Chagas' disease found that the presence of circulating *T. cruzi* by PCR in chronically infected persons correlated with typical cardiac manifestations of chronic cardiac damage, supporting an active role of the parasite in the pathophysiology of Chagas' cardiomyopathy [99].

Echocardiography in the early phase of the infection may be normal, but tissue Doppler may reveal changes in systolic and diastolic function of the right ventricle [100]. Echocardiography may demonstrate DCM with distinctive appearance of preserved ventricular septum function, posterior wall hypocontractility, and an apical aneurysm with possible thrombus [97]. A long indeterminate phase of the disease may follow the acute phase, during which electrocardiographic and radiologic abnormalities may not be present [16]. During this occult phase of the disease, dobutamine stress echocardiography can be used to evaluate the myocardial reserve. Acquatella *et al*. [101] studied a group of patients in the intermediate phase of the disease with stress echocardiography and found that both patients with and without wall motion abnormalities at baseline had chronotropic incompetence and a blunted contractile response to inotropy. Ten percent to 30% of patients will progress to the potentially fatal phase of the disease [16]. Chronic Chagas' cardiomyopathy may be caused by several factors: an intense allergic response to the parasite, an autoimmune response, microvascular pathology caused by an infection of endothelial cells and myocytes that alter synthetic function, an inflammatory response, and parasite-associated fibroblast stimulation and other factors [94].

The most common ECG changes in patients with chronic Chagas' disease are RBBB (found in 30% to 60% of cases) and left anterior hemiblock [102]. Ajmaline, a conduction-depressing antiarrhythmic agent, may evoke fascicular block in an infected patient before the disease is clinically manifest [103]. Atrial fibrillation and ventricular arrhythmias are common, the latter being a major cause of sudden death among patients with chronic Chagas' disease. The overall 10-year mortality is reported to be 36% and the reported incidence of sudden death is 17.6% [104].

Treatment of patients with Chagas' disease includes management of the clinical symptoms of congestive heart failure and anticoagulation and antiarrhythmic therapy when indicated. Analogues of primaquine may clear parasites from the blood in the early stage of infection but may have no impact on the inexorable development of the chronic phase. Current recommended antibiotic treatment is nifurtimox, 8 to 10 mg/kg by mouth in four divided doses for 120 days [105]. Amiodarone and mexiletine appear to be useful in treating the ventricular arrhythmias of Chagas' disease. Recently, Giniger et al. [106] reported that electrophysiologic studies may be valuable to guide treatment in Chagas' patients with significant ventricular tachycardia. The potential benefit of implantable antitachycardic devices requires further investigation. Future immune therapy may prove beneficial in halting this devastating disease. Interferon-gamma given to mother rats protected the offspring from acute T. cruzi infection [107]. Heart transplantation has been surprisingly successful. Long-term follow-up (34+38 months) of 10 patients with Chagas' heart disease with cyclosporine immunosuppression had seven alive in New York Heart Association class I. There were no signs of recurrence of Chagas' disease in the allograft [108]. A larger study of 22 patients who underwent orthotopic heart transplantation had a total actuarial survival at 24 months of 60%. However, Chagas' disease reactivation was seen in six patients [109].

Toxoplasmosis

Toxoplasmosis is a parasitic infection caused by *Toxoplasma gondii*. Three patterns of infection are seen: diffuse, miliary type; glandular, involving only the lymph nodes; and organ infiltration. *T. gondii* infection is a potentially severe disease in immunocompromised patients. Myocyte infection may be of little consequence until a cyst ruptures, causing myocytic necrosis, lymphocytic infiltration, and interstitial fibrosis [110]. Symptoms may include chest pain, arrhythmias, and heart failure. The diagnosis is confirmed by a *Toxoplasma* antibody titer greater than 1:256. Current recommended treatment is pyrimethamine 25 mg once a day and sulfadiazine 4 g/d in four divided doses for 3 to 4 weeks [105]. Antibiotic prophylaxis for prevention of donor-acquired *T. gondii* infection in transplant recipients is recommended.

Helminthic Myocarditis

Trichinosis, caused by *Trichinella spiralis* infection, is fatal in 5% of cases, primarily caused by myocardial involvement. Chest pain and heart failure may develop because of a lymphocytic and eosinophilic infiltration. Treatment includes mebendazole 200 to 400 mg orally three times daily for 3 days, then corticosteroids 400 to 500 mg three

times daily for 10 days [109]. Echinococcosis occurs primarily in sheep-raising areas of the world and is caused by *Echinococcus granulosus* infection. The dog is the primary host and sheep are the intermediate host; human infection is caused by accidental ingestion of infected feces. Infestation in the liver, lung, or heart may result in a hydatid cyst. Cysts developing in the left or right ventricle may obstruct flow, rupture, and embolize, or cause an anaphylactic reaction. A calcified cyst may be seen on a chest radiograph or by two-dimensional echocardiography. Careful surgical resection is recommended, if feasible. Medical therapy is with albendazole 400 mg orally twice daily for 28 days [98].

CONCLUSIONS

Myocarditis remains a challenging dilemma, both in its diagnosis and management. Endomyocardial biopsy may prove beneficial in patients with fulminant heart failure unresponsive to conventional therapy or in whom an opportunistic or unusual treatable infection is suspected. Management is supportive and is geared toward relieving symptoms; when available, treatment is geared to the specific infectious agent. Research to determine the specific antigens provoking the aggressive immune reaction and new genetic approaches to more accurate diagnosis coupled with new immunomodulating therapeutic approaches may significantly reduce the acute and chronic effects of infectious myocarditis.

REFERENCES AND RECOMMENDED READING

1. Woodruff JF: Viral myocarditis: a review. *Am J Pathol* 1980, 101:427–484.

2. Karjalainen J, Heikkila J, Nieminen M, *et al.*: Etiology of mild acute infectious myocarditis. *Acta Med Scand* 1983, 213:65–73.

3. Ridker PM, Hennekens CH, Buring JE, Rifai N: C-reactive protein to the markers of inflammation in the prediction of cardiovascular disease in women. *N Engl J Med* 2000, 342:836–843.

4. Maze SS, Adolph RJ: Myocarditis: unresolved issues in diagnosis and treatment. *Clin Cardiol* 1990, 13:69–79.

5. Sole MJ, Liu P: Viral myocarditis: a paradigm for understanding the pathogenesis and treatment of dilated cardiomyopathy. *J Am Coll Cardiol* 1993, 22 (suppl A):99–105.

6. Leslie K, Blay R, Haisch C, *et al.*: Clinical and experimental aspects of viral myocarditis. *Clin Microbiol Rev* 1989, 2:191–203.

7. Grist MR, Reid D; Epidemiology of viral infection of the heart. In *Viral Infections of the Heart*. Edited by Banatrala E. London: Hodder and Stoughton Ltd.; 1993:23–31.

8. Karjalainen J, Heikkila J: Incidence of 3 presentations of acute myocarditis in young men in military service: a 20 year experience. *Eur Heart J* 1999, 20:1120–1125.

9. Morgera T, Dilenarda A, Dreas L, *et al.*: Electrocardiography of myocarditis revisited. *Am Heart J* 1992, 124:456–467.

10. Wiles HB, Gillette PC, Harley RA, Upshur JK: Cardiomyopathy and myocarditis in children with ventricular ectopic rhythm. *J Am Coll Cardiol* 1992, 20:359–362.

11. Bowles N, Richardson P, Olsen E, Archard L: Detection of Coxsackie B virus specific RNA sequences in myocardial biopsy samples from patients with myocarditis and dilated cardiomyopathy. *Lancet* 1986, 1:1120–1123.

12. Akhtar N, Ni J, Stromberg D, *et al.*: Tracheal aspirate as a substrate for PCR detection of viral genome in childhood pneumonia and myocarditis. *Circulation* 1999, 99:2011–2018.

13. Chow LH, Radio SJ, Sears TD, *et al.*: Insensitivity of right ventricular myocardial biopsy in the diagnosis of myocarditis. *J Am Coll Cardiol* 1989, 14:915–926.

14. Pinamonti B, Alberti E, Cigalotto A, *et al.*: Echocardiographic findings in myocarditis. *Am J Cardiol* 1988, 62:285.

15. Chandraratna PA, Nomalasuriya A, Reid CL, *et al.*: Left ventricular asynergy in acute myocarditis: simulation of acute myocardial Infarction. *JAMA* 1983, 250:1428–1430.

16. Shirani J, Ilercil A, Chandra M, *et al.*: Cardiovascular imaging in clinical and experimental acute Infectious myocarditis. *Front Biosci* 2003, 8:323–336.

17. Pinamonti B, Alberti E, Cigalotto A, *et al.*: Echocardiographic findings in myocarditis. *Am J Cardiol* 1988, 62:285–291.

18. Nieminen MS, Heikkila J, Karjalainen J: Echocardiography in acute infectious myocarditis: relation to clinical and electrocardiographic findings. *Am J Cardiol* 1984, 53:1331–1337.

19. Hauser AM, Gordon S, Cieszkowski J *et al.*: Severe transient left ventricular "hypertrophy" occurring during acute myocarditis. *Chest* 1983, 83:275–277.

20. Lieback E, Hardouin I, Meyer R, *et al.*: Clinical value of echo tissue characterization in the diagnosis of myocarditis. *Eur Heart J* 1996, 17:135–142.

21. Quigley PJ, Richardson PJ, Meany BT, *et al.*: Long-term follow-up of acute myocarditis: correlation of ventricular function and outcome. *Eur Heart J* 1987, 8:39–42.

22. Lauer B, Schannwell M, Kuhl U, *et al.*: Antimyosin autoantibodies are associated with deterioration of systolic and diastolic left ventricular function in patients with chronic myocarditis. *J Am Coll Cardiol* 2000, 35:11–18.

23. Khaw BA, Gold HK, Yasuda T, *et al.*: Scintigraphic quantification of myocardial necrosis in patients after intravenous injection of myosin-specific antibody. *Circulation* 1986, 74:501–508.

24. Yasuda T, Palacios IF, Dec W, *et al.*: Indium 111 monoclonal antimyosin antibody imaging in the diagnosis of acute myocarditis. *Circulation* 1987, 76:306–310.

25. Wakafugi S, Kajiya S, Hayakawa M, *et al.*: Ga67 myocardial scintigraphy in patients with acute myocarditis. *Jpn Circ J* 1987, 51:1373.

26. O'Connell JB, Costanzo-Nordin MR, Subramanian R, *et al.*: Peripartum cardiomyopathy: clinical, hemodynamic, histologic and prognostic characteristics. *J Am Coll Cardiol* 1986, 8:52–56.

27. Di Cesare E: MRI of the cardiomyopathies. *Eur J Radiol* 2001, 38:179–184.

28. Gagliardi MG, Bevilacqua M, Di Renzi P, *et al.*: Usefulness of magnetic resonance imaging for the diagnosis of acute myocarditis In Infants and children, and comparison with endomyocardial biopsy. *Am J Cardiol* 1991, 68:1089–1091.

29. Sun Y, Ma P, Bax JJ: 99mTc-Mibi myocardial perfusion imaging in myocarditis. *Nucl Med Commun* 2003, 24:779–783.

30. Sutton DC, Sutton GC, Kent G: Needle biopsy of the human ventricular myocardium. *Q Bull Northwest Univ Med Sch* 1956, 30:213.

31. Sakakibara S, Konno S. Endomyocardial biopsy. *Jpn Heart J* 1962, 3:537–543.

32. Mason JW: Techniques for right and left ventricular endomyocardial biopsy. *Am J Cardiol* 1978, 41:887.

33. Fowles RE, Mason JW: Myocardial biopsy. *Mayo Clinic Proc* 1982, 57:459.

34. Miller LW, Labovitz AJ, McBride LA, *et al.*: Echocardiography guided endomyocardial biopsy: a 5 year experience. *Circulation* 1988, 78:99.

35. Pophal SG, Sigfusson G, Booth KL, *et al.*: Complications of endomyocardial biopsy in children. *J Am Coll Cardiol* 1999, 34:2105–2110.

36. Chow LH, Radio SJ, Sears TD, McManus BM: Insensitivity of right ventricular endomyocardial biopsy in the diagnoses of myocarditis. *J Am Coll Cardiol* 1989, 14:1915.

37. Mason JW, Billingham ME, Ricci DR: Treatment of acute inflammatory myocarditis assisted by endomyocardial biopsy. *Am J Cardiol* 1989, 45:1037–1044.

38. Dec GW Jr, Palacios IF, Fallon JT, *et al.*: Active myocarditis in the spectrum of acute dilated cardiomyopathies: clinical features, histologic correlates, and clinical outcome. *N Engl J Med* 1985, 312:885–890.

39. Zee-Cheng CS, Tsai CC, Palmer DC, *et al.*: High incidence of myocarditis by endomyocardial biopsy in patients with idiopathic congestive cardiomyopathy. *J Am Coll Cardiol* 1984, 3:63–70.

40. Nippoldt TB, Edwards WD, Holmes DR Jr, *et al.*: Right ventricular endomyocardial biopsy: clinicopathologic correlates in 100 consecutive patients. *Mayo Clin Proc* 1982, 57:407–418.

41. Aretz HT: Myocarditis: the Dallas Criteria. *Hum Pathol* 1987, 18:619–624.

42. Lieberman EB, Hutchins GM, Herskowitz A, *et al.*: Clinicopathologic description of myocarditis. *J Am Coll Cardiol* 1991, 18:1617–1626.

43. Waller BF, Slack JD, Orr CD, *et al.*: "Flaming," "smoldering" and "burned out": the fireside saga of myocarditis. *J Am Coll Cardiol* 1991, 18:1627–1630.

44. Rossen R, Birdsall H, Mann D: The enemy within: immunologic responses to cardiac tissue. *Cardiol Rev* 1996, 4:237–253.

45. McCarthy RE, Boehmer JP, Hruban RH, *et al.*: Long term outcome of fulminant myocarditis as compared to acute (nonfulminant) myocarditis. *N Engl J Med* 2000, 342:690–695.

46. Felker GM, Boehmer JP, Hruban RH, *et al.*: Echocardiographic findings in fulminant and acute myocarditis. *J Am Coll Cardiol* 2000, 36:227–232.

47. Dec GW, Palacios IF, Fallon JT: Cardiomyopathies: clinical features, histologic correlates, and clinical outcome. *N Engl J Med* 1985, 312:885–890.

48. Caforio ALP, Goldman JH, Baig MK, *et al.*: Cardiac autoantibodies in dilated cardiomyopathy become undetectable with disease progression. *Heart* 1997, 77:62–67.

49. Marti V, Coll P, Ballester M, *et al.*: Enterovirus persistence and myocardial damage detected by in-monoclonal antimyosin antibodies in patients with dilated cardiomyopathy. *Eur Heart J* 1996, 17:545–549.

50. Maron BJ, Isner JM, McKenna WJ: 26th Bethesda Conference: recommendations for determining eligibility for competition in athletes with cardiovascular abnormalities. *J Am Coll Cardiol* 1994, 24:880–890.

51. Dong R, Liu P, Wee I, Butany J, Sole MJ: Verapamil ameliorates the clinical and pathological course of murine myocarditis. *J Clin Invest* 1992, 90:2022–2030.

52. Peters NS, Poole-Wilson PA: Myocarditis: continuing clinical and pathologic confusion. *Am Heart J* 1991, 121:942–948.

53. Mason JW, O'Connell JB, Herskowtiz A, *et al.*: Myocarditis Treatment Trial Investigators: a clinical trial of immunosupportive therapy for myocarditis. *N Engl J Med* 1995, 333:269–275.

54. Nishio R, Matsumori A, Shioi T, *et al.*: Treatment of experimental viral myocarditis with interleukin-10. *Circulation* 1999, 100:1102–1108.

55. Bozkurt B, Villaneuva FS, Holubkor R, *et al.*: Intravenous immune globulin in the therapy of peripartum cardiomyopathy. *J Am Coll Cardiol* 1999:34, 177–180.

56. Miric M, Vasiljevic J, Milovan B, *et al.*: Long-term follow-up of patients with dilated heart muscle disease treated with human leukocytic inteferon alpha or thymic hormones. *Heart* 1996, 75:596–601.

57. Chen YS, Wang MJ, Chou NK, *et al.*: Rescue for acute myocarditis with shock by extracorporeal membrane oxygenation. *Ann Thorac Surg* 1999, 68:2220–2224.

58. O'Connell JB, Dec GW, Goldenberg IF *et al.*: Results of heart transplantation for active lymphocytic myocarditis. *J Heart Transpl* 1990, 9:351–356.

59. Pham JM, Kormos RL *et al.*: Cardiac transplantation in patients with active myocarditis. *J Heart Lung Transpl* 1993, 12(suppl A):146.

60. Maisih B, Herzum M, Hufnagel G, *et al.*: Immunosuppressive treatment for myocarditis and dilated cardiomyopathy. *Eur Heart J* 1995, 16(suppl):153–161.

61. Levy WS, Simon GL, Rios JC, Ross AM: Prevalence of cardiac abnormalities in human immunodeficiency virus infection. *Am J Cardiol* 1989, 63:86.

62. Bowles N, Ni J, Kearney D, *et al.*: Detection of viruses in myocardial tissue by polymerase chain reaction: evidence of adenovirus as a common cause of myocarditis in children and adults. *J Am Col Cardiol* 2003, 42:466–472.

63. Weiss MB, Marboe CC, Escala EL, *et al.*: Natural history of untreated chronic myocarditive (active myocarditis with fibrosis). *Eur Heart J* 1987, 8(suppl J):247.

64. Temesgen Z. Overview of HIV Infection. *Ann Allergy Asthma Immunol*, 1999. 83:1–5.

65. Kaul S, Fishbein MC, Siegel RJ: Cardiac manifestations of acquired Immune deficiency syndrome. *Am Heart J* 1991, 122:535–544.

66. Rekpattanapipat P, Wongraparut N, Jacobs LE, *et al.*: Cardiac manifestations of acquired Immune deficiency syndrome. *Arch Intern Med* 2000, 160:602–608.

67. Herskowitz A, Willoughby J, Wu T-C, *et al.*: Immunopathogenesis of HIV-1 associated cardiomyopathy. *Clin Immunol Immunopathol* 1993, 68:235–241.

68. Barbaro G, Di Lorenzo G, Grisorio B, Barbarini G, and the Gruppo Italiano per lo Studio Cardiologico dei pazienti affetti da AIDS Investigators: Cardiac involvement in the acquired immunodeficiency syndrome: a multicenter clinical-pathological study. *AIDS Res Hum Retroviruses* 1998, 14:1071–1077.

69. Reilly JM, Cunnion RE, Anderson DW, *et al.*: Frequency of myocarditis, LV dysfunction and ventricular tachycardia in AIDS. *Am J Cardiol* 1988, 62:789–793.

70. Herskowitz A, Willoughby SB, Vlahov D, *et al.*: Dilated heart muscle disease associated with HIV infection. *Eur Heart J* 1995, 16(Suppl O):50–55.

71. Baroldi G, Corallo S, Moroni M, *et al.*: Focal lymphocytic myocarditis in acquired immunodeficiency syndrome (AIDS): a correlative morphologic and clinical study in 26 consecutive fatal cases. *J Am Coll Cardiol* 1988, 12:463.

72. Anderson DW, Virmani R: Emerging patterns of heart disease in human immunodeficiency virus infection. *Hum Pathol* 1990, 21:253.

73. Barbaro G: Cardiovascular manifestation of HIV Infection. *J R Soc Med* 2001, 94:384–390.

74. Barbarini G, Barbaro G: Incidence of the involvement of the cardiovascular system in HIV infection. *AIDS* 2003, 17:S46–S50.

75. Bruno R, Sacchi P, Filice G: Overview on the incidence and the characteristics of HIV-related opportunistic infections and neoplasms of the heart: impact of highly active antiretroviral therapy. *AIDS* 2003, 17(Suppl 1):S83–S87.

76. Hadigan C, Meigs JB, Corcoran C, *et al.*: Metabolic abnormalities and cardiovascular disease risk factors in adults with human immunodeficiency virus and lipodystrophy. *Clin Infect Dis* 2001, 32:130–139.

77. Koppel K, Bratt G, Erikson M, Sandstorm E: Serum lipid levels associated with increased risk for cardiovascular disease is associated with HAART in Hiv-1 infection. *Int J STD AIDS* 2000, 11:451–455.

78. Rickerts V, Brodt H, Staszewski S, Stille W.: Incidence of myocardial infarctions in HIV-infected patients between 1983 an 1998: the Frankfurt HIV-cohort Study. *Eur J Med Res* 2000, 5:329–333.

79. Frustaci A, Chimenti C, Pieroni M, Gentiloni N: Giant cell myocarditis responding to immunosuppressive therapy. *Chest* 2000, 117:905–907.

80. Faisal W, Shuter J: Primary bacterial infection of the myocardium. *Front Biosci* 2003, 8:s228–s231.

81. Meininger G, Nadasdy T, Hruban R, *et al.*: Chronic active myocarditis following acute *Bartonella henselae* infection (cat scratch disease). *Am J Surg Pathol*, 2001: 25:1211–1214.

82. Wang G, Burczynski F, Hasinoff B, *et al.*: Infection of myocytes with chlamydiae. *Circulation* 2002, 148:3955–3959.

83. Behnam R., Walter S., Hanes V: Myocardial abscess complicating myocardial Infarction. *J Am soc Echocardiogr* 1995, 8:334–337.

84. Saphir O: Meningococcus myocarditis. *Am J Pathol* 1936, 12:677–687.

85. Bateman AC, Richards M, Pallett AP: Fatal myocarditis associated with a Lancefield Group B *Streptococcus. J Infect* 1998, 36:354–355.

86. Havaldar PV, Patil VD, Siddibhavi BM, *et al.*: Fulminant diphtheritic myocarditis. *Indian Heart J* 1989, 41:265.

87. Steere AC, Batsord WP, Wineberg M: Lyme carditis: cardiac abnormalities of Lyme disease. *Ann Intern Med* 1980, 93:8–16.

88. Steere AC: Lyme disease. *N Engl J Med* 1989, 321:586–596.

89. Ciesielski C, Markowitz LE, Horsley R, *et al.*: Lyme disease surveillance in the United States, 1983–86. *Rev Infect Dis* 1989, 11(Suppl 6):S1435–S1441.

90. McAlister HF, Klementowicz PT, Andrews C, *et al.*: Lyme carditis: an important cause of reversible heart block. *Ann Intern Med* 1989, 110:339–345.

91. Van der Linde MR: Lyme carditis: clinical characteristics of 105 cases. *Scand J infect Dis* 1991, 77(Suppl):81–84.

92. Sangha O, Phillips CB, Fleishmann KE, *et al.*: Lack of cardiac manifestations among patients with previously treated Lyme disease. *Ann Intern Med* 1998, 128:346–353.

93. Haddad F, Nadelman R: Lyme disease and the heart. *Front Biosci* 2003, 8:S769–S782.

94. Morris SA, Tannowitz HB, Wittner M, Bilezikian JP: Pathological physiological insights into the cardiomyopathy of Chagas' disease. *Circulation* 1990, 82:1900–1909.

95. Hudson L, Britten V: Immune response to South American trypanosomiasis and its relationhship to Chagas' disease. *Br Med Bull* 1985, 41:175.

96. Edwards WD, Holmes DR Jr, Reeder GS: Diagnosis of active lymphocytic myocarditis by endomyocardial biopsy: quantitative criteria for light microscopy. *Mayo Clin Proc* 1982, 57:419–425.

97. Oliveira JSM, Correa DA, *et al.*: Cardiac thrombosis and thromboembolism in chronic Chagas' heart disease. *Am J Cardiol* 1983, 52:147–151.

98. Belloti G, Bocchi E, Moraes A, Higuchi M, *et al.*: In vivo detection of *Trypanosoma cruzi* antigens in heart of patients with chronic Chagas' heart disease. *Am Heart J* 1996, 131:301–307.

99. Salomone OA, Turi D, Omelianiuk MO, *et al.*: Prevalence of circulating trypanosoma cruzi detected by polymerase chain reaction in patients with Chagas' cardiomyopathy. *Am J Cardiol* 2000:85, 1274–1276.

100. Barros MVL, Mchado FS, Ribeiro ALP, *et al.*: Detection of right ventricular dysfunction in Chagas' disease using Doppler tissue imaging. *J Am Soc Echocardiogr* 2002, 15:1197–1201.

101. Acquatella H, Perez JE, Condado JA: Limited myocardial contractile reserve and chronotropic Incompetence In patients with chronic Chagas disease. *J Am Coll Cardiol* 1999, 33:522–529.

102. Rosenbaum MB, Alvarez AJ: The electrocardiogram in chronic chagasic myocarditis. *Am Heart J* 1955, 50:492–527.

103. Chiale PA, Przybylski J, Laino RA, *et al.*: Electrocardiographic changes evoked by ajmaline in chronic Chagas' disease without clinical manifestations. *Am J Cardiol* 1982, 49:14–20.

104. McGuire JH, Hoff R, Sherlock I, *et al.*: Cardiac morbidity and mortality due to Chagas' disease: prospective electrocardiographic study of a Brazilian community. *Circulation* 1987, 75:1140–1145.

105. Mandell GL, Douglas RG Jr, Bennet JE: *Principles and Practice of Infectious Diseases: Antimicrobial Therapy.* New York: Churchill Livingstone; 1992.

106. Giniger AG, Retyk EO, Laino RA, *et al.*: Ventricular tachycardia in Chagas' disease. *Am J Cardiol* 1992, 70:459–462.

107. Davila HD, Revelli S, Didoli G, *et al.*: Protection of young rats from acute *T. cruzi* infection by interferon-gamma given to their mothers during pregnancy. *Am J Trop Med Hyg* 1996, 54:660–664.

108. Carvalho V, Sousa E, Vila J, *et al.*: Heart transplantation in Chagas' disease. *Circulation* 1996, 94:1815–1817.

109. Bocchi E, Bellotti G, Mocelin A, Uip D, *et al.*: Heart transplantation in chronic Chagas' disease. *Ann Thorac Surg* 1996, 61:1727–1733.

110. Leak D, Meghji M: Toxoplasmic infection in cardiac disease. *Am J Cardiol* 1979, 43:841–849.

Infectious Endocarditis
Gordon A. Ewy

29

> ### Key Points
> - The diagnostic criteria for infectious endocarditis now include echocardiographic features.
> - The classic triad of findings in patients with infectious endocarditis is fever, organic heart murmur, and positive blood culture.
> - Cardiac auscultation is important in the prevention, diagnosis, and assessment of severity in patients with infectious endocarditis.
> - Echocardiography is used to identify vegetations or perivalvular abscesses and to determine chamber size and function and condition of the valves.
> - Infectious endocarditis is a potentially lethal disease; patients should be referred when this diagnosis is seriously considered.

DIAGNOSTIC CRITERIA

Although infectious endocarditis is rare, the annual incidence varies from two to four per 100,00 people; failure to diagnose and treat appropriately results in excess mortality and morbidity. The Duke clinical criteria [1••] outlined in Table 1 make the task of diagnosis easier. The diagnosis is definitive when both, one major and three minor criteria, or five minor criteria are present. [1••].

One of the major criteria is a positive blood culture with typical organisms. Typical organisms include *Streptococcus viridans*, *Streptococcus bovis*, *Enterococcus*, *Staphylococcus*, or the HACEK group (*Haemophilus*, *Actinobacillus*, *Cardiobacterium*, *Eikenella*, and *Kingella* species). A single culture positive for any of these organisms fulfills the criterion of positive culture with a typical organism, except that the frequency of short-lived bacteremia in patients without endocarditis requires two positive cultures for *Streptococcus viridans*. If there is another focus of infection (*eg*, skin abscess, pneumonia), a positive blood culture becomes a minor criterion.

Persistently positive blood cultures (*see* Table 1) are two positive cultures at least 12 hours apart. Persistently positive cultures are necessary if the organism is not one typically associated with infectious endocarditis.

A study of the value and limitations of the Duke criteria for the diagnosis of infectious endocarditis has shown that the major cause of misclassification is the presence of negative blood cultures [2]. The most common cause of negative blood cultures was prior antibiotic therapy and Q-fever endocarditis [2].

The echocardiographic criteria are straightforward but cannot be preexistent if they are to be used as a major criterion. Nonoscillating masses are a minor echocardiographic criterion.

Predisposing conditions include the presence of an organic regurgitant cardiac murmur, prosthetic heart valves, immunologic compromise, intravenous drug use, and previous endocarditis. Vascular phenomena include embolus, Osler's nodes, Janeway lesions, and conjunctival petechiae; splinter hemorrhage or petechiae elsewhere are not specific enough. Immunologic phenomena include glomerulonephritis, positive rheumatoid factor, and C-reactive protein.

CLINICAL PRESENTATION

The classic triad of infectious endocarditis is fever, organic heart murmur, and positive blood culture; however, one, two, or (rarely) all three may be absent. Fever, the most frequent finding, may be absent in debilitated patients, but the most frequent cause of absent fever is previous antibiotic use. A heart murmur may be absent very early in the disease, especially when a normal valve is infected by a virulent organism. Murmurs of tricuspid or pulmonary valve involvement are often soft, low frequency, or atypical, and they can be easily overlooked. Patients who have undergone cardiac transplantation can have an infection at the atrial suture line. Other immunocompromised patients can have endocarditis without organic murmurs, as may occur with infection on a lead of a permanently implanted cardiac pacemaker. These are rarer causes of infectious endocarditis without a heart murmur. As discussed later, blood culture is negative in approximately 5% of patients with infectious endocarditis.

Constitutional symptoms of fatigue, malaise, anorexia, and weight loss are variable and relate to the state of the patient, the infecting organism, and (most importantly) to the duration of the infection. Peripheral manifestations, such as petechiae, splinter hemorrhages, Osler's nodes (vasculitis vs bacteremia), Janeway lesions, and Roth spots in the fundi, are directly related to the duration of the infection.

Other findings, such as splenomegaly, anemia, and embolic phenomena, are likewise related in part to the duration of the infection. Thromboembolic phenomena may be pulmonary (from right-sided endocarditis) or systemic (central nervous system, renal, or other peripheral sites) from left-sided endocarditis. Mycotic aneurysms result from peripheral infection of an arterial wall and may rupture.

AUSCULTATION

Cardiac auscultation plays an important role in infectious endocarditis. It not only allows for the identification of patients at increased risk for infectious endocarditis (those with regurgitant valvular lesions) but also identifies organic lesions and changing lesions in patients with endocarditis, helping to identify the state of cardiac function during the course of the illness.

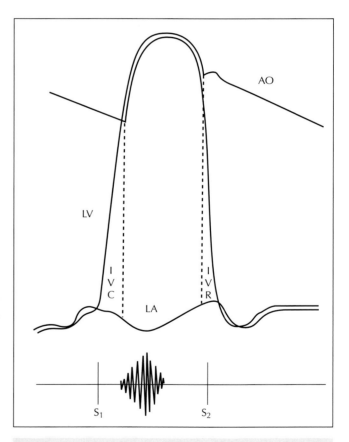

FIGURE 1 Flow murmurs have a distinct period of silence between the heart sounds and the murmur. During the isovolumetric contraction (IVC) period (the time between the closure of the atrioventricular [AV] valve and the opening of the semilunar valve), all valves are closed. Any murmur during this period must result from an abnormality. All valves are also closed during the isovolumetric relaxation (IVR) period (the time between the closure of the semilunar valves and the opening of the AV valves). This produces the silent periods right after the first heart sound (S_1) and right before the second heart sound (S_2). AO—aortic pressure; LA—left atrial pressure; LV—left ventricular pressure.

TABLE 1 PROPOSED CLINICAL CRITERIA FOR DIAGNOSIS OF INFECTIOUS ENDOCARDITIS*

Major

Positive blood culture (typical organism or persistently positive)

Echocardiographic (oscillating mass, abscess, or dehiscence of a prosthetic valve)

Minor

Predisposition

Fever greater than 38.0°C

Vascular phenomena

Immunologic phenomena

Echocardiographic (when not used as major criterion)

Microbiologic (one positive culture with typical organism)

*Both major criteria, one major criterion and three minor criteria, or five minor criteria are required for a definitive diagnosis.

Prevention

Patients with flow or ejection murmurs are not at risk for infectious endocarditis, but patients with regurgitant murmurs should have endocarditis prophylaxis. Therefore, it is important to identify by auscultation the presence of clinically significant regurgitant murmurs. The emphasis is on auscultation, because Doppler echocardiography frequently identifies valvular regurgitation that is not clinically significant, especially in elderly patients. Likewise, "echo-only" mitral valve prolapse without a murmur or a thickened mitral valve is a benign condition. Overdiagnosis of mitral valve prolapse by echocardiography is less frequent since Levine *et al.* [3] pointed out the saddle shape of the normal mitral ring and the fact that, in normal patients, apparent mitral valve prolapse is frequently present in the apical four-chamber view but not in the two-chamber view.

A flow murmur across the aortic or pulmonary valve is confined to the early and midsystolic period. There is a distinct period of silence between the first heart sound and the onset of the murmur, and another between the end of the murmur and the second heart sound (Fig. 1). Flow murmurs

during ventricular ejection are early systolic. In patients with normal ventricular function, two thirds of the left ventricular volume is ejected in the first one third of systole. Mild obstruction results in little change. Moderate to severe aortic or pulmonary valve obstruction prolongs the duration of maximal flow, and the duration of the murmur increases.

In contrast, regurgitant murmurs involve either the isovolumetric contraction period or the isovolumetric relaxation period, producing a murmur that begins coincident with the first heart sound (Fig. 2), the second heart sound (Fig. 3), or both. In the latter, the murmur is pan- or holosystolic (Fig. 4), because during the isovolumetric contraction period (the time between the closure of the atrioventricular [AV] valve and the opening of the semilunar valves) all valves are closed. Any murmur during this period must result from an abnormality. The same holds for the isovolumetric relaxation period, thus the silent periods right after the first heart sound and before the second heart sound.

As in systole, not all diastolic murmurs result from an organic abnormality of the heart. Diastolic murmurs

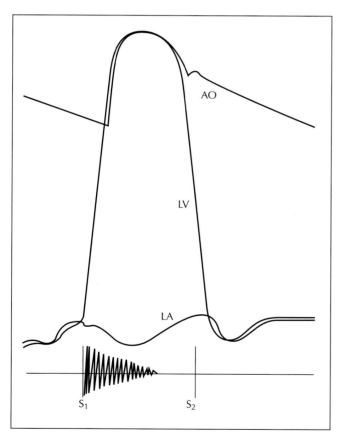

FIGURE 2 Murmurs that begin with the first heart sound (S_1) and therefore involve the isovolumetric contraction period (when all heart valves are closed) are regurgitant and therefore require endocarditis prophylaxis. AO—aortic pressure; LA—left atrial pressure; LV—left ventricular pressure; S_2—second heart sound.

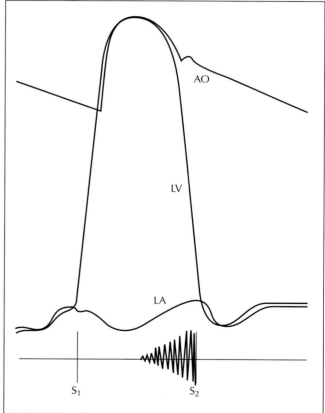

FIGURE 3 Systolic murmurs that are coincident with the second heart sound (S_2), and thus involve the isovolumetric relaxation period (a period when all heart valves are closed) and are regurgitant, require endocarditis prophylaxis. AO—aortic pressure; LA—left atrial pressure; LV—left ventricular pressure; S_1—first heart sound; S_2—second heart sound.

include regurgitation of the semilunar (aortic or pulmonic) valves, and obstruction of the AV (mitral or tricuspid) valves. Functional diastolic murmurs result from enhanced flow across the AV valves from another defect.

The technique of cardiac auscultation must be done carefully so as not to overlook murmurs that make the individual susceptible to infectious endocarditis. The room should be quiet, the stethoscope of top quality, and the patient examined in several positions. When listening for the murmur of aortic regurgitation, one must place the diaphragm of the stethoscope firmly against the chest wall in the third left intercostal space (Fig. 5). The patient should be auscultated in the supine, sitting, standing, and squatting (Fig. 6) positions during normal respiration and leaning forward during forced full expiration.

Likewise, when auscultating for mitral regurgitant murmurs, the patient must be examined with the stethoscope placed at the apex with the patient in the supine, left lateral, sitting, standing, squatting, and restanding positions. It is often only on restanding after squatting (Fig. 7) that the murmur of mitral valve prolapse or hypertrophic obstructive cardiomyopathy becomes apparent.

Is the presence of a single systolic click an indication for antibiotic prophylaxis? The opinion of cardiologists is divided. The current American Heart Association (AHA) guidelines [4] are not to recommend antibiotic prophylaxis

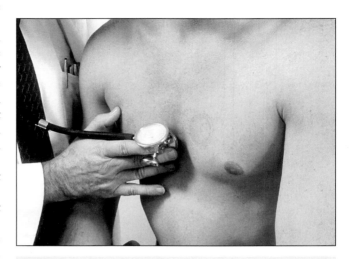

FIGURE 5 The pressure on the stethoscope should be such that an imprint from the stethoscope diaphragm remains on the skin when removed. One listens for a soft diastolic murmur; at times, this murmur is so soft that it simulates the sound of a gentle wind in the trees.

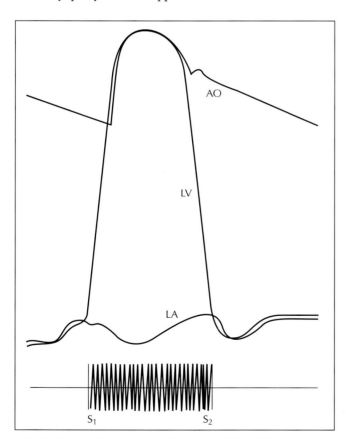

FIGURE 4 Pansystolic or holosystolic murmurs are always regurgitant, because they involve both isovolumetric periods (times when all of the heart valves are closed). AO—aortic pressure; LA—left atrial pressure; LV—left ventricular pressure; S_1—first heart sound; S_2—second heart sound.

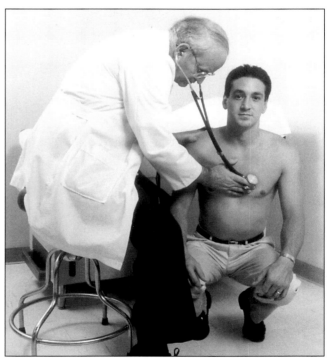

FIGURE 6 Auscultation with patient in the squatting position (note physician sitting on a stool) is an important maneuver, as squatting increases venous return (preload) and blood pressure (afterload), accentuates the murmur of aortic regurgitation, and decreases the murmur of hypertrophic obstructive cardiomyopathy.

Cardiology for the Primary Care Physician

for clicks only. The caveat is that the patient must be examined carefully and thoroughly in appropriate positions without eliciting a murmur. Although endocarditis has been described in patients with clicks only, these descriptions were from an era when patients were not routinely examined in the standing, squatting, and restanding positions.

In addition, there are a number of sounds that can be mistaken for clicks that do not originate from the mitral valve (Table 2). The characteristic of a systolic click of mitral valve prolapse is its variable position in systole depending on the left ventricular volume. The smaller the left ventricular volume (as with abrupt standing), the earlier the click; the larger the ventricular volume (as with squatting), the later the click. Endocarditis prophylaxis is also recommended for patients at very high risk without regurgitant murmur, such as those with prosthetic heart valves or severely immunocompromised patients.

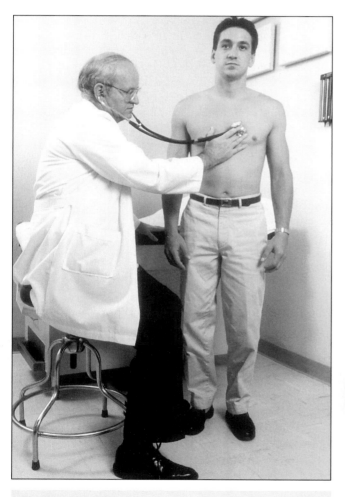

FIGURE 7 Auscultation of the patient standing after squatting is an important provocative maneuver, because this maneuver decreases venous return and thereby results in less filling of the left ventricle (decreased preload). This maneuver also decreases the blood pressure (decreased afterload). The resultant decrease in left ventricular volume increases or unmasks the murmur of mitral valve prolapse and hypertrophic obstructive cardiomyopathy.

Diagnosis

Cardiac auscultation is also an important aspect of the diagnosis of infectious endocarditis. Exact interpretation of auscultatory findings is not as critical for diagnosis as it is in prevention, because echocardiography is an essential diagnostic tool in the diagnosis of infectious endocarditis.

Rarely, a murmur will be absent in the early days of endocarditis, especially when endocarditis occurs on a normal valve, such as endocarditis from staphylococci. These virulent organisms soon destroy enough of the valve that a murmur appears.

In the appropriate clinical setting, the sudden appearance of a new regurgitant murmur is nearly diagnostic of infectious endocarditis. Regurgitant apical systolic murmurs in infectious endocarditis may result from AV valve perforation, rupture of chordae tendineae, destruction of the valve, or functional AV incompetence. Regurgitant diastolic murmurs are caused by aortic or pulmonary valve perforation or destruction secondary to aortic-ventricular or aortic-atrial connections resulting from abscess-induced connections.

The auscultatory findings of tricuspid valve incompetence are more subtle. The murmur may not be typically regurgitant. The murmur may increase with inspiration (the Caravallo sign) [5], but these diagnostic features are frequently absent. The jugular venous pulse should be carefully observed for the presence of regurgitant CV waves.

Low-frequency diastolic murmurs can result from inflow obstruction caused by large vegetations or flow from increased AV valve incompetence or nonpulmonary hypertensive pulmonary valve incompetence. Inflow obstructions are rare in infectious endocarditis and most commonly result from fungal vegetation or clot formation on vegetations. The development of an apical diastolic flow murmur in a patient with preexisting mitral regurgitation usually indicates an increased degree of mitral regurgitation. The diastolic murmur of pulmonary artery insufficiency in a patient with normal pulmonary artery pressures is also low frequency but is best heard along the left sternal border.

High-frequency diastolic murmurs from the pulmonary valve occur in patients with preexisting pulmonary hyper-

TABLE 2 CLICK-LIKE SOUNDS NOT CAUSED BY MITRAL OR TRICUSPID VALVE PROLAPSE	
Early systolic	**Early diastolic**
Pulmonic ejection sound	Opening snap
Aortic ejection sound	**Late diastolic**
Split first heart sound	Pacemaker chest wall sound
Late systolic	
Wide split second heart sound	**Variable systolic and diastolic**
Variable systolic	Extracardiac (pneumothorax)
Atrial septal aneurysm	

tension, such as in patients with Eisenmenger syndrome. The usual cause of a high-frequency diastolic murmur in infectious endocarditis is destruction or perforation of the aortic valve. These murmurs likewise are best heard along the left sternal border, but on occasion, perforation may lead to an eccentrically directed jet producing a high-frequency murmur best heard in the third or fourth right intercostal space compared with the third or fourth left intercostal space. Right-sided murmurs of aortic regurgitation suggest unusual causes of aortic regurgitation such as infectious endocarditis.

Determining Severity

Low-frequency third and fourth heart sounds indicate deterioration of ventricular function, usually from increasing severity of the lesions. Third heart sounds are heard with the development of heart failure. They occur at the peak of the rapid filling wave of the left ventricular pressure curve and the peak of the Doppler transmitral velocity wave (E point).

Development of a fourth heart sound suggests acute valvular incompetence, myocarditis, or a hyperkinetic state. This sound occurs at the height of the A wave in the left ventricular pressures trace and the *A* point on the Doppler transmitral velocity tracing. These low-frequency sounds are best heard with the bell of the stethoscope placed lightly on the skin, just making an air seal. Firm pressure stretches the skin, making it a diaphragm and filtering out low-frequency sounds.

The auscultatory findings of acute severe aortic and mitral regurgitation are quite different from those of chronic aortic and mitral regurgitation. These are described in Tables 3 and 4, respectively.

ECHOCARDIOGRAPHY

The sensitivity of echocardiography for identifying vegetations in patients with infectious endocarditis is approximately 55% for M-mode techniques, 70% to 80% for two-dimensional, and over 90% for transesophageal echocardiography [6]. The role of echocardiography is outlined in Table 5. Echocardiography can identify a vegetation or a perivalvular abscess, and it can document chamber size and function as well as the condition of the valves. Identification of a mobile or oscillating mass, an abscess, or dehiscence of a prosthetic valve are components of definite clinical criteria for the diagnosis of infectious endocarditis.

The echocardiographic size of the vegetation in some series has important prognostic significance. In right-sided endocarditis, lesions over 20 mm were associated with a 33% 6-month mortality rate, whereas 6-month mortality was only 1% if the mass was smaller [7].

The prognostic implications of vegetation size remain controversial. Some studies of left-sided endocarditis found a worse prognosis with large-sized vegetation. In some studies, emboli are more likely with large vegetation size [6] when they are mobile (*ie*, have a stalk) [7–9]. It appears that the mobility of the vegetation or those with a stalk have a higher risk on systemic emboli.

Emboli may depend on factors other than size and mobility. Some studies have implicated the organism (more common with *Streptococcus*), the antibiotic used, and the response of vegetation size to therapy.

TABLE 3 MANIFESTATIONS OF SEVERE AORTIC REGURGITATION		
	Acute	**Chronic**
First heart sound	Absent	Present
Diastolic murmur	Short	Long
Pulse pressure	Normal	Increased
Ejection sound	Absent	Present
Heart rate	Fast	Normal

TABLE 4 MANIFESTATIONS OF SEVERE MITRAL REGURGITATION		
	Acute	**Chronic**
Rhythm	Sinus	Atrial fibrillation
Left atrial size	Normal	Enlarged
Fourth heart sound	Present	Absent
Third heart sound	Present or absent	Present
Pulmonary component S_2	Increased	Normal
Murmur	Late systolic attenuation	Pansystolic
Pulmonary congestion	Early	Late

TABLE 5 ECHOCARDIOGRAPHY IN INFECTIOUS ENDOCARDITIS
Visualization of vegetations: evaluate valvular anatomy and function
Detect abscess, fistula, or perforation
Evaluate hemodynamic consequences
Negative transesophageal echocardiography, very high probability of not having infectious endocarditis
Bacteremia without endocarditis in patients with valvular heart disease is treated much differently
Transesophageal echocardiography should be repeated in patients; a negative study if the clinical course dictates

BLOOD CULTURES

Blood cultures are critically important to the diagnosis and management of infectious endocarditis. It is recommended that three blood cultures be taken 1 hour apart with at least 10 mL of blood for each. The reason for drawing the cultures 1 hour apart is that transient bacteremia from *Streptococcus viridans* endocarditis is not uncommon. Bacteremia from endocarditis is relatively constant, so most of the cultures are usually positive. Contamination is less likely if three separate cultures are taken.

Culture-Negative Endocarditis

Blood cultures are negative in 5% to 10% of patients with the infectious endocarditis. Common causes of culture-negative endocarditis are listed in Table 6. The major cause of negative blood cultures in patients with infectious endocarditis is prior antibiotic therapy. The longer the therapy with effective antibiotics before they are discontinued, the longer it takes for bacteremia to reappear.

TABLE 6 CATEGORIES OF CULTURE-NEGATIVE ENDOCARDITIS
Prior antimicrobial therapy before culture
Infection by fastidious microorganisms
HACEK group
Nutritionally deficient streptococci
Brucella spp.
Neisseria spp.
Anaerobes
Corynebacterium spp.
Legionella spp.
Fungi
Q fever (*Coxiella burnetii*)
Chlamydia sp.
Subacute right-sided endocarditis
HACEK—*Haemophilus, Actinobacillus, Cardiobacterium, Eikenella,* and *Kingella* species.

TABLE 7 NONINFECTIOUS ENDOCARDITIS OR MASSES
Myxoma
Papilloma
Acute rheumatic carditis
Lupus nonbacterial verrucous endocarditis
Marantic endocarditis
Endocardial fibroelastosis
Fibroblastic endocarditis (Löffler's endocarditis)
Carcinoid

Bacteremia Versus Endocarditis

A major diagnostic dilemma may occur in a patient with organic heart disease who presents with fever. The problem is compounded if there are positive blood cultures or the patient has an endocardial mass or endocarditis of noninfectious origin (Table 7).

ANTIBIOTIC PROPHYLAXIS

The AHA recommendations for who should and should not receive prophylactic therapy are outlined in Tables 8 and 9, respectively. Recommendations for antibiotic therapy for endocarditis prophylaxis are outlined in Table 10.

TABLE 8 PROCEDURES AND CONDITIONS FOR WHICH ENDOCARDITIS PROPHYLAXIS IS RECOMMENDED
Dental procedures likely to cause gingival bleeding
Surgical operations that involve intestinal or respiratory mucosa
Esophageal dilation
Gallbladder surgery
Cystoscopy
Urethral dilation
Prosthetic surgery
Incision and drainage abscess
Vaginal hysterectomy
Vaginal delivery during an infection
Prosthetic cardiac valves
Previous endocarditis
Rheumatic valve dysfunction
Mitral valve prolapse with mitral regurgitation
Hypertrophic cardiomyopathy

TABLE 9 PROCEDURES AND CONDITIONS FOR WHICH INFECTIOUS ENDOCARDITIS PROPHYLAXIS IS NOT RECOMMENDED
Dental procedures not likely to produce gingival bleeding
Bronchoscopy with flexible scope
Endoscopy without biopsy
Cesarean section
Cardiac catheterization
Isolated secundum atrial septal defect
Atrial septal defect, ventricular septal defect, and patent ductus arteriosus repair after 6 months
Coronary artery bypass surgery
Mitral valve prolapse without mitral regurgitation
Functional heart murmurs
Implanted pacemakers

WHEN TO REFER

Infectious endocarditis is a potentially lethal disease. Accordingly, patients should be referred whenever this diagnosis is seriously considered. All patients should be followed up by a team consisting of the patient's primary-care physician, cardiologist, infectious disease specialist, and cardiovascular surgeon.

INDICATIONS FOR SURGERY

Surgery is indicated when antibiotics fail to control endocarditis. Evidence of failure may be signs of progressive invasion of the myocardium with abscess formation, heart block, or development of fistulas; persistent sepsis; progressive hemodynamic instability; or repeated emboli [10]. Most fungal infections require surgery for cure. Surgery for persistent culture-positive active endocarditis is necessary at times. Although morality is high, averaging about 25% of patients, the long-term outcome of survivors is good [11].

COMPLICATIONS AND PROGNOSIS

Complications are not uncommon in infectious endocarditis. Table 11 lists the more common complications in order

TABLE 10 BACTERIAL ENDOCARDITIS PROPHYLAXIS IN ADULTS

Dental/oral/upper respiratory tract and esophageal procedures for patients at high risk
Amoxicillin 2.0 g orally 1 h before procedure

For amoxicillin/penicillin-allergic patients
Clindamycin 600 mg orally 1 h before procedure, then one half this dose 6 h after initial dose

Genitourinary/gastrointestinal procedures
Ampicillin 2.0 q IV plus gentamycin 1.5 mg/kg IV (not to exceed 120 mg) 30 min before procedure, followed by amoxicillin 1.0 g orally 6 h after the initial dose

TABLE 11 COMPLICATIONS OF INFECTIOUS ENDOCARDITIS

Cardiac
Neurologic
Septic
Associated with medical treatment
Renal
Extracranial systemic emboli
Septic pulmonary emboli
Complications related to surgery
Acute prosthetic heart valve insufficiency

of frequency [12]. Although cardiac complications are the most common, fatality rates may be higher from neurologic or septic complications.

SYSTEMIC EMBOLI

Systemic embolizations occur in 20% to 40% of patients with infectious endocarditis, most occurring with the first few weeks of therapy. The incidence decreases to 10% to 20% after initiation of antibiotic therapy. Embolization is silent in about 20% of patients. The larger the vegetation, the greater the incidence of systemic embolization. In general, surgical intervention to avoid systemic emboli has the greatest benefit if done in the early phase (within 2 weeks) when embolic rates are the highest, but should be considered only in patients where embolic rates are highest, *eg*, recurrent emboli, congestive heart failure, aggressive antibiotic-resistant organisms, or when prosthetic valve endocarditis is present. Surgery should also be considered in patients with vegetations over 15 mm and high mobility, vegetations that increase in size, or vegetations that fail to decrease in size with appropriate therapy. Surgery is also recommended in patients in whom the infection extends beyond the valve annulus.

KEY REFERENCES

Recently published papers of outstanding interest, as identified in *References and Recommended Reading*, have been annotated.

•• Durack DT, Luke AS, Bright DK, and the Duke Endocarditis Service: New criteria for diagnosis of infective endocarditis: Utilization of specific echocardiographic criteria. *Am J Med* 1994, 96:200–209.

New criteria for the diagnosis of endocarditis. This is a classic.

REFERENCES AND RECOMMENDED READING

Recently published papers of particular interest have been highlighted as:
- Of interest
- •• Of outstanding interest

1.•• Durack DT, Luke AS, Bright DK, and the Duke Endocarditis Service: New criteria for diagnosis of infective endocarditis: Utilization of specific echocardiographic criteria. *Am J Med* 1994, 96:200–209.

2. Habib G, Derumeaux G, Avierinos J-F, *et al.*: Value and limitations of the Duke Criteria for the diagnosis of infectious endocarditis. *J Am Coll Cardiol* 1999, 33:2023–2039.

3. Levine RA, Triulzi MO, Harrigan P, *et al.*: The relationship of mitral annular shape to the diagnosis of mitral valve prolapse. *Circulation* 1987, 75:756–767.

4. Dajani AS, Taubert KA, Wilson W, *et al.*: Prevention of bacterial endocarditis: recommendations by the American Heart Association. *Circulation* 1997, 96:358–366.

5. Gooch AS, Maranchao V, Scampardonis G, *et al.*: Prolapse of both mitral and tricuspid leaflets in systolic murmur-click syndrome. *N Engl J Med* 1972, 287:1218–1222.

6. Siddiq S, Missri J, Silverma DJ: Endocarditis in an urban hospital in the 1990s. *Arch Intern Med* 1996, 156:2454–2458.

7. Heinle SK, Durack DT, Longabaugh JP, *et al.*: Can echocardiography predict risk of embolic events in infectious endocarditis? *Choices Cardiol* 1992, 7:79–81.

8. Hecht SR, Berger M: Right-sided endocarditis in intravenous drug users. Prognostic features in 102 episodes. *Ann Intern Med* 1992, 117:560–566.

9. Khandheria BK: Suspected bacterial endocarditis: to TEE or not TEE. *J Am Coll Cardiol* 1993, 21:222–224.

10. Jamieson SW: Surgical therapy for infective endocarditis. *Mayo Clin Proc* 1995, 70:598–599.

11. Mullany CL, Chua YL, Schaff HV, *et al.*: Early and late survival after surgical treatment of culture-positive active endocarditis. *Mayo Clin Proc* 1995, 70:517–525.

12. Mansur AJ, Grinberg M, da Luz PL, *et al.*: The complications of infectious endocarditis: a reappraisal in the 1980s. *Arch Intern Med* 1992, 152:2428–2432.

SELECT BIBLIOGRAPHY

AHA Scientific Statement: Diagnosis and management of infective endocarditis and its complications. *Circulation* 1998, 98:2836–2948.

DiSalvo GD, Habib G, Pergola V, *et al.*: Echocardiography predicts embolic events in infective endocarditis. *J Am Coll Cardiol* 2001, 37:1069–1076.

Habib G: Embolic risk in subacute bacterial endocarditis: determinants and role of transesophageal echocardiography. *Curr Cardiol Rep* 2003, 5:129–136.

Kay D: *Infectious Endocarditis*, edn 2. New York: Raven Press; 1992.

Mugge A, Daniel WG: Echocardiographic assessment of vegetations in patients with infective endocarditis. *Echocardiography* 1995, 12:651–661.

Mylonakis E, Calderwood SB: Infective endocarditis in adults. *N Engl J Med* 2001, 345:1318–1330.

Reid CL, Chandraratna PAN, Rahimtoola SH: Infectious endocarditis: improved diagnosis and treatment. *Curr Probl Cardiol* 1985, 10:1–51.

Pericardial Disease
Jae K. Oh

30

Key Points

- Pericarditis is a disease of diverse origins; treatment consists of administering a combination of anti-inflammatory drugs and therapy directed at the specific underlying disease.

- Cardiac tamponade constitutes an emergency that requires prompt recognition and treatment. Pericardiocentesis is most safely performed under two-dimensional echocardiography guidance.

- Constrictive pericarditis is a curable disease that should be considered in patients with unexplained heart failure especially when ejection fraction is normal; evaluation with a combination of noninvasive testing and cardiac catheterization can accurately establish the diagnosis in most patients.

- Tissue Doppler imaging of the mitral annulus is very helpful in distinguishing constrictive pericarditis from myopathies responsible for heart failure.

- Constrictive pericarditis in a subset of patients is transient and can be fully recovered after medical management (*ie*, with diuretic therapy, steroids, or nonsteroidal anti-inflammatory agents).

The pericardium is not essential for sustaining life or health, as evidenced by a lack of cardiac dysfunction when it is congenitally absent or surgically opened. Normal functions of the pericardium include maintenance of an optimal cardiac shape, promotion of cardiac chamber interaction, restraint of overfilling of the heart, reduction of friction between the beating heart and adjacent structures, provision of a physical barrier to infection, and limitation of cardiac displacement during the cardiac cycle. Most often the clinical importance of the pericardium is seen through its involvement in a number of disease states.

ACUTE PERICARDITIS

Pathophysiology

Acute pericarditis is an inflammatory condition of the pericardium caused by a variety of agents and disease states (Table 1). The most common etiologic agents are viral and likely account for most cases of "idiopathic" pericarditis. With the recent epidemic of multiple drug–resistant tuberculosis in urban populations, tuberculous pericarditis may very well become an increasing problem after decades of declining incidence [1–3], but is still uncommon. Tuberculous pericarditis most commonly occurs in the absence of demonstrable pulmonary or extrapulmonary tuberculosis. Patients with AIDS can develop pericarditis or tamponade as a result of infection with the virus itself or a large number of opportunistic organisms [4,5]. Pericarditis can be clinically identified in 7% to 23% of patients with transmural myocardial infarction, and the risk for pericarditis is proportional to the size of the infarction [6,7]. Bacterial pericarditis often develops in the context of significant extracardiac infections, particularly intrathoracic infections [8].

Clinical Manifestations

The cardinal clinical features of acute pericarditis are chest pain, friction rub, and electrocardiographic (ECG) changes. Many patients relate prodromal symptoms suggestive of a viral infection. The chest pain of pericarditis varies in location, intensity, and character; it may be described as sharp or dull. Most often, it is precordial or retrosternal and may be referred to the trapezius ridge. It is often aggravated by inspiration, coughing, or recumbency, and it is lessened by sitting upright and leaning forward. Although typically taking 1 or 2 hours to develop fully, at times the pain can appear with remarkable abruptness. Patients with pericarditis may be febrile and tachycardic. The pericardial friction rub is the pathognomonic auscultatory finding. It is typically scratchy and characteristically has three components, although it is not unusual for only one or two components to be audible. The systolic component is most consistently present. The friction rub may be

evanescent or influenced by the patient's position; thus, repeated auscultation, and auscultation with the patient in several positions, is essential.

Bacterial pericarditis should be suspected in the presence of high fevers, chills, or night sweats. Patients with bacterial pericarditis frequently lack pleuritic chest pain or pericardial friction rubs.

Laboratory Findings

Evaluation of a patient with suspected pericarditis should include ECG, chest radiography, a complete blood count, and echocardiography. Echocardiography is the diagnostic procedure of choice when hemodynamically significant pericardial disease is suspected. Serial ECGs are valuable in establishing or confirming the diagnosis of pericarditis; four stages of ECG evolution have been described (Fig. 1). Although ECG abnormalities occur

---

TABLE 1 CAUSES OF PERICARDITIS

Idiopathic
Viral (Coxsackie B5, B6; echovirus; adenovirus; influenza, AIDs; others)
Purulent (Most common organisms in recent series are *Pneumococcus*, *Streptococcus*, *Staphylococcus*, gram-negative bacilli, and fungi)
Tuberculosis
Sarcoidosis
Amyloidosis
Uremia
Myocardial infarction
Acute pericarditis
Dressler's syndrome (postmyocardial infarction syndrome)
Dissection of the aorta
Neoplastic disease (lung, breast, melanoma, lymphoma, leukemia)
Radiation therapy
Autoimmune diseases (lupus, rheumatoid arthritis, etc.)
Trauma (cardiac or intravenous catheterization, chest trauma, pacemaker insertion, thoracic surgery)
Drugs (daunorubicin, diphenylhydantoin, hydralazine, isoniazid, methysergide, penicillin, phenylbutazone, procainamide)
Anticoagulants (warfarin, heparin)

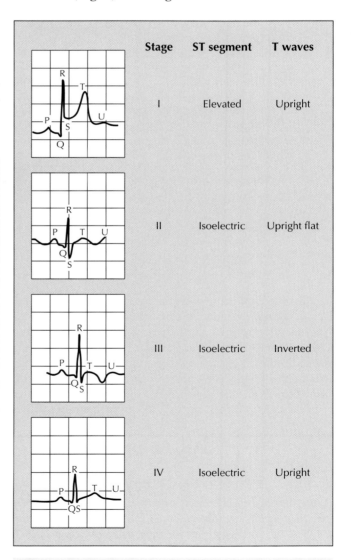

	Stage	ST segment	T waves
	I	Elevated	Upright
	II	Isoelectric	Upright flat
	III	Isoelectric	Inverted
	IV	Isoelectric	Upright

FIGURE 1 The four stages of electrocardiographic changes in acute pericarditis.

in 90% of cases, all four stages can be serially identified in approximately 50% of patients. Early ECG changes of pericarditis must be distinguished from the normal variant of early repolarization and from myocardial ischemia or infarction. In early repolarization, the distribution of the ST-segment elevation may be very similar to that in pericarditis, but the elevation remains unchanged and does not evolve through the serial changes seen in acute pericarditis. The ST:T ratio in lead V_6 can help in differentiating early repolarization from pericarditis. If the magnitude of ST-segment elevation is less than one-fourth of T-wave amplitude, early repolarization is more likely; if this ratio is greater than 1:4, pericarditis is more likely. The ST-segment elevation of pericarditis differs from that of myocardial infarction in that it is typically concave upward and present in all leads except aVR and V_1, where the ST segment frequently will be depressed. Furthermore, ST segments typically return to normal before the T waves become inverted in patients with pericarditis, whereas in those with myocardial infarction, T-wave inversion evolves while the ST segments are still elevated. Finally, the ECG in patients with pericarditis often demonstrates depression of the PR segment in those leads with ST elevation (Fig. 2), and the PR depression may precede ST elevation [3].

Mild leukocytosis and mild elevation of the erythrocyte sedimentation rate are common in viral or idiopathic pericarditis. These findings are less common in the pericarditis of uremia or connective tissue disorders. A significant leukocytosis with a shift to the left raises the possibility of bacterial pericarditis. Cardiac enzyme levels may be slightly elevated in cases where the inflammatory process involves subepicardial myocardium. Chest radiography usually reveals no abnormalities in uncomplicated pericarditis, but it may show an enlarged cardiac silhouette if a significant pericardial effusion is present. Echocardiography may reveal a pericardial effusion, but absence of an effusion by no means excludes the diagnosis.

When the suspicion of bacterial or tuberculous pericarditis is high, a diagnostic pericardiocentesis is indicated. The pericardial fluid should be examined with Gram and acid-fast bacillus stains and cultured for bacteria, mycobacteria, and fungi. Tubercle bacillus is demonstrated by stain or culture in only one third to one half of patients with tuberculous pericarditis. The diagnosis is often based on a history of contact or conversion of a purified protein derivative (PPD) skin test. The presence of increased levels of adenosine deaminase in pericardial fluid has been proposed as a specific test for tuberculous pericarditis [9]. Levels above 40 IU/L suggest tuberous pericarditis [9,10].

Management
Idiopathic and viral pericarditis
In most cases of idiopathic acute pericarditis, anti-inflammatory treatment with nonsteroidal anti-inflammatory agents usually suppresses the clinical manifestations within 24 hours. For patients in whom nonsteroidal agents fail to ameliorate symptoms, steroid therapy can be initiated with a caution. Relapsing pericarditis is often observed in patients who are treated with steroids early in their course of pericarditis. It is often very difficult to taper off the steroid therapy completely, and the only therapy in this situation may be pericardiectomy. In most patients, a single course of anti-inflammatory therapy controls the illness, and the pericarditis resolves without sequelae. In some patients (15% to 32%), the pericarditis may recur over weeks or months after the initial episode [11,12]. These episodes can be treated with repeated courses of nonsteroidal or steroidal anti-inflammatory agents. Colchicine (0.6 mg, twice daily) appears to be a promising adjunct to conventional treatment for cases of recurrent pericarditis [12], and immunosuppressive drugs (eg, azathioprine) have been used occasionally. In rare cases, frequent and severe recurrences despite aggressive drug therapy do require pericardiectomy [13].

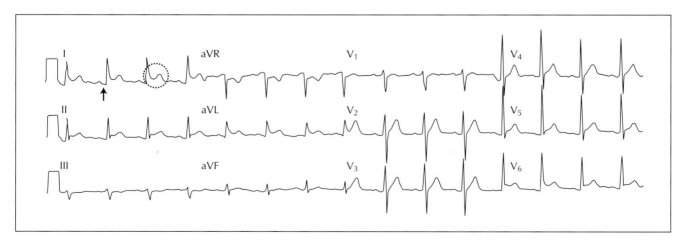

FIGURE 2 Typical electrocardiography of acute pericarditis with PR depression (*arrow*) and concave upward ST segment elevation (*circle*).

Bacterial and tuberculous pericarditis

Bacterial pericarditis is a medical emergency that must be treated with drainage and antibiotic agents. Mortality rates range from 56% to 77% [8]. The presence of gram-negative organisms indicates a poor prognosis. Untreated tuberculous pericarditis is associated with 80% mortality rates. Management involves administration of three antituberculous drugs for at least 9 months. The role of corticosteroid therapy and early surgical pericardiectomy in patients with tuberculous pericarditis has been a source of controversy [1]. In the only prospective controlled trial addressing this question, prednisolone therapy was associated with a reduction in mortality and the need for emergent repeat pericardiocentesis; the rates of subsequent constrictive pericarditis did not differ between patients receiving prednisolone and placebo [14]. Complete open drainage reduced the need for subsequent urgent pericardiocentesis but did not influence development of subsequent constriction or mortality [14].

Uremia

Uremic pericarditis prior to dialysis almost always responds to the initiation of dialysis. Pericarditis in patients already receiving chronic dialysis is a more complex challenge. The pericarditis may have an identifiable cause with a specific remedy in a significant proportion of these patients. In the majority of cases, however, no specific cause will be identified, and the pericarditis typically responds to intensification of the dialysis regimen [15]. Pericardial effusions, however, will not consistently resolve with intensive dialysis [16]. Lack of response to intensive dialysis may be predicted by several clinical variables (Table 2) [15]. Nonsteroidal anti-inflammatory agents can be used in these patients. Also, indomethacin has been successful in alleviating fevers but did not influence the duration of chest pain, pericardial rub, or the subsequent development of tamponade.

Transmural myocardial infarction and thrombolytic therapy

Pericarditis can be mistaken for acute myocardial infarction, leading to inappropriate administration of thrombolytic

agents with potentially catastrophic results [17]. Indeed, pericarditis is a relative contraindication to both thrombolytic therapy and anticoagulation treatment. Most cases of pericarditis complicating myocardial infarction, however, develop later in the illness and are not a confounding factor in the early hours, when decisions concerning thrombolytic therapy are being made. Thrombolytic therapy is associated with a reduced incidence of pericarditis, probably because it reduces the size of the infarction [6]. When pericarditis occurs after infarction, it usually resolves promptly and does not require therapy beyond the use of analgesic drugs. The incidence of Dressler's syndrome (postmyocardial infarction syndrome consisting of fever, malaise, and pleural and pericardial effusions associated with pleuropericardial pain) appears to have decreased, a trend some authorities attribute to decreased use of anticoagulation agents in patients who have had myocardial infarction [18].

PERICARDIAL EFFUSION AND CARDIAC TAMPONADE

Pericardial effusion may develop as a result of pericarditis or as a response to injury to the parietal pericardium. Once the relatively small reserve volume of the pericardium is filled, intrapericardial pressure rises precipitously with the addition of more fluid. Pericardial effusions may be encountered in the absence of pericarditis in many clinical settings, including uremia, cardiac trauma or chamber rupture, malignancy, AIDS, amyloid, scleroderma, and hypothyroidism. Clinical manifestations relate to the pressure in the pericardium, which in turn depends on the rapidity of accumulation and the absolute volume of the effusion because the stiffness of the pericardium determines fluid increments precipitating tamponade [19]. Rapid accumulation of even modest volumes can be associated with increased intrapericardial pressures and life-threatening hemodynamic compromise. This usually occurs in the setting of interventional therapy or myocardial biopsy. Another typical situation is in patients with aortic dissection that extends into the pericardial cavity because of proximal dissection of the aorta and the hemopericardium. With a slowly accumulating effusion, the pericardium can accommodate 1 to 2 L of fluid without a clinically significant elevation in intrapericardial pressure. Large idiopathic chronic pericardial effusion can be tolerated for long periods, but tamponade can develop unexpectedly [20]. Cardiac tamponade ensues when the accumulation of fluid compromises the filling of the heart and, consequently, impairs cardiac output.

Clinical Manifestations

The widespread availability of echocardiography has led to the identification of small effusions in asymptomatic patients in a wide variety of clinical settings. Small, incidentally discovered effusions rarely cause symptoms or complications. Large effusions may become clinically manifest by compressing adjacent structures, and they may

---

TABLE 2 FACTORS PREDICTING FAILURE OF INTENSIVE DIALYSIS IN TREATMENT OF UREMIC PERICARDITIS

Temperature > 102°F
Rales
Jugular venous distention
Peritoneal dialysis as sole modality
WBC > 15,000 mm^3
WBC shift to the left
Large pericardial effusion by echocardiography

WBC—white-blood-cell count

---

cause dysphagia, cough, dyspnea, hiccups, hoarseness, nausea, or a sense of abdominal fullness. Some patients may present with right upper quadrant pain caused by stretching of the hepatic capsule from increased right heart pressure. Signs of pericardial effusion are absent in patients with small effusions without increased pressure. Large effusions may muffle the heart sounds or cause rales or dullness on auscultation of the chest as a result of compression of the lung parenchyma. The typical signs of cardiac tamponade include high venous pressure, low systemic arterial pressure, diminished pulse pressure, tachycardia, tachypnea, and pulsus paradoxus. The jugular venous pressure is usually markedly elevated, with obliteration of the normal y-descent. The frequency of these physical findings is somewhat variable (Table 3). A paradoxic pulse may be absent in certain clinical situations (eg, tamponade coexisting with atrial septal defect or aortic insufficiency). This absence can be an important confounding variable in cases of proximal aortic dissection, which can cause both acute severe aortic insufficiency and cardiac tamponade.

Laboratory Findings

Chest radiography can demonstrate a number of findings in patients with pericardial effusion (Table 4, Fig. 3). Because these radiographic signs are inconsistently present, however, chest radiography cannot reliably confirm or exclude the diagnosis. Chest radiography also may offer clues to important coexisting conditions such as aortic dissection or malignancy. The ECG may be entirely normal or include changes typical of pericarditis; large effusions can cause a reduction in QRS voltage and electrical alternans.

Echocardiography is the most rapid and accurate means to diagnose a pericardial effusion. The effusion appears as an echo-free space between the moving epicardium and stationary pericardium. Small effusions tend to be imaged only posteriorly; however, a posterior echo-free space in some cases may reflect subepicardial fat rather than pericardial effusion. Larger effusions are distributed anteriorly as well as posteriorly. Large effusions can be associated with a swinging motion of the

TABLE 3 PHYSICAL FINDINGS IN CARDIAC TAMPONADE	
Physical finding	**Frequency, %**
Jugular venous distention	100
Tachypnea	80–97
Tachycardia	77–100
Pulsus paradoxus	77–89
Arterial pulse pressure < 40 mm Hg	46
Systolic blood pressure < 100 mm Hg	36–42
Diminished heart sounds	34–88
Pericardial friction rub	22–29

TABLE 4 CHEST RADIOGRAPHIC FINDINGS IN PERICARDIAL EFFUSION		
	Size of effusion	
Radiographic sign	**Moderate and large**	**Small**
Enlarged cardiac silhouette	78%	68%
Pericardial fat stripe	22%	8%
Left-sided pleural effusion	43%	12%
Increase in cardiac diameter since last chest radiograph	27%	54%

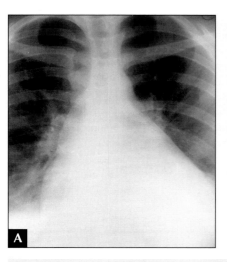
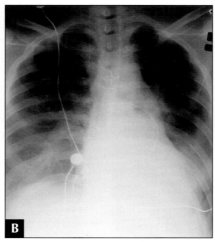
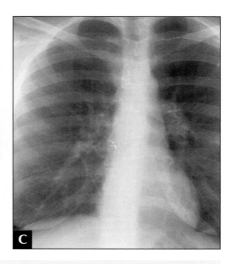

FIGURE 3 Chest radiographs illustrating the characteristic enlarged cardiac silhouette in a large pericardial effusion (**A**), after therapeutic pericardiocentesis (**B**), and several months later, after complete resolution of the pericardial effusion (**C**). The shape of the heart in the patient with the large effusion (**A**) has been likened to a water bottle.

heart within the fluid-filled pericardium—the mechanism of electrical alternans. Late diastolic collapse of the right atrium and early diastolic collapse of the right ventricle are useful echocardiographic signs indicating increased intrapericardial pressure. The hemodynamic significance of pericarditis effusion is best assessed by Doppler echocardiography. Cardiac tamponade results in a characteristic respiratory variation of mitral inflow, tricuspid inflow, and hepatic vein flow velocities similar to the changes observed in patients with constrictive pericarditis [21]. Cardiac catheterization in the setting of tamponade will reveal elevated and equal (or near-equal) filling pressures in all four chambers as well as a depressed cardiac output. Examination of the atrial pressure waveforms reveals the loss of the normal y-descent. The initial presentation and hemodynamic profile of tamponade may be altered by a concomitant state of intravascular volume depletion, a scenario termed *low-pressure cardiac tamponade*. In most cases of cardiac tamponade, however, cardiac catheterization is not necessary to establish the diagnosis.

Fluid obtained by pericardiocentesis should be sent for culture and cytologic examination except in the case of clear-cut traumatic tamponade. The gross appearance of the fluid is not helpful in establishing the cause, although malignant effusion is more likely bloody, and cell counts and chemistries are of limited value. Fluid cytologic smears will be abnormal in approximately 80% of malignant effusions; the remainder are usually identified via surgical biopsy of the pericardium.

Management

Management of pericardial effusions is largely dictated by the presence or absence of hemodynamic compromise from increased pericardial pressure and the nature of the underlying disorder. In most cases, a small or incidentally discovered effusion warrants no specific intervention. Once an

effusion of a certain magnitude is present, however, accumulation of even small additional amounts of fluid may result in a marked increase of intrapericardial pressure and rapid clinical deterioration. Thus, patients with any evidence of increased intrapericardial pressure or rapidly accumulating effusions must be monitored closely.

Drainage of pericardial fluid is the cornerstone of therapy for cardiac tamponade. Administration of fluids and vasopressor agents may be useful temporizing measures, but they are not a substitute for drainage and should never delay prompt removal of the pericardial fluid. Most commonly, drainage is achieved by percutaneous pericardiocentesis performed via the apical or subxiphoid route under echocardiographic guidance [22]. The procedure is effective and safe but may be complicated by laceration or puncture of the heart. Echocardiography can decrease the risk of cardiac puncture. At least 1 cm of an echo-free space anterior to the heart should be present before percutaneous pericardiocentesis is undertaken. Pericardiocentesis is ideally carried out in the special procedure room or the cardiac catheterization laboratory with echocardiographic or fluoroscopic guidance. Results of pericardiocentesis can be monitored by echocardiography in terms of the amount of fluid and the impact on hemodynamics. Although concomitant right heart cardiac catheterization or fluroscopic guidance were necessary in the past, these are rarely necessary if the procedure is guided by two-dimensional echocardiography. On occasion, emergency pericardiocentesis may need to be performed at the bedside. Rarely are circumstances sufficiently emergent to preclude confirmation of the diagnosis with echocardiography. Evacuation of the pericardial fluid also can be achieved via a subxiphoid surgical pericardiotomy; this procedure permits pericardial biopsy in cases of suspected malignant effusion.

In some cases, a single pericardiocentesis is effective in fully alleviating the effusion, but in most cases, consideration should be given to leaving a catheter temporarily in the pericardium for continued drainage [23]. Subsequent management of the patient is largely dictated by the specific cause of the effusion. For malignant effusions, potential treatment modalities include chemotherapy, radiation therapy, intrapericardial sclerosis, indwelling pericardial drainage catheters, surgery, or percutaneous balloon pericardiotomy [24]. No clinical trials have directly compared these various options, but success rates have been similar in individual reports [24]. The specific tumor type and the severity of hemodynamic compromise caused by the effusion must be taken into account when deciding among the various treatment options.

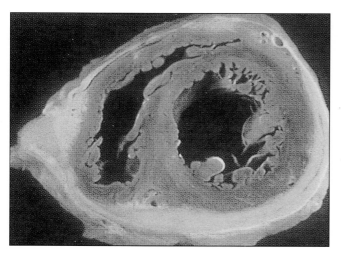

FIGURE 4 Pathology specimen of the heart in cross-section from a patient who died with constrictive pericarditis. (*See* Color Plate)

CONSTRICTIVE PERICARDITIS

The major perturbation of constrictive pericarditis is the abnormal, usually but not always thickened, pericardium encasing the heart in a solid, noncompliant envelope (Fig. 4), thereby impairing diastolic filling [25]. The rigid pericardium markedly increases intracardiac filling pressures. Effusive-constrictive pericarditis is a syndrome with features of both effusion and constriction. The patient initially presents with clinical symptoms most consistent with a pericardial effusion, but after the effusion is relieved, clinical and hemodynamic features of coexistent constriction appear. This syndrome may represent an intermediate step in the development of constrictive pericarditis.

Etiologies

Constrictive pericarditis is caused by various etiologies. In our initial report covering 47 years from 1935 to 1982, the etiology of constrictive pericarditis could not be determined in 73% of patients. However, with the increasing practice of cardiac bypass surgery and radiation treatment, the etiologies of constrictive pericarditis have changed (Fig. 5). The most commonly known etiology of constrictive pericarditis is cardiac bypass surgery followed by acute pericarditis and radiation therapy. Other etiologies include trauma, neoplasia, infection, collagen vascular disease, and tuberculosis. The interval between the onset of symptoms and the diagnosis of constriction is longest in patients with idiopathic constrictive pericarditis and shortest in patients with acute pericarditis after bypass surgery [26].

Clinical Manifestations

Many symptoms of constrictive pericarditis are nonspecific and relate to chronically elevated cardiac filling pressures and chronically depressed cardiac output. Patients usually develop ascites, peripheral edema, anorexia, and postprandial fullness. Cardiac cirrhosis may develop. Symptoms of left-sided congestion such as exertional dyspnea, orthopnea, and cough may occur, but these are much less prominent. The chronically low cardiac output results in fatigue and wasting.

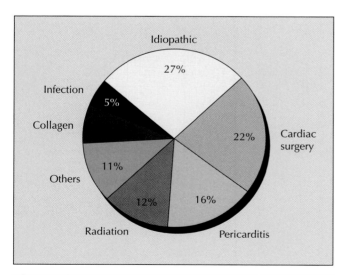

FIGURE 5 Etiologies of constrictive pericarditis from 1985 to 1998 at the Mayo Clinic (*n*=212).

Physical examination may reveal a massively swollen abdomen and edematous lower extremities combined with a cachectic, wasted upper torso. The liver is frequently enlarged. The presence of predominant right-sided failure or ascites out of proportion to peripheral edema may be clues to the presence of constriction rather than other causes of heart failure. When this abdominal process is a predominant presentation, a patient with constrictive pericarditis may undergo gastrointestinal evaluation such as liver biopsy, ultrasound of the abdomen, or even abdominal exploration before the diagnosis of constrictive pericarditis is considered.

Almost all patients with constrictive pericarditis have marked jugular venous distention [26] with prominent x- and y-descents, typically resulting in an M or W shape of the venous waves. Kussmaul's sign, which consists of the loss of normal inspiratory decrease in the jugular venous pressure with inspiration, may be present. Arterial pulse pressure may be diminished or normal, and a pulsus paradoxus is present in one third of cases. Auscultation of the heart can reveal a characteristic, early diastolic sound: the pericardial knock.

Laboratory Findings

In a substantial portion of patients with constrictive pericarditis, the diagnosis may not be apparent during the initial evaluation. Many patients are evaluated for liver function abnormalities, malignancy, or venous insufficiency. Therefore, it is not unusual that the patient may undergo extensive noncardiac work-up, such as liver biopsy, lymph node biopsy, hematologic work-up, or vascular evaluation, before the diagnosis of constrictive pericarditis. The ECG abnormalities seen in patients with constrictive pericarditis include low voltage, T-wave inversions, P mitrale, atrial fibrillation, atrioventricular and intraventricular conduction delays, and the development of Q waves, none of which is diagnostic. The cardiac silhouette on a chest radiograph may be small, normal, or enlarged. The presence of calcification on chest radiography is helpful in the diagnosis of constrictive pericarditis in patients with right heart failure and jugular venous pressure elevation. The patients with longer durations of symptoms of constrictive pericarditis are more likely to have a pericardial calcification on chest radiography. Only 24% of patients with constriction were found to have pericardial calcification on chest radiograph [27], however, and conversely, a calcified pericardium does not automatically connote constriction.

The suspicion of constrictive pericarditis in a patient with heart failure is sometimes first raised when the echo demonstrates preserved left ventricular systolic function. Other characteristic echocardiographic features can establish the diagnosis. These findings are abnormal septal motion, septal bounce, dilated inferior vena cava, thickened pericardium, and respiratory variation in Doppler velocities [28]. More recently, tissue Doppler imaging and velocity recording of early diastolic mitral annulus velocity has been shown to be helpful in diagnosing and distinguishing constrictive pericarditis from restrictive cardiomyopathy in patients with heart failure and normal systolic function [29,30].

Differentiation of constrictive pericarditis from restrictive cardiomyopathy is a major diagnostic challenge. Constrictive pericarditis is a treatable disease, whereas restriction usually carries a poor prognosis despite therapy. Restriction is most commonly caused by infiltrative disease of the myocardium such as amyloidosis. Both constrictive pericarditis and restrictive cardiomyopathy are characterized by impaired diastolic filling of the ventricles. A number of criteria have been employed to distinguish between constrictive pericarditis and restrictive cardiomyopathy [31], but there is a significant overlap in these indices. More recently, a characteristic hemodynamic feature of constrictive pericarditis was described by Hatle *et al.* [28] that is not present in patients with restriction. Ventricular filling varies with the phases of respiration in patients with constrictive pericarditis. This unique respiratory variation of diastolic filling can be shown by Doppler echocardiography and cardiac catheterization (Figs. 6 and 7). Early diastolic mitral annulus velocity becomes lower in myocardial disease, but increases in constrictive pericarditis (termed *annulus paradoxus*) [30]. CT and MRI are more accurate for detecting pericardial thickening than echocardiography; however, lack of pericardial thickening on CT and MRI scans does not rule out the presence of constrictive pericarditis. Up to 20% of patients with constrictive peri-

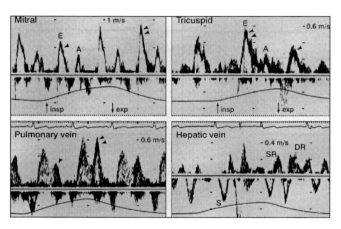

FIGURE 6 A composite of mitral inflow, pulmonary vein, tricuspid inflow, and hepatic vein Doppler recordings showing characteristic respiratory variation in flow velocities in patients with constrictive pericarditis.

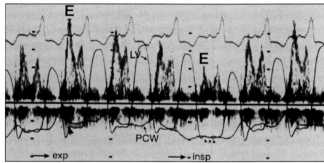

FIGURE 7 Simultaneous pressure recording from the left ventricle (LV) and pulmonary capillary wedge (PCW) along with mitral inflow Doppler velocities in constrictive pericarditis. There is reduced LV diastolic filling with inspiration.

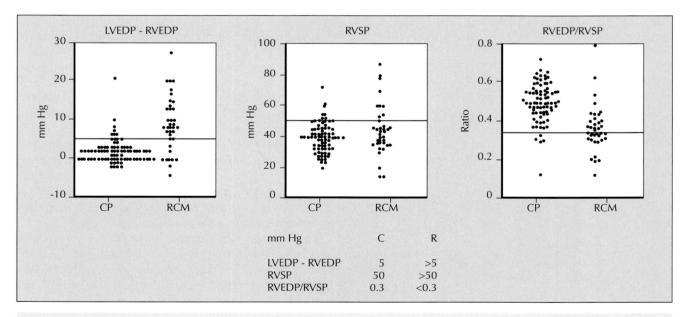

mm Hg	C	R
LVEDP - RVEDP	5	>5
RVSP	50	>50
RVEDP/RVSP	0.3	<0.3

FIGURE 8 Traditional hemodynamic criteria for constriction (C) and restriction (R). CP—constrictive pericarditis; LVEDP—left ventricular end-diastolic pressure; RCM—restrictive cardiomyopathy; RVEDP—right ventricular end-diastolic pressure; RVSP—right ventricular systolic pressure. (*Adapted from* Hatle *et al.* [28].)

carditis present with normal pericardial thickness on CT or MRI scans. This was confirmed by measurement of the thickness of the pericardium obtained from patients with surgically confirmed pericardiectomy [32].

The diagnostic criteria for constrictive pericarditis by cardiac catheterization was initially reported in 1946; it includes the elevation of the atrial pressures, the rapid increase in ventricular diastolic pressures, and the equalization of end-diastolic pressure of both ventricles [33]. Unfortunately, similar hemodynamic changes can occur in patients with restrictive cardiomyopathy. Although there are some differences in the hemodynamic criteria between restriction and constriction as a group, there is a large overlap between these two groups (Fig. 8). Hence, it is hard to make a definitive diagnosis of constrictive pericarditis or restrictive cardiomyopathy based on the traditional catheterization data. New cardiac catheterization criteria for constrictive pericarditis should include the evidence of ventricular interdependence and respiratory variation in ventricular filling. Cardiac catheterization also provides the opportunity to perform endomyocardial biopsy to search for evidence of infiltrative cardiomyopathy.

With the combined use of these diagnostic tests, it is possible to differentiate constrictive pericarditis from restrictive cardiomyopathy in the majority of cases. When the diagnosis remains ambiguous, it may be necessary to perform a thoracotomy to permit direct inspection of the pericardium.

Management

Pericardiectomy is a definitive treatment for those with constrictive pericarditis. In most cases, patients exhibit dramatic and sustained improvement, although several months may pass before complete improvement is noted. The outcome is not uniformly favorable, however, because of the hepatic or cardiac failure that may be irreversible with the myocardium atrophied because of the long-standing compression. In addition, patients with radiation-induced constrictive pericarditis have a very poor prognosis compared with the remainder of the patient group [26]. Overall, the surgical mortality has improved greatly, currently about 6% to 10%. In our experience, the surgical mortality could be predicted by patient age, New York Heart Association functional class before pericardiectomy, and radiation etiology as well as pericardial calcification shown on chest radiography. Constrictive physiology features and symptoms may also recur or remain persistent because of the involvement of the epicardial layer by the inflammatory and fibrotic process, most frequently in patients with radiation-induced constriction or in those with a long interval between their symptom development and the diagnosis [26]. In a subset of patients, constrictive physiology may be transient, especially in those with viral pericarditis, effusive constrictive pericarditis, postcardiotomy syndrome, and the collagen vascular etiology with a known onset. The constriction and the patient's heart failure symptoms can be completely resolved after intensive nonsteroidal or steroidal anti-inflammatory therapy for 2 to 3 months [34]. Effusive-constrictive pericarditis is a form of transient constrictive pericarditis. Although most patients with effusive-constrictive pericarditis recover spontaneously [35], an anti-inflammatory agent may facilitate their hemodynamic recovery and even avoid future pericardiectomy.

WHEN TO REFER

Because these various pericardial disorders can occur in a wide variety of clinical contexts, patients typically will first undergo evaluation by generalists or noncardiology subspecialists. The history, physical examination, ECG, and radiographic features of acute pericarditis, pericardial effusion, and tamponade should be familiar to all family practitioners, internists, and internal medicine subspecialists. Indeed, the primary-care physician will most often be the one who identifies the possibility of a pericardial emergency (tamponade and bacterial pericarditis). When percutaneous pericardial drainage procedures are contemplated, either for diagnostic or therapeutic reasons, echocardiographic evaluation should precede pericardiocentesis. Echocardiography and subsequent pericardiocentesis should ideally be performed by physicians experienced in these procedures. Pericardiocentesis is best performed in a special procedure room so as to permit the opportunity to obtain confirmatory hemodynamic measurements and any other adjuvant diagnostic information. It is also the setting best equipped to respond to complications.

The patient with suspected constriction should be referred to a cardiologist for evaluation. Although the diagnosis may be firmly established in some cases with radiographic imaging, the patient will often require further diagnostic evaluation in order to confirm the diagnosis and to evaluate the possibility of associated conditions before referral to a cardiothoracic surgeon for thoracotomy.

Constriction should be considered in all patients with heart failure and normal systolic function.

Management of the patient whose pericardial disease relates to a systemic illness (including uremia, connective tissue disorders, malignancy, or AIDS) will usually necessitate participation of the appropriate subspecialist. In most of these circumstances, treatment of the pericardial disease is but one component of managing a complicated illness, and management will frequently entail use of specialized procedures such as dialysis or antitumor therapy.

REFERENCES AND RECOMMENDED READING

1. Fowler NO: Tuberculous pericarditis. *JAMA* 1991, 266:99–103.
2. Bloom BR, Murray CJ: Tuberculosis: commentary on a reemergent killer. *Science* 1992, 257:1055–1064.
3. Spodick DH: Acute pericarditis: current concepts and practice. *J Am Med Association* 2003, 289:1150.

4. Acierno LJ: Cardiac complications in acquired immunodeficiency syndrome (AIDS): a review. *J Am Coll Cardiol* 1989, 13:1144–1154.

5. Estok L, Wallach F: Cardiac tamponade in a patient with AIDS: a review of pericardial disease in patients with HIV infection. *Mt Sinai J Med* 1998, 65:33–39.

6. Correlae E, Maggioni AP, Romano S, *et al.*: Comparison of frequency, diagnostic and prognostic significance of pericardial involvement in acute myocardial infarction treated with and without thrombolytics. *Am J Cardiol* 1993, 71:1377–1381.

7. Tofler GH, Muller JE, Stone PH, *et al.*: Pericarditis in acute myocardial infarction: characterization and clinical significance. *Am Heart J* 1989, 117:86–90.

8. Sagrista-Sauleda J, Barrabes JA, Permanyer-Miralda G, Soler-Soler J: Purulent pericarditis: review of a 20-year experience in a general hospital. *J Am Coll Cardiol* 1993, 22:1661–1665.

9. Koh KK, Kim EJ, Cho CH, *et al.*: Adenosine deaminase and carcinoembryonic antigen in pericardial effusion diagnosis, especially in suspected tuberculous pericarditis. *Circulation* 1994, 89:2728–2735.

10. Dogan R, Demircin M, Sarigul A, *et al.*: Diagnostic value of adenosine deaminase activity in pericardial fluids. *J Cardiovasc Surg* 1999, 40:501–504.

11. Fowler NO, Harbin AD: Recurrent acute pericarditis: follow-up study of 31 patients. *J Am Coll Cardiol* 1986, 7:300–305.

12. Adler Y, Finklestein Y, Guindo J, *et al.*: Colchicine treatment for recurrent pericarditis. *Circulation* 1998, 97:2183–2185.

13. Greason KL, Danielson GK, Oh JK, Nishimura RA: Pericardiectomy for chronic relapsing pericarditis. *J Am Coll Cardiol* 2001, 37:478A.

14. Strang JI, Gibson DG, Mitchison DA, *et al.*: Controlled clinical trial of complete open surgical drainage and of prednisolone in treatment of tuberculous pericardial effusion in Transkei. *Lancet* 1988, ii:759–764.

15. De Pace NL, Nestico PF, Schwartz AB, *et al.*: Predicting success of intensive dialysis in the treatment of uremic pericarditis. *Am J Med* 1984, 76:38–46.

16. Frommer JP, Young JB, Ayus JC: Asymptomatic pericardial effusion in uremic patients: effect of long-term dialysis. *Nephron* 1985, 39:296–301.

17. Renkin KJ, DeBruyne B, Benit E, *et al.*: Cardiac tamponade early after thrombolysis for acute myocardial infarction: a rare but not reported hemorrhagic complication. *J Am Coll Cardiol* 1991, 17:280–285.

18. Lichstein E, Arsura E, Hollander G, *et al.*: Current incidence of postmyocardial infarction (Dressler's) syndrome. *Am J Cardiol* 1982, 50:1269–1271.

19. Spodick DH: Current Concepts: acute cardiac tamponade. *N Engl J Med* 2003, 349:684–690.

20. Sagrista-Sauleda J, Angel J, Permanyer-Miralda G, Soler-Soler J: Long-term follow-up of idiopathic chronic pericardial effusion. *N Engl J Med* 1999, 341:2054–2059.

21. Burstow DJ, Oh JK, Bailey KR, *et al.*: Cardiac tamponade: characteristic Doppler observations. *Mayo Clin Proc* 1989, 64:312–324.

22. Tsang TS, Freeman WK, Sinak LJ, Seward JB: Echocardiographically guided pericardiocentesis: evolution and state-of-the-art technique. *Mayo Clin Proc* 1998, 73:647–652.

23. Tsang TS, Oh JK, Seward JB: Diagnosis and management of cardiac tamponade in the era of echocardiography. *Clin Cardiol* 1999, 22:446–452.

24. Vaitkus PT, Herrmann HC, LeWinter MM: Treatment of malignant pericardial effusion. *JAMA* 1994, 272:59–64.

25. Fowler NO: Constrictive pericarditis: Its history and current status. *Clin Cardiol* 1995, 18:341–350.

26. Ling LH, Oh JK, Schaff HV, *et al.*: Constrictive pericarditis in the modern era: evolving clinical spectrum and impact on outcome after pericardiectomy. *Circulation* 1999, 100:1380–1386.

27. Ling LH, Oh JK, Breen JF, *et al.*: Calcific constrictive pericarditis: is it still with us? *Ann Intern Med* 2000, 132:444–450.

28. Hatle LK, Appleton CP, Popp RL: Differentiation of constrictive pericarditis and restrictive cardiomyopathy by Doppler echocardiography. *Circulation* 1989, 79:357–370.

29. Garcia MJ, Rodriguez L, Ares M, *et al.*: Differentiation of constrictive pericarditis from restrictive cardiomyopathy: assessment of left ventricular diastolic velocities in longitudinal axis by Doppler tissue imaging. *J Am Coll Cardiol* 1996, 27:108–114.

30. Ha JW, Oh JK, Ommen SR, *et al.*: Diagnostic value of mitral annular velocity for constrictive pericarditis in the absence of respiratory variation in mitral inflow velocity. *J Am Soc Echocardiogr* 2002, 15:1468–1471.

31. Vaitkus PT, Kussmaul WG: Constrictive pericarditis versus restrictive cardiomyopathy: a reappraisal and update of diagnostic criteria. *Am Heart J* 1991, 122:1431–1441.

32. Talreja DR, Edwards WD, Danielson GK, *et al.*: Constrictive pericarditis in with histologically normal pericardial thickness. *Circulation* 2003, 108:1852–1857.

33. Bloomfield RA, Lauson HD, Cournand A, *et al.*: Recording of right heart pressures in normal subjects and in patients with chronic pulmonary disease and various types of cardiocirculatory disease. *J Clin Invest* 1946, 25:639–664.

34. Haley JH, Tajik AJ, Danielson GK, *et al.*: Transient constrictive pericarditis: causes and natural history. *J Am Coll Cardiol* 2004, 43:271-275.

35. Sagrista-Sauleda J, Angel J, Sanchez A, *et al.*: Effusive-constrictive pericarditis. *N Engl J Med* 2004, 350:469-475.

Congenital Heart Disease, Including Unrepaired Lesions in the Adult

31

Melvin D. Cheitlin
John A. Paraskos

> ### Key Points
>
> - More patients with congenital heart disease will be seen by the internist than ever in the past; patients with congenital heart disease are living to have children with congenital heart disease.
>
> - The increase in adults with congenital heart disease, corrected and uncorrected, is at a rate of 5% per year. At present, it is estimated that there are 1 million such patients in the United States.
>
> - In adult patients, congenital heart disease is frequently not recognized and is misdiagnosed.
>
> - Atrial septal defect is the most common significant congenital heart defect seen in the adult and is unrecognized because the physical findings are subtle.
>
> - The pregnant patient with Eisenmenger's syndrome has a high maternal and fetal mortality rate.
>
> - The most common cause of a continuous murmur is a patent ductus arteriosus; clinicians should remember that patent ductus arteriosus is not the *only* cause of continuous murmur.
>
> - With the exception of the patient with a septal defect or patent ductus arteriosus with pulmonary vascular disease, cyanotic congenital heart disease is very unusual and is unexpected in the adult. However, it can occur and, if recognized, the patient can benefit from surgery.
>
> - Doppler echocardiography is the single most important diagnostic tool in congenital heart disease and frequently makes cardiac catheterization unnecessary.

Congenital heart disease is usually the province of the pediatrician and the pediatric cardiologist. Most significant lesions are found in children and are identified or surgically "corrected" by the time the internist sees the patient. However, the condition of some patients is not discovered in childhood, and the internist sees congenital heart disease most often in the five ways listed in Table 1 [1]. This chapter deals with the first two categories of congenital cardiac lesions.

This chapter does not deal with congenital heart disease lesions not seen in adults without prior surgery. This includes two of the more common cyanotic lesions, tricuspid atresia and transposition of the great vessels, which is dealt with in the chapter on postsurgical congenital heart disease.

MINOR LESIONS

A good example of a minor lesion is the bicuspid aortic valve. Most bicuspid aortic valves of normal histology are competent or have only minor regurgitation; however, occasionally these valves can be severely incompetent. Of the complications seen with these valves, the most important is infective endocarditis. Antibiotic prophylaxis for dental procedures or surgery through contaminated areas is required to decrease the possibility of endocarditis developing. Other complications include the development of aortic insufficiency or calcification and severe aortic stenosis at 40 to 50 years of age. Patients with bicuspid aortic valves have an increased incidence of aortic dissection in later life, probably because of a connective tissue abnormality common to the aortic valve and the aortic media. A large proportion of people with bicuspid aortic valves never have any complications and can live a normal life span without problems.

Clues that the valve is bicuspid come from physical examination. Because the valve does not open properly, these patients can have an ejection click and a short systolic ejection murmur. The murmur is similar to an innocent ejection murmur, but if it is associated with an ejection click, a diagnosis of abnormal aortic valve is probable. Because there is difficulty with coaptation at the aortic leaflets, minimal aortic regurgitation may be present, the murmur of which can be increased in loudness by a hand-grip or by squatting. The diagnosis can be made with Doppler echocardiography. When this lesion is recognized, the major appropriate treatment is prophylaxis at the time of dental procedures and at other times of bacteremia to prevent endocarditis. Because of the abnormal aortic media, in some patients dilatation of the ascending aorta and even aneurysm can be seen.

Other lesions that may cause problems in differential diagnosis are 1) dextrocardia and situs inversus and 2) a pulmonary varix (or pulmonary varicose vein), which may appear as a solitary nodule on the chest roentgenogram. The varix presents as a rounded density in the lung, usually near the cardiac silhouette on the left or the right side and frequently in association with a disease that increases left atrial pressure, such as mitral stenosis. Under fluoroscopy, the lesion can be seen to collapse during a Valsalva maneuver.

Many other minor lesions are important to recognize, such as the right-sided aortic arch that can be mistaken for a paratracheal mass. The major challenge with most is recognizing the lesion, and thus, avoiding the mistake of diagnosing a more serious problem.

TABLE 1 MOST COMMON PRESENTATIONS OF CONGENITAL HEART DISEASE IN ADULTS

Minor lesions without hemodynamic consequence

Major lesions that were not diagnosed previously

Major lesions that were previously diagnosed but at present are not amenable to surgery, including irreversible pulmonary vascular disease and cyanotic patients with extremely small pulmonary arteries that would not support a shunt

Lesions recognized, operated on, and anatomically or physiologically "corrected"

Lesions operated on and "cured" —an extremely small category consisting of some secundum atrial septal defects and patent ductus arteriosus that are closed

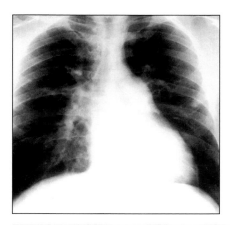

FIGURE 1 Chest x-ray, posterior-anterior projection of 40-year-old man with a secundum atrial septal defect with a pulmonary blood flow/systemic blood flow ratio of 2:1.

RECOGNITION OF COMMON CONGENITAL HEART DISEASE PROBLEMS

The unoperated, hemodynamically important congenital heart disease problems likely to be seen in the adult are relatively few. Adult patients with pulmonary atresia and tetralogy of Fallot can be seen previously undiagnosed. McNamara and Latson [2], looking at the number of children born with congenital heart disease, showed that atrial septal defect, interventricular septal defect, patent ductus arteriosus (PDA), tetralogy of Fallot, and coarctation of the aorta constituted approximately 60% of the cases of congenital heart disease in adults. If Ebstein's disease, aortic stenosis, pulmonic valve stenosis, and bicuspid aortic valve are added, the vast majority of the important congenital heart disease lesions seen in adulthood are accounted for.

Predominant Left-to-Right Shunts with Normal or Moderately Increased Pulmonary Vascular Resistance

Predominant left-to-right shunts with normal or moderately increased pulmonary vascular resistance can occur at the atrial level, the ventricular level, or the pulmonary artery level. All of these shunts result in the return of pulmonary venous blood to the right side of the heart. This increase in pulmonary blood flow increases pulmonary vascular markings on chest roentgenography (Fig. 1). If the shunt is large, ventricular enlargement along with pulmonary hypertension results, leading to right ventricular hypertrophy and finally right-sided heart failure.

Interatrial septal defect

Atrial septal defects are the most common congenital heart lesions seen in adults, accounting for about one third of cases. Atrial septal defects occur two or three times more commonly in women than in men.

Anatomy

Three types of atrial septal defects are 1) ostium secundum (about 75% of atrial defects), 2) ostium primum (results in a low-lying atrial septal defect where the atrial septum joins the confluence of the mitral and tricuspid rings; about 15%), and 3) sinus venosus defects (about 10%; it is most often either superior near the entrance of the superior vena cava or inferior near the inferior vena cava and the ostium of the coronary sinus).

Pathophysiology

Because the right ventricle is more compliant than the left ventricle, it fills more readily. In diastole, blood just returning from the lung to the left atrium goes through the defect into the right side of the heart, resulting in a right ventricular end-diastolic volume and subsequent stroke volume that are larger than those on the left. The blood flow through the lung is markedly increased. Right ventricular dysfunction and right heart failure may eventually occur. The pathophysiology is similar in the three types of atrial septal defects.

Additional lesions seen with ostium primum defects are clefting of the mitral or tricuspid valve with valvular insufficiency. With sinus venosus defects, anomalous drainage of one or more pulmonary veins into the right atrium or superior vena cava is common.

Physical, electrocardiographic, and roentgenographic findings

The physical, electrocardiographic, and chest roentgenographic findings in atrial septal defect are listed in Table 2.

Echocardiography

There is an increased right ventricular volume and a flattening of the interventricular septum at end-diastole, with systolic paradoxical motion of the septum. Doppler echocardiography shows a continuous flow across the atrial septum (Fig. 2). With the intravenous injection of agitated saline (intravenous contrast injection), microbubbles are seen filling the right atrium and right ventricle, and a negative-contrast jet may be seen flowing across the atrial septum from right to left.

Complications

Pulmonary hypertension. The most important complication of atrial septal defect is the development of severe pulmonary vascular disease, which occurs only with large atrial septal defects with large left-to-right shunts and produces a form of Eisenmenger's syndrome. It occurs in fewer than 10% of patients with large atrial septal defects. It almost always occurs after puberty, and if the patient reaches 30 to 40 years of age without developing

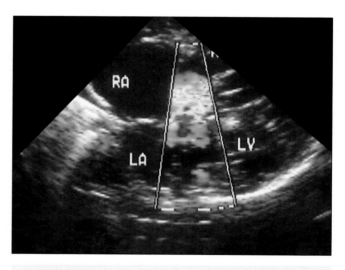

FIGURE 2 Echo-Doppler, subcostal view of a 40-year-old man with an ostium primum atrial septal defect. Doppler signal shows abnormal continuous jet from left atrium to right atrium across the low-lying atrial septal defect. RA—right atrium; RV—right ventricle; LA—left atrium; LV—left ventricle. (*See* Color Plate.)

TABLE 2 PHYSICAL, ELECTROCARDIOGRAPHIC, AND CHEST ROENTGENOGRAPHIC FINDINGS IN ATRIAL SEPTAL DEFECT	
Finding	**Comment**
Systolic ejection murmur in the second left intercostal space	Produced by the increased right ventricular stroke volume
Increase in the pulmonary vascular markings on chest roentgenography	Caused by the increased pulmonary blood flow
Diastolic flow rumble at the left sternal border	Produced by an increase in flow across the tricuspid valve
Wide, fixed splitting of the second heart sound	Caused by the increased right ventricular filling in diastole, which is unaffected by respiration
rSR' in V_1 on the electrocardiogram	Caused by the increased right ventricular diastolic filling, which increases the size of the right atrium and the right ventricle

pulmonary hypertension, the later development of pulmonary vascular disease is rare. There is an increase in right ventricular and pulmonary artery systolic pressure, with the subsequent development of right ventricular hypertrophy. Eventually, the shunt becomes right-to-left, and cyanosis occurs.

The pulmonary artery branches maintaining high, even systemic, pressures dilate, and they may become atherosclerotic and calcified. The patient now has the complications of systemic arterial desaturation, with polycythemia and the subsequent clotting and bleeding problems. In addition, the patient may develop syncopal episodes, probably from arrhythmias, dyspnea, hemoptysis, and anginal chest pain. Pregnancy is poorly tolerated, with fetal wastage high and the maternal mortality rate increased.

Congestive heart failure. With the increased volume load on the right ventricle, right ventricular dilatation and hypertrophy occur. Eventually, right ventricular systolic dysfunction supervenes, and the right ventricle dilates further, interfering with left ventricular filling in diastole. With failure, both the right and the left ventricle filling pressures rise together, as do the right and the left atrial pressures, which must remain equal because of the large connection between them.

Atrial arrhythmias. Atrial arrhythmias (ie, atrial fibrillation and atrial tachycardias) are not uncommon, especially in patients older than 40 years. Once they occur, surgical correction does not eliminate the possibility that they will recur.

Treatment
Young patients with an atrial septal defect of any type who have a pulmonary-to-systemic blood flow ratio of greater than or equal to 1.8:1 should have repair of their defect. If the right ventricle is dilated, even lesser-volume shunts should be repaired. The surgery is very low risk, and many of the complications mentioned will probably be avoided. In sinus venosus defects, the anomalous pulmonary veins can be redirected to drain into the left atrium.

Age is not a contraindication to repair. There is good evidence that repair, even after age 40, improves the patient's functional capacity and decreases symptoms [3•].

Because there is no jet formation to disrupt the endocardium and create a site for the development of infective endocarditis and if no associated lesions such as mitral valve prolapse or clefting of the mitral valve with mitral regurgitation are present, antibiotic prophylaxis to prevent endocarditis is not needed in patients with atrial septal defect [4••].

Alternatives to surgical closure of the secundum atrial septal defect are being developed. These approaches consist of patches, or "clam shells," which can be affixed by means of catheters. So far, this treatment is available at relatively few institutions. In many centers in which there has been enough experience with this technique, catheter closure for secundum atrial septal defects is the procedure of choice [5•].

Interventricular septal defect
Interventricular septal defect is the most commonly recognized congenital heart lesion in infants. A large percentage of these defects close in early infancy; therefore, only approximately 10% of adult patients with congenital heart disease have a large ventricular septal defect (VSD) [6,7••].

Pathophysiology
The effect of the VSD depends on its size, its position, and the relative ratio of pulmonary vascular resistance to systemic vascular resistance. Ventricular septal defects can be 1) perimembranous (70% of cases), 2) supracristal (or just below the aortic valve; 5% of cases), 3) a posterior or atrioventricular canal defect (5% of cases), or 4) muscular (20% of cases).

Small ventricular septal defect. With small VSDs, there is a connection between the high-pressure left ventricle and the low-pressure right ventricle. In systole, a high-velocity, small-volume jet of blood is directed from the left to the right ventricle. This left-to-right shunt adds little to the pulmonary blood flow. Therefore, the effect is to create a loud pansystolic murmur without any change in cardiac size or ventricular function. This type of defect, called *Roger's disease,* is commonly seen in the adult.

Moderate-sized ventricular septal defect. With the moderate-sized VSD, the left-to-right shunt is larger, but the defect is not large enough to create a common chamber with equal pressure between the right and the left ventricles. The right-to-left shunt is determined by the size of the VSD and the magnitude of the pulmonary vascular resistance relative to that of the systemic vascular resistance. With normal pulmonary vascular resistance, the left-to-right shunt can be large, with pulmonary blood flow two to three times systemic blood flow. The right ventricular pressure can be raised owing to the increased pulmonary blood flow, but it is not equal to the left ventricular pressure because the size of the defect is too small.

Large ventricular septal defect. With the large VSD, the area of the VSD is more than half of the area of the aortic ring, making the right ventricle and the left ventricle a common chamber. With the large VSD, the increased pulmonary blood flow and high pulmonary artery pressure result in irreversible pulmonary vascular disease and Eisenmenger's syndrome, usually by the end of the first or the second decade of life.

Physical findings
Small ventricular septal defect. Because the left-to-right shunt is small, there is no volume overload of the ventricles, no cardiac enlargement, and no increase in pulmonary vascular markings. The major finding is the presence of a loud pansystolic murmur along the left sternal border, usually in the third and fourth interspace and usually of grade IV to VI intensity.

The supracristal VSD murmur can simulate a pulmonic stenosis murmur, except that it is pansystolic and not ejection in type. If aortic regurgitation develops, a diastolic murmur comes directly off the second heart sound (S_2) and the systolic and diastolic murmur can be confused with the murmur of PDA and other lesions causing continuous murmurs.

Moderate-sized ventricular septal defect. In addition to the pansystolic murmur along the left sternal border, enlargement of the left atrium and dilatation and hypertrophy of the left ventricle may be noted on chest roentgenography and electrocardiography (ECG). The S_2 may be increased in intensity, and in adolescents and thin adults, a diastolic flow rumble of increased blood flow across the mitral valve may be heard at the apex. A ventricular gallop (S_3) resulting from an increased rate of left ventricular filling is not unusual.

Large ventricular septal defect. By the time patients reach adolescence or adulthood, they most often have severe pulmonary hypertension and pulmonary vascular disease. If they still have an appreciable left-to-right shunt, a pansys-

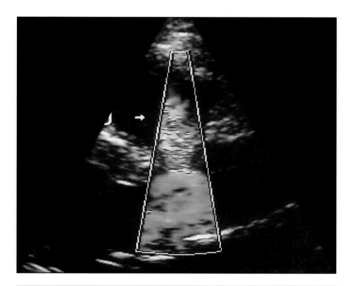

FIGURE 3 Echo-Doppler, parasternal long-axis view of a 32-year-old man with a moderate-sized ventricular septal defect. Systolic jet is seen through the ventricular septal defect from left ventricular outflow tract to right ventricle. (*See* Color Plate.)

TABLE 3 COMPLICATIONS OF VENTRICULAR SEPTAL DEFECT

Ventricular septal defect	Complication
Small VSD	Infective endocarditis
Supracristal VSD	Progressive aortic regurgitation
Moderate and large VSD	Congestive heart failure
	Infective endocarditis
	Pulmonary vascular disease

VSD—ventricular septal defect.

tolic murmur is still present. The pulmonic heart sound (P_2) is always increased and now may be coincident with the aortic second sound (A_2), so that there is a single loud S_2. The left ventricle is laterally displaced and hypertrophied, as is the right ventricle.

As the pulmonary vascular resistance increases relative to the systemic vascular resistance, the left-to-right shunt decreases. The size of the left ventricle decreases; the systolic murmur decreases in intensity and is no longer present throughout systole, finally disappearing altogether. At this point, predominant right ventricular hypertrophy may be present. With pulmonary hypertension, pulmonic valvular regurgitation causes a high-frequency blowing diastolic murmur that is heard along the left sternal border, similar to the murmur of aortic regurgitation. With right ventricular failure and dilatation, the tricuspid ring dilates and tricuspid regurgitation occurs, causing a systolic murmur along the left sternal border that may increase with inspiration.

Diagnosis
With the left-to-right shunt, the pansystolic murmur is the best clue to the diagnosis. The enlarged left ventricle and left atrium and increased pulmonary vascular markings are seen on chest roentgenography. Echocardiography identifies the chamber enlargement and the increased left ventricular stroke volume, and Doppler echocardiography demonstrates the position of the jet across the interventricular septum (Fig. 3). From the velocity of the jet, the gradient in systole can be estimated. With low pressure in the right ventricle, the jet is high velocity. The systolic gradient between the right and the left ventricles is smaller with the large VSD or as the pulmonary vascular resistance increases, and the velocity of the jet also is less.

Complications
The development of irreversible pulmonary vascular disease is the most common complication of the large VSD (Table 3). High pulmonary blood flow and pressure, and high shear forces damage the intima of the small pulmonary arteries and release endothelin, resulting in vasoconstriction, intimal hyperplasia, medial hypertrophy of the small pulmonary arteries, and fewer small pulmonary vessels. All of these changes, which are irreversible, result in pulmonary vascular disease and pulmonary hypertension with left-to-right shunting and cyanosis with its complications. Eventually, dilatation of the right ventricle occurs, as does severe left- and right-sided heart failure.

With large left-to-right shunts, left ventricular failure can occur. In my experience, the high-flow, low-pressure VSD, sufficient to cause heart failure, is extremely unusual in adults. With large VSDs, the most common presentation in the adult is that of Eisenmenger's syndrome.

In some patients, hypertrophy of the crista supraventricularis causes infundibular stenosis, converting the clinical picture to that of a "pink" tetralogy of Fallot. The severity of the obstruction caused by the infundibular stenosis is such that a right-to-left shunt may occur through the VSD, and the clinical picture becomes that of a tetralogy of Fallot.

Infective endocarditis. The high-velocity jet injures the endocardium. Vegetations occur on the right ventricular side of the VSD or on the tricuspid or pulmonic valve. Emboli therefore occur most often to the lungs.

Prolapse of the right coronary cusp of the aortic valve and aortic regurgitation with supracristal VSD.

Treatment

Small VSDs without hemodynamic significance need only antibiotic prophylaxis to prevent endocarditis. If infective endocarditis recurs in a patient with a small VSD despite adequate antibiotic prophylaxis, then consideration should be given to closing the VSD.

In patients with large VSDs with a large left-to-right shunt and with a pulmonary blood flow–to–systemic blood flow ratio of 2:1 or greater, surgical closure is indicated. This type of VSD is unusual in the adult. With pulmonary hypertension, if a left-to-right shunt is still present in the range of 1.8:1, the pulmonary vascular resistance is not greater than 7.5 Wood units, and the arterial saturation is greater than 90%, then closure can be considered. If vasodilators, the most successful of which is intravenous prostacyclin, reduces the pulmonary vascular resistance and increases the left-to-right shunt, then closure of the VSD is likely to be successful. Closure with catheter devices is being developed but is still in the investigational stage [8].

With Eisenmenger's syndrome and cyanosis, operative closure is contraindicated because it would require all the systemic venous return to go through the lungs and would precipitate severe right-sided heart failure. Phlebotomy is indicated only for a very high hematocrit level (> 65) or if the "polycythemic syndrome" of headache, lethargy, and excessive fatigue occurs. The only hope that these patients have is lung transplantation with or without heart transplantation. This approach is still available in only a few centers.

Patent ductus arteriosus

Patent ductus arteriosus accounts for 10% of congenital heart lesions in adults.

Anatomy

Patent ductus arteriosus completes the "big three" of left-to-right shunts. It is by far the most common cause of a continuous murmur and results from persistent patency of the fetal ductus arteriosus, which connects the proximal descending aorta just beyond the takeoff of the left subclavian artery with the pulmonary artery just to the left of the bifurcation [9].

Pathophysiology

With a small PDA, the high-pressure aorta is connected with the pulmonary artery, which results in a high-velocity jet of low volume into the pulmonary artery. The larger the ductus, the more the shunt is determined by the ratio of pulmonary vascular resistance to systemic vascular resistance. If the patent ductus is large enough, there is equalization of pressure in the pulmonary artery and the aorta; then, the size of the shunt depends completely on the ratio of pulmonary vascular resistance to systemic vascular resistance. As with the VSD, the high pressure and high flow result in irreversible changes in the pulmonary vasculature, an irreversible increase in pulmonary vascular resistance, and Eisenmenger's syndrome.

Physical findings

Small patent ductus arteriosus. The continuous jet from the aorta to the pulmonary artery results in a high-pitched, continuous murmur, with peaking of the murmur at the time of the S_2. The murmur is best heard in the second interspace to the left of the sternum and under the left clavicle. If the shunt is small, there is no increase in heart size and no increase in pulmonary vascular markings.

Moderate-sized patent ductus arteriosus. The volume of the left-to-right shunt is increased; the murmur becomes louder and coarser, still peaking at the S_2; and the pulmonary artery pressure may be increased, causing an increased P_2. Because of the increased flow across the mitral valve, there may be a mitral diastolic flow rumble and an S_3 at the apex. Left ventricular hyperactivity and possibly a right ventricular lift are present because of the high right ventricular pressure.

Patent ductus arteriosus with pulmonary hypertension. As the pulmonary artery and aortic pressures equalize, the left-to-right shunt is totally dependent on the ratio of pulmonary vascular resistance to systemic vascular resistance. As the pulmonary vascular resistance approaches the systemic vascular resistance, the murmur may be heard only in late systole. Finally, with a further increase in pulmonary vascular resistance, there is little left-to-right shunt and no murmur is heard. The P_2 is then loud and coincident with the A_2, creating a loud single S_2. The findings are those of pulmonary hypertension, frequently with a diastolic decrescendo murmur of pulmonic regurgitation. With right ventricular dilatation, right-sided heart failure and tricuspid regurgitation may result.

With pulmonary vascular disease, a right-to-left shunt occurs, with arterial desaturation occurring downstream from where the patent ductus enters. This event results in the finding of "differential cyanosis," pink fingers and cyanosis and clubbing of the toes (Fig. 4).

Diagnosis

The best clue to the presence of a PDA is the continuous murmur. With the larger shunts, the ascending aorta, the left atrium, and the left ventricle should be dilated and hypertrophied, which can be seen on both chest roentgenography and ECG. Echocardiography reveals the chamber enlargement, and Doppler echocardiography demonstrates the abnormal continuous high-velocity jet entering the main pulmonary artery, swirling down one side of the pulmonary artery and up the other, that is characteristic of a PDA (Fig. 5).

As pulmonary vascular resistance increases, the jet may be less obvious or even absent, and the findings are those of pulmonary hypertension and right ventricular failure, with an increased S_2, pulmonic regurgitation, tricuspid regurgitation, right-sided S_3 and atrial gallop (S_4) sounds, and an elevated jugular venous pressure. Here, the presence of differential cyanosis can make the diagnosis.

The differential diagnosis of a continuous murmur is important and consists of problems that create a continuous murmur at the base of the heart to the left of the sternum

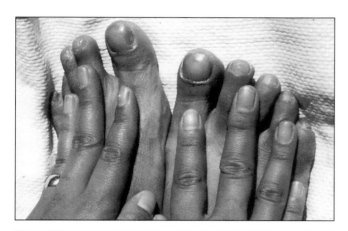

FIGURE 4 Hands and feet of a 20-year-old woman with patent ductus arteriosus and pulmonary vascular disease. Note cyanosis and clubbing of the toes, and pink nonclubbed fingers. (*See* Color Plate.)

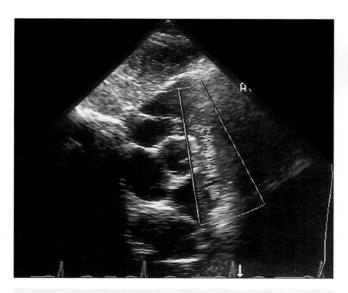

FIGURE 5 Echo-Doppler, short-axis view at level of aortic valve. The color of Doppler shows an abnormal jet in the main pulmonary artery which, on motion, showed that jet through the patent ductus entered at the bifurcation of the pulmonary artery and went down the main pulmonary artery. (*See* Color Plate.)

(Table 4). Four conditions must be considered when a continuous murmur is heard: 1) aorta–pulmonary artery window, in which a connection exists between the ascending aorta and the main pulmonary artery; 2) ruptured sinus of Valsalva aneurysm into the outflow tract of the right ventricle; 3) supracristal VSD with aortic regurgitation; and 4) coronary artery–pulmonary artery fistula. Of all of these conditions, PDA is by far the most common.

Another lesion that is important to exclude is a venous hum loud enough to be heard in the second interspace on the left. The murmur can be obliterated by pressing firmly over the internal jugular vein and occluding it. In addition, a mammary souffle in the pregnant or postpartum woman with lactating breasts can be confusing. Blood flow to the breasts is markedly increased, creating continuous bruits; here, finding the position of the loudest bruit and pressing firmly with the stethoscope can obliterate the bruit. Other causes of continuous murmur, such as coronary arteriovenous fistulas, coronary-cameral fistulas, pulmonary arteriovenous fistulas, and systemic arteriovenous fistulas, are usually loudest in different areas of the chest and are usually not confused.

Complications

The complications of PDA are similar to those of VSD, although a large left-to-right shunt and a lower-pressure pulmonary artery are more often seen in adults with PDA than in those with VSD. The danger of a small PDA is the development of infective endarteritis, and its presence requires antibiotic prophylaxis at the time of dental or other procedures causing bacteremias.

Treatment

At present, the procedure of choice for closure of a small- to medium-sized ductus arteriosus is catheter embolization

TABLE 4 DIFFERENTIAL DIAGNOSIS OF A CONTINUOUS MURMUR
Confusion with PDA
Aortic-pulmonary window
Sinus of Valsalva aneurysm rupturing into the right atrium or right ventricle
Supracristal VSD with aortic regurgitation
Coronary artery to pulmonary artery fistula
Venous hum
Other causes of continuous murmurs
Mammary souffle in pregnant women with lactating breasts
Coronary arteriovenous fistula
Coronary cameral fistula
Pulmonary arteriovenous fistula
Systemic arteriovenous fistula
PDA—patent ductus arteriosus; VSD—ventricular septal defect.

with coils or other devices [10•]. This is successful in closing the ductus and is a lesser problem for the patient than is thoracotomy. However, in the large patent ductus, surgical closure is usually still the best approach because of the problem of embolization of the coils or devices into the pulmonary artery. Because of the life-long danger of infective endarteritis (about 0.5% annually after the second decade of life) and the low mortality for the procedure, closure of even a small patent ductus arteriosus is indicated. If surgical closure is necessary as the patient gets older, the ductus becomes atherosclerotic and is therefore more easily torn at surgery, increasing the danger of a surgical mishap. In patients older than 60 years, the danger of the surgery is similar to or greater than the danger of developing infective endarteritis, and I do not recommend surgery. With a large PDA and a large shunt, especially in a symptomatic patient, I recommend surgery at any age.

In a patient with pulmonary vascular disease and little or no left-to-right shunt, surgical closure is contraindicated, and lung transplantation is the patient's only hope.

Pure Valvular Lesions
Aortic stenosis
Anatomy
Congenital aortic stenosis can occur at any level of the left ventricular outflow tract and ascending aorta. The most common type is caused by valvular abnormalities. If its histology is normal, the bicuspid aortic valve does not create severe aortic stenosis, but it may be incompetent, resulting in aortic regurgitation. Severe aortic stenosis may occur with the bicuspid valve early in infancy if the valve is dysplastic. If the histology of the valve is normal, a minority of patients with bicuspid aortic valve will develop fibrosis and calcification and severe aortic stenosis between 40 and 50 years of age [11].

The aortic valves that are congenitally stenotic in childhood are those with only one commissure; the bicuspid valve with a fused commissure or a unicuspid valve; and those without any normally formed commissures, the so-called acommissural valves. Much less often, left ventricular outflow tract obstruction above (supravalvular) or below (subvalvular) the aortic valve occurs. Supravalvular aortic stenosis can be caused by a discrete membrane, an hourglass constriction, or a hypoplastic ascending aorta. These obstructions are usually above the takeoff of the coronary arteries. The subvalvular obstructions can be discrete and membranous, caused by abnormal hypertrophy (so-called hypertrophic cardiomyopathy), or caused by a fibromuscular tunnel involving both the interventricular septum and the anterior leaflet of the mitral valve. These problems are more difficult to treat surgically.

Pathophysiology
The obstruction to the left ventricular outflow tract results in a systolic afterload burden to the left ventricle, which causes left ventricular hypertrophy, and the pathophysiologic consequences are similar in all ways to those seen in the adult with acquired aortic stenosis.

The increase in left ventricular mass, the high left ventricular systolic pressure, the relatively low aortic diastolic pressure, and the high extramural pressure on the intramural coronary arteries all result in an increase in myocardial oxygen demand and a decrease in coronary blood supply. The pathophysiologic factors result in myocardial ischemia, which can lead to angina pectoris and myocardial infarction.

Ventricular arrhythmia and sudden death can result from myocardial ischemia. Exertional syncope can be caused by an inability to increase stroke volume with exercise and therefore a decrease in systolic blood pressure, but it may be caused by sudden self-limited ventricular arrhythmias or inappropriate reflexes that cause vasodilation and bradycardia at a time when the aortic systolic pressure is falling.

Physical findings
The systolic ejection murmur at the base, which radiates into the carotid arteries, is the most valuable diagnostic sign of aortic stenosis. With valvular aortic stenosis, because the valve is flexible in the young adult, there is frequently a systolic ejection click. In half of the patients, minimal aortic regurgitation is audible. If the chest wall has a normal configuration and the cardiac output is normal, the murmur is usually loud enough to create a systolic thrill. Therefore, in a young person, the absence of a thrill is powerful evidence against severe aortic stenosis. However, in an older person, who may have decreased cardiac output and an increased anteroposterior diameter of the chest, the absence of a systolic thrill is less valuable in predicting the absence of severe aortic stenosis.

Left ventricular hypertrophy is the natural compensation for severe aortic stenosis, so a sustained point of maximal impulse and an S_4 are also good evidence of the increased severity of aortic stenosis. With left ventricular failure, there is dilatation of the left ventricle and an S_3, but they are present very late in the natural history of the disease. The absence of a systolic ejection click should lead the clinician to suspect calcification of the aortic valve or an unusual type of aortic stenosis, either supravalvular or subvalvular.

Diagnosis
The systolic ejection murmur is the best clue to the diagnosis of aortic stenosis. Chest roentgenography usually shows poststenotic dilatation of the ascending aorta, but the cardiac silhouette is usually normal. The ECG in severe aortic stenosis usually demonstrates left ventricular hypertrophy (Fig. 6), although approximately 15% to 20% may show only ST-T wave changes or be within normal limits. In these situations, echocardiography shows left ventricular hypertrophy if the aortic stenosis is severe, usually without dilatation of the left ventricle. In young adults, left ventricular contractility is usually preserved. Supravalvular aortic stenosis, subvalvular aortic stenosis, and hypertrophic cardiomyopathy can be diagnosed with echocardiography, which is the best way to visualize the discrete membranous

type of subaortic stenosis. Doppler echocardiography can reliably measure the systolic gradient across the stenotic aortic valve and, by estimation of the area of the left ventricular outflow tract, the area of the stenotic aortic valve. In patients with mild to moderate aortic stenosis, periodic Doppler echocardiography is an excellent way to detect an increase in the severity of the obstruction.

Complications and treatment

The complications of congestive heart failure, angina pectoris including non–Q wave myocardial infarction, exertional syncope, arrhythmias, sudden death, and infective endocarditis are all similar to those seen with acquired aortic stenosis. In adolescents and young adults, the presence of severe aortic stenosis with a systolic gradient of 50 mm Hg, or an aortic valve area of less then 0.8 cm^2, is an indication for surgical correction. With commissurial fusion and an uncalcified valve, correction can be achieved by repair rather than by replacement. In children and some young adults, balloon valvotomy can be just as effective as surgical valve repair. If the valve is calcified, as it is in almost all patients older than 40 years, valvular replacement is necessary.

When valve repair is possible, it is highly likely that a second surgical procedure, and even replacement of the valve, will be necessary after 15 to 20 years [12••].

Valvular pulmonary stenosis

Anatomy

Valvular pulmonary stenosis is a relatively uncommon problem in adults. Although stenosis of the right ventricular outflow tract can be at, below, or above the pulmonic valve, valvular pulmonary stenosis is by far the most common as an isolated lesion. Infundibular stenosis without a VSD and supravalvular pulmonary stenosis are rare.

Pathophysiology

Valvular pulmonary stenosis is caused by an abnormally formed pulmonic valve. The valve has three cusps with pliable leaflets, fused commissures, and a central orifice.

The obstruction to right ventricular outflow causes an afterload burden on the right ventricle, resulting in right ventricular hypertrophy. There is a large gradient across the pulmonic valve, and the jet causes poststenotic dilatation of the main pulmonary artery and frequently of the left pulmonary artery but not of the right. With severe valvular pulmonary stenosis, secondary hypertrophy of the crista supraventricularis can occur, resulting in infundibular obstruction, which resolves after relieving the pulmonary valvular stenosis.

Physical findings

The obstruction across the pulmonic valve results in a high-velocity jet created by the entire stroke volume. This jet results in a loud ejection murmur, best heard in the second intercostal space to the left of the sternum. It radiates into the lung fields and less well into the neck. The flexible stenotic valve and poststenotic dilatation result in an ejection click, which typically decreases in intensity with inspiration. The murmur, on the other hand, may increase in intensity on inspiration.

Right ventricular hypertrophy results in a systolic precordial lift. A prominent "A" wave may also be present in the jugular venous pulse. If there is a right-to-left shunt through a patent foramen ovale, cyanosis may be present.

Diagnosis

The systolic ejection murmur in the second interspace to the left of the sternum is the first clue to the diagnosis. The characteristic ejection click is an excellent clue to the pulmonary valvular abnormality. With severe pulmonic valve stenosis, right ventricular hypertrophy is seen on the ECG. The chest radiograph shows the poststenotic dilatation of the main pulmonary artery, and the cardiac silhouette is usually not enlarged. Only with right ventricular failure does the right ventricle dilate and the cardiac silhouette enlarge. Doppler echocardiography demonstrates right ventricular hypertrophy and the high-velocity jet across the pulmonic valve, allowing for an estimation of the systolic gradient.

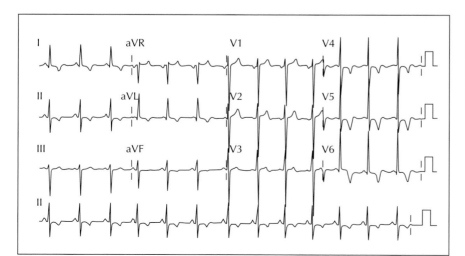

FIGURE 6 Electrocardiogram showing left ventricular hypertrophy and left atrial abnormality in a 45-year-old man with a calcified bicuspid aortic valve and a mean systolic gradient across the aortic valve of 80 mm Hg.

Complications

Valvular pulmonary stenosis is a rare disease in adults. If it occurs in adults severely enough to cause right ventricular hypertrophy then relief of the pulmonary stenosis is indicated. At present, balloon valvotomy is the preferred method of opening the valve, and only if the valve is dysplastic or calcified, or if marked pulmonic regurgitation is present, is valve replacement necessary. If the patient has signs of right ventricular failure, the valve should be dilated at any age. If pulmonic valvular stenosis is present, even if it is mild, antibiotic prophylaxis to prevent endocarditis is indicated, although infective endocarditis with this lesion is rare. In asymptomatic patients with valvular pulmonic stenosis and good right ventricular function in which a valvotomy has been done, prognosis is excellent, with 94% still alive 20 years after diagnosis [13].

Coarctation of the aorta

Anatomy

In adults, coarctation of the aorta constitutes approximately 5% of cases of congenital cardiovascular disease, occurring two to five times more often in males than in females. The most common form consists of a relatively short constriction of the descending aorta just beyond the takeoff of the left subclavian artery at the level of the ligamentus arteriosus. Occasionally, the aorta proximal to this point can be markedly hypoplastic, resulting in a longer length of constriction. Less commonly, the coarctation occurs proximal to or at the takeoff of the left subclavian artery, resulting in lower systolic blood pressure in the left arm compared with the right.

A bicuspid aortic valve is the most commonly associated abnormality and may be present in up to 80% of patients. In addition, associated congenital aneurysms may be present in the aorta either proximal or distal to the coarctation or in arteries of the circle of Willis (so-called berry aneurysms). Associated abnormalities such as PDA, aortic valve and subvalvular stenosis, and mitral valve abnormalities are not uncommon.

Pathophysiology

Coarctation of the aorta results in higher blood pressure in the aorta and arteries proximal to the obstruction and lower blood pressure distally. With severe coarctation of the aorta, collateral circulation develops that bypasses the obstruction. This collateral circulation involves the branches of the subclavian and cervical arterial system, the intercostal arteries, and the internal mammary and periscapular arteries, all of which have connections to arteries arising distal to the coarctation. These vessels dilate and elongate, becoming enlarged and tortuous.

The variables that determine the clinical picture depend on the severity of the obstruction. Minor obstructions cause almost no collateral formation and produce only a dampening of the distal aortic pressure, whereas severe to total occlusion of the aorta causes marked damping of the pulse beyond the coarctation and decreases in distal arterial blood pressure. The size and number of collaterals are also important. The collaterals can be so large and extensive that distal aortic flow is not impaired, and even distal pulse pressure and mean blood pressure may be only mildly decreased. However, the proximal aortic hypertension results in left ventricular hypertrophy and can eventually cause congestive heart failure.

Physical findings

The diagnosis of coarctation of the aorta is easily made by noting a decreased or an absent femoral arterial pulse compared with the brachial pulse. In some patients, the femoral pulses may be difficult to feel; in this case, the diagnosis can be made by comparing the systolic blood pressure in the right arm with the blood pressure in the leg, with both being taken with appropriately sized cuffs. It is important to take the blood pressure in both arms to pick up the unusual coarctation that begins proximal to or at the takeoff of the left subclavian artery. Normally, the indirect systolic blood pressure by cuff should be 10 mm Hg or higher in the leg than in the arm. If the systolic blood pressure is lower in the leg than in the arm, a diagnosis of aortic obstruction is made; in the proper setting, the etiology is coarctation of the aorta.

The murmur generated by flow past the obstruction is a late systolic bruit heard at the base of the heart anteriorly and as well or better in the interscapular area to the left of the spine. If the patient has a bicuspid aortic valve, an ejection click, a blowing diastolic murmur of aortic regurgitation, or both may also be heard. With the patient leaning forward with the arms crossed over the chest, intercostal and periscapular arterial pulsations can be palpated over the posterior chest wall, and systolic bruits may be heard over the enlarged, tortuous collateral vessels.

Diagnosis

The ECG can be within normal limits or show left ventricular hypertrophy. On chest roentgenography, the ascending aorta is frequently dilated; there is a large aortic "knob" because of the lateral displacement of the left subclavian artery. At times, notching of the descending aorta can be seen at the point of the constriction, and poststenotic dilatation can be noted below the coarctation. Rib notching, especially of the third rib and lower, is seen because of the enlarged tortuous intercostal arteries. On barium swallow, a proximal and distal impingement on the barium-filled esophagus of the aorta above and below the coarctation can be seen. On two-dimensional echocardiography, only hypertrophy of the left ventricle and abnormalities of the aortic valve may be seen. With transesophageal echocardiography, the area of the coarctation can be visualized and Doppler echocardiography can reveal the high-velocity jet of blood across the coarctation.

Complications and treatment

Eventually, left-sided heart failure can occur, as can infective endarteritis distal to the coarctation and infective endocarditis on the bicuspid aortic valve. Berry aneurysm rupture can cause a cerebrovascular bleed, and dissection of the aorta proximal to the coarctation has been reported. Aneurysms can develop proximal or distal to the coarctation or in arteries away from the coarctation.

In coarctation of the aorta that is severe enough to cause an increase in proximal aortic blood pressure and the development of collateral circulation, usually with a transcoarctation gradient of 30 mm Hg or more, resection of the coarctation should be done, especially in young people. Balloon dilatation is increasingly being reported, mainly in children [14]. There is increasing reports of experience in adults, and the incidence of developing postdilatation aneurysms is disturbing. At present, surgical resection or repair is the treatment of choice for adults. If the coarctation is mild, without collateral formation and with minimal difference in blood pressure proximal and distal to the coarctation, there is little evidence that resection of the coarctation is better than treatment with antihypertensive agents.

Even after coarctation repair, antibiotic prophylaxis to prevent infective endocarditis is recommended. After repair, there is evidence of reduced vascular reactivity and hypertension can persist or recur. Left ventricular hypertrophy may persist and together with hypertension is an important predictor of morbidity and mortality [15]. Dissection of the aorta can occur even after repair of the coarctation, and there is an increased early incidence of coronary artery disease in these patients.

Cyanotic Lesions
(Lesions with Right-to-Left Shunts)

Cyanotic lesions are characterized by a right-to-left shunt large enough to cause arterial desaturation. For a patient to be cyanotic, the reduced hemoglobin concentration must be at least 5 g/dL. Lesser concentrations, for instance in patients with anemia, will not result in cyanosis. The right-to-left shunting can occur at any cardiac level. Table 5 lists examples of lesions in this group and the cardiac level at which shunting occurs.

Although several congenital heart lesions are included in this group, relatively few are seen in the adult without previous surgery.

Eisenmenger's syndrome

Eisenmenger's syndrome lesions have already been discussed under the section dealing with atrial septal defects, VSDs, and PDA. When pulmonary hypertension occurs, it is clinically difficult to make a distinction between these lesions. All are characterized by the findings of pulmonary hypertension (ie, a loud P_2, right ventricular hypertrophy, possibly pulmonic valve regurgitation, right-sided heart failure, dilatation of the right ventricle with tricuspid regurgitation, and right-sided S_3 and S_4 sounds). The murmurs are no longer characteristic, the proximal pulmonary arteries are large, and often calcified, and the peripheral lung fields are clear because of extreme narrowing of the more distal pulmonary

vessels, or so-called pruning (Figs. 7 and 8). The definitive differential diagnosis can be made with two-dimensional Doppler echocardiography. With careful management, patients with Eisenmenger's syndrome can live for 20 to 30 years after diagnosis, into the sixth and seventh decades of life [16••]. Symptomatology occurs because of hyperviscosity because of the erythrocytosis caused by hypoxemia and is manifested by exercise intolerance, headache, backache,

TABLE 5 RIGHT-TO-LEFT SHUNTS CLASSIFIED BY CARDIAC LEVEL	
Level at which shunting occurs	**Examples of lesions**
Venous	Total anomalous pulmonary venous drainage; anomalous drainage of the superior vena cava into the left atrium
Atrial	Atrial septal defect with pulmonary hypertension; tricuspid atresia; Ebstein's disease; valvular pulmonary stenosis with blown-open foramen ovale
Ventricular	Ventricular septal defect with pulmonary hypertension; tetralogy of Fallot; pulmonary atresia
Arterial	Transposition of the great vessels; truncus arteriosus; double-outlet right ventricle; pulmonary arteriovenous fistula; patent ductus with pulmonary hypertension

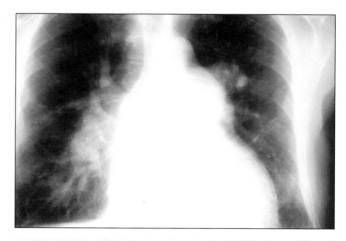

FIGURE 7 Chest x-ray, posteroanterior projection of a 50-year-old man with a large ventricular septal defect, pulmonary hypertension, and pulmonary vascular disease. Note huge main pulmonary artery, large right and left proximal pulmonary arteries, and absence of pulmonary vascular markings in the lateral one third of lung fields ("pruning"). The cardiac silhouette is enlarged, with dilated left ventricle.

visual disturbance, dizziness, and paresthesias. Hemoptysis occurs frequently because of rupture of collaterals. There is an abnormal hemostasis, with bleeding and thrombosis. Cerebrovascular accidents occur because of paradoxical embolization and cerebral venous thrombosis, intracerebral hemorrhage, and brain abscess. Syncope is related to the marked sudden decrease in cardiac output or to arrhythmias [17••]. Sudden death is frequent and is related to arrhythmias or pulmonary arterial rupture. Pulmonary artery thrombosis occurs in 20% to 30% of patients. The role of anticoagulation in this disease, considering the increased bleeding tendency, remains to be determined [18].

Pregnancy has a high morbidity and mortality, both maternal and fetal, and should be avoided in these patients. Noncardiac surgery is also accompanied by high morbidity and mortality. If either pregnancy or noncardiac surgery must occur, avoidance of intravascular fluid depletion, including blood loss, and maintenance of systemic vascular resistance during anesthesia are essential [19•,20••].

Patients with Eisenmenger's syndrome should undergo catheterization to quantitate pulmonary vascular resistance and magnitude of shunt. Attempts at reducing pulmonary vascular resistance with vasodilators, including inhalation of 100% O_2, nitric oxide, and prostacyclin, should be done, but the degree of reversibility is usually small. Chronic infusion of prostacyclin has been reported to reduce pulmonary vascular resistance minimally but to improve cardiac output and New York Heart Association functional class [17••,21].

Poor outcome in patients with Eisenmenger's syndrome is indicated by a history of syncope, clinical right ventricular failure, decreased cardiac output, and severe hypoxemia. At this point, lung transplantation and repair of the shunt defect, or heart–lung transplant, is the patient's only option. The survival after heart-lung transplant has improved, with 30-day survival at 81% and 1-year survival at 71% [22•].

Tetralogy of Fallot

Anatomy
Beyond infancy, tetralogy of Fallot is the most common lesion causing cyanosis. It is characterized by obstruction in the right ventricular outflow tract and a VSD, usually proximal to the outflow obstruction. The right ventricular obstruction is usually infundibular, with or without valvular pulmonic stenosis. Least common is valvular pulmonic stenosis alone. The other two lesions inferred from the "tetralogy" are right ventricular hypertrophy and an aortic root that overrides the VSD.

Pathophysiology
The clinical picture depends on the severity of the right ventricular outflow tract obstruction, the size of the VSD, and the systemic vascular resistance. As mentioned in the section on VSD, in patients with large VSDs and pulmonary hypertension, right ventricular hypertrophy is at times accompanied by hypertrophy of the crista supraventricularis, which can form an acquired infundibular obstruction. In

many of these patients, the obstruction is mild enough so that left-to-right shunting still occurs, and although a systolic gradient is present across the infundibular obstruction, there is still a predominant left-to-right shunt.

With the congenital malformation of the right ventricular outflow tract that defines the true tetralogy of Fallot, the right ventricular outflow tract is severely stenotic, and the shunt through the VSD is from right to left. The murmur is therefore that of infundibular pulmonary stenosis and not that of VSD.

Physical findings and diagnosis
In infundibular pulmonary stenosis with hypertrophy of the crista supraventricularis and VSD, the murmur may still be pansystolic, loudest at the left sternal border. With obstruction, the predominant systolic murmur is that of infundibular pulmonary stenosis: in other words, a loud ejection murmur frequently with a systolic thrill. The pulmonary arteries may still be large on roentgenography and echocardiography. In this disease, the magnitude of a right-to-left shunt is usually small at rest.

With tetralogy of Fallot, the right ventricular outflow tract is severely obstructed, the pulmonary blood flow is never increased, and the main pulmonary artery and its branches are small. There is a loud systolic ejection murmur at the base, often with a systolic thrill. An ejection click may be present if there is valvular pulmonic stenosis or a dilated ascending aorta. It is common for patients with these lesions from infancy to have cyanosis of the mucous membranes of the mouth, nail beds, and conjunctiva and to have clubbing of the fingers and toes. Right ventricular hypertrophy is invariably noted on ECG. On chest radiography, the cardiac silhouette is not dilated, the apex is rounded and tipped upward off the diaphragm ("boot-shaped heart"), the pulmonary vessels are dimin-

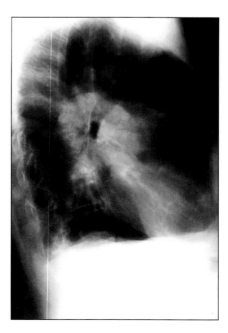

FIGURE 8 Chest x-ray, right lateral view. Same patient as in Figure 7.

ished, and there is concavity in the area of the main pulmonary artery. About 15% of patients with tetralogy of Fallot have a right-sided aortic arch. Although a definitive diagnosis can be made with two-dimensional Doppler echocardiography, it is recommended that these patients have catheterization, mainly to look at the size of the pulmonary artery and its branches and at the origin and disposition of the coronary arteries. In 15% of cases, the left anterior descending coronary artery anomalously arises from the right coronary artery or the anterior sinus of Valsalva and crosses the right ventricular outflow tract.

Without surgery, only about 10% of patients would live to adulthood. Shunt procedures such as the Blalock-Taussig or Pott's shunt markedly improve the prognosis. The complications of erythrocytosis already mentioned occur in these unoperated patients. Most patients with tetralogy of Fallot seen in adulthood have had corrective surgery.

Treatment

In most cases in which tetralogy of Fallot is found in the adult, complete correction is indicated. This is true even if the patient is doing well with a Blalock-Taussig (subclavian artery-to-pulmonary artery), Potts (descending aorta-to-left pulmonary artery), or Waterston-Cooley (ascending aorta-to-right pulmonary artery) shunt. Patients with systemic-to-pulmonary artery shunts have a high incidence of infective endocarditis, and all can eventually develop pulmonary vascular disease. Patients with complete correction of tetrology of Fallot have a good prognosis. Most have residual pulmonic valve regurgitation, and when this is severe, right ventricular dilatation and failure can result. At present, at the time of surgery avoidance of pulmonic valve regurgitation is ideal. In those patients with severe pulmonic regurgitation and right ventricular dilatation, especially if the right ventricular function is decreasing, elimination of the pulmonic regurgitation by construction of a pulmonic valve baffle or replacement is recommended [23].

Pulmonary arteriovenous fistula

Anatomy
Pulmonary arteriovenous fistulas can be single, multiple, or even microscopic in number and size. They are often associated with hereditary hemorrhagic telangiectasia (Rendu-Osler-Weber disease).

Pathophysiology
A right-to-left shunt exists because the arteriovenous fistula bypasses the pulmonary capillary bed. Because these arteriovenous fistulas are low-resistance shunts in the low-resistance pulmonary circuit, there is no afterload or preload burden on either the right or the left ventricle. The main problem is arterial desaturation and its consequences: polycythemia, clubbing, and the possibility of endarteritis. The heart itself is not abnormal from the pulmonary arteriovenous fistulas per se.

Physical findings
Telangiectasis on the mucous membranes and a personal or family history of gastrointestinal bleeding can be seen in patients with Rendu-Osler-Weber disease. The cardiac examination may be normal. The fistulas are subpleural, and if they are at the lung surface and have a large flow, they create a continuous murmur. At times, this murmur can be difficult or impossible to hear. The murmur may be mainly systolic. Because most of these fistulas are in the lower lobes, the murmur is usually in the anterior or lateral chest. Findings of cyanosis and clubbing are present [24•].

Diagnosis
The lesions are commonly seen on plain chest films. The ECG is normal. The chest radiograph may show the AV fistulae as solitary pulmonary lesions. Frequently, vascular markings can be traced to and from these nodules. With the roentgenographic findings and cyanosis, even without the diagnostic continuous murmur, a diagnosis can be made. Doppler echocardiography is of help in ruling out the other, more common causes of continuous murmurs and central cyanosis. With the injection of microbubbles, bubbles can be seen to rapidly fill the left side of the heart after filling the right side. It may not be possible to tell how the microbubbles get into the left side of the heart by transthoracic echocardiography.

Angiocardiography is essential in defining how many arteriovenous fistulas exist and where they are located (Fig. 9).

Complications
These fistulas create cyanosis and its complications. Hemoptysis is not uncommon. Gastrointestinal bleeding associated with Rendu-Osler-Weber syndrome can be seen. Finally, endarteritis caused by infection of arteriovenous fistulas has occurred. Systemic embolization through arteriovenous fistulas has been described, as have brain abscess and meningitis.

Treatment
A single fistula or a limited number of pulmonary arteriovenous fistulas that create a large right-to-left shunt can be surgically excised by partial lobectomy. Catheter embolization of pulmonary arteriovenous fistulas can be accomplished, with elimination of or marked diminution in the shunt. This approach may be preferable to surgical excision, even with a single fistula. It is the preferred technique for multiple arteriovenous fistulas.

Ebstein's disease
Anatomy
Ebstein's disease is a congenital lesion that is characterized by displacement of a portion of the tricuspid valve attachment into the anatomic right ventricle. The posterior and septal leaflets are usually involved, and the displacement varies from mild to severe, resulting in enlargement of the

chamber above the tricuspid valve (the "right atrium") and compromise of the chamber below (the "right ventricle"). The anterior leaflet is large and redundant and has frequent abnormal attachments to the right ventricular wall. There is frequently an atrial septal defect or an open foramen ovale.

Pathophysiology

The tricuspid valve is usually incompetent, resulting in a varying degree of tricuspid regurgitation. The "right atrium" is enlarged. If the tricuspid regurgitation is sufficient, the right atrial pressure is abnormally high, and if an atrial septal defect is present, a right-to-left shunt at the atrial level can cause arterial desaturation and cyanosis.

There is frequently a muscle connection between the right atrium and the right ventricle, or a bundle of Kent; therefore, the anatomic substrate for Wolff-Parkinson-White syndrome exists in approximately 20% of patients.

Physical findings

The patient may have a precordial lift in the area of the outflow tract of the right ventricle. There may be signs of tricuspid regurgitation with an increased "V wave." The large anterior leaflet may move toward the atrium one or more times during ventricular systole, causing one or more nonejection clicks ("sail sign"). The murmur of tricuspid regurgitation with its enhancement on inspiration is common as is a short diastolic inflow murmur. The S_1 and S_2 are frequently widely split, so that it often sounds as if there are several systolic clicks. Frequently, there are S_3 and S_4 sounds. The patient may be cyanotic, with clubbing. The patient may be cyanotic with clubbing.

Approximately 20% of patients have supraventricular tachycardias.

Diagnosis

The chest roentgenogram shows a wide sweep of the right atrial border. The heart looks globular, but the pulmonary vascular markings are always normal or diminished, never plethoric. The ECG usually shows a right bundle branch block with a low-voltage rSR′ or a qR in V_1 and occasion-ally demonstrates first-degree atrioventricular block or Wolff-Parkinson-White syndrome, usually with a posteriorly directed delta wave. Two-dimensional Doppler echocardiography can make the diagnosis because the attachment of the posterior or septal leaflet, which is displaced toward the apex, is clearly visualized on echocardiography (Fig. 10).

Complications

Most patients with Ebstein's disease who survive to adulthood do quite well. Cyanosis in childhood is a bad prognostic sign. Symptoms are related to the degree of tricuspid regurgitation and the presence and magnitude of a right-to-left shunt. The most troublesome problem that many people experience is with paroxysmal atrial tachycardia. Evidence indicates that the bundle of Kent can be interrupted by radiofrequency catheter ablation, which

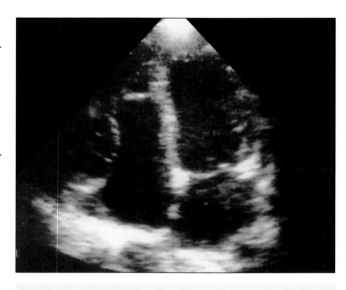

FIGURE 10 Two-dimensional echocardiogram, four-chamber view of a 50-year-old man with Ebstein's anomaly. Note displacement of the septal leaflet of the tricuspid valve down into the right ventricle almost to the apex.

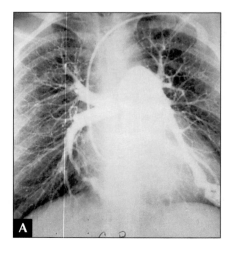

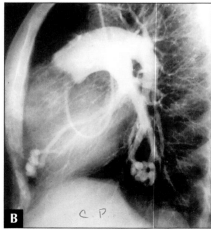

FIGURE 9 **A**, Angiocardiogram, pulmonary artery injection in the posteroanterior projection of a 30-year-old woman with pulmonary vascular disease who suddenly developed a continuous murmur lateral to the cardiac apex. Two pulmonary arteriovenous fistulae are visible, one in the right middle lobe and one on the left lower lobe. **B**, Angiocardiogram, pulmonary artery injection in the left lateral projection. Note the filling of the retrosternal space by the enlarged right ventricle as well as the two arteriovenous fistulae. Same patient as in *A*.

should be accomplished for those with recurrent paroxysmal atrial tachycardia.

For patients who are symptomatic and have easy fatigability, cyanosis, or shortness of breath, surgical correction should be considered. Various techniques of plication of the portion of the right ventricle above the tricuspid valve have been advocated, together with closing of the atrial septal defect, and tricuspid valve replacement has also been described [25]. In patients who are minimally symptomatic or are asymptomatic, no surgery or ablation techniques are indicated [26••,27].

Corrected Transposition of the Great Vessels

Corrected transposition of the great vessels, also known as l-transposition with levocardia, is the result of the embryologic cardiac tube's bending to the left instead of to the right. This results in ventricular inversion, with the right ventricle and aortic root positioned to the left of the left ventricle and pulmonary artery root. This, in turn, results in the systemic veins draining into an anatomic right atrium through a bicuspid valve into an anatomic left ventricle, from which the pulmonary artery arises. The pulmonary venous blood drains into an anatomic left atrium through a tricuspid valve into an anatomic right ventricle, from which arises the aorta. The blood circulation is therefore physiologically correct, but the ventricles are inverted so that the systemic ventricle, the ventricle supporting the systemic arterial circulation, is an anatomic right ventricle.

This anomaly usually exists with other congenital heart anomalies, such as ventricular septal defect and subpulmonic stenosis. The tricuspid valve, functioning as the left-sided atrioventricular valve, is often displaced into the anatomic right ventricle (left-sided Ebstein's disease) and is regurgitant.

Physical findings

Without associated defects, there may be no abnormal findings. The second sound in the second interspace to the left of the sternum may often be loud and may be confused with the snapping second sound of pulmonary hypertension. This results from the aortic valve's being to the left of the pulmonic valve. The other findings are those of the associated lesions (*eg*, the systolic murmur of a ventricular septal defect or systolic ejection murmur of subpulmonic stenosis).

Chest radiography

The heart size is usually normal. The left border of the heart may be curved, without indentation, representing the ascending aorta as it arises on the left.

Electrocardiography

Because the conduction system is reversed, there may be a QS in V_1 and no Q wave in V_6. Varying degrees of atrioventricular block are frequent.

Diagnosis

Unless there are other anomalies, this lesion is often missed. Patients with atrioventricular block and a characteristic chest radiograph should have an echocardiogram, with which inversion of the ventricles can be noted.

Complications

With no other lesions, some patients have lived into the seventh and eighth decades of life. However, more often the anatomic right ventricle cannot sustain the systemic circulation for a normal lifespan, and frequently these patients have right ventricular dysfunction, dilatation, and failure, resulting in "left heart failure." Failure can be precipitated or accentuated by left-sided atrioventricular valve regurgitation, and a high degree of atrioventricular block may require a pacemaker. Surgery is usually considered to correct accompanying congenital heart defects. However, the anatomic right ventricle (the systemic ventricle) will frequently dilate and fail in the fourth to sixth decade, and the "tricuspid valve," acting as the systemic atrioventricular valve, may become severely regurgitant. Surgery in these patients can convert the anatomic left ventricle into the systemic ventricle and the anatomic right ventricle into the pulmonic ventricle, thus establishing the normal anatomic correction. Obviously, the systemic and pulmonary venous returns must be redirected through a Senning or Mustard procedure [28].

References and Recommended Reading

Recently published papers of particular interest have been highlighted as:
• Of interest
•• Of outstanding interest

1. Cheitlin MD: Congenital heart disease in the adult. *Mod Concepts Cardiovasc Dis* 1986, 55:20–24.

2. McNamara DG, Latson LA: Long-term follow-up of patients with malformations for which definitive surgical repair has been available for 25 years or more. *Am J Cardiol* 1982, 50:560–568.

3.• Konstantinides S, Geibel A, Olschewski M, *et al.*: A comparison of surgical and medical therapy for atrial septal defect in adults. *N Engl J Med* 1995; 333:469–473.

4.•• Li W, Somerville J: Infective endocarditis in the grown-up congenital heart (GUCH) population. *Eur Heart J* 1998, 19:166–173.

5.• Staniloae CS, El-Khally Z, Ibrahim R, *et al.*: Percutaneous closure of secundum atrial septal defect in adults: a single center experience with the amplatzer septal occluder. *J Invasive Cardiol* 2003,15:393–397.

6. Ellis JH IV, Moodie DS, Sterba R, *et al.*: Ventricular septal defect in the adult: natural and unnatural history. *Am Heart J* 1987, 114:115–120.

7.•• Pieroni DR, Nishimura RA, Bierman FZ, *et al.*: Second natural history study of congenital heart defects. Ventricular septal defect: echocardiography. *Circulation* 1993, 87(suppl):I80–188.

8. Thanopoulos BD, Karanassios E, Tsaousis G, *et al.*: Catheter closure of congenital/acquired muscular VSDs and perimembranous VSDs using the Amplatzer devices. *J Interv Cardiol* 2003, 16:399–407.

9. Morgan JM, Gray HH, Miller GA, *et al.*: The clinical features, management and outcome of persistence of the arterial duct presenting in adult life. *Int J Cardiol* 1990, 27:193–199.

10.• Wang JK, Liau CS, Huang JJ, *et al.*: Transcatheter closure of patent ductus arteriosus using Gianturco coils in adolescents and adults. *Catheter Cardiovasc Interv* 2002, 55:513–518.

11. Fenoglio JJ Jr, McAllister HA Jr, DeCastro CM, *et al.*: Congenital bicuspid aortic valve after age 20. *Am J Cardiol* 1977, 39:164–169.

12.•• Brown JW, Ruzmetov M, Vijay P, *et al.*: Surgery for aortic stenosis in children: a 40-year experience. *Ann Thorac Surg* 2003, 76:1398–1411.

13. Hayes CJ, Gersony WM, Driscoll DJ, *et al.*: Second natural history study of congenital heart defects: results of treatment of patients with pulmonary valvar stenosis. *Circulation* 1993, 87(suppl I):28–37.

14. Zabal C, Attie F, Rosas M, *et al.*: The adult patient with native coarctation of the aorta: balloon angioplasty or primary stenting? *Heart* 2003, 89:77–83.

15. de Divitiis M, Pilla C, Kattenhorn M, *et al.*: Ambulatory blood pressure, left ventricular mass, and conduit artery function late after successful repair of coarctation of the aorta. *J Am Coll Cardiol* 2003, 41:2259–2265.

16.•• Cantor WJ, Harrison DA, Moussadji JS, *et al.*: Determinants of survival and length of survival in adults with Eisenmenger syndrome. *Am J Cardiol* 1999, 84:677–681.

17.•• Berman EB, Barst RJ: Eisenmenger's syndrome: current management. *Prog Cardiovasc Dis* 2002, 45:129–138.

18. Silversides CK, Granton JT, Konen E, *et al.*: Pulmonary thrombosis in adults with Eisenmenger syndrome. *J Am Coll Cardiol* 2003, 42:1982–1987.

19.• Daliento L, Somerville J, Presbitero P, *et al.*: Eisenmenger syndrome: factors relating to deterioration and death. *Eur Heart J* 1998, 19:1845–1855.

20.•• Weiss BM, Zemp L, Seifert B, Hess OM: Outcome of pulmonary vascular disease in pregnancy: a systematic overview from 1978 through 1996. *J Am Coll Cardiol* 1998, 31:1650–1657.

21. Rosenzweig EG, Kerstein D, Barst RJ: Long-term prostacyclin for pulmonary hypertension with association congenital heart defects. *Circulation* 1999, 99:1858–1865.

22.• Waddell TK, Bennett L, Kennedy R, *et al.*: Heart-lung or lung transplantation for Eisenmenger syndrome. *J Heart Lung Transplant* 2002, 21:731–737.

23. de Ruijter FT, Weenink I, Hitchcock FJ, *et al.*: Right ventricular dysfunction and pulmonary valve replacement after correction of tetralogy of Fallot. *Ann Thorac Surg* 2002, 73:1794–1800.

24.• Swanson KL, Prakash UB, Stanson AW: Pulmonary arteriovenous fistulas: Mayo Clinic experience, 1982-1997. *Mayo Clin Proc* 1999, 74:671–680.

25. Di Russo GB, Gaynor JW: Ebstein's anomaly: indications for repair and surgical technique. *Semin Thorac Cardiovasc Surg Pediatr Card Surg Annu* 1999, 2:35–50.

26.•• Celermajer DS, Bull C, Tiss JA, *et al.*: Ebstein's anomaly: presentation and outcome from fetus to adult. *J Am Coll Cardiol* 1994, 23:170–176.

27. Younoszai AK, Brook MM, Silverman NH: Ebstein's malformation. *Curr Treat Options Cardiovasc Med* 1999, 1:363–372.

28. Mavroudis C, Backer CL: Physiologic versus anatomic repair of congenitally corrected transposition of the great arteries. *Semin Thorac Cardiovasc Surg Pediatr Card Surg Annu* 2003, 6:16–26.

SELECT BIBLIOGRAPHY

Brickner ME, Hillis LD, Lange RA: Congenital heart disease in adults: first of two parts. *N Engl J Med* 2000, 342:256–263.

Brickner ME, Hillis LD, Lange RA: Congenital heart disease in adults: second of two parts. *N Engl J Med* 2000, 342:334–342.

Cheitlin MD, Sokolow M, McIlroy MB: Congenital heart disease (with special references to adult cardiology). In *Clinical Cardiology*, edn 6. Norwalk, CT: Appleton & Lange; 1993:358–406.

Deanfield J, Thaulow E, Warnes C, *et al.*: Task Force on the Management of Grown Up Congenital Heart Disease, European Society of Cardiology; ESC Committee for Practice Guidelines. Management of grown up congenital heart disease. *Eur Heart J* 2003, 24:1035–1084.

Liberthson RR: *Congenital Heart Disease: Diagnosis and Management in Children and Adults*. Boston: Little Brown; 1989.

Congenital Heart Disease in the Adult Postoperative Patient

John S. Child
Joseph S. Alpert

32

Key Points

- Cardiac operations for congenital heart disease have resulted in the survival of many previously operated infants and children to adulthood.

- Understanding of the basic malformation, the nature of the surgical operation, and any potential residua, sequelae, and complications is mandatory for proper care of adults with operated congenital heart disease.

- Residua and sequelae generally can be categorized as electrophysiologic or as anatomic with attendant hemodynamic consequences.

- Superimposed, adult acquired diseases such as hypertension, aortic stenosis, or coronary artery disease may result in deterioration of ventricular function despite a good operative outcome, and they require proper diagnosis and treatment.

- It is important for a physician to know how to integrate sophisticated imaging and hemodynamic assessment, the mainstay being echocardiography, into the care of the patient.

Because of advances in cardiovascular surgical techniques during the past 25 years, there are many long-term survivors of cardiac operations during infancy and childhood, and physicians are faced with caring for an increasing number of patients with congenital heart disease [1••,2,3]. Caring for adults with congenital heart disease requires knowledge of the original defect, the hemodynamic and anatomic problems caused by that defect, and the progressive age-related changes in anatomy and physiology. Proper patient care after catheterization or surgical palliation or repair requires intimate knowledge of the nature and effects of the intervention and of the postoperative residua, sequelae, and complications (Table 1) [1••,2,3].

The success of these interventions is judged by the patient's quality of life, survival time, and need for reoperation. The general practitioner must be knowledgeable about currently applied techniques and materials as well as outmoded techniques previously applied during infancy and childhood. Adults who underwent surgery 20 or more years ago are alive because of their operations, but they may have had inadequate myocardial protection or have degenerating prosthetic materials.

GENERAL POSTOPERATIVE CONSIDERATIONS

Except for ligation of an uncomplicated patent ductus arteriosus and suture closure of a secundum atrial septal defect, all other surgery for cardiac anomalies leaves behind or causes some obligatory abnormality, ranging from trivial to serious (Tables 1 and 2). Postoperative residua and sequelae can be broadly categorized as electrophysiologic or anatomic (valvular, myocardial, vascular), or related to the durability of prosthetic materials and valves.

Electrophysiologic Sequelae

Electrophysiologic sequelae include atrial and ventricular arrhythmias caused by scar or aneurysm formation after atrial or ventricular incisions or patch suturing. Insertion of intracardiac patches or conduits may cause disruption of the conduction system. For example, repair of tetralogy of Fallot includes a right ventricular outflow tract incision and ventricular septal defect patch. If the right ventricular outflow tract or pulmonary artery obstruction is inadequately relieved by the operation, the resultant right ventricular pressure overload superimposed on the right ventricular outflow tract scar or aneurysm may cause ventricular arrhythmias.

Anatomic Sequelae and Residua

Important anatomic sequelae and residua must be sought. Bicuspid aortic valves are often associated with aortic coarctation and continue to pose risks of progressive stenosis, regurgitation, and endocarditis after coarctation repair. Variations on a parachute mitral valve, often found in conjunction with coarctation and other stenoses in sequence on the left-sided circulation, may have gone undetected. Repair of an ostium primum atrial septal defect includes cleft mitral valve repair; residual mitral regurgitation may exist and is occasionally progressive. Subaortic, discrete stenosis may coexist and should be recognized.

Repaired tetralogy of Fallot is often associated with pulmonary regurgitation because of a valvulotomy or a transannular incision and patch. Isolated mild to moderate low-pressure pulmonary regurgitation is common and well-tolerated. Severe pulmonary regurgitation may cause right ventricular failure and tricuspid regurgitation, particularly if there is any residual right ventricular outflow, pulmonary valvular, or arterial (eg, branch stenosis) obstruction. Also, muscular ventricular septal defects may have been missed preoperatively. Postoperative aortic regurgitation is common in the adult whose malformation was associated with a dilated aortic root or trunk (eg, tetralogy of Fallot, transposition of the great arteries, single ventricle in association with pulmonic stenosis, truncus arteriosus). Atrioventricular valve regurgitation is common preoperatively in candidates for the Fontan procedure and may progress postoperatively. These valvular lesions pose a continuing risk for endocarditis and may affect long-term ventricular performance.

Prosthetic Materials

Use of prosthetic materials such as septal patches, mechanical or bioprosthetic valves, and intracardiac and extracardiac conduits may have long-term consequences. Prosthetic valves are associated with a risk for thrombus formation and infective endocarditis. Bioprosthetic valves may undergo premature degeneration and calcification. External conduits may kink or develop internal intimal thickening ("peel formation"), and valved conduits frequently undergo valvular degeneration that may result in severe obstruction.

TABLE 1 REPRESENTATIVE RESIDUA AND SEQUELAE AFTER INTRACARDIAC REPAIR FOR CONGENITAL HEART DISEASE

Residua (defects only partially or not corrected)	Sequelae (defects caused by the form of operative intervention)
Bicuspid aortic valve (coarctation)	Mechanical—ventricular function (ventriculotomy), intraventricular or venous baffle obstruction (eg, Mustard or Rastelli repair)
Cleft mitral leaflet (ostium primum atrial septal defect)	
Residual ventricular outflow obstruction	
Atrioventricular valve regurgitation (after Fontan procedure for tricuspid atresia or single ventricle)	Electrophysiologic—atrial arrhythmias and sinus node dysfunction (atrial septal defect, Mustard intra-atrial baffle, Fontan), conduction defects (central right bundle branch block or left anterior fascicular block after ventricular septal patch, eg, tetralogy of Fallot), ventriculotomy-induced ventricular arrhythmias or conduction defects
Systemic hypertension (coarctation) or pulmonary hypertension (shunts)	
Myocardial function—long-term ability of right ventricle (transposition) or single ventricle to function as systemic ventricle; effects of previous volume/pressure overload, prolonged cyanosis and erythrocytosis on coronary reserve and myocardial contractility	Valvular—aortic or pulmonic regurgitation (valvotomy, tetralogy of Fallot), mitral regurgitation or stenosis after repair of cleft mitral leaflet (primum atrial septal defect)
	Prosthetic materials—patches (deterioration with time, ventricular septal patch leaks), conduits (kinking or progressive intraluminal obstruction), valves (bioprosthetic deterioration with stenosis/regurgitation) or disk valves with thrombosis, fracture, or stenosis; anticoagulant complications
Cyanosis—residual left superior vena cava to left atrium with or without coronary sinus atrial septal defect	Cyanosis—pulmonary arteriovenous fistulae (Glenn shunt)

An internal conduit holds a risk for conduit leaks, internal obstruction, and kinking, or it may partially obstruct the chamber within which it sits. Examples of procedures using external and internal conduits include the Fontan repair with an external conduit from the right atrium to the pulmonary artery (for tricuspid atresia or single ventricle with pulmonic stenosis), and the Rastelli repair with an external conduit from the right ventricle to the pulmonary artery (for D-transposition or double-outlet right ventricle) and an intraventricular conduit to route the left ventricle to the aorta via the ventricular septal defect.

Transthoracic echocardiography with Doppler and color-flow imaging is the main procedure for detailed anatomic and hemodynamic postoperative evaluation of patients with congenital heart disease. These studies are best done in laboratories having extensive experience with these abnormalities [4]. Transesophageal echocardiography (TEE) is needed when transthoracic echocardiography is not technically adequate and structures are not readily accessible to surface echocardiography (*eg*, aortic coarctation) [5]. Magnetic resonance imaging (MRI) is complementary for imaging abnormalities of the great vessels. If

TABLE 2 POTENTIAL RESIDUA AND SEQUELAE AFTER REPAIR OF SPECIFIC COMMONLY OPERATED CONGENITAL HEART DEFECTS

Original defect	Residua	Sequelae
Bicuspid aortic valve	Aortic regurgitation or stenosis (if valvotomy) Left ventricular enlargement or left ventricular hypertrophy	Prosthetic valve malfunction Anticoagulation
Coarctation	Bicuspid aortic valve Hypertension Residual coarctation Left ventricular hypertrophy Coronary disease Intracranial aneurysm	Recurrent coarctation
Atrial septal defect secundum	Atrial arrhythmias Mitral prolapse/mitral regurgitation Right atrial and right ventricular enlargement Right ventricular failure Tricuspid regurgitation Pulmonary hypertension	Atrial fibrillation/stroke
Atrial septal defect primum	Residual cleft mitral valve/mitral regurgitation Discrete subaortic stenosis (missed) Right ventricular, right atrial, left atrial enlargement Tricuspid regurgitation Pulmonary hypertension Atrial arrhythmias	Mitral stenosis Subaortic stenosis caused by chordal attachments to ventricular septum and suture of mitral valve cleft Patch leak Atrial arrhythmias
Tetralogy of Fallot	Right ventricular outflow tract obstruction Ventricular septal defect patch leak Branch pulmonary stenosis Right ventricular hypertrophy Aortic regurgitation (dilated aorta)	Ventricular septal defect patch: right bundle branch block, aortic regurgitation Right ventricular outflow tract incision Pulmonary regurgitation Ventricular arrhythmias Conduit obstruction
Transpositions	Decreased systemic right ventricular function Aortic regurgitation	Intracardiac conduit leak/obstruction Extracardiac conduit obstruction Intra-atrial baffle leak or obstruction Caval or pulmonary venous obstruction Atrial and ventricular arrhythmias, sinus node dysfunction
Univentricular hearts (tricuspid atresia, single ventricle)	Atrioventricular valve regurgitation Myocardial dysfunction Aortic regurgitation	Fontan conduit obstruction/thrombus Atrial patch leak Atrial and ventricular arrythmias Pulmonary arteriovenous fistulae (Glenn shunt)

the echocardiographic and MRI data are not definitive, they conflict with the clinical picture, or reoperation is indicated, goal-directed diagnostic cardiac catheterization may be necessary. Intraoperative TEE improves results by detecting unexpected anomalies, refining known anatomic details, or allowing detection and re-repair of unsatisfactory results while the patient is still in the operating room.

SPECIFIC POSTOPERATIVE LESIONS

Congenital aortic stenosis caused by a bicuspid aortic valve is one of the most common congenital cardiac malformations, although it may go unrecognized early in life. It may be directly repaired in younger patients (< 21 years old) by valvotomy or balloon dilation using percutaneous catheter techniques if the valve is pliant and noncalcified with obstruction caused by congenital fusion of the commissures. There is often some degree of aortic regurgitation after valvotomy or balloon valvuloplasty, and the inherently abnormal valve remains a site for recurrent stenosis or infective endocarditis. Aortic regurgitation usually progresses gradually but can suddenly increase because of infective endocarditis. Generally, recurrent aortic stenosis progresses slowly, and reoperation is often necessary. Echocardiographic quantitation of aortic valve area, aortic regurgitation, and left ventricular size and ejection fraction should be done routinely on a yearly basis. For the older patient, direct valve replacement is often preferable. Surgically important aortic regurgitation may require valve replacement to remove the left ventricular volume overload and to preserve ventricular function. Despite the best attempts at selecting patients, some may exhibit late myocardial dysfunction and ventricular arrhythmias. The type of aortic prosthesis used affects its long-term durability, and the need for anticoagulation therapy and possible reoperation. Antibiotic endocarditis prophylaxis is required for life.

Valvular pulmonic stenosis (isolated) can usually be repaired with excellent results. Minimal residua and sequelae are expected if the valve repair is performed when the patient is young (< 21 years old), even if mild degrees of pulmonic stenosis and regurgitation remain. If severe pulmonic stenosis is operated on after 21 years of age, the outlook is excellent; however, the longstanding right ventricular pressure overload and hypertrophy can result in right ventricular failure. Balloon dilation has largely replaced surgical valvotomy, except for dysplastic valves, and short-term results have been excellent.

Ebstein's anomaly is the most common cause of surgically important congenital tricuspid valvular regurgitation. If the anterior tricuspid leaflet is shown by echocardiography to be long and mobile, a surgeon experienced with this anomaly can achieve a good repair. Residual, mild to moderate, low-pressure tricuspid regurgitation is usually well tolerated. Valvular reconstruction reduces right ventricular volume overload and improves right ventricular function. An interatrial communication (a commonly associated defect) should be closed at the same time to eliminate cyanosis and to avoid future risk of paradoxic embolization. Wolff-Parkinson-White syndrome is a common association. During the same operation, right-sided atrioventricular bypass tracts are surgically interrupted to prevent the accelerated ventricular response to supraventricular arrhythmias. Postoperative supraventricular arrhythmias may still recur but usually respond to pharmacologic treatment with antiarrhythmic agents. If amiodarone therapy or radiofrequency ablation becomes necessary, consultation with a specialist is needed. Valve replacement has a long-term mortality rate of 10% to 15%. Tissue valves are preferred because of concerns about the risk of pulmonary embolization from mechanical prostheses despite anticoagulation. Improvement after surgical intervention notwithstanding, there are obligatory residual abnormalities of ventricular size and function.

Isolated, left-sided, atrioventricular valve incompetence may occur with congenital transposition of the great arteries. The left-sided tricuspid valve may have an Ebstein-like malformation, with severe left atrioventricular valve regurgitation initially mistaken for mitral regurgitation until echocardiographic study elucidates the inverted ventricles. Valve replacement is usually required when regurgitation is severe. The possibility of complete heart block (approximately 2% accrued incidence per year) and right ventricular failure (the systemic subaortic ventricle) warrants annual electrocardiograms and echocardiograms.

SURGICAL PROCEDURES

Intra-atrial Surgery

Atrial septal defects, particularly the secundum variety, are some of the most common congenital heart defects. Early closure of these defects prevents subsequent right ventricular dysfunction or pulmonary hypertension. Surgical closure achieves excellent long-term results, particularly if performed by the age of 40 years. Nonetheless, even patients older than 60 years benefit symptomatically and prognostically from repair, but they do experience more arrhythmias and pulmonary problems than patients operated on before age 40 [6••,7,8].

Removal of the left-to-right shunt usually decreases the right ventricular size to normal if done during childhood, whereas adults who undergo repair usually have some residual right ventricular enlargement. Long-term right ventricular dysfunction is infrequent. Even if a patient has preoperative tricuspid regurgitation and right ventricular failure, right ventricular function usually improves postoperatively. Significantly increased pulmonary vascular resistance decreases long-term improvement and survival.

The incidence of atrial arrhythmias increases with each decade in adults with unrepaired atrial septal defect. The later the operation is performed, the less preventable these arrhythmias. With repair after age 40, as many as 50% of patients with preoperative sinus rhythm will have late postoperative atrial fibrillation.

Intra-atrial "switch" surgery has primarily been performed for complete transposition of the great arteries (Fig. 1). Such procedures redirect the systemic venous blood flow to the left ventricle (which supplies blood to the lungs via the pulmonary artery) and the pulmonary venous flow to the right ventricle (which ejects blood to the body via the aorta). Currently, the trend is to perform an arterial switch procedure during infancy, but a large number of today's young adults have previously had a Mustard or Senning atrial switch procedure. Although approximately 80% of these patients survive to adulthood, long-term complications are the rule (Tables 1 and 2) [9,10]. Routine follow-up electrocardiograms should be obtained. Atrial arrhythmias are common; injury to the sinus node may cause bradycardias and junctional escape rhythms, which may require inserting a permanent pacemaker. Because of the unusual intracardiac pathways, the pacemaker should be inserted by a physician experienced in dealing with these patients.

Long-term concerns about the functioning of the right ventricle in the systemic subaortic position persist, with some patients developing cardiomyopathy and ventricular failure. Echocardiography should be performed at least yearly to detect this complication. Afterload reduction with angiotensin-converting enzyme (ACE) inhibitors may be needed if the right ventricular ejection fraction is decreased or systemic arterial hypertension is detected.

Intraventricular Surgery

Intraventricular surgery includes repair of ventricular septal defects and tetralogy of Fallot as well as Rastelli procedures. Intraventricular surgery may be performed via a right atriotomy or ventriculotomy. Long-term outcome is affected by the adequacy of myocardial protection, degree of residual ventricular pressure or volume overload, subsequent electrophysiologic sequelae, and durability of prosthetic conduits, valves, and patches.

The most representative malformation is tetralogy of Fallot. Patients who received palliative aortopulmonary shunts (Blalock-Taussig, Pott's, or Waterston) and subsequent intracardiac repair at approximately 2 years of age have a nearly 90% survival rate 20 years after operation. Before complete repair, these shunts may gradually obstruct and result in increased cyanosis because of decreased pulmonary blood flow, or they may be too large and either result in left ventricular volume overload or increased pulmonary vascular resistance and pulmonary hypertension. Adults who received palliative shunts as children benefit from complete repair. Although patients older than 40 years at the time of repair have a late mortality rate of approximately 15%, long-term survival is enhanced by intracardiac repair, and most of these patients lead essentially normal lives [11,12].

Approximately 15% of persons with tetralogy of Fallot require reoperation for residua and sequelae of the previous intracardiac repair, including residual right ventricular outflow tract obstruction and ventricular septal defect patch leaks (Figs. 2 and 3). Severe pulmonary regurgitation may occur if the pulmonary valve is excised and can result in right ventricular failure and tricuspid regurgitation requiring reoperation to insert a bioprosthetic valve. In patients with severe hypoplasia of the pulmonary valve or pulmonary atresia, a right ventricular–to–pulmonary artery conduit may be necessary. As previously noted, this can result in late obstruction because of intimal buildup or degeneration of a tissue valve within the conduit. Such hemodynamic abnormalities cause pressure and volume overload of a right ventricle with an incisional scar and, occasionally, a right ventricular aneurysm. This is the substrate for ventricular arrhythmias and sudden death. Bundle branch blocks or high-grade heart block may result

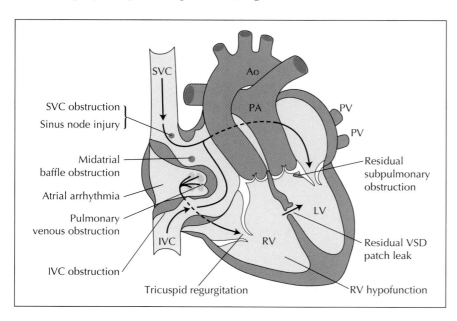

FIGURE 1 Postoperative Mustard repair procedure for D-transposition of the great arteries. The intra-atrial baffle can be seen to connect the superior and inferior vena cavae (SVC, IVC) to the left ventricle (LV), which directs deoxygenated blood to the lungs via the pulmonary artery (PA). Pulmonary veins (PV) are routed to the right ventricle (RV), which directs oxygenated blood to the body via the aorta (Ao). As such, the circulation in series is reconstituted. This schematic diagram displays the various potential sequelae or complications. VSD—ventricular septal defect.

from incision and resection of the right ventricular outflow tract and insertion of the ventricular septal defect patch.

Late postoperative left ventricular function relates to the adequacy of myocardial protection at operation, age at time of repair, and degree of left-side heart volume overload from prior palliative shunt procedures. There are also concerns that the duration of cyanosis before repair may relate to progressive myocardial fibrosis and late ventricular dysfunction. Patients with severe cyanotic tetralogy of Fallot may have reduced left ventricular volume and ejection fraction.

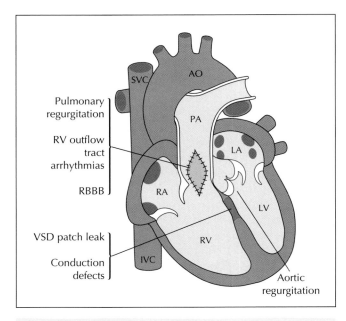

FIGURE 2 Representative corrective repair for tetralogy of Fallot. The misaligned ventricular septal defect (VSD) has been closed with a patch. Obstruction to flow from the right ventricle (RV) to the pulmonary artery (PA) may occur in the right ventricular outflow tract, pulmonary annulus or valve, or the PA. Here, a transannular patch is enlarging the right ventricular outflow tract and annulus after resection of obstructing right ventricular outflow tract muscle via the right ventricular incision. Potential sequelae or complications of the VSD patch and transannular incision and patch are shown. The aortic root, once overriding the VSD, may be affected by chronic aortic regurgitation. AO—aorta; IVC—inferior vena cava; LA—left atrium; LV—left ventricle; RA—right atrium; RBBB—right bundle branch block; SVC—superior vena cava.

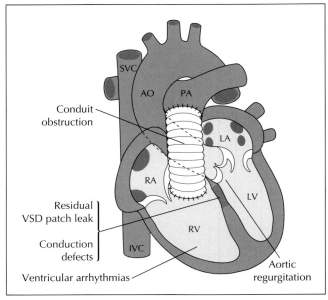

FIGURE 3 Rastelli repair of severe tetralogy of Fallot/pulmonary atresia. The ventricular septal defect (VSD) is patched, and the right ventricle (RV)–to–pulmonary artery (PA) connection is made by a conduit, usually containing a bioprosthetic valve. Potential sequelae, residua, and complications are noted. AO—aorta; IVC—inferior vena cava; LA—left atrium; LV—left ventricle; RA—right atrium; SVC—superior vena cava.

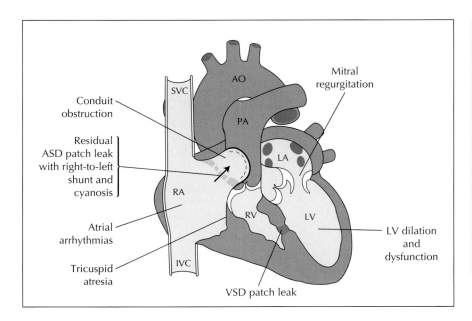

FIGURE 4 Right atrium (RA)–to–pulmonary artery (PA) connection for tricuspid atresia, functionally a univentricular heart, is a common variation on the Fontan connection seen in patients operated on within the last few years. (Now, a total cavopulmonary connection with a lateral tunnel is more commonly performed.) The obligatory atrial septal defect (ASD) is closed. Flow from the left ventricle (LV) to the PA is removed by closing a ventricular septal defect (VSD) as shown or by oversewing the pulmonary valve. Potential residua, sequelae, and complications also are depicted. AO—aorta; IVC—inferior vena cava; LA—left atrium; RV—right ventricle; SVC—superior vena cava.

Repair after 2 years of age leaves residual left ventricular dysfunction, even though volumes increase postoperatively. Because of concerns about long-term left dysventricular function in adults with repaired tetralogy of Fallot, systemic arterial hypertension must be treated, preferably with afterload-reducing agents (ACE inhibitors). Aortic regurgitation (common in the adult with tetralogy of Fallot) may become severe and cause ventricular failure. These patients are also susceptible to infective endocarditis and require lifelong prophylaxis. Two-dimensional echocardiography and Doppler evaluation are necessary to evaluate the right ventricular outflow tract and pulmonary artery anatomy for obstruction and to measure right ventricular systolic pressure and ventricular septal patch leaks.

Central Arterial Surgery

Central arterial surgery includes palliative aortopulmonary shunts and repair of patent ductus, coarction of the aorta, or sinus of Valsalva aneurysms. Surgical division of an isolated small patent ductus arteriosus in a child is an extracardiac operation and as close to a curative cardiac operation as can be performed. Currently, a potentially competing technique is transcatheter closure. If the ductus is moderate to large, surgical division in childhood usually allows for regression of the left atrial and ventricular size. If a large ductus is not closed early, pulmonary hypertension and pulmonary vascular disease may occur.

Surgical repair of coarctation of the aorta relieves the obstructive gradient in most instances [13]. A bicuspid aortic valve often coexists and requires endocarditis prophylaxis. Even in the well-repaired aortic coarctation, yearly follow-up for late hypertension is needed. Patients should undergo treadmill stress testing with the specific goal of detecting an inordinate rise in arterial blood pressure that may occur despite normal resting blood pressure. Resting and immediate postexercise blood pressures should be taken in both the arms and legs to detect any residual coarctation gradient. Recurrent coarctation may require repeat surgery or balloon dilation if severe. Residual coarctation should be quantified by TEE or MRI of the descending thoracic aorta.

Caval to Pulmonary Arterial Connections

Fontan or Glenn shunts are performed to increase pulmonary blood flow in malformations with a functional "univentricular heart" with pulmonic stenosis and intracardiac shunts (Fig. 4). Cyanosis is relieved, and symptoms are improved or alleviated [14]. Long-term problems relate mainly to arrhythmias and ventricular function; atrial fibrillation or flutter is poorly tolerated. Cardiac output and systemic venous congestion decrease. Ventricular function can deteriorate over time and may cause or be compounded by atrioventricular valve regurgitation. Routine echocardiographic evaluation of ventricular function and valvular regurgitation is necessary. The caval and right atrial connections to the right ventricle or pulmonary artery can be imaged by transesophageal echocardiography.

Infective endocarditis prophylaxis is necessary for patients with valvular regurgitation. Hypertension must be corrected with afterload reduction (ACE inhibitors) to decrease the workload of the ventricle. Ventricular dysfunction occasionally becomes sufficiently severe to require orthotopic cardiac transplantation.

KEY REFERENCES

Recently published papers of outstanding interest, as identified in *References and Recommended Reading*, have been annotated.

•• Perloff JK, Child JS: *Congenital Heart Disease in Adults*, edn 2. Philadelphia: WB Saunders; 1998.

Most complete and current in-depth review of the spectrum of issues in these patients; excellent overall reference or for specific questions and detailed bibliography.

•• Konstantinides S, Geibel A, Olschewski M, *et al.*: A comparison of surgical and medical therapy for atrial septal defect in adults. *N Engl J Med* 1995, 333:469–473.

This retrospective study shows that closure of an atrial septal defect in adults over 40 years old improves survival and prevents functional deterioration and heart failure but does not prevent atrial arrhythmias. As such, these patients require continued follow-up for atrial arrhythmias in order to reduce the risk of thromboembolic complications.

REFERENCES AND RECOMMENDED READING

Recently published papers of particular interest have been highlighted as:
• Of interest
•• Of outstanding interest

1.•• Perloff JK, Child JS: *Congenital Heart Disease in Adults*, edn 2. Philadelphia: WB Saunders; 1997.

2.   Care of the adult with congenital heart disease. *J Am Coll Cardiol* 2001, 37:1167–1198.

3.   Morris CD, Menashe VD: Twenty-five year mortality after surgical repair of congenital heart defect in childhood. *JAMA* 1991, 266:3447–3542.

4.   Child JS: Echocardiographic evaluation of adults with postoperative congenital heart disease. In *The Practice of Clinical Echocardiography*, edn 2. Edited by Otto CM. Philadelphia: WB Saunders; 2002:901–921.

5.   Child JS: Congenital heart disease. In *Multiplane Transesophageal Echocardiography*. Edited by Roelandt JRTC, Pandian NG. New York: Churchill Livingstone; 1996:173–198.

6.•• Konstantinides S, Geibel A, Olschewski M, *et al.*: A comparison of surgical and medical therapy for atrial septal defect in adults. *N Engl J Med* 1995, 333:469–473.

7.   Attie F, Rosas M, Granados N, *et al.*: Surgical treatment for secundum atrial septal defects in patients > 40 years old. A randomized clinical trial. *J Am Coll Cardiol* 2001, 38:2035–2042.

8.   Steele PM, Fuster V, Cohen M, *et al.*: Isolated atrial septal defect with pulmonary vascular obstructive disease—long term followup and prediction of outcome after surgical correction. *Circulation* 1987, 76:1037–1042.

9.   Gelatt M, Hamilton RM, McCrindle BW, *et al.*: Arrhythmia and mortality after the Mustard procedures: a 30-year single-center experience. *J Am Coll Cardiol* 1997, 29:194–201.

10. Warnes CA, Somerville J: Transposition of the great arteries: late results in adolescents and adults after the Mustard operation. *Br. Heart J* 1987, 58:148–155.

11. Murphy JG, Gersh BJ, Mair DD, *et al.*: Long-term outcome in patients undergoing surgical repair for tetrology of Fallot. *N Engl J Med* 1993, 329:593–599.

12. Waien SA, Liu PP, Ross BL , *et al.*: Serial follow-up of adults with repaired tetralogy of Fallot. *J Am Coll Cardiol* 1992, 295–300.

13. Cohen M, Fuster V, Steele PM, *et al.:* Coarctation of the aorta. Long-term follow-up and prediction of outcome after surgical correction. *Circulation* 1989, 80:840-845.

14. Gates RN, Laks H, Drinckwater DC Jr, *et al.*: The Fontan procedure in adults. *Ann Thorac Surg* 1997, 63:1085–1090.

Pulmonary Hypertension
Stuart Rich

33

Key Points
- The accurate diagnosis of pulmonary hypertension requires multiple tests to evaluate all possible contributing factors.
- General treatment measures appear to be helpful for patients with pulmonary hypertension of many etiologies.
- The assessment of drug effects and drug initiation should be left to experienced specialists.
- The prognosis of patients with severe pulmonary hypertension may markedly improve with appropriately focused, aggressive treatments.
- There is now a broad spectrum of treatments available to treat pulmonary arterial hypertension.

Although not common, pulmonary hypertension usually overwhelms the clinical course of a patient when it develops. For this reason, early diagnosis of pulmonary hypertension could have important implications for patients regarding their responsiveness to treatment and clinical course. There are many causes of pulmonary hypertension that can affect the pulmonary vascular bed in similar ways. Injury to the pulmonary vascular endothelium produces a cascade of effects including pulmonary vasoconstriction and thrombosis that is self-perpetuating and can lead to extreme pulmonary hypertension and right-side heart failure. Some patients have pulmonary hypertension from more than one cause, such as chronic obstructive pulmonary disease as well as pulmonary thromboembolism. For these patients, distinguishing the relative contribution of each underlying disease to the overall clinical state can be quite difficult.

Many physicians are confused when a patient has pulmonary hypertension that appears to be out of proportion to the underlying disease. The response of the pulmonary vascular bed to all types of stimuli is markedly variable, however. Some patients may have only minimal elevations in pulmonary hypertension when exposed to hypoxia; other patients may have a pronounced effect. Appreciating the variability of the pulmonary vascular response to injury explains why many patients have pulmonary hypertension that appears to be more severe than the extent of the underlying disease process.

ROLE OF THE GENERALIST
Patients suspected of having pulmonary hypertension should be referred to a specialist in the field because of the complexity of pulmonary hypertensive disease and the morbidity associated with both diagnostic testing and therapies. Early diagnosis of pulmonary hypertension is fundamental to successfully treating the patient, however, and in this regard, heightened suspicion by the primary

care physician is critical in making an early diagnosis. Echocardiography can be helpful in detecting pulmonary hypertension at earlier stages. After patients with pulmonary hypertension have been evaluated and placed on long-term treatment, the generalist should be able to manage the patient, with periodic consultation from the cardiologist or pulmonologist. Because there are so few centers of excellence in this area, it is essential for the generalist to reassume day-to-day care.

DIAGNOSIS

A new clinical classification of pulmonary hypertension has been established (Table 1) [1•]. Because the underlying cause of pulmonary hypertension may not be readily apparent, a physician needs to assess all possible etiologies, even when there is no clinical history or there are no overt signs of an underlying disease process.

TABLE 1 CLASSIFICATION OF PULMONARY HYPERTENSION
Pulmonary arterial hypertension
Pulmonary venous hypertension
Pulmonary hypertension associated with disorders of the respiratory system and/or hypoxemia
Pulmonary hypertension due to chronic thrombotic and/or embolic disease
Pulmonary hypertension due to disorders directly affecting the pulmonary vasculature

Chest radiography is helpful in evaluating parenchymal lung disease. Pulmonary hypertension often manifests with cardiomegaly and enlarged central pulmonary arteries (Fig. 1). Tapering of the pulmonary vasculature and oligemia are nonspecific findings. The lung fields on the chest radiograph film may appear normal in spite of interstitial lung disease; hence, if interstitial lung disease is suspected, a high-resolution chest computed tomographic (CT) scan is the test of choice. Its sensitivity for detecting interstitial abnormalities may preclude the need for open-lung biopsy.

Patients with pulmonary hypertension generally have limited exercise tolerance and may have exercise-induced syncope. Exercise tolerance is an important prognostic indicator, however, and assessing it may help in the early detection of patients with mild pulmonary hypertension when symptoms are manifest primarily with effort. The concomitant measurement of systemic oxygen saturation with pulse oximetry will confirm abnormal cardiopulmonary performance and help guide the physician toward the need for oxygen therapy. Patients whose history suggests limited effort tolerance should be studied using low-level treadmill protocols or a 6-minute walk test.

Pulmonary Function Testing and Echocardiography

Pulmonary function tests are necessary to establish whether an obstructive airways disease or restrictive lung disease is present. Patients who develop pulmonary hypertension from obstructive airways disease should have associated clinical findings, but restrictive lung disease can be more difficult to ascertain. Increased pulmonary artery pressure

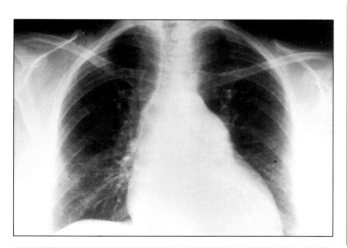

FIGURE 1 Chest radiographic (posteroanterior view) of a patient with unexplained pulmonary hypertension. Cardiomegaly with a large central pulmonary artery, prominent right descending pulmonary artery, and tapering of the vessels toward the periphery. The lung fields are clear. This could be a radiograph of a patient with pulmonary hypertension from almost any etiology.

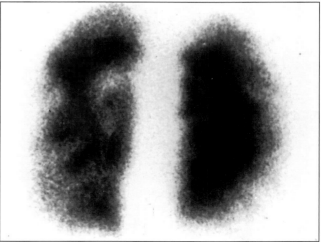

FIGURE 2 Perfusion lung scan (posterior upright view) of a patient with primary pulmonary hypertension. Patchy distribution of tagged albumin is marked but not in any anatomic segmental or subsegmental distribution suggesting pulmonary thromboembolism. This lung-scan pattern also may be seen in patients with pulmonary hypertension of other etiologies.

produces restrictive changes in the lungs to a moderate degree. Thus, the diagnosis of restrictive lung disease requires a combination of restrictive changes on pulmonary function testing and evidence of parenchymal lung disease either by chest radiography, high-resolution CT scan, or lung biopsy. Although diffusion capacity from carbon monoxide may be reduced with pulmonary hypertension of any etiology, extremely low levels may reflect interstitial lung disease when it is not obvious from other tests [2].

The ventilation-perfusion lung scan will reveal patients with a high likelihood of having thromboembolism. Because thromboembolism that produces pulmonary hypertension is usually silent, this lung scan needs to be performed on every patient regardless of a history of deep-vein thrombosis or previous pulmonary embolism. Patients with primary pulmonary hypertension also may have abnormal, patchy distribution of radionuclide (Fig. 2). Contrast-enhanced spiral CT scans may reveal the extent and location of thromboemboli in affected patients.

Echocardiography is very helpful in revealing underlying congenital heart disease. Use of saline contrast and color Doppler will aid in detecting intracardiac shunts, which usually are bidirectional or reversed in patients with pulmonary hypertension. When in doubt, transesophageal echocardiography can be instrumental in differentiating an atrial septal defect from a patent foramen ovale.

Pulmonary Angiography and Cardiac Catheterization

Although pulmonary angiography carries increased risk in patients with pulmonary hypertension, it is mandatory for patients whose lung scan suggests the possibility of pulmonary thromboembolism. Hypotensive episodes after pulmonary angiography may be vagally mediated, and pretreating patients with 1 mg of atropine and using low-osmolar, nonionic agents may make the procedure safer in this regard.

Because the clinical management of the patient with pulmonary hypertension can be complex, cardiac catheterization is advised for every patient in whom the diagnosis of pulmonary hypertension is suspected. In addition to confirming the etiology, catheterization will help to establish the prognosis by directly measuring cardiac output and pulmonary artery saturation, both of which predict survival. It is also essential to accurately determine pulmonary-capillary wedge pressure to assess left ventricular end-diastolic pressure. The pulmonary-capillary wedge pressure may be difficult to obtain in these patients, but a conclusion that the patient had a "falsely elevated wedge pressure" is unacceptable. Catheterization of patients with advanced disease can be quite difficult; these patients should be referred to physicians with considerable experience. The response to acute vasodilator testing is helpful in determining the optimal treatments.

CAUSES OF PULMONARY HYPERTENSION AND TREATMENT

Pulmonary Arterial Hypertension

Pulmonary arterial hypertension can be primary (idiopathic) or associated with other conditions (Table 2). The natural history of primary pulmonary hypertension is poor, with a mean survival of 2.8 years from the time of diagnosis [3]. As many as 20% of these patients however, can return to a normal lifestyle and have improved survival if they are diagnosed early and respond to high doses of calcium channel blockers [4]. The use of calcium blockers at high doses should be limited to patients who respond to acute vasodilator testing and should be initiated by physicians with established experience and expertise. Patients with mild to moderate symptoms who are not candidates for calcium blockers may be treated with oral bosentan, an endothelin receptor blocker [5•]. Patients with moderate to severe symptoms may be treated with a prostacyclin, either subcutaneous treprostinil or intravenous epoprostenol [6•]. Epoprostenol has been shown to improve quality of life and survival (Fig. 3) [7•]. Patients who continue to deteriorate in spite of medical management should be considered for lung transplantation [8]. The use of single-bilateral lung or heart–lung transplantation are all acceptable.

Collagen Vascular Disease

Pulmonary arterial hypertension complicating collagen vascular disease is becoming increasingly recognized since virtually all of the collagen vascular diseases have been reported to be associated with pulmonary hypertension. The mechanism may be associated interstitial lung disease, direct effects on the pulmonary vasculature causing vasoconstriction, or both.

These patients may respond well to endothelin receptor blockers or prostacyclins, depending on the presence and extent of associated interstitial fibrosis [9]. The high prevalence of pulmonary hypertension in patients with scleroderma justifies periodic screening with echocardiography.

TABLE 2 CLINICAL SPECTRUM OF PULMONARY ARTERIAL HYPERTENSION

Primary pulmonary hypertension
  Sporadic
  Familial
Related to
  Collagen vascular disease
  Congenital systemic to pulmonary shunts
  Portal hypertension
  HIV infection
  Anorexigens
  Persistent pulmonary hypertension of the newborn

Congenital Heart Disease

Pulmonary arterial hypertension secondary to congenital heart disease is well recognized in infants and children and is occasionally seen in adults. The fundamental principle in managing congenital heart disease with pulmonary hypertension is surgical correction before the pulmonary vascular disease becomes advanced. A patent intracardiac shunt associated with pulmonary hypertension usually results in right-to-left shunting with systemic hypoxemia. Patients with pulmonary hypertension and reversed shunting (Eisenmenger's syndrome) are considered inoperable. The efficacy of vasodilators in these patients is variable. The prostacyclins appear to be quite effective in these patients [10]. Patients who continue to deteriorate should be evaluated for heart–lung or lung transplantation.

Obstructive Lung Disease

The development of pulmonary hypertension in patients with chronic obstructive pulmonary disease results in increased mortality. The only established, effective treatment of pulmonary hypertension in these patients has been chronic supplemental oxygen therapy. Although it rarely reduces pulmonary artery pressure in the short term, oxygen retards progression of the pulmonary hypertension. Monitoring the response to oxygen therapy with arterial blood gases is important to check for carbon dioxide retention.

Vasodilators have been tested in patients with pulmonary hypertension from chronic obstructive pulmonary disease, but little documentation of their effectiveness exists. More importantly, however, vasodilators may worsen gas exchange, reduce arterial oxygen saturation, and cause pronounced systemic hypoxemia. Vasodilators are not recommended, but if they are given to patients with lung disease, careful monitoring of the arterial blood gases before and after their administration is important.

Mitral Valve Stenosis

Pulmonary hypertension is a common complication of mitral valve stenosis because of the increased left atrial pressure transmitted backward into the pulmonary vascular bed. The severity of pulmonary hypertension in mitral stenosis varies and it results from reactive vasoconstriction occurring in addition to the increased left atrial pressure. The definitive treatment for these patients has been mitral valve surgery. Although operative mortality increases among patients with severe pulmonary hypertension, no level of pulmonary artery pressure precludes mitral valve replacement or valvotomy, because pulmonary artery pressure should regress by at least 50% postoperatively. The experience using balloon valvuloplasty for mitral stenosis has been quite similar—the level of pulmonary hypertension usually falls to a modest degree initially and continues to fall over time [11].

Left Ventricular Diastolic Dysfunction

Physicians are familiar with the concept of pulmonary hypertension as a result of increased left atrial pressure from mitral stenosis. It is less well appreciated that similar levels of pulmonary hypertension can develop in patients with hypertensive or ischemic heart disease (or both) who have increased left ventricular end-diastolic pressure [12]. This may be the most common cause of pulmonary hypertension in adults. The correct diagnosis can be established by cardiac catheterization demonstrating high left ventricular end-diastolic filling pressures. The treatment of these patients (as for patients with other secondary forms of pulmonary hypertension) is focused on the underlying cause. Thus, patients with hypertensive heart disease should have their systemic blood pressures aggressively treated, because the pulmonary artery pressures would be expected to respond accordingly. Similarly patients with ischemic heart disease should have the left ventricular ischemia aggressively managed. Once these patients develop right ventricular failure, managing the left ventricular dysfunction becomes extraordinarily difficult.

Pulmonary Thromboembolism

Chronic thromboembolic obstruction of the proximal pulmonary arteries is an established treatable cause of pulmonary hypertension with pulmonary thromboen-

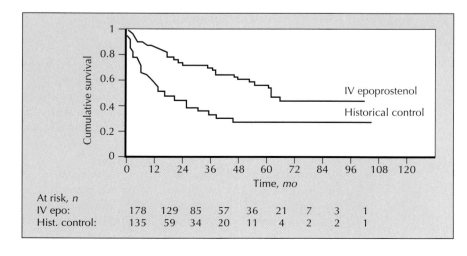

FIGURE 3 The long-term survival of patients with primary pulmonary hypertension followed up to 9 years and treated with intravenous (IV) epoprostenol is compared with historical controls. Survival was markedly improved. (*Adapted from* Sitbon *et al.* [14].)

At risk, n									
IV epo:	178	129	85	57	36	21	7	3	1
Hist. control:	135	59	34	20	11	4	2	2	1

darterectomy. Patients who undergo successful pulmonary thromboendarterectomy may return to a relatively normal lifestyle [13].

General Treatment Measures

General treatment measures for patients with pulmonary arterial hypertension are indicated in Table 3. Digitalis has been shown to have similar effects for the treatment of pulmonary hypertension as it does for left heart failure. Diuretics will help to relieve venous congestion and reduce dyspnea. Oxygen is of unproven benefit for treating pulmonary hypertension without chronic obstructive pulmonary disease, but it may be useful for patients with resting or exercise-induced hypoxemia. Warfarin anticoagulation therapy improves survival in patients with primary pulmonary hypertension. Low-dose anticoagulation therapy, to prolong the international normalized ratio to two to three times the control value, appears to be effective and is associated with a minimal risk of bleeding. Patients with liver dysfunction from venous congestion may be very sensitive to anticoagulants and need particularly close monitoring.

Because patients with pulmonary hypertension often have a limited cardiac output, they need to be advised regarding changes in their lifestyle. Isometric activities in particular should be avoided as they may induce syncope. On the other hand, patients with advanced pulmonary hypertension may lead productive lives as they learn to limit their stress, and these patients should be encouraged to be as active as possible.

WHEN TO REFER

Diagnosing and managing pulmonary hypertension is highly specialized and associated with increased risks.

TABLE 3 GENERAL TREATMENT MEASURES FOR PATIENTS WITH PULMONARY HYPERTENSION

Treatment	Comments
Daily activity	General activity advised, isometric and strenuous activity should be avoided
Supplemental oxygen	Continuous in hypoxic lung disease, supplemental in instances of profound hypoxemia (exercise/altitude)
Cardiac glycosides	May be helpful in overt right ventricular failure
Diuretics	Relieve venous congestion and edema; may require large doses or multiple drugs
Anticoagulants	Improve survival in some patients, low doses effective

Specifically, commonly used tests such as CT scanning and echocardiography may show subtle abnormalities that are difficult to accurately interpret for patients with severe pulmonary hypertension. Other tests, such as exercise testing, pulmonary angiography, and right-side heart catheterization are associated with increased morbidity. Therefore, patients with the clinical features of pulmonary hypertension should be referred to specialists with expertise in this area for an accurate diagnosis.

Even more important, however, is the need for referring patients with a confirmed diagnosis of pulmonary hypertension to recognized experts for treatment. Given the rapidly developing therapies, it may be difficult to determine which treatment is best suited for a given patient. Similarly, surgical interventions requiring mitral valve replacement, repair of congenital heart disease, or thromboendarterectomy require particular expertise, because operative morbidity and mortality are clearly increased in patients with pulmonary hypertension. These patients must be referred to institutions with proven experience in these specialized areas.

As pulmonary hypertension is probably more common than we appreciate, the generalist retains a critical role in making the initial diagnosis, initiating the workup, and the ongoing management of patients on therapy. Many treatment measures are both new and complex, so frequent communication between the generalist and the specialist is important to maintain a high level of day-to-day care.

REFERENCES AND RECOMMENDED READING

Recently published papers of particular interest have been highlighted as:
• Of interest

1.• Fishman AP: Clinical classification of pulmonary hypertension. *Clin Chest Med* 2001, 22:385–391.

2. Steen V, Medsger TA Jr: Predictors of isolated pulmonary hypertension in patients with systemic sclerosis and limited cutaneous involvement. *Arthritis Rheum* 2003, 48:516–522.

3. D'Alonzo GG, Barst RJ, Ayres SM, et al.: Survival in patients with primary pulmonary hypertension: results from a national prospective registry. *Ann Intern Med* 1991, 115:343–349.

4. Rich S, Kaufmann E, Levy PS: The effect of high doses of calcium-channel blockers on survival in primary pulmonary hypertension. *N Engl J Med* 1992, 327:76–81.

5.• Rubin LJ, Badesch DB, Barst RJ, et al.: Bosentan therapy for pulmonary arterial hypertension. *N Engl J Med* 2003, 346:896–903.

6.• Simonneau G, Barst RJ, Galie N, et al.: Continuous subcutaneous infusion of treprostinil, a prostacyclin analogue, in patients with pulmonary arterial hypertension: a double-blind randomized controlled trial. *Am J Respir Crit Care Med* 2002, 165:800–804.

7.• McLaughlin VV, Shillington A, Rich S: Survival in primary pulmonary hypertension: the impact of epoprostenol therapy. *Circulation* 2002, 106:1477–1482.

8. Mendeloff EN, Meyers BF, Sundt TM, et al.: Lung transplantation for pulmonary vascular disease. *Ann Thorac Surg* 2002, 73:209–219.

9. Badesch DB, Tapson VF, McGoon MD, *et al.*: Continuous intravenous epoprostenol for pulmonary hypertension due to the scleroderma spectrum of disease. *Ann Intern Med* 2000, 132:425–434.

10. Rosenzweig EB, Kerstein D, Barst RJ: Long-term prostacyclin for pulmonary hypertension with associated congenital heart defects. *Circulation* 1999, 99:1858–1865.

11. Ribeiro PA, Al Zaibag M, Abdullah M: Pulmonary artery pressure and pulmonary vascular resistance before and after mitral balloon valvotomy in 100 patients with severe mitral valve stenosis. *Am Heart J* 1993, 125:1110–1113.

12. Kessler KM, Willens HJ, Mallon SM: Diastolic left ventricular dysfunction leading to severe reversible pulmonary hypertension. *Am Heart J* 1993, 126:234–235.

13. Williamson TL, Kim NH, Rubin LJ: Chronic thromboembolic pulmonary hypertension. *Prog Cardiovasc Dis* 2002, 45:203–212.

14. Sitbon O, Humbert M, Nunes H, *et al.*: Long-term intravenous epoprostenol infusion in primary pulmonary hypertension: prognostic factors and survival. *J Am Coll Cardiol* 2002, 40:780–788.

SELECT BIBLIOGRAPHY

Runo JR, Loyd JE: Primary pulmonary hypertension. *Lancet* 2003, 3618:1533–1544.

Sitbon O, Humbert M, Simonneau G: Primary pulmonary hypertension: current therapy. *Prog Cardiovasc Dis* 2002, 45:115–128.

34

Pulmonary Embolism

Paul D. Stein
Russell D. Hull

Key Points

- Anticoagulant therapy is the primary treatment for deep venous thrombosis and pulmonary embolism; for treatment, intravenous or subcutaneous heparin should be administered in doses sufficient to prolong the activated partial thromboplastin time to a range that corresponds a plasma heparin level of 0.2 to 0.4 IU/mL by the protamine sulfate method or heparin level of 0.3 to 0.6 IU/mL by an amidolytic anti-Xa assay. Heparin and warfarin therapy can be started together, and warfarin should be administered to achieve an international normalized ratio of 2.0 to 3.0 and continued for at least 3 months.

- Low molecular weight heparin is at least as safe and effective as unfractionated heparin for the treatment of deep venous thrombosis.

- The bedside evaluation of pulmonary embolism is meaningful and helps determine the extent to which diagnostic tests should be pursued; a sound bedside impression also contributes strongly to formulating a noninvasive diagnosis of pulmonary embolism.

- The diagnostic validity of ventilation-perfusion lung scanning is enhanced when this technique is combined with prior clinical assessment.

- Strategies of diagnosis based on diagnosing and treating deep venous thrombosis as an alternative to the diagnosis of pulmonary embolism spare many patients the necessity of pulmonary angiography.

- Contrast-enhanced spiral computed tomography is a nearly noninvasive technique that may replace conventional pulmonary angiography, but it has not yet been fully evaluated.

- Transvenous inferior vena cava occlusion is indicated if there is a contraindication to anticoagulant use, a continuing predisposition to pulmonary embolism, or a recurrence of pulmonary embolism on full-dose anticoagulants.

- Thrombolytic therapy for pulmonary embolism is indicated if the patient is hypotensive or hypoxic on high levels of oxygen or otherwise unstable.

Pulmonary embolism (PE) is a complication of deep venous thrombosis (DVT). The most frequent predisposing factor for PE (and for DVT) is bed rest, usually following surgery (Table 1).

DEEP VENOUS THROMBOSIS

Diagnosis

Deep venous thrombosis of the thigh veins is more likely to cause PE than thrombosis of the veins of the calves. Techniques for diagnosing DVT include impedance plethysmography, B-mode ultrasonography, magnetic resonance imaging (MRI), contrast-enhanced spiral computed tomography (CT), conventional venography, and radionuclide scanning. Radionuclide fibrinogen uptake scanning is more sensitive for detecting venous thrombosis in the calves than venous thrombosis in the thighs. Therefore, in view of the greater danger of DVT of the thighs, the value of radionuclide scanning of the legs is limited. Impedance plethysmography is sensitive for the detection of DVT of the thighs [1,2], and B-mode ultrasonography using compression has a sensitivity equal to or higher than that of impedance plethysmography for the detection of DVT [3–5]. Both methods are valid alternatives to contrast venography [5]. Most centers employ B-mode ultrasonography; impedance plethysmography is rarely used. Sparse data suggest that MRI is sensitive and specific, but expensive; its role requires confirmation by further testing [6•]. Technetium labeling of activated platelets may show acute DVT, but its sensitivity and specificity are not yet fully evaluated [7]. Contrast-enhanced spiral CT of the legs when done by injection of contrast material into a dorsal vein of the foot, has shown a good sensitivity and specificity in a limited number of patients [8]. Venous phase imaging, following injection of contrast material into a peripheral vein appears promising [9,10], but requires further evaluation. Conventional venography, which is an invasive procedure, generally does not need to be performed in view of the excellent results shown with noninvasive techniques.

Prevention and Treatment

Fatal PE resulting from untreated, clinically symptomatic DVT occurs more frequently (37%) than fatal PE in patients with asymptomatic, early DVT diagnosed by refined techniques (5%) [11,12]. Detailed recommendations for the prevention of DVT were made by the American College of Chest Physicians Consensus Conference on Antithrombotic Therapy [13••]. Recommendations depend on the level of risk of DVT and the risk of bleeding. Prophylaxis includes unfractionated heparin or low molecular weight heparin, intermittent pneumatic compression, and elastic stockings, alone or in combination. Antithrombotic prevention of DVT differs from anticoagulant therapy in that the dose of heparin is lower. Intermittent pneumatic compression is beneficial in preventing DVT. Graded-pressure elastic stockings also may be beneficial, but aspirin is generally not [13••].

Anticoagulant therapy for DVT, based on recommendations by the American College of Chest Physicians Consensus Conference on Antithrombotic Therapy, is outlined in Table 2 [14••]. An attempt should be made to achieve a critical therapeutic heparin level within the first 24 hours [15]. Heparin is administered to increase the activated partial

TABLE 1 PREDISPOSING FACTORS FOR ACUTE PULMONARY EMBOLISM

Factor	Patients with positive angiographic findings, %*
Immobilization (≤ 3 mo)	54
Surgery (≤ 3 mo)	42
Coronary artery disease (ever)	20
Thrombophlebitis (ever)	19
Malignancy	18
Myocardial infarction	13
Trauma (lower extremities)	12
Congestive heart failure (right or left)	12
Chronic obstructive pulmonary disease	10
Stroke (ever)	10
Asthma	7
Pneumonia (acute)	7
History of pulmonary embolism	6
Collagen vascular disease	4
Postpartum (≤ 3 mo)	2
Interstitial lung disease	2
Sickle cell disease	1
Vasculitis	1
Self-administered drug use	1

*Patients may have more than one predisposing factor; n = 383.

TABLE 2 RECOMMENDATIONS FOR THE TREATMENT OF PULMONARY EMBOLISM (PE) OR DEEP VENOUS THROMBOSIS (DVT)

Low molecular weight heparin is recommended over unfractionated heparin

If unfractionated heparin is used, prolong the activated partial thromboplastin time to a range that corresponds to a plasma heparin level to 0.2 to 0.4 IU/mL by protamine sulfate or 0.3 to 0.6 IU/mL by an amidolytic anti-Xa assay

Start warfarin and heparin together

Heparin or low molecular weight heparin should be continued at least 5 days

Discontinue heparin on day 5 or 6 if international normalized ratio (INR) has been therapeutic 2 consecutive days

Continue heparin 10 days if massive PE or severe iliofemoral thrombosis

Treat with warfarin at least 3 months (INR 2.0–3.0); long-term low molecular weight heparin or unfractionated heparin may be used if warfarin is contraindicated or inconvenient

If reversible or time-limited risk factor, treat at least 3 months

If a first episode of idiopathic DVT or PE, treat at least 6 months

If a recurrent DVT or PE, or a continuing risk factor, treat at least 12 months or longer

If isolated calf vein thrombosis, treat 6 to 12 weeks or obtain serial noninvasive leg tests over 10 to 14 days to assess for proximal extension

Adapted from Hyers *et al.* [14••].

thromboplastin time (APTT) to 1.5 to 2.5 times the mean of the control value. This value corresponds to a heparin blood level of 0.2 to 0.4 IU/mL by the protamine sulfate titration assay and 0.3 to 0.6 IU/mL by the factor Xa assay. However, there is wide variability in the APTT and heparin blood levels with different reagents and even with different batches of the same reagent [16]. It is therefore vital for each laboratory to establish the therapeutic level of heparin, as measured by the APTT, that will provide a heparin blood level of at least 0.2 IU/mL by the protamine titration assay for each batch of thromboplastin reagent used, particularly if the reagent is provided by a different manufacturer [16]. Therapeutic levels of heparin should be maintained for 5 or 6 days. Warfarin should be administered to maintain the international normalized ratio (INR) at 2.0 to 3.0 [14••,17]. Heparin should be continued until the INR is within this therapeutic range for two consecutive days. Low molecular weight heparins have several advantages over unfractionated heparin: 1) low molecular weight heparins have a greater bioavailability when given by subcutaneous injection; 2) the duration of the anticoagulant effect is greater, permitting once- or twice-daily administration; and 3) the anticoagulant response (anti-Xa activity) is highly correlated with body weight, permitting administration of a fixed dose [18]. Laboratory monitoring is not necessary. Low molecular weight heparin can be used for the outpatient treatment of DVT [19,20]. It may replace unfractionated heparin in the initial management of patients with thromboembolism. Warfarin therapy should be continued for 3 to 6 months. Warfarin should be continued longer if a continuing predisposition to DVT exists. It is helpful to obtain a noninvasive image of the legs at the time that anticoagulants are about to be discontinued to be certain that no continuing DVT is present.

PULMONARY EMBOLISM

Clinical Diagnosis

It is useful to consider PE in terms of the syndrome of presentation: the syndrome of pulmonary hemorrhage or infarction, of uncomplicated PE (ie, PE not complicated by pulmonary hemorrhage or infarction and not complicated by circulatory collapse), and of circulatory collapse or shock [17]. The PE is least severe in patients with the pulmonary infarction syndrome, and most severe in patients with circulatory collapse [21]. One-third of patients with PE die within 1 or 2 hours after the onset of clinical findings [22]. The diagnosis of PE is unsuspected in about 70% [22]. Most patients who survive long enough for a diagnosis to be made have the syndrome of pulmonary infarction (pleuritic pain or hemoptysis).

Among patients with no prior cardiopulmonary disease in whom a clinical diagnosis was made, the vast majority had either dyspnea or tachypnea, or pleuritic pain (Table 3) [23].

Pleuritic pain is more common than hemoptysis among patients with no prior cardiopulmonary disease, and almost all have dyspnea, tachypnea, pleuritic pain, unexplained evidence of atelectasis, or a parenchymal abnormality on the chest radiograph [24]. Conversely, clinically detectable PE is rare in patients without one of these findings. Signs of pulmonary hypertension or right ventricular failure (eg, an accentuated pulmonary component of the second sound or a right ventricular lift) are uncommon. Qualitative signs of DVT, including erythema, palpable cord, tenderness, Homans' sign, or edema, occur in less than one third of patients with PE, but the addition of calf asymmetry of 1 cm or more to these signs increased the prevalence of a detectable abnormality of the lower extremities from 27% to 56% [25]. Nevertheless, DVT is the cause of PE in most patients [26].

Sudden, unexplained shortness of breath in a patient who is a likely candidate for PE (a patient who has had recent surgery, is debilitated, or is immobilized) is a finding that leads to a diagnosis. The electrocardiogram is usually abnormal [23,27]. The typical electrocardiographic abnormalities

TABLE 3 SYMPTOMS AND SIGNS OF ACUTE PULMONARY EMBOLISM IN PATIENTS WITH NO PRE-EXISTING CARDIAC OR PULMONARY DISEASE	
Symptoms or signs	Patients with symptom or sign, %*
Dyspnea	73
Pleuritic pain	66
Cough	37
Leg swelling	28
Leg pain	26
Hemoptysis	13
Palpitations	10
Wheezing	9
Anginalike pain	4
Tachypnea (> 20/min)	70
Rales (cackles)	51
Tachycardia (> 100/min)	30
Fourth heart sound	24
Increased pulmonary component of second sound	23
Deep venous thrombosis	11
Diaphoresis	11
Temperature > 38.5° C	7
Wheezes	5
Homans' sign	4
Right ventricular lift	4
Pleural friction rub	3
Third heart sound	3
Cyanosis	1

*n = 117.

are nonspecific ST-segment or T-wave changes (> 40% of patients) (Table 4) [23,27]. Right ventricular hypertrophy, right bundle branch block, right-axis deviation, P pulmonale, and an $S_1Q_2T_3$ pattern are uncommon [23,27]; in fact, new left-axis deviation occurs more often than right-axis deviation. Rhythm disturbances are uncommon [23,27].

The chest radiograph frequently shows unexplained parenchymal abnormalities, small pleural effusions, or elevation of a hemidiaphragm (Table 5) [23]. Vascular signs on chest radiography (decreased pulmonary vascularity, a prominent central pulmonary artery, or both) are uncommon or difficult to recognize.

In view of difficulties in making a clinical diagnosis of acute PE, objective point score systems have been developed. Wells et al. [28] showed PE in seven of 357 patients (2%) with suspected PE who had a low probability clinical assessment based on their scoring system, shown in Table 6. Others have also developed an objective scoring system with good results [29].

D-dimer

A D-dimer level below 500 ng/mL measured by the quantitative rapid enzyme-linked immunosorbent assay (ELISA) method gives a high certainty for the exclusion of DVT and of PE if the clinical probability is low or moderate [30]. It is as useful as a nearly normal lung scan or negative duplex ultrasound for the exclusion of PE or DVT [30]. A negative D-dimer by other techniques, in combination with a low probability clinical assessment, is also useful for the exclusion of PE [31–34].

Ventilation-Perfusion Lung Scan

Pulmonary embolism is present in 87% of patients whose ventilation-perfusion lung scan shows a high probability of

---

TABLE 4 ELECTROCARDIOGRAPHIC MANIFESTATIONS IN PATIENTS WITH PULMONARY EMBOLISM AND NO PRIOR CARDIAC OR PULMONARY DISEASE

Electrocardiographic finding	Patients with finding, %*
Normal electrocardiographic findings	30
Rhythm disturbances	
Atrial flutter	1
Atrial fibrillation	4
Atrial premature contractions	4
Ventricular premature contractions	4
P wave	
P pulmonale	2
QRS abnormalities	
Right-axis deviation	2
Left-axis deviation	13
Incomplete right bundle branch block	4
Complete right bundle branch block	6
Right ventricular hypertrophy	2
Pseudoinfarction	3
Low voltage (frontal plane)	3
ST segment and T wave	
Nonspecific ST segment or T-wave abnormalities	49

*Some patients had more than one abnormality; n = 89.

TABLE 5 CHEST RADIOGRAPHIC FINDINGS IN PULMONARY EMBOLISM IN PATIENTS WITH NO PREVIOUS CARDIAC OR PULMONARY DISEASE

Chest radiographic finding	Patients with finding, %†
Atelectasis or pulmonary parenchymal abnormality	68
Pleural effusion	48
Pleural-based opacity	35
Elevated diaphragm	24
Decreased pulmonary vascularity	21
Prominent central pulmonary artery	15
Cardiomegaly	12
Westermark's sign*	7

*Prominent central pulmonary artery and decreased pulmonary vascularity.
†n = 117.

TABLE 6 CLINICAL SCORING SYSTEM

Clinical feature	Score*
Signs and symptoms of deep venous thrombosis (DVT) (objectively measured leg swelling plus pain with palpation in the deep vein region)	3.0
Malignancy (patients receiving cancer therapy within the last 6 months or receiving palliative care)	1.0
Heart rate > 100/min	1.5
Immobilization (bed rest except bathroom for > 3 consecutive days) or surgery in last 4 weeks	1.5
Previous objectively diagnosed DVT or pulmonary embolism (PE)	1.5
Hemoptysis	1.0
PE as likely or more likely than an alternative diagnosis	3.0

*Interpretation of clinical assessment score: low probability of PE if score is < 2.0; moderate probability of PE if score is 2 to 6; high probability of PE if score is > 6.
Adapted from Wells et al. [28].

PE [35] (Fig. 1). If lung scan findings are normal, PE is excluded (Table 7) [35]. If the probability is intermediate, there is no information, with PE being present in approximately 30% of patients. If the probability is low, PE is present in 14%. Therefore, a low-probability ventilation-perfusion lung scan does not exclude PE [35]. Prior clinical assessment combined with interpretation of the ventilation-perfusion lung scan improves the diagnostic validity (Table 7) [35]. If the ventilation-perfusion scan is interpreted as high probability for PE, and if the clinical impression is concordantly high, then the prevalence of PE is 96%. If the ventilation-perfusion scan is low probability and the clinical suspicion is concordantly low, then pulmonary embolism is excluded in 96% of patients [35].

The probability of PE can be determined based on the number of mismatched perfusion defects [36,37]. A further refinement of probability can be made if the ventilation-perfusion lung scan is interpreted after patients are stratified according to prior cardiopulmonary disease (Fig. 2) [36]. Fewer mismatched perfusion defects are required to diagnose PE in patients with no prior cardiopulmonary disease. Adding clinical assessment to the stratification results in a more accurate evaluation [38].

Pulmonary Angiography

Pulmonary angiography (Fig. 3) is associated with serious complications in approximately 1% of patients [39]. When needed, pulmonary angiography is useful, and it remains the diagnostic "gold standard" for PE. Patients in whom the risk of complications from PE are greatest are those referred for angiography from the medical intensive care unit. Frequently, such patients are receiving respiratory

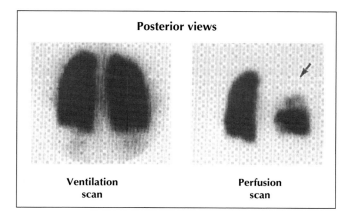

Posterior views

Ventilation scan   Perfusion scan

FIGURE 1 Posterior views of ventilation lung scan (*left*) and perfusion lung scan (*right*) showing normal ventilation with absent perfusion in the right upper lobe (*arrow*).

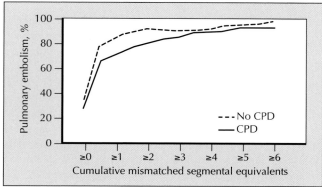

FIGURE 2 Predictive value of pulmonary embolism relative to the cumulative number of mismatched segmental equivalent perfusion defects among patients with no prior cardiopulmonary disease (CPD) and those with prior CPD. Significant differences occurred with 0.5 or more and 1.0 or more segmental equivalents (*P* < 0.01) and with 1.5 or more segmental equivalents (*P* < 0.05). (*Adapted from* Stein *et al.* [36].)

TABLE 7 PROBABILITY OF PULMONARY EMBOLISM (PE) USING CLINICAL ASSESSMENT IN COMBINATION WITH VENTILATION-PERFUSION LUNG SCANS

Ratio of PE-positive patients to total patients, *n/n (%)**

Scan category	CP of 80%–100%	CP of 20%–79%	CP of 0%–19%	All probabilities
High probability	28/29 (96)	70/80 (88)	5/9 (56)	103/118 (87)
Intermediate probability	27/41 (66)	66/236 (28)	11/68 (16)	104/345 (30)
Low probability	6/15 (40)	30/191 (16)	4/90 (4)	40/296 (14)
Near-normal to normal	0/5 (0)	4/62 (6)	1/61 (2)	5/128 (4)
Total	61/90 (68)	170/569 (30)	21/228 (9)	252/887 (28)

*PE positive indicates an angiographic reading that shows PE or the determination of PE by the outcome classification committee on review. PE status is based on angiographic interpretation for 713 patients, on angiographic interpretation and outcome classification committee reassignment for four patients, and on clinical information alone (without definitive angiography) for 170 patients.

CP—clinical probability.

support and are in an unstable condition. The presence or absence of PE and the magnitude of pulmonary hypertension does not relate to the frequency of morbidity from angiography [39]. Elderly patients (*ie*, 70 years of age or older) are at greater risk for renal impairment from the injection of contrast material than younger patients [40].

Contrast-enhanced Spiral Computed Tomography

Contrast-enhanced spiral CT permits visualization of PE after the injection of contrast material into a peripheral vein [41,42]. Imaging with contrast-enhanced spiral CT compared with conventional pulmonary angiography or autopsy, based on pooled data, shows a sensitivity of 72% and a specificity of 95% [6•]. These investigations were performed with single detector helical CT scanners. Multidetector helical CT systems, combined with improved software and multiplanar image reconstruction, are likely to improve the sensitivity and specificity of imaging for PE.

Published data on spiral CT limited to central pulmonary arteries suggest that the diagnosis of PE is reliable if PE is limited to the main or lobar pulmonary arteries or even segmental branches [43–47]. Pooled data show a sensitivity of 85/90 (94%). Specificity, based on pooled data, was 99/105 (94%). However, a more recent study showed a 38% false positive in segmental arteries [48]. Until further data become available, we recommend that the diagnostic criteria for contrast-enhanced spiral CT should be conservative and require that an intraluminal filling defect be shown in a main or lobar pulmonary artery for a positive diagnosis of PE.

The probability of a significant recurrence of PE is small if the spiral CT does not show PE and lung scan is not high probability, or venous ultrasound of the lower extremities is negative. Pooled data from three investigations, all of which used 3-mm collimation, showed symptomatic recurrent PE on follow-up in untreated patients in three of 364 (0.8%) [49–51]. There was no fatal recurrent PE. An additional investigation using earlier techniques (5-mm collimation) showed PE on follow-up in three of

109 (2.8%) [52]. One of these PE was fatal. For practical purposes, therefore, a negative contrast-enhanced spiral CT using 3-mm collimation or smaller rules out PE if supplemented by one other test.

Strategy for Diagnosis

Several strategies have been proposed to reduce the number of pulmonary angiograms that may be required [26,53,54••,55]. Since the publication of these strategies, additional effective methods for the diagnosis or exclusion of PE have been developed.

Pulmonary embolism may be considered to be excluded if any of the following apply:

- Negative D-dimer (< 500 ng/mL) performed by the quantitative rapid ELISA method combined with a low- or moderate-probability clinical assessment.
- Negative D-dimer by the whole blood agglutination method in combination with a low-probability clinical assessment and negative venous ultrasound.
- Normal V/Q lung scan. Acute PE is extremely rare in the presence of a normal V/Q lung scan.
- Low pretest clinical assessment for PE and a low probability interpretation of the V/Q lung scan. This combination showed PE on 3-month follow-up in zero of 113 patients (0%) [28]. In PIOPED I, patients with a low-probability clinical assessment and a low-probability V/Q scan showed PE in four of 90 (4%) [35].
- Low-probability clinical assessment, low-probability V/Q, and negative bilateral venous ultrasound. This combination of tests showed PE in one of 41 (2.4%) on 3-month follow-up [56].
- Low or moderate pretest probability of PE, and low or intermediate (nondiagnostic) V/Q scan in combination with a single negative bilateral venous ultrasound. This combination of tests showed PE on 3-month follow-up in 17 of 665 (2.6%) [28].
- Negative contrast-enhanced spiral CT in combination with another test. Pooled data from three investigations, all of which used 3-mm collimation, showed symptomatic recurrent PE on follow-up in untreated patients in three of 364 (0.8%) [49–51].
- Negative pulmonary angiogram.

A patient may be considered to have PE if any of the following applies:

- Main or lobar pulmonary artery filling defect on contrast-enhanced spiral CT. (This criterion may be revised when the results of a large multicenter trial [PIOPED II] become available.)
- High probability interpretation of V/Q lung scan in a patient with no prior PE.
- Intraluminal filling defect on pulmonary angiogram.
- In a patient in whom the V/Q or spiral CT is not normal, a surrogate diagnosis of PE may be based on a positive venous ultrasound if there is no history of prior DVT or DVT at a different site. The requirement that the patient have either no history of prior DVT or they

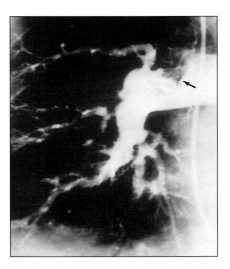

FIGURE 3
Pulmonary arteriogram of right pulmonary artery showing multiple intraluminal filling defects, one of which occludes the artery to the right upper lobe (*arrow*).

have prior DVT in a different location reduces the possibility of detecting chronic DVT rather than acute DVT. These requirements are more restrictive than in the application to clinical prognostic strategies [54••,57–64].

With the large number of combinations of diagnostic tests that are useful, there are several possible diagnostic pathways. It may be economical to initiate the diagnostic pathway with an objective clinical evaluation that uses a point score system in combination with a D-dimer, preferably by the quantitative rapid ELISA method. If PE remains a diagnostic possibility after these, then either a V/Q lung scan or contrast-enhanced spiral CT would be the next diagnostic test. In recent years the spiral CT seems to be the most popular. Some, however, find it faster and more economical to obtain a venous ultrasound to detect DVT, which would serve as a surrogate diagnosis. If the V/Q scan or spiral CT is nondiagnostic, and/or single venous ultrasound is negative, one could obtain serial ultrasounds, or a pulmonary angiogram. The latter would be particularly recommended in patients with poor cardiorespiratory reserve, or in patients in whom the clinical suspicion is high. In patients with good cardiorespiratory reserve, serial objective leg tests are safe, and the risk of PE is low among patients in whom serial investigations of the legs shown no DVT [54••,56,57]. It may be more economical or convenient to obtain studies of the legs before ventilation-perfusion lung scans or spiral CT.

TREATMENT

Antithrombotic therapy for PE is the same as antithrombotic therapy for DVT (Table 3). Low molecular weight heparin is preferred over unfractionated heparin for the treatment of DVT or PE [14••]. Outpatient treatment of DVT with low molecular weight heparin is approved. Outpatient treatment of PE with low molecular weight heparin is not approved.

Thrombolytic therapy is indicated if the patient is hypotensive or hypoxic on 100% oxygen or otherwise unstable. Thrombolytic therapy is not indicated for the routine treatment of PE. It is generally recommended that pulmonary angiograms be obtained in patients with suspected PE who may be candidates for thrombolytic therapy. Pulmonary angiography, however, markedly increases the risk of major bleeding with thrombolytic therapy. Therefore, thrombolytic therapy perhaps may be administered to unstable patients on the basis of a strong clinical impression and a high-probability ventilation-perfusion lung scan or positive spiral CT [65,66].

KEY REFERENCES

Recently published papers of outstanding interest, as identified in References and Recommended Reading, have been annotated.

••Geerts WH, Jeit JA, Clagett GP, et al.: Prevention of venous thromboembolism. Chest 2001, 119(suppl):132S–175S.

Detailed recommendations for the prevention of deep venous thrombosis are given in this paper.

••Hyers TM, Agnelli G, Hull RD, et al.: Antithrombotic therapy for venous thromboembolic disease. Chest 2001, 119(suppl):176S–193S.

Fundamentally important authoritative guideline for therapy.

••Stein PD, Hull RD, Pineo G: Strategy that includes serial noninvasive leg tests for diagnosis of thromboembolic disease in patients with suspected acute pulmonary embolism based on data from PIOPED. Arch Intern Med 1995, 155:2101–2104.

Strategy of diagnosis that combines the traditional angiographic approach with the Canadian approach of diagnosing "thromboembolic disease." The strategy incorporates serial noninvasive leg tests.

REFERENCES AND RECOMMENDED READING

Recently published papers of particular interest have been highlighted as:

• Of interest
•• Of outstanding interest

1. Moser KM, LeMoine JR: Is embolic risk conditioned by location of deep venous thrombosis? Ann Intern Med 1981, 94:439–444.

2. Hull RD, Hirsh J, Carter CJ, et al.: Pulmonary angiography, ventilation lung scanning, and venography for clinically suspected pulmonary embolism with abnormal perfusion lung scan. Ann Intern Med 1983, 98:891–899.

3. White RH, McGahan JP, Daschbach MM: Diagnosis of deep-vein thrombosis using duplex ultrasound. Ann Intern Med 1989, 111:297–304.

4. Becker DM, Philbrick JT, Abbitt PL: Real time ultrasonography for the diagnosis of lower extremity deep venous thrombosis. Arch Intern Med 1989, 149:1731–1734.

5. Heijboer H, Cogo A, Buller HR, et al.: Detection of deep vein thrombosis with impedance plethysmography and real-time compression ultrasonography in hospitalized patients. Arch Intern Med 1992, 152:1901–1903.

6.• ACCP Consensus Committee on Pulmonary Embolism: Second report opinions regarding the diagnosis and management of venous thromboembolic disease. Chest 1998, 113:499–504.

7. Taillefer R, Therasse E, Turpin S, et al.: Comparison of early and delayed scintigraphy with ^{99m}Tc-apcitide and correlation with contrast-enhanced venography in detection of acute deep vein thrombosis. J Nucl Med 1999, 40:2029–2035.

8. Baldt MM, Zontsich T, Fleischmann D, et al.: Deep venous thrombosis of the lower extremity: efficacy of spiral CT venography compared with conventional venography in diagnosis. Radiology 1996, 200:423–428.

9. Cham MD, Yankelevitz DF, Shaham D, et al., for the Pulmonary CT Angiography-Indirect CT Venography Cooperative Group: Deep venous thrombosis: detection by using indirect CT venography. Radiology 2000, 216:744–751.

10. Loud PA, Katz DS, Klippenstein DL, et al.: Combined CT venography and pulmonary angiography in suspected thromboembolic disease: diagnostic accuracy for deep venous evaluation Am J Roentgenol 2000;174:61–65.

11. Byrne JJ: Phlebitis: a study of 748 cases at the Boston City Hospital. N Engl J Med 1955, 253:579–586.

12. Collins R, Scrimgeour A, Yusuf S, Peto R: Reduction in fatal pulmonary embolism and venous thrombosis by perioperative administration of subcutaneous heparin. N Engl J Med 1988, 318:1162–1173.

13.•• Geerts WH, Jeit JA, Clagett GP, *et al.*: Prevention of venous thromboembolism. *Chest* 2001, 119(suppl):132S–175S.

14.•• Hyers TM, Agnelli G Hull RD, *et al.*: Antithrombotic therapy for venous thromboembolic disease. *Chest* 2001, 119(suppl):176S–193S.

15. Hull RD, Raskob GE, Hirsch J, *et al.*: Continuous heparin compared with intermittent subcutaneous heparin in the initial treatment of proximal-vein thrombosis. *N Engl J Med* 1986, 315:1109–1114.

16. Brill-Edwards P, Ginsberg S, Johnston M, *et al.*: Establishing a therapeutic range for heparin therapy. *Ann Intern Med* 1993, 119:104–109.

17. Hirsh J, Dalen JE, Deykin D, Poller L: Oral anticoagulants: mechanism of action, clinical effectiveness, and optimal therapeutic range. *Chest* 1992, 102(suppl):312S–326S.

18. Hirsh J, Levine MN: Low molecular weight heparin. *Blood* 1992, 79:1–17.

19. Koopman MMW, Prandoni P, Piovella F, *et al.*: Treatment of venous thrombosis with intravenous unfractionated heparin administered in the hospital as compared with subcutaneous low-molecular-weight heparin administered at home. *N Engl J Med* 1996, 334:682–687.

20. Levine M, Gent M, Hirsh J, *et al.*: A comparison of low-molecular-weight heparin administered primarily at home with unfractionated heparin administered in the hospital for proximal deep vein thrombosis. *N Engl J Med* 1996, 334:677–681.

21. Stein PD, Willis PW III, DeMets DL: History and physical examination in acute pulmonary embolism in patients without preexisting cardiac or pulmonary disease. *Am J Cardiol* 1981, 47:218–223.

22. Stein PD, Henry JW: Prevalence of acute pulmonary embolism among patients in a general hospital and at autopsy. *Chest* 1995, 108:978–981.

23. Stein PD, Terrin ML, Hales CA, *et al.*: Clinical, laboratory, roentgenographic and electrocardiographic findings in patients with acute pulmonary embolism and no pre-existing cardiac or pulmonary disease. *Chest* 1991, 100:598–603.

24. Stein PD, Saltzman HA, Weg JG: Clinical characteristics of patients with acute pulmonary embolism. *Am J Cardiol* 1991, 68:1723–1724.

25. Stein PD, Henry JW, Godalakrishnan D, Relyea B: Asymmetry of the calves in the assessment of patients with suspected acute pulmonary embolism. *Chest* 1995, 107:936–939.

26. Stein PD, Hull RD, Saltzman HA, Pineo G: Strategy for diagnosis of patients with suspected acute pulmonary embolism. *Chest* 1993, 103:1553–1559.

27. Stein PD: Acute pulmonary embolism. *Dis Month* 1994, 40:465–524.

28. Wells PS, Ginsberg JS, Anderson DR, *et al.*: Use of a clinical model for safe management of patients with suspected pulmonary embolism. *Ann Intern Med* 1998, 129, 997–1005.

29. Wicki J, Perneger TV, Junod AF, *et al.*: Assessing clinical probability of pulmonary embolism in the emergency ward. A simple score. *Arch Intern Med* 2001, 161:92–97.

30. Stein PD, Hull RD, Patel KC, *et al.*: D-dimer for the exclusion of acute deep venous thrombosis and pulmonary embolism: a systematic review. *Ann Intern Med* 2004, 140:589–602.

31. Wells PS, Anderson DR, Rodger M, *et al.*: Evaluation of D-dimer in the diagnosis of suspected deep-vein thrombosis. *N Engl J Med* 2003, 349:1227–1235.

32. Kraaijenhagen RA, Piovella F, Bernardi E, *et al.*: Simplification of the diagnostic management of suspected deep vein thrombosis. *Arch Intern Med* 2002, 162:907–911.

33. Bates SM, Kearon C, Crowther M, *et al.*: A diagnostic strategy involving a quantitative latex D-dimer assay reliably excludes deep vein thrombosis. *Ann Intern Med* 2003, 138:787–795.

34. Wells PS, Anderson DR, Rodger, *et al.*: Excluding pulmonary embolism at the bedside without diagnostic imaging: management of patients with suspected pulmonry embolism presenting to the emengency deparment by using simple clinical model and D-dimer. *Ann Intern Med* 2001, 135;99–107.

35. A Collaborative Study by the PIOPED Investigators: Value of the ventilation/perfusion scan in acute pulmonary embolism: results of the Prospective Investigation of Pulmonary Embolism Diagnosis (PIOPED). *JAMA* 1990, 263:2753–2759.

36. Stein PD, Gottschalk A, Henry JW, Shivkumar K: Stratification of patients according to prior cardiopulmonary disease and probability assessment based upon the number of mismatched segmental equivalent perfusion defects: approaches to strengthen the diagnostic value of ventilation/perfusion lung scans in acute pulmonary embolism. *Chest* 1993, 104:1461–1467.

37. Stein PD, Henry JW, Gottschalk A: Mismatched vascular defects: an easy alternative to mismatched segmental equivalent defects for the interpretation of ventilation/perfusion lung scans in pulmonary embolism. *Chest* 1993, 104:1468–1472.

38. Stein PD, Henry JW, Gottschalk A: The addition of clinical assessment to stratification according to prior cardiopulmonary disease further optimizes the interpretation of ventilation/perfusion lung scans in pulmonary embolism. *Chest* 1993, 104:1472–1476.

39. Stein PD, Athanasoulis C, Alavi A, *et al.*: Complications and validity of pulmonary angiography in acute pulmonary embolism. *Circulation* 1992, 85:462–469.

40. Stein PD, Gottschalk A, Saltzman HA, Terrin ML: Diagnosis of acute pulmonary embolism in the elderly. *J Am Coll Cardiol* 1991, 18:1452–1457.

41. Rathbun SW, Raskob GE, Whitsett TL: Sensitivity and specificity of helical computed tomography in the diagnosis of pulmonary embolism: a systematic review. *Ann Intern Med* 2000, 132:227–232.

42. Mullins MD, Becker DM, Hagspiel KD, Philbrick JT: The role of spiral volumetric computed tomography in the diagnosis of pulmonary embolism. *Arch Intern Med* 2000, 160:293–298.

43. Goodman LR, Curtin JJ, Mewissen MW, *et al.*: Detection of pulmonary embolism in patients with unresolved clinical and scintigraphic diagnosis: helical CT versus angiography. *Am J Roentgenol* 1995, 164:1369–1374.

44. Blum AG, Delfau F, Grigon B, *et al.*: Spiral computed tomography versus pulmonary angiography in the diagnosis of acute pulmonary embolism. *Am J Cardiol* 1994:74:96–98.

45. Teigen CL, Maus TP, Sheedy PF, *et al.*: Pulmonary embolism: diagnosis with contrast enhanced electron-beam CT and comparison with pulmonary angiography. *Radiology* 1995, 194:313–319.

46. Remy-Jardin M, Remy J, Wattinne L, Giraud F: Committee pulmonary thromboembolism: diagnosis with spiral volumetric CT with the single-breath-hold technique-comparison with pulmonary angiography. *Radiology* 1992, 185:381–387.

47. Remy-Jardin M, Remy J, Dechildre F, *et al.*: Diagnosis of pulmonary embolism with spiral CT: comparison with pulmonary angiography and scintigraphy. *Radiology* 1996, 200:699–706.

48. Perrier A, Howarth N, Didler D, et al.: Performance of helical computed tomography in unselected outpatients with suspected pulmonary embolism. *Ann Intern Med* 2001, 135:88–97.

49. Goodman LR, Lipchik RJ, Kuzo RS, *et al.*: Subsequent pulmonary embolisms: risk after a negative helical CT pulmonary angiogram: prospective comparison with scintigraphy. *Radiology* 2000, 215:535–542.

50. Lomis NNT, Yoon H-C, Moran AG, Miller FJ: Clinical outcomes of patients after a negative spiral CT pulmonary arteriogram in the valuation of acute pulmonary embolism. *JVIR* 1999, 10:707–712.

51. Garg K, Sieler H, Welsh CH, et al.: Clinical validity of helical CT being interpreted as negative for pulmonary embolism: implications for patient treatment. Am J Roentgenol 1999, 172:1627–1631.

52. Ferretti GR, Bosson J-L, Buffaz P-D, Ayanian D, et al.: Acute pulmonary embolism: role of helical CT in 164 patients with intermediate probability at ventilation-perfusion scintigraphy and normal results at duplex US of the legs. *Radiology* 1997, 205:453–458.

53. Dalen JE: When can treatment be withheld in patients with suspected pulmonary embolism? *Arch Intern Med* 1993, 153:1415–1418.

54.•• Stein PD, Hull RD, Pineo G: Strategy that includes serial noninvasive leg tests for diagnosis of thromboembolic disease in patients with suspected acute pulmonary embolism based on data from PIOPED. *Arch Intern Med* 1995, 155:2101–2104.

55. Wells PS, Ginsberg JS, Anderson DR, et al.: Use of a clinical model for safe management of patients with suspected pulmonary embolism. *Ann Intern Med* 1998, 129:997–1005.

56. Wells PS, Anderson DR, Rodger M, et al.: Excluding pulmonary embolism at the bedside without diagnostic imaging: management of patients with suspected pulmonary embolism presenting to the emergency department by using a simple clinical model and D-dimer. *Ann Intern Med* 2001, 135:98–107.

57. Hull RD, Raskob GE, Coates G, et al.: A new noninvasive management strategy for patients with suspected pulmonary embolism. *Arch Intern Med* 1989, 149:2549–2555.

58. Stein PD, Hull RD, Saltzman HA, Pineo G. Strategy for diagnosis of patients with suspected acute pulmonary embolism. *Chest* 1993, 103:1553–1559.

59. Kelley MA, Carson JL, Palevsky HI, Schwartz JS: Diagnosing pulmonary embolism: new facts and strategies. *Ann Intern Med* 1991, 114:300–306.

60. Hull RD, Hirsh J, Carter CJ, et al.: Pulmonary angiography, ventilation lung scanning, and venography for clinically suspected pulmonary embolism with abnormal perfusion lung scan. *Ann Intern Med* 1983, 98:891–899.

61. Hull RD, Hirsh J, Carter CJ, et al.: Diagnostic value of ventilation-perfusion lung scanning in patients with suspected pulmonary embolism. *Chest* 1985, 88:819–828.

62. Huisman MV, Buller HR, Ten Cate JW, Vreeken J: Serial impedance plethysmography for suspected deep venous thrombosis in outpatients. *N Engl J Med* 1986, 314:823–828.

63. Hull RD, Raskob GE, Carter CJ: Serial impedance plethysmography in pregnant patients with clinically suspected deep-vein thrombosis. *Ann Intern Med* 1990, 112:663–667.

64. Hull RD, Raskob GE, Ginsberg JS, et al.: A noninvasive strategy for the treatment of patients with suspected pulmonary embolism. *Arch Intern Med* 1994, 154:289–297.

65. Stein PE, Dalen JD: Thrombolytic therapy in acute pulmonary embolism. In *Harrison's Online*. McGraw Hill; 2003, http://harrisons.accessmedicine.com/serverjava/Arknoid/amed/harrisons/ex_editorials/ed13.

66. Stein PE, Dalen JD: Thrombolytic therapy in acute pulmonary embolism. In *Venous Thromboembolism*. Edited by Dalen JE. New York: Marcel Dekker; 2003:253–256.

SELECT BIBLIOGRAPHY

Dalen JE: *Venous Thromboembolism*. New York: Marcel Dekker; 2003.

Hull RD, Raskob GE, Pineo GF: *Venous Thromboembolism: An Evidence-Based Atlas*. Armonk, NY: Futura Publishing; 1996.

Official Statement of the American Thoracic Society: The diagnostic approach to acute venous thromboembolism. *Am J Respir Crit Care Med* 1999, 160:1043–1066.

Stein PD: *Pulmonary Embolism*. Media, PA: Williams & Wilkins; 1996.

Cardiac Tumors

Adafisayo Oduwole
Elizabeth O. Ofili
Navin C. Nanda

Key Points

- Although most primary cardiac tumors are histologically "benign," clinical manifestations can be devastating and include cerebrovascular and peripheral emboli, cardiac arrhythmias, valvular obstruction, pericardial constriction or tamponade, and death.
- Fibroelastomas are usually incidental findings at autopsy.
- Rhabdomyomas are the most common benign tumor in infants and children and are often associated with tuberous sclerosis.
- A high index of suspicion is necessary for early diagnosis. Echocardiography usually provides rapid and accurate diagnosis; chest radiography tends to be nonspecific.
- Surgical excision is curative in most cases, although some myxomas may recur. Periodic postoperative clinical and echocardiographic surveillance is important.
- Metastatic tumors are uniformly fatal; surgery is largely palliative.

PRIMARY CARDIAC TUMORS

Cardiac tumors can be primary or metastatic and can involve the heart or pericardium. Advances in diagnostic imaging now allow accurate diagnosis in most patients. Clinical manifestations and hemodynamic features of cardiac tumors can mimic virtually all other forms of heart disease. Thus, a high index of suspicion is necessary for making an accurate diagnosis.

Primary tumors of the heart and pericardium are rare, with an incidence of 0.002% to 0.250% in autopsy series [1]. Figure 1 shows the relative incidence of primary tumors of the heart. Although 75% of primary cardiac tumors are histologically benign, clinical manifestations can be quite devastating, with complications such as death caused by arrhythmia, pericardial constriction or tamponade, valvular obstruction, and cerebral arterial embolism.

Benign Tumors

Myxomas are the most common cardiac tumors, accounting for 30% to 50% of benign cardiac tumors in most series [2]. Over 90% of myxomas occur sporadically. Women are more commonly affected, with a typical age range of 30 to 60 years; however, patients as young as 3 years and as old as 80 years have also been reported [2]. Most myxomas are solitary tumors and are often pedunculated and attached to the limbus of the fossa ovalis of the left atrium by a short stalk. Myxomas are noted for their protean clinical manifestations. Constitutional signs and symptoms, obstructive manifestations, and embolic phenomena are the classic triad of myxoma presentation [3,4]. Presenting symptoms may include syncope, episodic dizziness, episodic dyspnea, and weight loss

(Table 1). Symptoms may vary with positional change. Syncope is particularly ominous and not infrequently associated with sudden death. Multiple systemic emboli may mimic systemic vasculitis or infective endocarditis, particularly when associated with fever, weight loss, and arthralgias. The neurologic consequences of embolization include transient ischemic attacks, seizures, syncope, and cerebral infarction.

Atrial myxomas may mimic mitral or tricuspid valve disease on physical examination (Table 2). The sudden movement of tumor from atrium to the ventricle has been associated with an early diastolic sound or "tumor plop." This high-frequency diastolic sound, in addition to a diastolic murmur and (in some cases) a systolic murmur of a valvular regurgitation, has been described. Left atrial myxomas frequently mimic mitral stenosis. Right atrial myxomas may present with recurrent pulmonary emboli and right heart failure. Right atrial myxomas have been reported to mimic the carcinoid syndrome, constrictive pericarditis, tricuspid stenosis, or Ebstein's anomaly.

Familial myxomas make up 7% of all myxomas and are transmitted by an autosomal dominant trait. Compared with patients with sporadic myxomas, patients presenting with familial myxomas are usually younger (mean age in the twenties), more likely to have multiple myxomas involving chambers other than the left atrium, and more likely to have

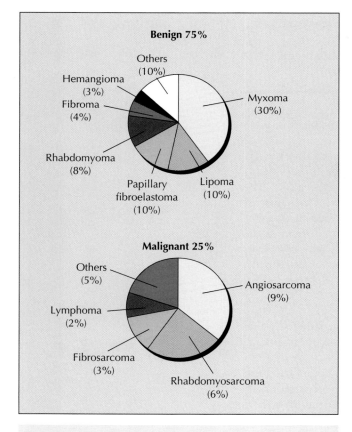

FIGURE 1 Relative incidence of primary cardiac tumors.

TABLE 1 CARDIAC MYXOMAS

Clinical manifestations

Symptoms	Incidence, %
Dyspnea on exertion	>75
Fever	50
Weight loss	50
Dizziness or syncope	20
Sudden death	15
Hemoptysis	15

Clinical presentation of cardiac myxoma in 130 patients	Patients, n
Signs and symptoms of mitral valve disease	57
Embolic phenomena	36
Incidental finding	16
Signs and symptoms of tricuspid valve disease	6
Sudden death	5
Pericarditis	4
Myocardial infarction	3
Signs and symptoms of pulmonary valve disease	2
Fever of unknown origin	2

Location of cardiac myxomas

Site	Incidence, %
Left atrium	75.0
Right atrium	20.0
Left ventricle	2.5
Right ventricle	2.5
Multiple myxomas	<5.0

TABLE 2 CONDITIONS MIMICKED BY ATRIAL MYXOMAS

Left atrium
Rheumatic mitral valve disease (stenosis, insufficiency)
Pulmonary hypertension
Cerebral emboli
Endocarditis
Myocarditis
Vasculitis

Right atrium
Rheumatic tricuspid valve disease (stenosis, insufficiency)
Pulmonary hypertension
Pulmonary emboli
Constrictive pericarditis
Ebstein's anomaly
Carcinoid heart disease

a recurrence of myxoma postoperatively [5,6]. In Carney syndrome, myxomas arise in noncardiac location (usually breast or skin), pigmentation of the skin occurs (usually lentigines or pigmented levi), and associated endocrine tumors (pituitary adenomas, adrenocortical or testicular tumors) may develop. Other syndromes include the NAME syndrome (nevi, atrial myxoma, myxoid neurofibroma, and ephelides) and the LAMB syndrome (lentigines, atrial myxoma, and blue nevi). Because cardiac myxomas may be familial, routine echocardiographic screening of first-degree relatives is appropriate, particularly in young patients who have multiple or right-sided tumors [7].

Papillary fibroelastomas are usually an incidental finding at autopsy and seldom associated with symptoms. Detection of these tumors has been enhanced by transesophageal echocardiography that has sensitivity, specificity, and overall accuracy of 89%, 88%, and 88%, respectively [8••]. They are usually single, mobile, and pendunculated in about 40% of cases and located on the aortic or mitral valve, and may be a source of emboli [9•].

Other benign tumors, such as rhabdomyomas, are the most common benign tumor in infants and children and are often associated with tuberous sclerosis [10]. These neoplasms are usually mutliple and involve the ventricular myocardium. Other benign tumors are shown in Figure 1. Clinical manifestations of other benign cardiac tumors are listed in Table 3.

Malignant Tumors

Malignant cardiac tumors account for 25% of all primary heart tumors. They include mesotheliomas, which typically involve the pericardium. Sarcomas involve the myocardium, and malignant vascular tumors can affect both the pericardium and the myocardium (Table 4).

There have been some recently reported cases [11,12] of primary lymphoma of the heart with good response to chemotherapeutic agents and disease-free survival between 21 and 34 months.

For right-sided tumors, transvenous biopsy is helpful in confirming the diagnosis. Figure 2 shows autopsy specimens and microscopy of a lymphoma. Premortem echocardiography suggested probable myxoma.

METASTATIC OR SECONDARY CARDIAC TUMORS

Metastatic tumors of the heart are 25 times more common than primary cardiac tumors. All major types of tumors can

TABLE 3 COMMON MANIFESTATIONS OF OTHER BENIGN CARDIAC TUMORS

Tumor	Manifestations
Rhabdomyoma	Most common childhood benign primary tumor; associated with systemic tuberous sclerosis; ventricular tachyarrhythmia
Fibroma	Second most common childhood tumor; may cause left ventricular outflow obstruction
Lipomas	Left ventricle, right atrium, and atrial septum affected in that order; rarely cause problems (valvular obstruction and conduction abnormalities)
Lipomatous hypertrophy	Adipose tissue accumulation in atrial septum; not true neoplasm; most common in the obese, elderly, and women; usually not pathologic
Papillary fibroelastoma	Affects heart valves; may embolize rarely or cause valvular dysfunction
Hemangioma and lymphangioma	Rare vascular tumors; may cause heart block and sudden death
Bronchogenic cysts, pericardial cysts, teratomas, and dermoid cysts	Most common benign pericardial tumor; usually in young children; can compress great vessels and rupture into pericardium

TABLE 4 COMMON MANIFESTATIONS OF MALIGNANT PRIMARY CARDIAC TUMORS

Tumor	Manifestations
Sarcomas	Affect young adults; right side of heart common; rapid downhill course; death within 2 years of symptoms; local infiltration and metastases to lungs, lymph nodes, sternum and vertebral column; cardiac tamponade, right heart failure, and vena caval obstruction may occur
Angiosarcomas	Including Kaposi's sarcoma and malignant hemangioendotheliomas; 2:1 male:female ratio; usually from right atrium, attached to septum; course and clinical manifestations as for other sarcomas, including rapid downhill course
Pericardial mesothelioma	Usually affects in third to fifth decade; more in men; no association with asbestos exposure; symptomatic late in course; survival less than 1 year after diagnosis

metastasize to the heart, with an average frequency of 10% in autopsy series. The highest percentages of metastases to the heart occur with melanoma (64%), leukemia (43%), and malignant lymphoma (35%). Lung and breast cancers predominate as the major sites of origin for cardiac metastases because of their high prevalence and contiguous anatomic location. Pericardial metastases are most frequent, and endocardial metastases occur rarely. Discrete nodules or diffuse infiltration may occur as a result of pericardial metastases. Fibrinous pericarditis and pericardial effusion usually are present. The effusion may not be bloody. Pericardial metastases may be diffuse or present as discrete nodules. Leukemic involvement typically causes effusion because of infiltration of the interstitium by leukemic cells. Mural thrombi and embolization secondary to metastatic cardiac tumors are quite rare. Metastatic cardiac tumors do not interfere with cardiac function until myocardial involvement is extensive. Cardiac metastases are almost always associated with widespread metastatic involvement in other organs.

The vast majority of patients with cardiac involvement because of metastatic tumor have few or no cardiac symptoms (Table 5) [1]. Despite autopsy evidence of cardiac metastases in 10% to 20% of patients with widespread metastatic disease, antemortem symptoms or physical findings of cardiac involvement occur only in approximately 8% of the cases [13]. This may be because cardiac abnormalities are often overlooked by clinicians in the presence of widespread neoplastic disease.

DIAGNOSTIC TECHNIQUES

Noninvasive diagnostic cardiac evaluation is increasingly used to confirm a suspected intracardiac tumor. As a result, it is not unusual for cardiac tumors to be diagnosed and cured in patients who are totally asymptomatic or without signs of cardiovascular disease. Chest radiography tends to be nonspecific but may provide important diagnostic clues (Table 6). Careful use of noninvasive modalities such as two-dimensional echocardiography, transesophageal echocardiography, and in some instances, magnetic resonance imaging help in the preoperative localization and assessment of tumor extent; invasive procedures such as cardiac catheterization are therefore unnecessary. Table 7 summarizes a diagnostic and surveillance algorithm for evaluation of cardiac tumors. Patients presenting with clinical manifestations of cardiogenic emboli should be referred for echocardiography. A high index of suspicion is necessary for early diagnosis, particularly in patients with nonspecific symptoms such as dyspnea, atypical chest pain, or palpitations.

Echocardiography

Two-dimensional echocardiography, when carefully performed, provides adequate information regarding the

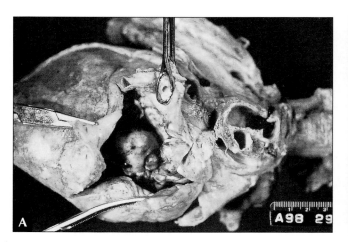

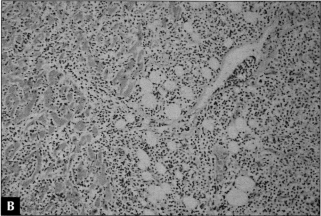

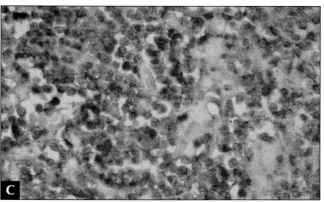

FIGURE 2 A 44-year-old man with AIDS admitted for syncope caused by primary cardiac lymphoma. **A,** Autopsy specimen showing a right atrial mass, confirmed to be a lymphoma on histology. **B,** Hematoxylin and eosin stain with infiltration by myocytes and lymphocytes. **C,** Immunoperoxidase stain of B-type lymphocytes. (*See* Color Plate)

presence or absence of an intracardiac tumor as well as its size, attachment, and mobility to allow for operative resection without preoperative angiography (Figs. 3 and 4). This technique is sensitive for detecting small tumors and is especially useful in the diagnosis of atrial and ventricular tumors. Furthermore, color Doppler flow studies allow for the assessment of the hemodynamic consequences of valvular obstruction or insufficiency caused by cardiac tumors [14].

Transesophageal Echocardiography

Transesophageal echocardiography provides an unimpeded view of both atria and interatrial septum. It allows a more accurate evaluation of the attachment of atrial myxomas and differentiation of atrial thrombi from cardiac tumors [15]. Transesophageal echocardiography is complementary to the transthoracic approach in providing additional visualization and superior resolution. It should be requested when the transthoracic echocardiogram is suboptimal or additional information regarding the tumor attachment and extent of involvement is needed. Transesophageal echocardiography is superior for the evaluation of right heart tumors and involvement of the vena cava [16,17•].

Computed Tomography

Computed tomography (particularly ultrafast computed tomography and electron beam computed tomography) may allow tissue discrimination with definition of the degree of intramural tumor extension. It is useful for assessing the degree of myocardial invasion and involvement of pericardial and extracardiac structures [18,19•].

Magnetic Resonance Imaging

This technique may be of considerable value in the detection and delineation of cardiac tumors, and in some cases, it may

---

TABLE 5 CLINICAL MANIFESTATIONS OF CARDIAC METASTATIC TUMORS

Manifestation	Description
Pericardial effusion and tamponade	Most common manifestations of metastatic disease (less common but may occur with benign tumors); cytologic examination of fluid or pericardial biopsy may be diagnostic; effusive constrictive pericarditis can occur if prior irradiation
Heart failure	May be dilated or restrictive right, left, or biventricular failure; leukemic infiltration and irradiation can cause restrictive cardiomyopathy; doxorubicin cardiomyopathy is dose related (> 400–500 mg/m^2); sudden onset; resistant to conventional treatment
Myocardial ischemia and infarction	May be from large transmural tumor nodules or, rarely, tumor embolization; usually widespread metastases and poor prognosis; death within several weeks
Embolization	Most common with benign atrial myxomas but can be seen with metastatic tumors
Conduction defects and arrhythmias	Heart block is common in mesothelioma of the atrioventricular node; arrhythmias are common with metastatic myocardial disease

---

TABLE 6 RADIOLOGIC FINDINGS IN CARDIAC TUMORS

Cardiac enlargement (chamber enlargement; pericardial effusion)

Mediastinal widening (hilar-mediastinal adenopathy)

Calcification (rhabdomyoma, fibroma, teratoma, myxoma)

TABLE 7 DIAGNOSTIC WORK-UP OF CARDIAC TUMORS

History and physical examination (may be nonspecific)

Chest radiography

Transthoracic two-dimensional or Doppler echocardiography (left ventricular tumors, left atrial, and right atrial myxomas)

Transesophageal echocardiography (if suboptimal, inconclusive, or nondiagnostic transthoracic echocardiogram)

Computed tomography and magnetic resonance imaging (extent of myocardial invasion; pericardial or extracardiac extension)

Coronary angiography (for coronary anatomy)

Surgical exclusion or biopsy

Periodic two-dimensional echocardiogram for follow-up after surgery

show the size, shape, and surface characteristics of the tumor more clearly than two-dimensional echocardiography [20]. The larger field-of-view with magnetic resonance imaging also may provide a better definition of tumor prolapse, secondary valve obstruction, and cardiac tumor size than two-dimensional echocardiography [18]. Spin echo and cine magnetic resonance images may allow morphologic and histologic characterization of cardiac myxomas [21].

Angiography

Cardiac catheterization and selective angiocardiography are not necessary in all cases of cardiac tumors, especially with the use of transesophageal echocardiography, ultrafast and electron beam tomography, and magnetic resonance imaging. Cardiac tumors that are amenable to surgery frequently can be diagnosed by these noninvasive techniques. In some cases, however, cardiac catheterization

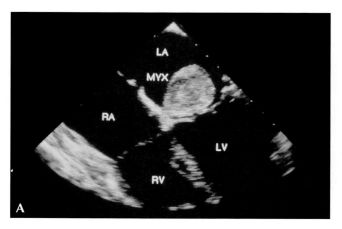

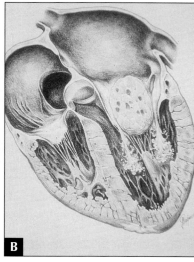

FIGURE 3 Transesophageal echocardiogram in a patient with left atrial myxoma. **A,** A large left atrial myxoma (MYX) attached to the base of interatrial septum is viewed in four-chamber view. **B,** Schematic of *panel A*. LA—left atrium; LV—left ventricle; RA—right atrium; RV—right ventricle. (*From* Nanda and Mahan [30]; with permission.)

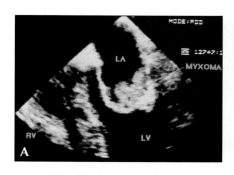

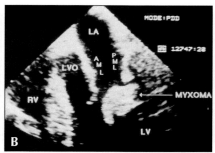

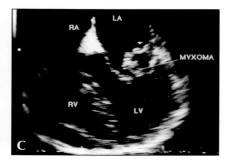

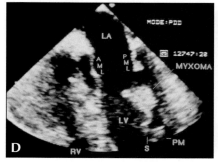

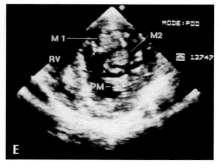

the tumor in the left atrium. The *arrowhead* points to the thinner portion of the mass in contact with the LA free wall (**C**). There is no evidence in **A, B,** or **C** to suggest (LV) attachment of the tumor. In (**D**), the attachment of the tumor to a papillary muscle (PM) head in LV by a long stalk (S) is clearly delineated. The long stalk makes it possible for the tumor to prolapse into LA in systole and move back into LV in diastole as well as for trapping in LA to occur. In the transgastric LV short-axis view (**E**), two separate tumors (M_1, M_2) with their stalks (*arrows*) are seen in the vicinity of the papillary muscles. AML—anterior mitral leaflet; PML—posterior mitral leaflet; RA—right atrium; RV—right ventricle. (*From* Samdarshi *et al.* [31]; with permission.)

FIGURE 4 Transesophageal echocardiogram in a patient with multicentric left ventricular myxomas mimicking a left atrial tumor. In systole (**A**), a large tumor mass is seen within the left atrium (LA) behind the closed position of the mitral leaflets imaged in the four-chamber plane. In diastole (**B**), the mass has moved from LA into the left ventricle (LV), mimicking the motion pattern of a left atrial tumor. Intermittently, especially during the transesophageal study in the awake state, the mass was also visualized in LA in diastole, suggesting intermittent trapping of

may allow visualization of the vascular supply of the tumor and identify the source of its blood supply and its relationship to the coronary arteries. The major risk of angiography is embolization resulting from dislodgement of tumor fragment or associated thrombus [22]. Therefore, its use before surgery is becoming increasingly less common, except perhaps for the sole purpose of assessing the coronary anatomy.

TREATMENT AND PROGNOSIS

Benign Tumors

Operative excision is the treatment of choice for most benign tumors (Table 8) and in many cases results in complete cure [23•]. Despite the histologically benign nature of these cardiac tumors, they are potentially lethal because of clinical manifestations of valvular obstruction, embolization, cardiac-rhythm disturbances, conduction defects, or sudden death. It is not uncommon for patients to die or experience a major complication while awaiting surgery. It is therefore mandatory to carry out the operation promptly after the diagnosis has been established [24]. Open heart surgery with cardiopulmonary bypass is required in most cases, with adequate inspection and removal of all tumor fragments. Some cases of successful removal of left ventricular myxoma by video assisted cardioscopy have been reported. The dislodgement of tumor fragments represents a major risk during surgery and may result in embolization. Because early surgery is curative, patients with recurrent unexplained, albeit nonspecific cardiac symptoms should undergo echocardiographic evaluation. The high sensitivity of this technique permits adequate screening in most patients provided that the technical quality is adequate for diagnosis.

Numerous reports have documented complete cure of left and right atrial myxomas during a follow-up of up to 22 years [24,25]. Causes of recurrent atrial myxomas include incomplete resection of the original tumor with regrowth or intracardiac implantation from the original tumor. Castells *et al.* [26] reported a low recurrence rate of 4.7%. Patients with a familial history of cardiac myxoma or features of a complex myxoma syndrome may have tumor recurrence in 12% to 22% of cases as opposed to 1% of cases with sporadic atrial myxoma. Echocardiographic follow-up is important for detecting recurrent tumors in such patients. Following resection of myxoma, it is generally recommended that all patients have periodic follow-up by two-dimensional echocardiography for detection of recurrence. Although no criteria have been established, echocardiographic follow-up every 2 to 5 years is reasonable depending on patient symptomatology; suspected complex myxoma requires closer follow-up.

Other benign tumors also have been excised with a high degree of success. These include rhabdomyoma, hamartoma, fibroma, hemangioma, and papillary fibroelastomas (Table 8). Spontaneous resolution occurs in some childhood rhabdomyomas [27•].

Malignant Tumors

Surgery is not an effective treatment for the great majority of primary malignant tumors of the heart, either because of the large mass of cardiac tissue involved or the presence of metastases [23•]. A major role for surgery in such cases may be to establish the diagnosis and to explore the possibility of a curable benign tumor. Transesophageal echocardiography–guided transvenous biopsy may preclude surgery in some cases [28•]. Survival times from 1 to 3 years have been reported following partial resection with additional chemotherapy or radiation therapy. Lymphosarcoma of the heart frequently responds to chemotherapy, radiation therapy, or both [29]. Most reports indicate a failure to alter the course of cardiac sarcomas even with various combinations of surgery, chemotherapy, and radiation therapy. Surgery for metastatic cardiac tumors is largely palliative; surgically placed pericardial windows are commonly used to treat large pericardial effusions and cardiac tamponade.

ACKNOWLEDGMENT

We thank Ms. Yumekia Merkerson for assistance in manuscript preparation.

TABLE 8 TREATMENT AND PROGNOSIS OF CARDIAC TUMORS

Type of tumor	Treatment	Prognosis
Benign primary tumor	Usually surgical excision (lipomatous hypertrophy of atrial septum is benign and does not need any treatment)	Excellent; recurrence rare
Malignant primary tumor	Surgery not effective in the majority of patients because of extensive cardiac involvement or metastases; partial resection plus chemotherapy or radiotherapy may prolong survival in a few patients	Generally poor
Metastatic-secondary tumors	Surgery only palliative; almost always associated with widespread metastatic involvement of other organs	Poor

KEY REFERENCE

A recently published paper of outstanding interest, as identified in *References and Recommended Reading*, has been annotated.

•• Sun JP, Asher CR, Yang XS, *et al.*: Clinical and echocardiographic characteristics of papillary fibroelastomas: a retrospective study in 162 patients. *Circulation* 2001, 103:2687.

Detection of papillary fibroelastomas has been enhanced by transesophageal echocardiography.

REFERENCES AND RECOMMENDED READING

Recently published papers of particular interest have been highlighted as:
• Of interest
•• Of outstanding interest

1. Fine G: Primary tumors of the pericardium and heart. *Cardiovasc Clin* 1973, 5:207–238.

2. Bulkley BH, Hutchins GM: Atrial myxomas: a fifty year review. *Am Heart J* 1979, 97:639–643.

3. Peters MN, Hall RJ, Cooley DA, *et al.*: The clinical syndrome of atrial myxoma. *JAMA* 1974, 230:695–701.

4. McDevitt HO, Bodomer WF: Protean clinical manifestations of primary tumors of the heart. *Am J Med* 1972, 52:1–8.

5. Farah MG: Familial cardiac myoxoma. A study of relatives of patients with myxoma. *Chest* 1994, 105:65–68.

6. McCarthy PM, Piehler JM, Schaff HV, *et al.*: The significance of multiple recurrences and "complex" cardiac myxomas. *Thorac Cardiovasc Surg* 1986, 91:389–396.

7. Carney JA: Difference between nonfamilial and familial cardiac myxomas. *Am J Surg Pathol* 1983, 9:53–55.

8.•• Sun JP, Asher CR, Yang XS, *et al.*: Clinical and echocardiographic characteristics of papillary fibroelastomas: a retrospective study in 162 patients. *Circulation* 2001, 103:2687.

9.• Brown RD, Khandheria BJ, Edwards WD: Cardiac papillary fibroelastomas: a treatable cause of transient ischemic attack and ischemic stroke detected by transesophageal echocardiography. *Mayo Clin Proc* 1995, 70:863.

10. Chan HSL, Sonley MJ, Moes CAF, *et al.*: Primary and secondary tumors of childhood involving the heart, pericardium, and great vessels: a report of 75 cases and review of the literature. *Cancer* 1985, 56:825–836.

11. Miyashita T, Miyazawa I, Kawaguchi T, *et al.*: A case of primary cardiac B cell lymphoma associated with ventricular tachycardia, successfully treated with systemic chemotherapy and radiotherapy: a long-term survival case. *Jpn Circ J* 2000, 64:135–138.

12. Skalides El, Parthenakis Fl, Sacharis EA, *et al.*: Pulmonary tumor embolism from primary cardiac B-cell lymphoma. *Chest* 1999, 116:1489–1490.

13. Roberts WC, Glancy DL, DeVita VT Jr: Heart in malignant lymphoma (Hodgkin's disease, lymphosarcoma, reticulum cell sarcoma and mycosis fungoides). A study of 196 autopsy cases. *Am J Cardiol* 1968, 22:149–153.

14. Panidis IP, Mintz GS, McAllister MO: Hemodynamic consequence of left atrial myxoma assessed by Doppler ultrasound. *Am Heart J* 1986, 111:927–931.

15. Ofili EO, Labovitz AJ: Transesophageal echocardiography in the evaluation of cardiac source of embolus and intracardiac masses. *J Invasive Cardiol* 1992, 4:349–358.

16. Leibowitz G, Keller NM, Daniel WG, *et al.*: Transesophageal versus transthoracic echocardiography in the evaluation of right atrial tumors. *Am Heart J* 1995, 130:1224–1227.

17.• Lynch M, Clements SD, Shenewise JS: Right-sided cardiac tumors detected by transesophageal echocardiography and its usefulness in differentiating the benign from the malignant ones. *Am J Cardiol* 1997, 79(6):781–784.

18. Jack CM, Cleland J, Geddes JS: Left atrial rhabdomyosarcoma and the use of digital gated computed tomography in its diagnosis. *Br Heart J* 1986, 55:305–307.

19.• Mousseaux E, Hernigou A, Azencot M, *et al.*: Evaluation by electron beam computed tomography of intracardiac masses suspected by transesophageal echocardiography. *Heart* 1996, 76(3):256–263.

20. Freedberg RS, Kronzon I, Rumancik WM, Liebeskind D: The contribution of magnetic resonance imaging to the evaluation of intracardiac tumors diagnosed by echocardiography. *Circulation* 1988, 77:96–103.

21. Matsuoka H, Hamada M, Honda T, *et al.*: Morphologic and histologic characterization of cardiac myxomas by magnetic resonance imaging. *Angiology* 1996, 47:693–698.

22. Pindyck F, Pierce EC, Baron MG, Lukban SB: Embolization of left atrial myxoma after transeptal cardiac catheterization. *Am J Cardiol* 1972, 30:569–571.

23.• Perchinsky MJ, Lichtenstein SV, Tyers GF: Primary cardiac tumors: forty years' experience with 71 patients. *Cancer* 1997, 79(9):1809–1815.

24. Semb BK: Surgical considerations in the treatment of cardiac myxoma. *J Thorac Cardiovasc Surg* 1984, 87:251–259.

25. Ernesto Greco, Mestres CA, Cartana R, *et al.*: Video assisted cardioscopy for removal of primary left ventricular myxoma. *Cardiothorac Surg* 1999, 16:677–678.

26. Castells E, Ferran V, Octavio de Toledo MC, *et al.*: Cardiac myxomas: surgical treatment, long term results and recurrence. *J Cardiovasc Surg* 1993, 34:49–53.

27.• DiMario FJ Jr, Diana D, Leopold H, Chameides L: Evolution of cardiac rhabdomyoma in tuberous sclerosis complex. *Clin Pediatr* 1996, 35(12):615–619.

28.• Malouf JF, Thompson RC, Maples WJ, Wolfe JT: Diagnosis of right atrial metastatic melanoma by transesophageal echocardiographic-guided transvenous biopsy. *Mayo Clin Proc* 1996, 71(12):1167–1170.

29. Vergnon JM, Vincent M, Perinett M, *et al*: Chemotherapy of metastatic primary cardiac sarcomas. *Am Heart J* 1985, 110:682–684.

30. Nanda NC, Mahan EF III: Transesophageal echocardiography. American Heart Association Council Clinical Cardiology Newsletter; Summer, 1990:3–22.

31. Samdarshi TE, Mahan EF III, Nanda NC, *et al.*: Transesophageal echocardiography diagnosis of multicentric left ventricular myxomas mimicking a left atrial tumor. *J Thorac Cardiovasc Surg* 1992, 103:471–474.

SELECT BIBLIOGRAPHY

Amano T, Kono T, Wada Y, *et al.*: Cardiac myxoma: its origin and tumor characteristics. *Ann Thorac Cardiovasc Surg* 2003, 9:215–221.

Odim J, Reehal V, Laks H, *et al.*: Surgical pathology of cardiac tumors. Two decades at an urban institution. *Cardiovasc Pathol* 2003, 12:267–270.

Nonpenetrating Cardiac Trauma

Steven B. Johnson
A. James Liedtke
Joseph S. Alpert

Key Points

- Rapid deceleration impact injuries to the anterior chest are a major cause of myocardial contusion.
- A 12-lead electrocardiogram is the initial screening test for diagnosing myocardial contusion.
- Current assessment of outcome statistics of cardiac complications secondary to myocardial contusion provides prospective clues to identifying high- and low-risk patients.
- It is now possible to develop a triage algorithm for managing patients with myocardial contusion.
- Direct injury to coronary arteries threatens myocardial perfusion and viability.
- Therapeutic strategies for coronary artery disease may be applicable to lesions resulting from coronary trauma.

Cardiac injury secondary to severe, nonpenetrating, chest-wall injury is a perilous, unpredictable consequence of deceleration impact injuries. It commonly occurs in motor vehicle accidents but can also occur in other types of blunt trauma such as falls and direct blows, *ie*, baseballs, to the anterior chest. Nonpenetrating cardiac injury can present at any point on a continuum of severity from minimal symptoms to life-threatening complications or death. It can be difficult to diagnose, particularly if accompanied by more obvious injuries of other organ systems. Parmley *et al.* [1], in one of the initial reviews on this topic, noted that cardiovascular involvement (most commonly contusion and rupture) in nonpenetrating trauma was not infrequent but was routinely unrecognized. Hospitals and trauma centers throughout the United States have dedicated increasingly greater staff and resources to the triage and management of trauma victims with suspected cardiac lesions.

This dedication has resulted in impressive results—in patients with even the most morbid of injuries, such as cardiac chamber rupture, survival following surgical repair is now possible [2]. Nevertheless, debate is still ongoing as how best to diagnose and manage patients with potential or actual cardiac injury. Some trauma experts have argued that current strategies for evaluation of the majority of these patients may be excessive and have argued that diagnostic and management systems be reevaluated to justify their cost. They further propose critically reviewing and possibly revamping utilization criteria for those triage algorithms, which necessitate intensive care facilities and expensive diagnostic and therapeutic procedures. This chapter focuses on two cardiac lesions: myocardial contusion and direct coronary artery trauma.

36

MYOCARDIAL CONTUSION
Diagnostic Criteria

Myocardial contusion has nonspecific diagnostic criteria and an uncertain clinical outcome, including major cardiac complications and, occasionally, cardiac death. The concept that myocardial contusion is analogous to myocardial infarction is probably inaccurate and not supported by the literature. Evidence in 1973 [3] was biased by the more dramatic expressions of myocardial trauma and contusion. With a more complete database developed from recent observations, the spectrum of injury expression is more complete. It now appears that the majority of myocardial contusions are transient abnormalities in cardiac performance that do not result in long-term complications [4••]. Intramuscular hemorrhage and edema are typically present and ischemia is an unusual finding. Exceptions to this concept are when direct injury results in chamber or valvular disruptions.

Myocardial contusion is an injury of the twentieth century. Most cases occur because of rapid deceleration events (before the era of air bags) secondary to motor-vehicle accidents or auto–pedestrian accidents (Table 1, Fig. 1). Typically, myocardial contusion presents as either electrocardiographic abnormalities or cardiac dysfunctions with wall motion abnormalities, valvular abnormalities, or pericardial effusions. There can be either immediate or delayed presentation of these findings, including normal hemodynamics and ECG findings at the time of presentation to the emergency department. Representative diagnostic clinical criteria for patients with suspected myocardial contusion are listed in Table 2. These criteria

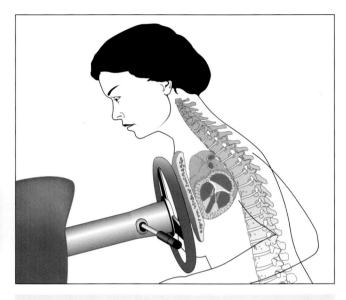

FIGURE 1 Typical impact injury to the anterior chest wall when the driver is thrust against the fixed steering column. Myocardial contusion results from high-speed deceleration accidents, most typically experienced by motor-vehicle and motorcycle crashes and auto–pedestrian accidents.

TABLE 1 MECHANISM OF INJURY IN PATIENTS WITH SUSPECTED MYOCARDIAL CONTUSION FOLLOWING BLUNT CHEST TRAUMA

Mechanism	Patients, n
Car or truck accident	214
Pedestrian accident	30
Motorcycle accident	16
Fall	26
Other	26
Total (227 men; 85 women)	312

TABLE 2 REPRESENTATIVE DIAGNOSTIC CLINICAL CRITERIA OF PRESUMPTIVE MYOCARDIAL CONTUSION*

Study	Criteria
Foil *et al.* [12]	Presence of chest pain, chest-wall contusion or tenderness, or sternal tenderness; a likely mechanism of injury such as rapid deceleration injury, bent or broken steering wheel, or a blow to the chest; dysrhythmias or ECG abnormalities (exclusive of sinus tachycardia)
Norton *et al.* [13]	ECG pattern consistent with evolving or resolving pattern of acute injury; CK-MB isoenzyme fraction ≥5 % of the total CK concentration, or an elevated CK concentration with a "positive" MB fraction; an abnormal echo (hypokinesis, pericardial effusion, acute valvular injury; apical thrombus; wall thickening with edema or hemorrhage)
Miller *et al.* [9]	History of direct blows to the chest, broken steering-wheel accidents; likely mechanism of injury; physical evidence of anterior chest-wall injury, precordial bruising, fractured sternum, or anterior rib fractures
Ross *et al.* [10]	ECG and CK-MB isoenzyme assay monitored over the first 72 hours
	ECG criteria: arrhythmias, atrial or ventricular ectopy, conduction defects, any ischemic changes; CK-MB percentage >2.5%

*Exclusive of autopsy results.
CK—creatine kinase; ECG—electrocardiogram; echo—echocardiogram.

reflect the lack of specific diagnostic signs, symptoms, and laboratory parameters while heightening awareness of the possible presence of cardiac injuries. Jugular venous distension may be a critical finding associated with injury to the heart, characterizing cardiac tamponade, valvular rupture, and right heart failure due to contusion. Noncardiac physical findings may include anterior chest wall tenderness, ecchymosis, or evidence of pulmonary injury. Sternal fractures, particularly in the lower half of the sternum, may be associated with myocardial contusion in up to 62% of patients [5,6] but clinical significance has been questioned [7]. Patients with a high-risk mechanism of injury (such as rapid deceleration or direct blows); anterior chest wall tenderness (especially if associated with lower sternal fractures); anterior chest pain; or demonstrating ECG changes or cardiac dysfunction should undergo further evaluation for myocardial contusion.

The definitive diagnosis of myocardial contusion is hindered by lack of an accepted "gold standard" diagnostic test. The heterogeneity of clinical presentation and the realization that myocardial injury without any clinical consequences may occur contributes to the problem as well [8].

Current literature encompasses a large population of patients studied with detailed workups [4–11]. At present the most reliable means of establishing the diagnosis of clinically significant myocardial contusion is by 12-lead electrocardiogram in conjunction with echocardiography. Recent work has emphasized that elevated blood tropinin levels occur in patients with myocardial contusion. Since blood tropinin levels can identify very small myocardial injuries, many patients with minor degrees of myocardial contusion are identified by this latter test.

An algorithm based on the results of selected 12-lead electrocardiography and echocardiography can be used to establish the diagnosis of clinically significant myocardial contusions (Fig. 2).

Updated outcome statistics of cardiac complications secondary to myocardial contusion confirm its reputation as a potentially life-threatening condition, both as a primary consequence of blunt chest-wall injury and as a disorder associated with other complications. For example, in traumatic thoracic aortic rupture, myocardial contusion worsens perioperative morbidity and mortality by promoting cardiac instability and cardiac arrest [17]. Deaths have also been reported [9,15,18] (Table 3). This complication is infrequent, however, and typically occurs with severe injury to other organ systems. Other complications are more frequent and include pericardial tears and effusions, nonlethal and lethal cardiac ruptures, acute myocardial infarction, transient myocardial ischemia, congestive heart failure, pulmonary edema and atrial thrombus, and cardiac dysrhythmias [9–13,15,16,18] (Table 4). Cardiac dysrhythmias include atrial premature beats, atrial fibrillation, sinoatrial nodal arrest, ventricular premature beats, ventricular tachycardia, ventricular fibrillation, nodal rhythm, atrioventricular conduction block, and intraventricular conduction delay. These rhythm disturbances at times require medical treatment or pacemaker insertion.

The most common rhythm disturbance is sinus tachycardia, which is uniformly nonspecific in the setting of acute trauma. Other rhythm disturbances may be more specific, including evidence of acute ST-T wave changes and intraventricular conduction delays. Any young trauma patient without a previous cardiac history who presents with evidence of chest trauma and a new right bundle branch block should be presumed to have a myocardial contusion, and an echocardiogram is recommended.

Blunt chest wall injury can also precipitate sudden cardiac death. Maron *et al.* [19,20] reviewed a registry of 25 children and young adults who died in sporting activities due to chest impact trauma. Cardiopulmonary resuscitation

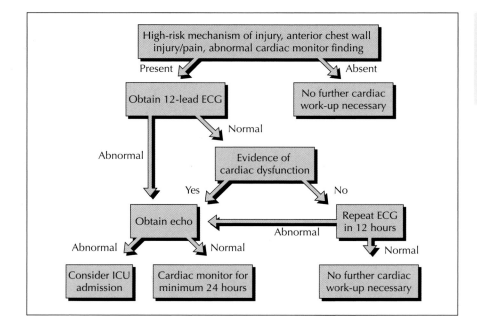

FIGURE 2 Results of selected 12-lead electrocardiography and echocardiography can be used to establish the diagnosis of clinically significant myocardial contusions. ICU—intensive care unit.

performed in 19 of these victims was unsuccessful. Autopsies were obtained in 22 of the 25 patients. Twelve victims had small chest contusions; most were located directly over the left ventricle. Also described were bruises, lacerations, and puncture wounds involving the chest wall, heart, pericardium, and lungs. The authors speculated that the sudden chest blow "presumably delivered at an electrically vulnerable phase of ventricular excitability," affected cardiac arrest due to ventricular dysrhythmias.

Updated statistics confirm that myocardial contusion is hazardous and requires careful diagnostic and electrical monitoring, dedicated professional staff, and the availability

TABLE 3 OUTCOME STATISTICS OF PATIENTS WITH NONPENETRATING BLUNT CHEST-WALL INJURY

Study	Patients reviewed, n	Patients with presumed or suspected MC, n	Deaths secondary to MC, n	Other cardiac complications
Wisner et al. [18]	3010	110	27*	19 Dysrhythmias (4 required treatment) 2 Cardiac rupture
Foil et al. [12]	1936	524	0	23 Dysrhythmias (19 required treatment) 3 Myocardial infarctions 2 Pericardial effusions 4 Hemodynamic instability
Cachecho et al. [16]	336	336	0	13 Atrial fibrillation (4 required treatment) 12 Supraventricular tachycardia/sinoatrial node dysfunction (7 required treatment) 24 Ventricular irritability (4 required treatment for ventricular tachycardia or ventricular bigeminy/trigeminy) 19 BBB or atrioventricular block 18 Ischemia 4 Congestive heart failure (all required treatment)
McLean et al. [15]	312	312	35 (at least 4 had MC)	27 With ventricular ectopic score > 3, including 17 ventricular tachycardia (2 required treatment) 14 Atrial fibrillation or sinus arrest or both (at least 5 treated) 11 New Q waves (4 died)
Dubrow et al. [11]	243	172	1 (MC not causal)	1 Ventricular ectopy 4 Ventricular tachycardia (2 required treatment) 3 Atrial ectopy 1 Atrial fibrillation 1 right BBB 1 Ischemia 1 Myocardial infarction
Miller et al. [9]	172	28	At least 3 (MC not necessarily causal in 2)	12 Dysrhythmias (4 required treatment) 4 Pericardial effusions
Norton et al. [13]	88	27	0	2 Atrial dysrhythmias 6 Ventricular dysrhythmias (5 required treatment) 8 Conduction delays 3 Myocardial infarctions (all required treatment) 3 Cardiogenic shock (all required treatment) 1 Apical thrombus (required treatment)
Ross et al. [10]	64	58	0	25 ECG changes with ST-T wave abnormalities 10 Ventricular ectopy 9 right BBB 3 Atrioventricular block 2 Atrial ectopy 3 Atrial fibrillation 4 Operative complications: ventricular ectopy, ventricular fibrillation, nodal rhythm, pulmonary edema

*Includes cardiac rupture, pericardial tear, coronary arterial injury.
BBB—bundle branch block; ECG—electrocardiogram; MC—myocardial contusion.

of sophisticated resources to conduct complex diagnostic and rapid therapeutic intervention; however, is this labor-intensive and costly triage algorithm mandatory for all patients with presumed myocardial contusion? Several reports agree on the markers defining a high-risk population of patients with myocardial contusion [9,13,15,16]. Cardiac complications strongly correlate with the presence and severity of multiorgan injuries as defined by the Injury Severity Score (ISS) [21]. This score derives from the Abbreviated Injury Scale, which was created by the Committee on Medical Aspects of Automotive Injury of the American Medical Association [22], revised in 1985 [23], and subsequently rendered "user-easy" [24].

Using multivariant analysis, Norton et al. [13] proposed that an abnormal electrocardiogram on admission and an ISS of 10 or higher were highly predictive of a clinically significant myocardial contusion, and that in their absence an important contusion (1%) was virtually excluded. Probability estimates from their analysis are shown in Table 4. They further noted that because these two predictive markers are easily acquired in the emergency department, a patient population at high risk for myocardial contusion could be rapidly identified and triaged to the appropriate intensive care unit or monitored bed.

Cachecho et al. [16] also observed a relationship between ISS and cardiac complications in a stable group of young patients with asymptomatic myocardial contusion. Increasing the ISS from 6.6 ± 6.1 to 23.5 ± 16.2 led to an increase in the occurrence of cardiac complications and dysrhythmias from 0% to 29%. Other important prognosticators were electrocardiogram abnormalities, which were either present on arrival at the emergency department or developed within the first 4 to 24 hours [9,12]; an adverse clinical course including hemodynamic shock [9]; and the occurrence or presence of atrial fibrillation, which in one study [15] was shown to be an increased risk factor for predicting cardiac deaths. Also important was the identity of patients at low risk for either the diagnosis of contusion or its complications. Foil et al. [12] noted that a normal electrocardiogram on admission and the lack of development of cardiac dysrhythmias in the first 4 hours of obser-vation virtually excluded significant cardiac sequelae, even in patients with physical findings of chest-wall contusion. They further proposed that these patients did not warrant hospitalization. These findings were again confirmed by Cachecho et al. [16], who observed in their patients that a normal or only minimally abnormal electrocardiogram did not require sophisticated cardiac monitoring during hospitalization and that the hospital stay strongly correlated with ISS.

Illig et al. [25] found similar results and noted that, based on the electrocardiogram obtained in the emergency department, patients could be effectively triaged to either home or hospital admission.

Dubrow et al. [11] defined their entrance criteria based on radionuclide angiography. This technique is insensitive to smaller lesions and is only diagnostic for those injuries with observably decreased global left ventricular ejection fraction or induced abnormalities in segmental wall motion. The ISS range was correspondingly higher (12.7 to 30.7) in three patient subgroups. Despite the higher absolute ISS values, mortality rates were lower than those predicted by their ISS ranking. This disparity was so wide (10% to 20% predicted vs 0.58% observed) that the authors concluded that in stable patients, "myocardial contusion does not by itself increase the risk of complication, does not necessitate intensive care unit monitoring, should be devalued when computing ISS scores, may account for lengthy and often unnecessary hospitalization, and in patients at risk for complications may be (more easily) identified by ECG abnormalities on arrival to the Emergency Department" [11].

Similar results were reached by Paone et al. [26]. They evaluated 159 cases of major blunt chest injury using several forms of diagnostic testing, including ECG monitoring, cardiac isoenzyme patterns and lactate dehydrogenase, and two-dimensional echocardiograms. They concluded that laboratory testings had "poor predictive value," and that clinical "observations with ECG monitoring" plus treatment of any symptomatic dysrhythmias were "an adequate and cost-conscious" approach. A meta-analysis survey by Maenza et al. [27] also concluded that the ECG and the creatine kinase (CK)-MB isoenzyme were the diagnostic

TABLE 4 CALCULATION OF THE PROBABILITY OF MYOCARDIAL CONTUSION USING ISS AND ECG IN 88 PATIENTS

Predictors of myocardial contusion			
ISS>10	Abnormal ED ECG	Probability of myocardial contusion	Patients with myocardial contusion, n
Yes	Yes	0.8656	9
No	Yes	0.3538	12
Yes	No	0.0396	4
No	No	0.0396	0

ECG—electrocardiogram; ED—emergency department; ISS—Injury Severity Score.

parameters of most merit in evaluating patients with clinically significant myocardial contusion.

However, the value of CK-MB isoenzyme analysis is contested. Fabian *et al.* [28] reported that in 140 of 1110 patients suffering nonpenetrating trauma and at increased risk for blunt cardiac injury, 56 had likely evidence for myocardial contusion as estimated either by increased CK-MB concentrations in blood or by abnormalities on the admission electrocardiogram. The authors cautioned, however, that elevated isoenzymes were transient and required careful sampling (at admission and every 6 hours for the first 24 hours). If these sampling times were missed, up to 75% of their patients with myocardial contusion would not have been so diagnosed. Other data, however, have not been confirmatory. In one study of 138 patients with severe injury, including possible myocardial contusion [16], only 1.4% had positive isoenzymes compared with 32% who had diagnostic electrocardiographic changes. Another study [12] found no significant association between CK isoenzyme changes and the occurrence of cardiac-related complications, and a third [9] observed that combined findings of electrocardiogram abnormalities and elevated CK isoenzymes were of no higher predictive value in defining patients at higher risk than using the electrocardiogram alone. In a final report of 182 patients with significant blunt chest wall trauma [29], the authors concluded that "CK-MB determinations in patients with suspected blunt myocardial injury were unjustifiably expensive and added confusion to an already vague clinical area." The problem of enzyme analysis is compounded in trauma cases by the presence of skeletal muscle injury, which almost always occurs in severe blunt chest-wall injury and lowers the CK-MB fraction (< 3%) relative to the total CK concentration in blood [30]. It is now generally accepted at most trauma centers that CK and CK-isoenzyme determinations are not indicated in the diagnosis and management of myocardial contusion and should not be obtained unless concern for acute myocardial infarction is present.

Recently, the use of cardiac troponin level determinations has been proposed as a less ambiguous diagnostic modality [31]. Others, however, have demonstrated low sensitivity (31%) and moderate specificity (91%) for elevated troponins in the diagnosis of myocardial contusion [32]. At this time, the role of cardiac troponin determinations in the diagnosis of myocardial contusion is still being defined but, like other biochemical markers, it appears likely to have a limited role. Truponin may, however, have a significant role in diagnosing acute myocardial infarction in the acute trauma patient who has significant skeletal muscle injury.

Imaging Modalities

The various imaging modalities available for the diagnosis and management of myocardial contusion provide an assessment of the functional status of the heart. Echocardiography has become the most frequently used modality,

with radionuclide angiography being less frequently employed. Echocardiography, either by transthoracic or transesophageal routes, can be useful in determining the site of injury and functional derangement of the injury. In addition, it is useful for detecting pericardial fluid, valvular injuries, and, in the case of transesophageal echo, can be used to detect associated thoracic aortic injuries [33,34]. A suggested limitation of echocardiography may be its inability to detect small areas of functional compromise but, due to the lack of clinical sequela of this type of minimal injury, clinicians should not be dissuaded from using this modality. An association has been described among patients with positive radionuclear imaging and mortality [15], but when a more complete population of trauma patients is surveyed, the sensitivity and specificity of this testing mode is reduced.

Transthoracic echocardiography

Rapid bedside echocardiography has become an important tool in the initial assessment of blunt chest trauma. The hallmark findings on echocardiography of myocardial contusion include increased end-diastolic wall thickness, increased echo brightness, and impaired regional systolic function [35]. These findings may be present to varying degrees requiring expertise in the diagnostic interpretation and knowledge of clinical consequences of the findings. Technical problems, most commonly related to imaging impediments such as subcutaneous emphysema, bandages, and obesity, may preclude complete evaluation with the transthoracic approach in 7% to 15% of patients. Varying results have been reported regarding the accuracy of transthoracic echocardiography in diagnosing myocardial contusion, with inability to accurately diagnose in 49% to 86% of cases [9,18,27,36,37]. Recently, however, increased experience and use of transthoracic echo in acute trauma has improved results, and many centers have adopted a key role for its use in this injury process [36]. At this time, transthoracic echocardiography should be used as the diagnostic modality if suspicion is high for myocardial contusion or if ECG changes are present or if cardiac dysfunction exists.

Transesophageal echocardiography

Transesophageal echocardiography (TEE) is a new imaging strategy in patients with blunt chest trauma. The modality has a better signal-to-noise ratio and imaging capability than transthoracic echocardiography. Transesophageal echocardiography is not limited by many of the physical constraints incurred by the transthoracic approach and, coupled with the better resolution of the higher frequency TEE probe, provides better evaluation of the heart and aorta. Nineteen prospective patients with severe chest-wall injury were evaluated by transesophageal echocardiography [31]. Patients were studied within 12 hours of trauma. No procedural complications were reported. Investigations were undertaken for widened mediastinum (> 8 cm on chest film), and a variety of lesions were noted, including tricuspid, mitral, and aortic insufficiency; pericardial effusions; myocardial contusions; and aortic hematoma. In five of 19 patients with hypokinetic motion abnormalities compatible with myocardial contusion, isoenzyme analysis was negative.

In another study of 132 patients suspected of having injury to the thoracic aortic, TEE accurately diagnosed all aortic injuries as well as found 24% of patients to have an associated cardiac abnormality [38,39]. The value of TEE in the diagnosis of thoracic aortic injuries has been supported by others [40]. In addition, it was deemed critical in determining the correct course of therapy in a patient with trauma-induced mitral regurgitation due to leaflet prolapse [41]. In summary, TEE has an important role in evaluating blunt chest trauma and is more accurate than transthoracic echo at detecting cardiac and aortic injuries. Due to its more invasive nature and potentially limited availability, TEE should be used when transthoracic is inadequate or nondiagnostic or in situations when concern over associated aortic injury is present.

Radionuclide angiography

McLean *et al.* [14] performed radionuclear angiography in 163 patients who suffered thoracic trauma. Only seven patients had abnormal studies; five of them died. Postmortem findings in four patients showed evidence of prior infarction in three and one new anterior infarction in the fourth. Another report [15] noted that a radionuclear study performed 1 week after injury showed normal wall motion and ejection fractions in a patient with biventricular contusions who died late. A third study reported a positive relationship between the extent of blunt trauma estimated by ISS and cardiac-gated, blood-pool scintigraphy using labeled technetium-99m, but with much less accuracy than with using electrocardiographic abnormalities [16].

The results of a small series of patients studied by coronary perfusion imaging using thallium-201 are more encouraging [42]. Approximately 70% of these patients with blunt chest trauma had scintigraphic defects related to areas of myocardial contusion, and all patients with these defects had either paroxysmal dysrhythmias or electrocardiogram abnormalities. Godbe *et al.* [43] reported that thallium-201 imaging with single-photon emission computed tomography is useful in predicting those patients suffering severe chest-wall trauma at increased risk for developing cardiac dysrhythmias. Another approach has used indium-111 antimyosin scintigraphy as the imaging probe. However, in one report [44], focal antimyosin uptake was uncommon in a series of 17 patients with severe multisystem trauma and suspected myocardial contusion. In general, radionuclide angiography is considered too sensitive to be practical and is not commonly used.

CORONARY ARTERY TRAUMA

In 1973, the question of coronary artery trauma in blunt chest-wall injury was speculative because of a deficiency in essential information and too few unequivocal cases with direct documentation of the diagnosis using coronary cineangiography [3]. This literature is still not available in large series comparable to those described for myocardial contusion. In 1979, Allen and Liedtke [45] listed five categories to characterize the case material:

1. Cardiac contusion (or myocardial infarction) in the absence of sustained injury to a major coronary artery,
2. Cardiac contusion (or myocardial infarction) associated with perfusion abnormalities of a major coronary artery,
3. Coronary artery fistula formation,
4. Coronary artery rupture, and
5. Animal experiments evaluating the effect of blunt trauma on the coronary vasculature.

It is difficult to separate myocardial infarction from myocardial contusion without mechanisms that specifically relate tissue injury with flow abnormalities in the major coronary vessels, particularly for contusions or infarctions in the presence of normal coronary arteries. In this instance, tissue damage may reflect primary myocardial injury, including trauma to the microcirculation; transient epicardial arterial spasm; or clot formation with secondary lysis, which cannot be adequately described by subsequent arteriography. Literature is limited to several case reports that detail the relationship between arterial damage and tissue necrosis. Chest injury has resulted from sporting accidents, accidents of childhood, and workplace events, as well as from traffic accidents [45–51]. In almost every circumstance in which coronary trauma was established or suspected, there were electrocardiographic findings of acute myocardial infarction.

In contrast to recommendations developed for the early triage of patients with myocardial contusion, myocardial infarct occurred 3 and 15 days after the initial traumatic event in two patients in these reports [49,51]. Either delayed vasomotor spasm or a hypercoagulopathy may contribute to the late clinical development of infarction. Accompanying these coronary injuries were examples of hypotension or shock, intra-arterial clot formation, post-traumatic angina with an abnormal exercise tolerance evaluation, severe myocardial injury with depressed left ventricular ejection fraction and left ventricular aneurysm formation, tachyarrhythmias (nonsustained ventricular tachycardia), and complete heart block requiring temporary pacemaker insertion [47–51]. This latter finding confirms previous observations of complete heart block noted in the setting of blunt chest-wall trauma [52].

Therapy

Coronary injuries are well-suited to the therapeutic strategies developed for managing acute myocardial infarction. For example, intracoronary urokinase was infused for 2 hours in a patient with left anterior descending coronary arterial thrombus that had occluded both the anterior descending artery and first diagonal branch of that perfusion system [47]. Also, Lijoi *et al.* [51] attempted percutaneous transluminal coronary angioplasty of a totally obstructed left anterior descending coronary artery and were initially successful. The vessel reoccluded at 24 hours, and the patient was subsequently managed with surgical revascularization. Current therapeutic intervention in such cases would almost invariably involve the use of coronary arterial stenting. In a 6-year-old boy with complicated

cardiac trauma from a crush injury, cardiac surgery was employed to excise a left ventricular aneurysm that extended from the coronary sulcus to the apex of the heart and was filled with thrombus [48]. The operation was successful, and symptoms of heart failure that had developed before surgery resolved.

Coronary artery rupture secondary to blunt chest-wall injury is life-threatening. Heyndricks *et al.* [53] reported a 62-year-old patient involved in a car accident who presented with acute inferior myocardial infarction and hypotension. The patient received several supportive maneuvers, including assisted ventilation, pacemaker insertion, resuscitation, and pericardiocentesis. Treatment was unsuccessful, and the patient died 9 hours after injury. Autopsy revealed 13 rib

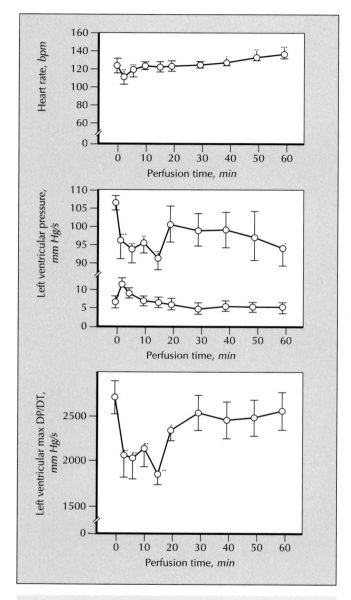

FIGURE 3 Changes in various parameters in global hemodynamic function in traumatized hearts. The major interval of mechanical dysfunction occurs early after the impact injury. **Middle panel**, *bottom open circles* represent left ventricular end-diastolic pressure; *top circles* represent left ventricular peak systolic pressure. *Dots* represent statistical significance by paired Student's *t*-test comparisons with pretrauma values: .—$P < 0.05$; ..—$P < 0.01$; ...—$P < 0.005$. *Bars* represent $\pm$ 1 SEM. Max DP/DT—maximum rate of pressure development during isovolumic contraction.

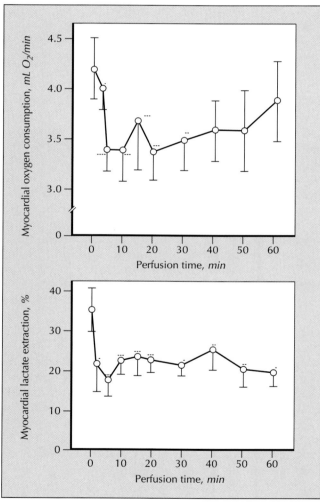

FIGURE 4 Changes in regional metabolism for oxygen consumption and lactate extraction in the perfusion distribution of the traumatized artery. The metabolic consequences of coronary injury, particularly for depressed lactate extraction, appear to last longer than for mechanical dysfunction. *Dots* represent statistical significance by paired Student's *t*-test comparisons with pretrauma values: .—$P < 0.05$; ..—$P < 0.01$; ...—$P < 0.005$. *Bars* represent $\pm$ 1 SEM.

fractures and the presence of blood bilaterally in both pleural spaces. One bone splinter had perforated the left pleura, lacerated the pericardium, and torn the right coronary artery from its origin on the aorta. There was also a smaller, transverse tear of the intima of the left coronary artery as well as a nonperforating tear of the aorta distal to the left subclavian artery. Histologic and histochemical examination confirmed the presence of an extensive, inferior myocardial infarction.

Consequences of Coronary Injury

In animal studies with controlled injuries to the coronary arteries, Sabbah and coworkers [54,55] described multiple coronary lesions by either microscopic examination or selective coronary arteriograms. They noted complete and partial obstructions to major coronary vessels, extravasation of blood from traumatic vascular wounds, accompanying extravascular hemorrhages, and a small arteriovenous fistula. Despite the angiographic severity of these lesions, which were evident by the third day after trauma, almost all findings resolved to near-normal or normal by 2 to 5 weeks of follow-up.

Even in the absence of demonstrable anatomic lesions, (ie, no spasm, thrombosis, hemorrhage, or laceration), functional consequences of direct coronary injury occur [56]. Other coronary abnormalities included a reduction in reactive hyperemia reflective of decreased coronary flow reserve and concomitant declines in regional systolic shortening, left ventricular pressure development, and left ventricular maximum rate of pressure development during isovolumic contraction. Metabolically, myocardial oxygen consumption and lactate extraction were decreased.

One unifying interpretation of these data is that there is an adverse reflex pattern of coronary perfusion with distribution of flow away from the subendocardial zone. This flow is sufficient to decrease coronary oxygen delivery and mechanical performance and to alter glucose metabolism, suggestive of early myocardial ischemia (Figs. 3 and 4, Table 5). These data *in toto* suggest that the coronary vasculature is not immune from direct injury after blunt chest-wall trauma; that consequences of this trauma may be expressed in a variety of clinical conditions, including life-threatening myocardial infarction or contusion; and that even without anatomic obstruction, derangements in coronary flow, which are functionally adverse (particularly to the subendocardium) may occur with subsequent mechanical and metabolic sequelae.

KEY REFERENCE

A recently published paper of outstanding interest, as identified in *References and Recommended Reading*, has been annotated.

•• Pretre R, Chilcott M: Blunt trauma to the heart and great vessels. *N Engl J Med* 1997, 336:626–632.

This article provides data on the nature and consequences of blunt chest trauma including aspects of diagnosis and management. The role of echocardiography is emphasized.

REFERENCES AND RECOMMENDED READING

Recently published papers of particular interest have been highlighted as:
•• Of outstanding interest

1. Parmley FF, Manion WC, Mattingly TW: Nonpenetrating traumatic injury of the heart. *Circulation* 1958, 18:371–396.

2. Fenton J, Myers ML, Lane P, Casson AG: Blunt cardiac trauma: survival after bichamber rupture. *Ann Thorac Surg* 1993, 55:1256–1257.

3. Liedtke AJ, DeMuth WE: Nonpenetrating cardiac injuries: a collective review. *Am Heart J* 1973, 86:687–697.

4.•• Pretre R, Chilcott M: Blunt trauma to the heart and great vessels. *N Engl J Med* 1997, 336:626–632.

5. Buckman R, Trooskin SZ, Flancbaum L, *et al.*: The significance of stable patients with sternal fractures. *Surg Gyn Obstet* 1987, 164:261–265.

6. Brookes JG, Dunn RJ, Rogers IR: Sternal fractures: A retrospective analysis of 272 cases. *J Trauma* 1993, 35:46–54.

7. Chiu WC, D'Amelio LF, Hammond JS: Sternal fractures in blunt chest trauma: A practical algorithm for management. *Am J Em Med* 1997, 15:252–255.

8. Mattox KL, Flint LM, Carrico CJ, *et al.*: Blunt cardiac injury. *J Trauma* 1992, 33:649–650.

9. Miller FB, Shumate CR, Richardson JD: Myocardial contusion: when can the diagnosis be eliminated? *Arch Surg* 1989, 124:805–808.

10. Ross P, Degutis L, Baker CC: Cardiac contusion: the effect on operative management of the patient with trauma injuries. *Arch Surg* 1989, 124:506–507.

11. Dubrow TJ, Mihalka J, Eisenhauer DM, *et al.*: Myocardial contusion in the stable patient: what level of care is appropriate? *Surgery* 1989, 106:267–274.

12. Foil MB, Mackersie RC, Furst SR, *et al.*: The asymptomatic patient with suspected myocardial contusion. *Am J Surg* 1990, 160:638–643.

TABLE 5 PERFUSION DATA IN FOUR TRAUMATIZED ANIMALS INJECTED WITH MICROSPHERE			
	Epicardial/endocardial flow ratio		
	Impact	**LAD**	**LCF**
Pretrauma			
Mean	0.94	0.97	1.36
SEM	0.15	0.09	0.24
5 Min after trauma			
Mean	1.60	1.30	1.42
SEM	0.36	0.07	0.36
P	< 0.025	< 0.005	NS
55 Min after trauma			
Mean	1.54	1.25	1.17
SEM	0.26	0.06	0.16
P	< 0.005	< 0.001	NS

Impact—LAD perfusion system directly beneath and around the impact site; LAD—left anterior perfusion system; LCF—left circumflex perfusion system; NS—not significant; *P*—statistical comparisons with pretrauma data; SEM—standard error of the mean.

13. Norton MJ, Stanford GG, Weigelt JA: Early detection of myocardial contusion and its complications in patients with blunt trauma. *Am J Surg* 1990, 160:577–582.

14. McLean RF, Devitt JH, Dubbin J, McLellan BA: Incidence of abnormal RNA studies and dysrhythmias in patients with blunt chest trauma. *J Trauma* 1991, 31:968–970.

15. McLean RF, Devitt JH, McLellan BA, *et al.*: Significance of myocardial contusion following blunt chest trauma. *J Trauma* 1992, 33:240–243.

16. Cachecho R, Grindlinger GA, Lee VW: The clinical significance of myocardial contusion. *J Trauma* 1992, 33:68–73.

17. Kram HB, Appel PL, Shoemaker WC: Increased incidence of cardiac contusion in patients with traumatic thoracic aortic rupture. *Ann Surg* 1988, 208:615–618.

18. Wisner DH, Reed WH, Riddick RS: Suspected myocardial contusion: triage and indications for monitoring. *Ann Surg* 1990, 212:82–86.

19. Maron BJ, Poliac LC, Kaplan JA, Mueller FO: Blunt impact to the chest leading to sudden death from cardiac arrest during sports activities. *N Engl J Med* 1995, 333:337–342.

20. Maron BJ, Gohman TE, Kyle SB, *et al.*: Clinical profile and spectrum of commotio cordis. *JAMA* 2002, 287:1142–1146.

21. Copes WS, Champion HR, Sacco WJ, *et al.*: The Injury Severity Score revisited. *J Trauma* 1988, 28:69–77.

22. Committee on Medical Aspects of Automotive Safety: Rating the severity of tissue damage. 1. The Abbreviated Injury Scale. *JAMA* 1971, 215:277–280.

23. *The Abbreviated Injury Scale (AIS)—1985 revision*. Des Plaines, IL: American Association for Automotive Medicine; 1985.

24. Civil ID, Schwab CW: The Abbreviated Injury Scale, 1985 revision: a condensed chart for clinical use. *J Trauma* 1988, 28:87–90.

25. Illig KA, Swierzewski MJ, Feliciano DV, *et al.*: A rational screening and treatment strategy based on the electrocardiogram alone for suspected cardiac contusion. *Am J Surg* 1991, 162:537–543.

26. Paone RF, Peacock JB, Smith DLT: Diagnosis of myocardial contusion. *South Med J* 1993, 86:867–870.

27. Maenza RL, Seaberg D, D'Amico F: A meta-analysis of blunt cardiac trauma: ending myocardial contusion. *Am J Emerg Med* 1996, 14:237–241.

28. Fabian TC, Mangiante EC, Patterson CR, *et al.*: Myocardial contusion in blunt trauma: clinical characteristics, means of diagnosis, and implications for patient management. *J Trauma* 1988, 28:50–57.

29. Keller KD, Shatney CH: Creatine phosphokinase-MB assays in patients with suspected myocardial contusion: diagnostic test or test of diagnosis? *J Trauma* 1988, 28:58–63.

30. Sobel BE, Jaffe AS: The value and limitations of cardiac enzymes in the recognition of acute myocardial infarction. *Heart Dis Stroke* 1993, 2:26–32.

31. Adams JE III, Dávila-Román VG, Bessey PQ, *et al.*: Improved detection of cardiac contusion with cardiac tropinin I. *Am Heart J* 1996, 131:308–312.

32. Ferjani M, Droc G, Dreux S, *et al.*: Circulating cardiac troponin T in myocardial contusion. *Chest* 1997, 111:427–433.

33. Johnson, SB, Sisley, A: The surgeon's use of transesophageal echocardiography. *Surg Clin North Am* 1998, 78:311–336.

34. Smith MD, Cassidy JM, Souther S, *et al.*: Transesophageal echocardiography in the diagnosis of traumatic rupture of the aorta. *N Engl J Med* 1995, 332:356–362.

35. Pandian NG, Skorton DJ, Doty DB, Kerber RE: Immediate diagnosis of acute myocardial contusion by two-dimensional echocardiography: studies in a canine model of blunt chest trauma. *J Am Coll Cardiol* 1983, 2:488–496.

36. Van Wijngaarden MH, Karmy-Jones R, Talwar MK, *et al.*: Blunt cardiac injury: a 10 year institutional review. *Injury* 1997, 28:51–55.

37. Reid CL, Kawanishi DT, Rahimtoola SH, Chandraratna PAN: Chest trauma: evaluation by two-dimensional echocardiography. *Am Heart J* 1987, 113:971–976.

38. Shapiro MJ, Yanofsky SD, Trapp J, *et al.*: Cardiovascular evaluation in blunt thoracic trauma using transesophageal echocardiography (TEE). *J Trauma* 1991, 31:835–840.

39. Kearney, PA, Smith, DW, Johnson, SB, *et al.*: The use of transesophageal echocardiography in the evaluation of traumatic aortic injury. *J Trauma* 1993, 34:696–703.

40. Brooks SW, Cmolik BL, Yong JC, *et al.*: Transesophageal echocardiographic examination of a patient with traumatic aortic transection from blunt chest trauma: a case report. *J Trauma* 1991, 31:841–845.

41. Turabian M, Chan K-L: Rupture of mitral chordae tendineae resulting from blunt chest trauma: diagnosis by transesophageal echocardiography. *Can J Cardiol* 1990, 6:180–182.

42. Bodin L, Rouby J-J, Viars P: Myocardial contusion in patients with blunt chest trauma as evaluated by thallium-201 myocardial scintigraphy. *Chest* 1988, 94:72–76.

43. Godbe D, Waxman K, Wang FW, *et al.*: Diagnosis of myocardial contusion: quantitative analysis of single photon emission computed tomographic scans. *Arch Surg* 1992, 127:888–892.

44. Hendel RG, Cohn S, Aurigemma G, *et al.*: Focal myocardial injury following blunt chest trauma: a comparison of indium-111 antimyosin scintigraphy with other noninvasive methods. *Am Heart J* 1992, 123:1208–1215.

45. Allen RP, Liedtke AJ: The role of coronary artery injury and perfusion in the development of cardiac contusion secondary to nonpenetrating chest trauma. *J Trauma* 1979, 19:153–156.

46. de Feyter PJ, Roos JP: Traumatic myocardial infarction with subsequent normal coronary arteriogram. *Eur J Cardiol* 1977, 6:25–31.

47. Ledley GS, Yazdanfar S, Friedman O, Kotler MN: Acute thrombotic coronary occlusion secondary to chest trauma treated with intracoronary thrombolysis. *Am Heart J* 1992, 132:518–521.

48. Cizmarova E, Simkovic I, Zelenay J, Masura J: Post-traumatic coronary occlusion and its consequences in a young child. *Pediatr Cardiol* 1988, 9:117–120.

49. Foussas SG, Athanasopoulos GD, Cokkinos DV: Myocardial infarction caused by blunt chest injury: possible mechanisms involved—case reports. *Angiology* 1989, 40:313–318.

50. Pringle SD, Davidson KG: Myocardial infarction caused by coronary artery damage from blunt chest injury. *Br Heart J* 1987, 57:375–376.

51. Lijoi A, Tallone M, Parodi E, *et al.*: Coronary occlusion secondary to blunt chest trauma: a first attempt at balloon angioplasty. *Tex Heart Inst J* 1992, 19:291–293.

52. Brennan JA, Field JM, Liedtke AJ: Reversible heart block following nonpenetrating chest trauma. *J Trauma* 1979, 19:784–788.

53. Heyndricks G, Vermeire P, Goffin Y, Van den Bogaert P: Rupture of the right coronary artery due to nonpenetrating chest trauma. *Chest* 1974, 65:577–579.

54. Sabbah HN, Stein PD, Hawkins ET, *et al.*: Extrinsic compression of the coronary arteries following cardiac trauma in dogs. *J Trauma* 1982, 22:937–943.

55. Sabbah HN, Mohyi J, Stein PD: Coronary arteriography in dogs following blunt cardiac trauma: a longitudinal assessment. *Cathet Cardiovasc Diagn* 1988, 15:155–163.

56. Liedtke AJ, Allen RP, Nellis SH: Effects of blunt cardiac trauma on coronary vasomotion, perfusion, myocardial mechanics, and metabolism. *J Trauma* 1980, 20:777–785.

37

Diseases of the Aorta

Kathryn L. Bates
Gregg M. Yamada

Key Points

- Seventy-five percent of arteriosclerotic aortic aneurysms involve the infrarenal abdominal aorta.

- Thoracic aneurysms most commonly result from atherosclerosis; most involve the descending thoracic aorta.

- Abdominal aortic aneurysms 4 cm or more in diameter may require surgical repair, and thoracic aortic aneurysms more than 6 to 7 cm in diameter require surgical repair.

- Magnetic resonance imaging, computed tomography, and transesophageal echo-cardiography are highly sensitive and specific for the diagnosis of aortic dissection.

- Untreated aortic dissections are associated with a high mortality.

- Arteritis syndromes including Takayasu's arteritis, giant cell arteritis, and the seronegative spondyloarthropathies are associated with varying degrees of aortic involvement.

- Most aortoiliac emboli are cardiac in origin.

- Embolization of small cholesterol crystals may follow surgical or catheter manipulation, leading to the cholesterol emboli syndrome.

A complex array of diseases, either congenital or acquired, may affect the aorta (Table 1). This chapter reviews the pathogenesis, clinical manifestations, and therapy of the most common aortic processes, including arteriosclerotic aneurysms, dissection, arteritis, and thromboembolic disease.

ARTERIOSCLEROTIC AORTIC ANEURYSMS

Arteriosclerotic aortic aneurysms include both abdominal and thoracic aortic aneurysms.

Abdominal Aortic Aneurysms

Pathophysiology

Seventy-five percent of aortic aneurysms involve the abdominal aorta distal to the origin of the renal arteries. Approximately 25% occur within the thoracic aorta. Most of these aneurysms are fusiform and result from arteriosclerotic weakening of the elastic media; other causes of aortic aneurysms are listed in Table 2. Aneurysmal dilatation leads to increased aortic wall tension, which results in further enlargement of the aneurysm. The normal diameter of an abdominal aorta is approximately 2.0 cm; a diameter greater than 3.0 cm is considered aneurysmal. Risk factors associated with abdominal aortic aneurysms include age, smoking, male sex, white race, atherosclerosis, peripheral vascular disease, hypertension, family history, and aneurysms of the femoral or popliteal arteries.

Presentation

Most patients who present with abdominal aortic aneurysms are asymptomatic. The diagnosis is suspected when routine physical examination reveals a pulsatile mid-epigastric mass or when aortic calcification is seen on abdominal radiographs (Fig. 1).

Diagnosis

The diagnosis may be confirmed with computed tomography (CT), magnetic resonance imaging (MRI), angiography, or ultrasonography. Abdominal ultrasonography is the most practical and cost-effective method for determining and monitoring aneurysm size [1,2], although CT provides additional preoperative information, delineating possible suprarenal extension or other abdominal abnormalities [3,4].

Treatment and prognosis

In general, the risk of abdominal aortic aneurysm rupture and prognosis is related to the size of the aneurysm, with larger aneurysms (> 5 cm in diameter) expanding more rapidly and being more likely to rupture than smaller aneurysms [5–7]. Aneurysm expansion rate is approximately 0.3 to 0.4 cm per year [8,9]. However, a small aneurysm that expands greater than 0.5 cm over a 6-month follow-up period is considered high risk for rupture and surgical consideration should be entertained. Special consideration should be given to women, who have smaller normal diameters than men. In this patient population, a diameter of 5.0 cm to 5.5 cm represents a greater degree of dilatation [10].

General indications for surgery

Elective resection should be considered for patients with asymptomatic abdominal aortic aneurysms greater than 5.5 cm in diameter, when a small aneurysm (less than 4.9 cm) increases in diameter greater than 0.5 cm within a 6-month interval, or when an aneurysm becomes symptomatic. Recommendations for the management of asymptomatic small to medium-sized aneurysms (4.0 cm–5.5 cm) are based on two large randomized trials [9,11,12]. Surveillance at 6-month intervals with abdominal ultrasonography or CT scan can be used as an alternative to surgery in certain patient populations [13]. However, patient preference should be taken into account with operative mortalities considered in each case. In this group, the likelihood of requiring surgery is 60% to 65% at 5 years and 70% to 75% at 8 years [9,11,12]. Similar surveillance should be used for small aneurysms (less than 4.0 cm). The operative mortality rate for elective repair is approximately 3% to 6% [10].

Endovascular stent grafting is a more recent treatment option for both abdominal and thoracic aortic aneurysms in patients who are poor candidates for surgical repair. Further investigation in this area is pending [11,14].

Medical therapy

Risk factor modification, especially smoking cessation, blood pressure control, and lipid lowering may be useful in patients with small to medium-sized aneurysms not treated surgically. Smoking has been shown to increase the rate of aneurysms by 20% to 25% [10]. Therefore, smoking cessation should be strongly reccomended. While beta-blocker

TABLE 1 DISEASES OF THE AORTA

Arteriosclerotic aortic aneurysms
Aortic dissection
Aortic arteritis
   Takayasu's arteritis
   Giant cell arteritis
   Ankylosing spondylitis
   Psoriatic arthritis
   Reiter's syndrome
Aortic thromboembolic disease
Aortic bacterial infection (syphilis, tuberculosis)
Traumatic injuries of the aorta
Aortic tumors
Coarctation and pseudocoarctation of the aorta
Hypoplastic aortic syndromes

TABLE 2 CAUSES OF AORTIC ANEURYSMS

Acquired
Atherosclerosis
Cystic medial degeneration
Infection (syphilis, tuberculosis)
Aortitis (infectious)
Trauma

Congenital
Aortitis (noninfectious)
Aneurysms associated with coarctation and patent ductus arteriosus

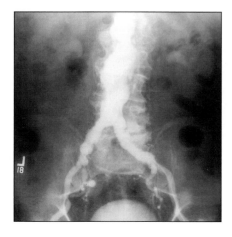

FIGURE 1
Abdominal aortogram demonstrating a fusiform infrarenal abdominal aortic aneurysm [36].

therapy has been shown to lower aneurysm expansion rate, randomized trial evidence to support their routine use is not available [8,15]. However, there may be a role for beta-blocker therapy as adjunctive treatment in patients not treated with surgery. Additionally, the routine use of cholesterol-lowering drugs, such as statins, and antibiotic therapy for the prevention or reduction in aneurysm expansion are still being investigated.

Usefulness of screening

At the present time, broad screening of an asymptomatic population with abdominal ultrasonography or abdominal palpation is not recommended. These recommendations are based on two large task force conclusions [16,17]. However, a targeted abdominal examination and ultrasound may be useful in men over age 60 years with high-risk profiles (smokers, hypertension, other vascular diseases).

Thoracic Aortic Aneurysms
Pathophysiology

Atherosclerosis is the most common cause of thoracic aortic aneurysms. Less common causes include annuloaortic ectasia, syphilis or other infections, and aortic valve disease. Arteriosclerotic thoracic aneurysms occur most frequently in the descending aorta and are typically fusiform, with the ascending aorta and the aortic arch less commonly involved. Patients with descending thoracic aortic aneurysms also may have associated abdominal aortic aneurysms [18]. Syphilitic aneurysms, which have a predilection for the ascending aorta, are often saccular. Aneurysms caused by cystic medial degeneration may involve the aortic sinuses and aortic valve, resulting in myocardial ischemia and valvular insufficiency.

Presentation

Descending aortic aneurysms are usually asymptomatic. In contrast, ascending aortic aneurysms are more likely to be symptomatic because of their impingement on adjacent thoracic structures. Patients may complain of a deep, aching anterior chest discomfort. Less common symptoms include dyspnea, cough, and hoarseness.

Palpable pulsations may be present along the anterior chest wall at either sternal border, the sternoclavicular borders, or the suprasternal notch. Aortic insufficiency and signs of Marfan's syndrome may be noted. Tracheal deviation, hoarseness, superior vena cava syndrome, and discrepant pulses and blood pressure also may be found.

Diagnosis

Thoracic aortic aneurysm may be suspected from routine posteroanterior and lateral radiographs, and it may be confirmed by angiography in patients requiring surgical resection (Fig. 2). CT, MRI, and transesophageal echocardiography (TEE) are sufficient to make the diagnosis, however, if surgery is not being considered.

Treatment and prognosis

Less information is available on the natural history of thoracic aortic aneurysms than for abdominal aneurysms. However, the most important determinant of rupture is size. Symptomatic thoracic aneurysms are associated with a 5-year survival rate of 27%, compared with 58% in asymptomatic patients. Symptomatic thoracic aneurysms, those over 6 to 7 cm in diameter in either the ascending or descending thoracic aorta, or accelerated growth greater than 10 cm per year in aneurysms less than 5.0 cm, require prompt surgical attention [19]. In another study of 133 patients, asymptomatic aneurysms greater than 4.0 to 5.9 cm and greater than 6.0 cm are associated with a 16% and 31% risk of rupture, respectively [20]. Because of the high prevalence of associated cardiovascular disease (eg, coronary artery disease), patients must be carefully selected for surgery. Early surgical mortality is approximately 5% to 10% and most often results from myocardial infarction, congestive heart failure, stroke, renal failure, or sepsis [21].

AORTIC DISSECTION
Pathophysiology

Aortic dissection results from a sudden intimal rupture followed by the formation of a dissecting hematoma along or within the aortic media separating the intima from the adventitia. Two thirds of all aortic dissections occur in the ascending aorta 2 to 5 cm above the aortic valve. The descending aorta, just distal to the origin of the left subclavian artery, is the second most common site of aortic dissection.

Cystic degenerative changes of the elastic and smooth muscle elements of the aortic media predispose the patient to the development of aortic dissection [22]; other factors associated with aortic dissection are listed in Table 3. Aortic dissection is more common in men, and hypertension is present in most patients with descending aortic dissection. Aortic dissection occurs in various connective tissue disorders associated with prominent, congenital cystic medial degeneration (eg, Marfan's syndrome, Ehlers-Danlos

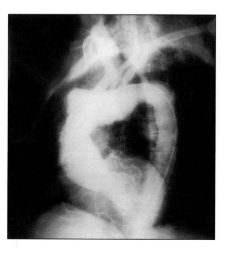

FIGURE 2
Thoracic aortogram demonstrating a saccular thoracic aortic aneurysm [36].

syndrome). An increased frequency of aortic dissection is also seen in patients with aortic coarctation, congenital bicuspid aortic valve, aortic stenosis, and pregnancy. Iatrogenic causes include cardiac catheterization, cardiac surgery, intra-aortic balloon counterpulsation, cardiopulmonary bypass, and prosthetic valve surgery.

The most widely cited classification for aortic dissection is that of DeBakey [23], which uses the location of the intimal tear and the extent of the aortic dissection as points of classification (Table 4). Type I dissections arise just above the aortic valve and extend into the descending aorta. Type II dissections are localized within the ascending aorta. Type III dissections originate in the descending aorta just distal to the origin of the left subclavian artery and extend into the abdominal aorta (Fig. 3).

A simpler classification (ie, the DeBakey classification) identifies the DeBakey types I and II dissections as proximal or ascending (type A) dissections and DeBakey type III dissections as distal or descending (type B) dissections (Fig. 4) [24]. Acute aortic dissections are those present for less than 2 weeks.

TABLE 3 FACTORS PREDISPOSING TO AORTIC DISSECTION
Primary or secondary cystic medial degeneration combined with:
Atherosclerosis
Hypertension
Advanced age
Aortic valve disease
Coarctation of the aorta
Aortic trauma, including iatrogenic trauma
Pregnancy

TABLE 4 DEBAKEY CLASSIFICATION OF AORTIC DISSECTION	
Classification	Description
I	Originates in the ascending aorta and propagates distal to the brachiocephalic artery
II	Originates in and is confined to the ascending aorta
III	Originates in the descending aorta near the ligamentum arteriosum
IIIA	Dissection does not extend below the diaphragm
IIIB	Dissection extends below the diaphragm

Presentation

Severe chest pain described as "stabbing," "ripping," or "tearing" in character is present in most patients. Unlike the presentation of myocardial ischemia, which often develops over several minutes, the intensity of the pain is extreme at onset. The site of dissection may be suggested by the location of the pain, but the pain commonly migrates into the neck, back, and extremities as the dissection extends along the aorta.

Aortic insufficiency, pulse abnormalities, neurologic deficits, and evidence of cardiac tamponade may be present in patients with ascending aortic dissection. Pulse deficits are less common in distal aortic dissections but if present may involve the femoral and left subclavian arteries. Although most patients present with hypertension, hypotension may signify aortic rupture, cardiac tamponade, or subclavian artery dissection.

Diagnosis

The diagnosis of aortic dissection may be suspected from the history and physical examination, and is confirmed with the CT scan, spiral CT scan, TEE, MRI, or angiography. Spiral CT and MRI may be more specific in identifying aortic arch and ascending dissections. The chest radiograph may reveal progressive mediastinal widening (Fig. 5). TEE is particularly useful in unstable patients. Additionally, TEE is a favored diagnostic modality because it can be obtained quickly and is readily available in most institutions. However, limitations in visualization of the ascending aorta and aortic arch are present. Spiral CT, MRI, and TEE are equally highly sensitive in the detection of thoracic aneurysms. Their sensitivity approaches 100% [25–28].

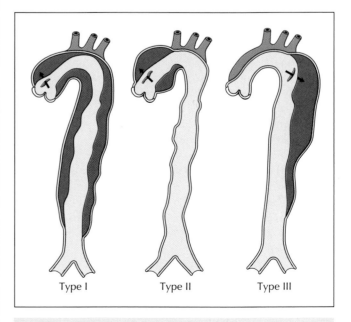

Type I   Type II   Type III

FIGURE 3 The DeBakey classification of aortic dissection. (*Adapted from* Eagle and De Sanctis [37].)

Treatment and Prognosis

Acute type A (ascending) aortic dissections (Fig. 6) almost invariably require immediate surgical therapy. Acute type B (descending) aortic dissections and chronic dissections of any location are first managed medically; surgery is reserved for complications such as rupture, expansion, continued pain, or distal ischemia. Untreated aortic dissections are associated with a 21% mortality at 24 hours, a 37% mortality at 48 hours, a 74% mortality at 2 weeks, and a 90% mortality at 3 months.

All patients with suspected aortic dissection require intensive monitoring for cardiac arrhythmias, hypotension, declining renal function, and other signs of systemic hypoperfusion before definitive diagnostic procedures are performed. The aim of medical therapy is to decrease both systemic arterial pressure and the rate of rise in aortic pressure. Analgesics and sedatives should be administered as needed. Intravenous beta-blockers (*eg*, metoprolol) in combination with vasodilators (*eg*, sodium nitroprusside) should be administered to all patients with hypertension.

Patients with hypotension require transfusion and emergent surgical correction. The surgical technique used depends on the location of the dissection.

Endovascular stent grafts (surgical or percutaneous) are a more recent treatment option for thoracoabdominal aneurysms and abdominal aortic dissections. This less invasive procedure is particularly attractive in patients who are poor operative candidates. Further investigation is needed to define the precise role and long-term effectiveness of this technique [29–31].

Penetrating Aortic Ulcer and Intramural Hematoma

Two additional conditions occur that are related to aortic dissection, penetrating atherosclerotic ulcers and intramural hematomas. A penetrating aortic ulcer occurs when an atherosclerotic plaque penetrates the internal elastic lamina, allowing a hematoma to form within the vessel media. No intimal flap is present. These penetrating ulcers typically occur in elderly, hypertensive patients, predominantly in the descending aorta. An intramural hematoma results from a hemorrhage within the vasa vasorum.

Presentation

Both conditions have similar clinical presentations, but may represent two distinct entities.

Diagnosis and Treatment

Diagnosis is made with MRI, TEE, or CT scan. Because these lesions may lead to aortic rupture, the present treatment strategies of both lesions are similar to that of aortic dissections. Ascending lesions are treated surgically, while descending lesions are medically managed unless deemed unstable. Endovascular stenting has also been proposed as a treatment method, but further investigation is needed [32••,33–35].

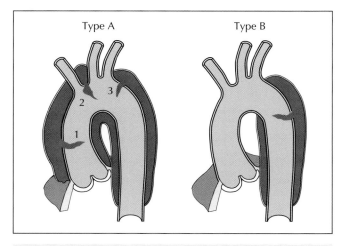

FIGURE 4 The DeBakey classification of aortic dissection. (*Adapted from* Miller *et al.* [38].)

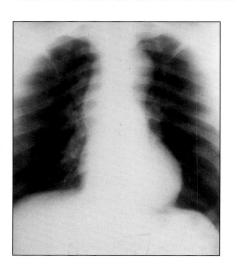

FIGURE 5 Posteroanterior chest radiograph demonstrating mediastinal widening caused by aortic dissection of the ascending aorta [39].

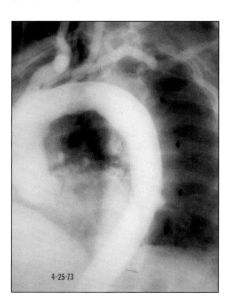

FIGURE 6 Ascending aortogram demonstrating type A aortic dissection [40].

WHEN TO REFER

Patients who are suspected of having aortic aneurysms or dissections should be referred to a cardiologist who specializes in vascular disease. Cardiac risk stratification will be needed in all patients, as many will have associated coronary artery disease. In the acute presentation of aortic dissection, the cardiology consultant will be needed to perform transesophageal echocardiography and, possibly, catheter-based diagnostic (angiography) and therapeutic (stent graft) procedures. Triage to vascular surgery will also be performed if surgical correction is warranted.

KEY REFERENCE

•• Coady MA, Rizzo JA, Elefteriades JA: Pathologic variants of thoracic aortic dissections. Penetrating atherosclerotic ulcers and intramural hematomas. *Cardiol Clin* 1999, 17:637–657.

Comprehensive review of penetrating aortic ulcers and intramural hematoma.

REFERENCES AND RECOMMENDED READING

Recently published papers of particular interest have been highlighted as:
•• Of outstanding interest

1. Littooy FN, Steffan G, Greisler HP, *et al.*: Use of sequential B-mode ultrasonography to manage abdominal aortic aneurysms. *Arch Surg* 1989, 124:419–421.

2. Shapira OM, Pasik S, Wassermann JP, *et al.*: Ultrasound screening for abdominal aortic aneurysms in patients with peripheral vascular disease. *J Cardiovasc Surg* 1990, 31:170–172.

3. Gomes MN, Choyke PL: Pre-operative evaluation of abdominal aortic aneurysms: ultrasound or computed tomography. *J Cardiovasc Surg* 1987, 28:159–166.

4. Pillari G, Chang JB, Zito J, *et al.*: Computed tomography of abdominal aortic aneurysm. *Arch Surg* 1988, 123:727–732.

5. Sterpetti AV, Schultz RD, Feldhaus RJ, *et al.*: Abdominal aortic aneurysm in elderly patients: selective management based on clinical status and aneurysmal expansion rate. *Am J Surg* 1985, 150:772–776.

6. Naevoid MP, Ballad DJ, Hailed J: Prognosis of abdominal aortic aneurysms: a population-based study. *N Engl J Med* 1989, 321:1009–1014.

7. Ernest CB: Abdominal aortic aneurysm. *N Engl J Med* 1993, 328:1167–1172.

8. Gadowski GR, Pilcher DB, Ricci MA: Abdominal aortic aneurysm expansion rate: Effect of size, beta-adrenergic blockade. *J Vasc Surg* 1994, 19:727.

9. Mortality results for randomized controlled trial of early elective surgery or ultrasonographic surveillance for small abdominal aneurysms. The UK Small Aneurysm Trial Participants. *Lancet* 1998, 352:1649–1655.

10. Powell JT, Greenhalgh RM: Small abdominal aortic aneurysms. *N Engl J Med* 2003, 348:1895.

11. Long-term outcomes of immediate repair compared with surveillance of small abdominal aortic aneuryms. *N Engl J Med* 2002, 346:1445–1452.

12. Lederle FA, Johnson GR, Wilson SE, *et al.*: Immediate repair compared with surveillance of small abdominal aortic aneurysms. *N Engl J Med* 2002, 346:1437–1444.

13. Brown LC, Powell JT: Risk factors for aneurysm rupture in patients kept under surveillance. UK Small Aneurysm Trial Participants. *Ann Surg* 1999, 230:289.

14. Blum U, Vosage G, Lammer J, *et al.*: Endoluminal stent-grafts for infrarenal abdominal aortic aneurysms. *N Engl J Med* 1997, 336:13.

15. Propranolol for small abdominal aortic aneurysms: results of a randomized trial. *J Vasc Surg* 2001, 35:72.

16. U.S. Preventive Services Task Force: *Guide to Clinical Preventive Services*, edn 2. Baltimore: Williams & Wilkins; 1996:67.

17. Scott RA: The Multicentre Aneurysm Screening Study (MASS) into the effect of abdominal aortic aneurysm screening on mortality in men: a randomised controlled trial. *Lancet* 2002, 360:1531.

18. Crawford ES, Cohen ES: Aortic aneurysm. A multifocal disease. *Arch Surg* 1982, 117:1393–1400.

19. Crawford ES, Crawford JL, Hazim SJ, *et al.*: Thoracoabdominal aortic aneurysms: preoperative and intraoperative factors determining immediate and long-term results of operations in 605 patients. *J Vasc Surg* 1986, 3:389–404.

20. Clouse WD, Hallet JW Jr, Schaff HV, *et al.*: Improved prognosis of thoracic aortic aneurysms: a population-based study. *JAMA* 1998 280:1926–1929.

21. Moreno-Cabral CE, Miller C, Mitchell S, *et al.*: Degenerative and atherosclerotic aneurysms of the thoracic aorta. *J Thorac Cardiovasc Surg* 1984, 88:1020–1032.

22. Dale JR, Pape LA, Cohn LH, *et al.*: Dissection of the aorta: pathogenesis, diagnosis, and treatment. *Prog Cardiovasc Dis* 1980, 23:237–242.

23. DeBakey ME, McCollum CH, Crawford ES, *et al.*: Dissection and dissecting aneurysms of the aorta: twenty year follow-up of five hundred twenty seven patients treated surgically. *Surgery* 1982, 92:1118–1134.

24. Erbel R, Delert H, Meyer J, *et al.*: Effect of medical and surgical therapy on aortic dissection evaluated by transesophageal echocardiography: implications for prognosis and therapy. *Circulation* 1993, 87:1604–1615.

25. Sommer T, Fehske W, Holzknecht N, *et al.*: Aortic dissection: a comparative study of diagnosis with spiral CT, multiplanar transesophageal echocardiography, and MR imaging. *Radiology* 1996, 19:347–352.

26. Masani ND, Banning AP, Jones RA, *et al.*: Follow-up of chronic thoracic aortic dissection: comparison of transesophageal echocardiography and magnetic resonance imaging. *Am Heart J* 1996, 131:1156–1163.

27. Chu VF, Chow CM, Stewart J, *et al.*: Transesophageal echocardiography for ascending aortic dissection: is it enough for surgical intervention? *J Card Surg* 1998, 13:250–265.

28. Losi MA, Betocchi S, Briguori C, *et al.*: Determinants of aortic artifacts during transesophageal echocardiography of the ascending aorta. *Am Heart J* 1999, 137:967–972.

29. Grabenwoger M, Hutschala D, Ehrlich MP, *et al.*: Thoracic aortic aneurysms: treatment with endovascular self-expandable stent grafts. *Ann Thorac Surg* 2000, 69:441–445.

30. Mitchell RS, Miller DC, Dake MD, *et al.*: Thoracic aortic aneurysm repair with an endovascular stent graft: the "first generation." *Ann Thorac Surg* 1999, 67:1971–1974.

31. Dake MD, Kato N, Mitchell RS, *et al.*: Endovascular stent-graft placement for the treatment of acute aortic dissection. *N Engl J Med* 1999, 340:1546–1552.

32.•• Coady MA, Rizzo JA, Elefteriades JA: Pathologic variants of thoracic aortic dissections. Penetrating atherosclerotic ulcers and intramural hematomas. *Cardiol Clin* 1999, 17:637–657.

33. Brittenden J, McBride K, McInnes G, *et al.*: The use of endovascular stents in the treatment of penetrating ulcers of the thoracic aorta. *J Vasc Surg* 1999, 30:946–949.

34. Vilacosta I, San Roman JA, Aragoncillo P, *et al.*: Penetrating atherosclerotic aortic ulcer: documentation by transesophageal echocardiography. J Am Coll Cardiol 1998, 32:83–89.

35. Coady MA, Rizzo JA, Hammond GL, *et al.*: Penetrating ulcer of the thoracic aorta: what is it? How do we recognize it? How do we manage it? *J Vasc Surg* 1998, 27:1006–1115.

36. Ciprano PR, Alonso DR, Baltaxe HA, Gay WA: Multiple aortic aneurysms in relapsing polychondritis. *Am J Cardiol* 1976, 37:1097–1102.

37. Eagle KA, De Sanctis RW: Aortic dissection. In *Current Problems in Cardiology*. Chicago: Year Book Medical Publisher; 1989:227–278.

38. Miller DC, Stinson EB, Oyer PE, *et al.*: Operative treatment of aortic dissections: experience with 125 patients over a sixteen-year period. *J Thorac Cardiovasc Surg* 1979, 78:365–369.

39. Kidd JN, Reul GJ, Cooley DA, *et al.*: Surgical treatment of aneurysms of the ascending aorta. *Circulation* 1976, 54(suppl 3):111–119.

40. Cigarroa JE, Isselbacher EM, DeSanctis RW, Eagle KA: Diagnostic imaging in the evaluation of suspected aortic dissection: old standards and new directions. *N Engl J Med* 1993, 328:35–43.

Diseases of Peripheral Arteries and Veins

John A. Spittell, Jr.
Peter C. Spittell

Key Points

- In addition to the evaluation of peripheral arterial pulsations, elevation-dependency tests provide confirmation of occlusive arterial disease in an extremity and a rough estimation of the degree of any ischemia.

- The most sensitive indicator of occlusive arterial disease in a lower extremity is an abnormal ankle:brachial index 1 minute after standard exercise.

- Arteriography is not necessary for the diagnosis of atherosclerotic occlusive peripheral arterial disease; it is indicated when restoration of pulsatile flow is planned.

- In the nondiabetic person with only intermittent claudication, restoration of pulsatile flow is elective.

- Features that suggest an uncommon type of occlusive peripheral arterial disease include a young person, involvement of the upper extremity and/or digits, and presentation as acute ischemia without prior symptoms of occlusive peripheral arterial disease.

- Atheroembolism (blue toes and livedo reticularis) may occur spontaneously from an atherosclerotic aorta or aneurysm, with the initiation of anticoagulant therapy, or follow arterial interventions or surgery.

- When venous thromboembolism recurs in the face of adequate anticoagulant effect, a secondary cause should be strongly suspected.

- Chronic indurated cellulitis (*ie*, lipodermatosclerosis), a complication of inadequately controlled chronic venous insufficiency, may mimic infection but can be relieved by adequate elastic support to the affected limb.

When symptomatic, diseases of peripheral arteries and veins cause pain, swelling, changes in skin color, or ulceration of the extremities or digits. The ease with which arterial and venous circulation of the extremities can be evaluated by physical examination and noninvasive methodology makes clinical diagnosis an office or bedside exercise in many cases.

DISEASES OF PERIPHERAL ARTERIES

Peripheral arterial disease is common and can present as either an acute or a chronic disorder, the latter being more common. Because occlusive and aneurysmal diseases are principally atherosclerotic in origin, they are the most frequently encountered disorders, but the less common types present the generalist with interesting diagnostic problems. Although the abnormalities presented by peripheral arterial disorders usually can be identified by a careful patient history and physical examination, noninvasive diagnostic studies are readily available to provide objective confirmation of clinical findings.

Occlusive Peripheral Arterial Disease

Occlusive peripheral arterial disease can be chronic or acute. The lower extremities are much more frequently involved than the upper extremities. Acute arterial occlusion can be thrombotic or embolic. Chronic occlusive arterial disease is most often caused by atherosclerosis, but thromboangiitis obliterans (Buerger's disease), giant cell arteritis, trauma, and external arterial compression (entrapment), although less common, are important for the clinician to keep in mind [1•,2].

Diagnosis

The classic feature of symptomatic occlusive arterial disease in the lower extremities is intermittent claudication, which is characterized by aching, cramping, or tiredness that occurs with walking and is relieved by standing still. It may be mimicked by musculoskeletal disorders, chiefly pseudo-claudication from lumbar spinal stenosis (Table 1). When more severe ischemia develops, the patient experiences pain at rest (ischemic rest pain) and, with even minor trauma, ischemic ulceration (Fig. 1, Table 2) occurs.

Reduced or absent pulsation of the extremity arteries is the classic physical finding in occlusive arterial disease. Arterial narrowing proximally may cause audible systolic bruits over large arteries, and when the lumen becomes more narrowed (usually > 80%) creating a gradient in diastole, the bruit may extend into diastole. A useful clinical estimate of the degree of ischemia can be obtained by observing development of pallor on elevation of the extremity and then the time required for return of color to the skin and the superficial veins to fill on dependency of the extremity or extremities after elevation (Table 3). In the

TABLE 1 CONDITIONS CONFUSED WITH INTERMITTENT CLAUDICATION

Site of claudication	Confused conditions
Foot	Foot strain
	Tight shoes
	Plantar neuroma
Calf	Muscle strain
	Flat feet
	Osteoarthritis of knee
Thigh	Sciatica
	Pseudoclaudication caused by spinal stenosis
Hip	Osteoarthritis of hip
	Pseudoclaudication caused by spinal stenosis

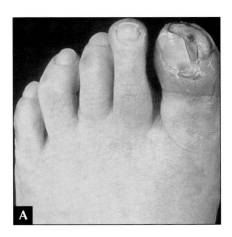 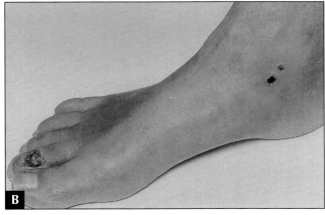

FIGURE 1 A, Ischemic ulceration, first toe. **B,** Ischemic ulceration, second toe and medial aspect of ankle.

TABLE 2 CHARACTERISTICS OF ISCHEMIC AND VENOUS STASIS ULCERATION

	Ischemic	Venous stasis
Location	Toe, heel, foot	Medial distal leg
Pain	Severe	Only when infected
Surrounding skin	± inflamed	Stasis pigmentation
Ulcer edge	Discrete	Shaggy
Ulcer base	Pale, eschar	Healthy

TABLE 3 OFFICE ESTIMATION OF THE DEGREE OF ISCHEMIA

Degree	Elevation pallor, *sec**	CR, *sec†*	VFT, *sec‡*
None	None in 60	10	15
Moderate	Pallor in 30–60	15–20	20–30
Severe	Pallor in < 30	40+	40+

*Elevation of extremity at an angle of 60° above level.
†Color return (CR) to skin of foot on dependency after elevation.
‡Superficial venous filling time (VFT) on dependency after elevation.

upper extremity, the Allen test (Fig. 2) to evaluate circulation in the hand and the thoracic outlet maneuvers (Fig. 3) are useful when occlusive arterial disease is present.

When taken with the patient supine using a standard blood pressure cuff and a handheld continuous-wave Doppler, the systolic brachial and ankle blood pressures provide an objective measure of lower extremity arterial circulation. Normally, the systolic blood pressure at the ankle exceeds that at the brachial level. When these pressures are determined before and after standard exercise (Table 4), functional as well as semiquantitative assessment of the

occlusive arterial disease can be made. In the office, as an alternative to a treadmill exercise study, one can determine the ankle:brachial index (ABI) before and after having the patient perform up to 50 consecutive plantar flexions in the erect posture [3]. Arteriography is usually not needed unless restoration of pulsatile flow is being considered or an unusual type of occlusive arterial disease is suspected.

Differential diagnosis

As noted, arteriosclerosis is by far the most common cause of occlusive peripheral arterial disease. Uncommon types of

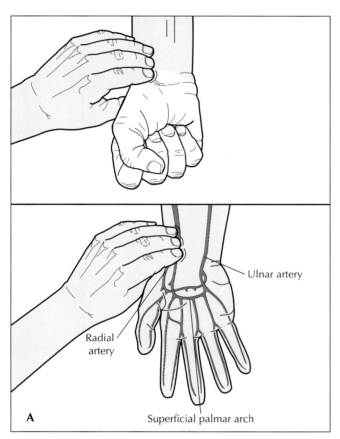

A

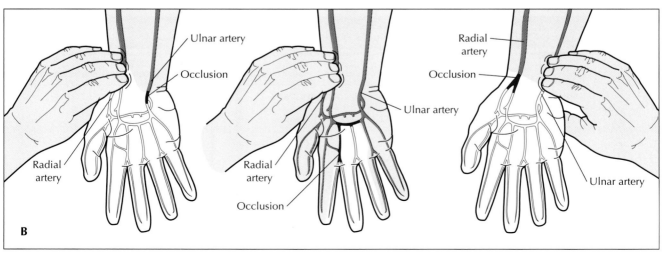

B

FIGURE 2 Allen test. **A,** Normal (negative) result, indicating patency of ulnar artery and superficial palmar arch. **B,** Abnormal (positive) results caused by occlusion of ulnar artery (*left*), superficial palmar arch (*bottom center*), and radial artery (*right*). (*Adapted from* Spittell [21].)

occlusive arterial disease are suggested by their occurrence in young persons, acute (often digital) ischemia, or associated systemic symptoms.

Atherosclerosis is more common in men over 40 years of age, particularly those with the risk factors of tobacco use, hyperlipidemia, or diabetes mellitus. It affects large and

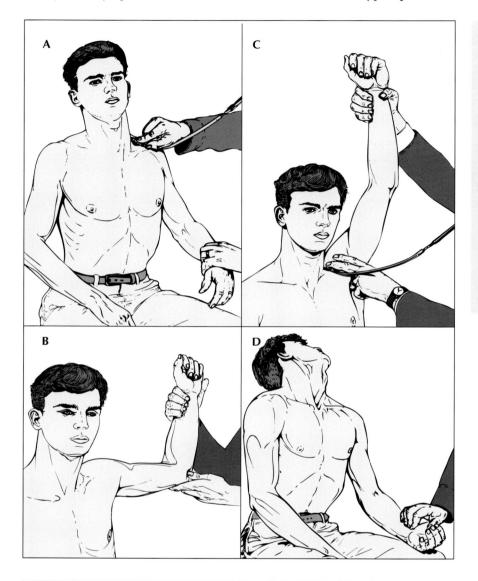

FIGURE 3 **A,** Costoclavicular maneuver, active. Auscultation over subclavian artery, above or below midportion of clavicle, may reveal systolic bruit as artery is compressed. Radial pulse and bruit over subclavian artery disappear when complete compression of subclavian artery occurs. **B,** Costoclavicular maneuver, passive. **C,** Hyperabduction maneuver. Axillary artery may be completely or incompletely compressed. In the latter case, bruit may be heard above or below the clavicle or, on occasion, deep in the axilla. **D,** Scalene or Adson maneuver. This test is used in both cervical rib or anomalous first thoracic rib syndrome and scalenus anticus syndrome. Auscultation over subclavian artery being tested may reveal bruit when the artery is partially compressed. (*Adapted from* Fairbairn [22].)

TABLE 4 NONINVASIVE LABORATORY ASSESSMENT OF ARTERIAL INSUFFICIENCY OF LEGS

	Standard exercise		Systolic blood pressure index*	
Degree of insufficiency	**Claudication**	**Duration,** *min*	**Before exercise**	**After exercise**
Minimal	0	5	Normal to mildly abnormal	Abnormal
Mild	Present	5	> 0.8	> 0.5
Moderate	Present	< 5	< 0.8	< 0.5
Severe†	Present	< 3	< 0.5	< 0.15

*Systolic pressure index is obtained by dividing the systolic ankle blood pressure by the systolic brachial blood pressure, both measured with the patient supine (normal, 0.95 or greater).
†Often, the systolic ankle blood pressure is less than 50 mm Hg.

Cardiology for the Primary Care Physician

medium-sized extremity arteries as well as the coronary and cerebral arteries.

Less common types of occlusive peripheral arterial disease include thromboangiitis obliterans (Buerger's disease), traumatic (repetitive, blunt-type) occlusive arterial disease in the hand, occlusive disease caused by compression of a peripheral artery (popliteal artery entrapment [Table 5] and thoracic outlet compression of the subclavian artery), and the arteritides (giant cell arteritis and connective tissue disorders). In connective tissue disorders, the occlusive disease is usually digital. Giant cell (temporal, cranial) arteritis affects persons over 50 years of age whose dominant symptoms are headache and those of a systemic illness, but at times it affects principally the subclavian arteries and other large arteries [4], whereas Takayasu's arteritis typically affects the branches of the aortic arch in young women.

Prognosis

Survival of persons with atherosclerosis is shortened due to associated coronary and cerebral artery disease. The risk of limb loss for the person without diabetes whose only symptom is intermittent claudication is approximately 5% in 5 years; when the ischemia is more severe (ischemic pain at rest or ischemic ulcer), the risk is approximately 12% in 5 years [5]. When arteriosclerosis obliterans (ASO) is symptomatic in the person with diabetes, the prognosis for limb loss is approximately fourfold that of the person without diabetes [6].

In thromboangiitis obliterans, the risk of limb loss is greater than in ASO. It depends mainly on the severity of the ischemia at the time of diagnosis and whether the patient stops using tobacco permanently.

In chronic occlusive arterial disease caused by repetitive, blunt trauma to the hand, loss of digits can occur if the cause is not recognized and corrected (Fig. 4). Limb or digital loss can occur with arterial compression syndromes as a result of embolization from mural thrombus that develops in the poststenotic aneurysm caused by chronic arterial compression. In occlusive arterial disease due to arteritis, frequency of limb loss depends on the severity of ischemia at the time of diagnosis and how much control over the arteritis is achieved.

Management

Definitive management of chronic occlusive arterial disease should be individualized according to its etiology, severity,

---

TABLE 5 CLINICAL FEATURES OF LESS COMMON TYPES OF OCCLUSIVE PERIPHERAL ARTERIAL DISEASE
Thromboangiitis obliterans (Buerger's disease)
Men affected more than women
Tobacco use
Age < 30 y
Small arteries upper and lower extremities involved
Claudication of arch or calf
Migratory superficial phlebitis common
Occlusive arterial disease of hands from repetitive blunt trauma
Often occupational—tools, "hammerhand"
Dominant hand
Tobacco use (predisposing factor)
Popliteal artery entrapment
Young men affected more than women
Symptoms unilateral
Calf pain with walking not running
Decreased or absent pedal pulses
Diagnosis by magnetic resonance angiography
Thoracic outlet compression
Clinical presentations
Mass, supraclavicular area
Unilateral Raynaud's
Unilateral digital ischemia
Axillary-subclavian vein thrombosis

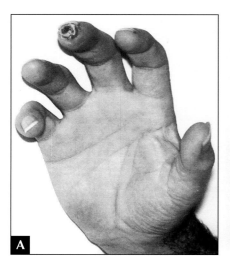
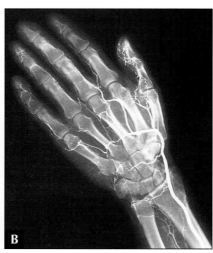

FIGURE 4 Right hand of a 42-year-old, right-handed millwright. **A,** Ischemic ulceration of the finger. **B,** Arteriogram showing a narrowed ulnar artery and occlusion of the ulnar portion of the superficial palmar arch.

disability, and prognosis, but the physician should have all patients take general measures to protect the ischemic limb from trauma and avoid vasoconstrictive influences. These general measures include the following:

1. Stop tobacco use,
2. Avoid trauma,
3. Wear proper footwear,
4. Attend to regular foot care and hygiene,
5. Walk on a regular basis,
6. Avoid vasoconstriction, and
7. Control atherosclerosis risk factors.

For all persons, conservative measures are indicated; control of risk factors (hyperlipidemia, hypertension, and diabetes) is indicated to delay progression of the atherosclerosis. The importance of discontinuing tobacco use should be emphasized. Continued smoking increases the risk of limb loss tenfold [5]. A regular walking program may increase the walking distance [7], and pharmacotherapy [8,9] may provide additional symptomatic relief of intermittent claudication. Careful attention to foot care and hygiene as well as selection of proper footwear is important. In the management of associated coronary disease and hypertension, drugs that may cause vasoconstriction are best avoided when alternative agents can be safely used. An antiplatelet agent should be used by all patients with intermittent claudication unless contraindicated.

In persons with traumatic occlusive disease, measures to protect the hand (regular use of gloves and avoiding blunt trauma) in addition to general measures are important to prevent progression. If ischemic ulceration has already occurred, an α-blocking agent or sympathectomy can be used to hasten healing and may provide longer-term protection of the ischemic digit [10]. When occlusive arterial disease is caused by arteritis, management should include therapy of the systemic process and general measures to protect the ischemic limb.

When to refer

In symptomatic atherosclerosis obliterans, restoration of pulsatile flow by either arterial surgery or percutaneous intervention can be used to relieve disabling claudication in the nondiabetic person. It is also indicated (when feasible) for the management of ischemic rest pain, ischemic ulceration, and symptomatic occlusive arterial disease in persons with diabetes. The frequency of coronary artery disease as a comorbid condition must always be kept in mind during preoperative evaluation and risk stratification if restoration of pulsatile flow is planned for persons with atherosclerotic occlusive peripheral arterial disease [11,12]. The appropriate management of arterial compression syndromes is surgical relief.

Acute Peripheral Arterial Occlusion

Acute occlusion of a peripheral artery can be thrombotic or embolic. Symptoms can be dramatic with one or all of the five *P*'s (pain, pallor, paresthesia, paralysis, and pulseless) or may be more subtle (*eg*, abrupt onset of intermittent claudi-

cation or shortening of walking distance in a person with existing claudication). The distinction between embolic and thrombotic arterial occlusion is frequently inferential (Table 6) but may be important, as either type can be a clue to an otherwise occult systemic or cardiovascular disorder.

Differential diagnosis

The differential diagnosis of acute peripheral arterial occlusion includes arterial spasm from drugs (*eg*, ergotism) or associated with extensive, acute, deep venous thrombosis (Table 6).

Management

Initial management of acute arterial occlusion should include protection of the ischemic limb (do not heat, cool, or elevate) and heparin therapy to protect the collateral circulation while the etiology is being determined. Definitive management options include thrombolytic therapy, surgical thromboembolectomy, or antithrombotic therapy. Factors influencing the choice of therapy include size of the artery occluded, condition of the limb, etiology of the occlusion, and the general and cardiac status of the patient. Atheroembolism from proximal aortic or arterial atherosclerotic plaques or aneurysms is now being recognized with increasing frequency as a result of improving noninvasive imaging techniques, particularly transesophageal echocardiography [13].

Features suggestive of atheroembolism include livedo reticularis, cyanotic digits, hypertension, renal insufficiency, transient eosinophilia, and an elevated sedimentation rate. In addition to hypertension, atherosclerotic disease, and a history of smoking, an elevated level of C-reactive protein (CRP) is associated with an increased incidence of atheroembolism complicating cardiac catheterization, so that determining CRP before the procedure may identify patients with soft, friable atherosclerotic plaques who are at increased risk of postprocedure atheroembolism [14].

TABLE 6 ACUTE ARTERIAL OCCLUSION
Conditions suggesting embolic arterial occlusion
Heart failure
Atrial fibrillation
Recent myocardial infarction
Proximal atherosclerosis
Proximal arterial aneurysm
Conditions suggesting thrombotic arterial occlusion
Symptomatic peripheral arterial disease
Acute arterial trauma
Myeloproliferative disease
Active arteritis
Acute aortic dissection

When to refer
Management is difficult unless the origin of the atheroembolic material can be surgically removed.

Peripheral Arterial Aneurysm
Like occlusive peripheral arterial disease, arterial aneurysms are most often atherosclerotic, more frequent in lower than in upper extremity arteries, and much more common in men than in women.

Diagnosis
Until an aneurysm becomes symptomatic as a result of complications (Table 7), the diagnosis depends on a careful physical examination or incidental recognition on radiography or ultrasonography performed for some other reason. Iliac artery aneurysms are usually associated with abdominal aortic aneurysms. Symptomatic iliac artery aneurysms may cause groin or perineal pain, iliac vein obstruction, or obstructive urologic symptoms [15].

Aneurysms of the femoral and popliteal arteries rarely occur in women. Popliteal aneurysms are bilateral approximately 50% of the time, and in over 40% of cases, they are associated with aneurysms elsewhere in the body, most often the abdominal area.

Differential diagnosis
Peripheral artery aneurysm may be confused with other types of mass, but differentiation is readily made with ultrasonography.

When to refer
Untreated peripheral artery aneurysms frequently produce complications, most often thromboembolic, that may threaten the limb, so elective surgical treatment before complications occur gives the best results. Arteriography before surgery is needed to evaluate the arterial circulation proximal and distal to the aneurysm.

DISEASES OF VEINS
Clinicians are appropriately most interested in acute deep venous thrombosis because of its embolic potential, but other disorders of veins (varicose veins and chronic venous insufficiency) are frequent causes of complications and morbidity, much of which can be prevented by proper management.

TABLE 7 COMPLICATIONS OF ANEURYSMS

Pressure on surrounding structures
Thrombosis
Distal embolization
Rupture
Infection

Venous Thrombosis
Both superficial and deep venous thrombosis are important clinical events from the diagnostic and therapeutic aspects.

Diagnosis
Superficial thrombophlebitis, presenting as a reddened, tender nodule or cord in the course of a superficial vein, is readily diagnosed on physical examination; however, if there is concern about the diagnosis of superficial thrombophlebitis, it can be confirmed or excluded by ultrasound. Deep venous thrombosis, however, is notorious for its variable clinical manifestations depending on the location and extent of the venous occlusion. Symptoms may include pain or swelling in the limb, and findings on physical examination may include tenderness over the involved vein and, when proximal to the calf, pitting edema distally and increased superficial (collateral) venous pattern.

The variability of clinical findings have made duplex ultrasonography the diagnostic procedure of choice in proximal deep vein thrombosis [16], but when only calf veins are involved, contrast venography remains the diagnostic gold standard. Impedance plethysmography is a useful noninvasive diagnostic test for deep vein obstruction, particularly in cases of recurrent proximal deep venous thrombosis.

Differential diagnosis
Superficial thrombophlebitis is easily differentiated from acute lymphangitis, because the latter is accompanied by chills and high fever. Occasionally, nodular conditions (erythema nodosum or vasculitis) require biopsy to confidently differentiate them.

Deep venous thrombosis involves a much more complicated differential diagnosis that includes nonthrombotic (chronic) venous obstruction, sciatica, muscle strain or tear, and acute lymphangitis and cellulitis. Unless physical findings, noninvasive diagnostic studies or duplex ultrasonsgraphy permit confident differential diagnosis, contrast venography is necessary.

Management
Therapy of superficial thrombophlebitis is basically symptomatic: local warm moist packs, analgesics, and elevation of the extremity. If the process extends despite such treatment, a short course of oral anticoagulant therapy may be used to effect resolution.

Therapy for acute deep venous thrombosis continues to be heparin initially, followed by oral anticoagulant therapy for 3 or preferably 6 months [17]. Treatment of selected patients with proximal deep vein thrombosis with low-molecular weight heparin on an outpatient basis is an alternative [18,19]. Thrombolytic therapy is usually reserved for acute, extensive, deep venous thrombosis (*eg*, axillary subclavian vein thrombosis or phlegmasia cerulea dolens [Fig. 5] in young persons to obtain rapid resolution and lessen the chances of venous valvular damage). Anticoagulant therapy must be instituted as soon as thrombolytic

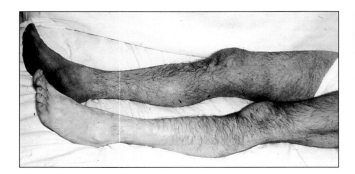

FIGURE 5 Phlegmasia cerulea dolens (extensive venous thrombosis of the whole right lower extremity).

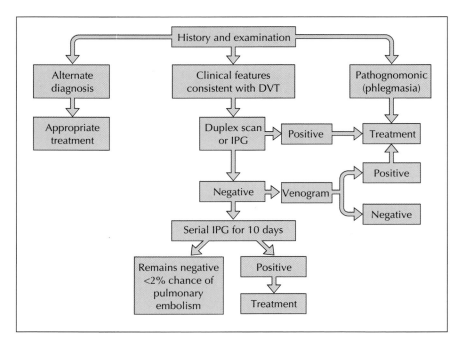

FIGURE 6 Algorithm for clinically suspected deep venous thrombosis (DVT). IPG—impedance plethysmography.

TABLE 8 RECURRENT VENOUS THROMBOSIS	
Primary (idiopathic)	**Coagulation disorders**
Familial	Hereditary
Nonfamilial	Activated protein C
	resistance [23]
Secondary	Antithrombin III deficiency
Thromboangiitis obliterans	ciency
Ulcerative bowel disease	Protein C deficiency
Myeloproliferative disease	Protein S deficiency
Connective tissue disease	Dysfibrinoginemia
Oral contraceptives	20210A allele of
Neoplasms	prothrombin gene [24]
Hyperhomocysteinemia	Acquired antiphospholipid
	antibody syndromes
	Circulating anticoagulant
	with systemic lupus
	Nonlupus types

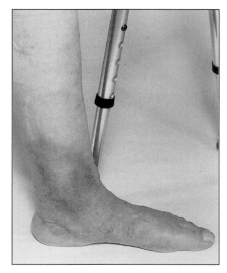

FIGURE 7 Chronic indurated cellulitis.

therapy ends so as to prevent rethrombosis. An algorithm for management of the patient with suspected deep venous thrombosis is shown in Figure 6.

Recurring superficial or deep venous thrombosis is an important clinical problem, both diagnostically and therapeutically. Causes that need to be considered are shown in Table 8. Oral anticoagulant therapy provides effective management of the primary types and coagulation disorders, but particularly in secondary types, recurrences may occur despite adequate oral anticoagulant therapy. Long-term anticoagulant therpay is generally indicated for persons whose initial thromboembolic episode was life threatening, for persons with more than one allelic coagulation abnormality (such as a combination of heterozygous Leiden mutation for factor V and the prothrombin G 20210A mutation), and for persons who experience two or more episodes of venous thromboembolism [20].

When to refer
Recurrent superficial phlebitis of a varicose vein is generally an indication for surgical removal.

Chronic Venous Insufficiency
An important and often neglected sequel of deep venous thrombosis is chronic deep venous insufficiency resulting from postphlebitic venous stasis. Regular use of properly fitted, adequate (30 to 40 mm Hg compression at the ankle) elastic stockings can prevent complications of chronic venous insufficiency.

The generalist is likely to be consulted by the patient who develops chronic tender induration of the medial distal leg because of uncontrolled chronic deep venous insufficiency (Fig. 7). The reddened, tender, indurated features of this complication (termed *lipodermatosclerosis* or *chronic indurated cellulitis*) suggest infection, but the problem is chronic venous stasis and its management the use of adequate support (Fig. 8) when the patient is ambulatory. The process gradually recedes with use of good elastic support over a foam pad for a period of several weeks. When resolved, recurrence can be prevented by the regular, daily use of adequate elastic support when ambulatory.

Venous stasis ulceration (Fig. 9), when early and small (< 1.0 cm), often can be managed on an ambulatory basis with the same type of elastic support described for chronic indurated cellulitis applied over a sterile dressing. Larger stasis ulcers are best managed by rest and elevation with moist dressings (sterile normal saline or 0.25% aluminum subacetate) until clean and, if needed, skin grafting. After healing, adequate elastic support (described earlier), often with the addition of a foam pad over the previously ulcerated area, should be used when ambulatory.

Varicose Veins
Varicose veins are the most common venous disorder seen by the generalist. They may be primary or secondary to postphlebitic chronic deep venous insufficiency. Obesity, pregnancy, and right heart failure are aggravating factors.

Frequently, the only complaint of the patient with varicose veins is cosmetic. Others may complain of "heaviness" in the affected leg or dependent edema.

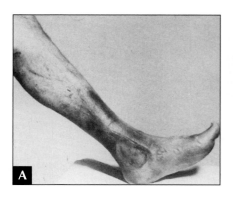
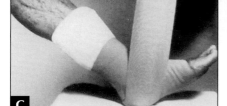
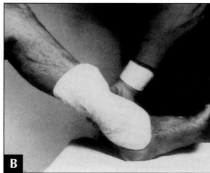
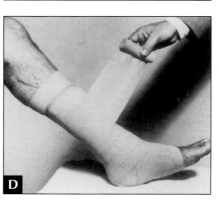

FIGURE 8 A–D, Application of foam pad under bandage for treatment of chronic indurated cellulitis or small venous stasis ulceration (*From* Juergens and Lofgren [25]; with permission.)

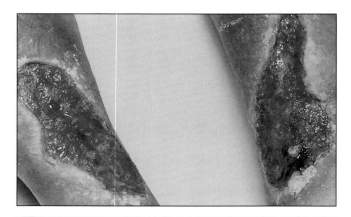

FIGURE 9 Large venous stasis ulcerations of both lower extremities.

Distinction between primary and secondary varicose veins is important if surgical treatment is being considered. Associated chronic deep venous insufficiency can be identified by Doppler ultrasonography of deep veins if surgical treatment of the varicose veins is an option.

Management

Use of adequate elastic support is indicated for asymptomatic primary varicose veins and for those associated with chronic deep venous insufficiency. Sclerotherapy may be used for minor primary varicose veins and for cutaneous venous stars.

When to refer

Surgical treatment (stripping) is indicated for primary varicose veins causing symptoms and when there is recurrent acute superficial varicose vein thrombophlebitis. Surgery is also indicated to remove large varicosities for cosmetic reasons.

REFERENCES AND RECOMMENDED READING

Recently published papers of particular interest have been highlighted as:

• Of interest

1.• Spittell JA Jr: Peripheral arterial disease. *Dis Mon* 1994, 40:641–704.

2. Spittell JA Jr: Some uncommon types of occlusive peripheral arterial disease. *Curr Probl Cardiol* 1983, 8:3–35.

3. McPhail IR, Spittell PC, Weston SA, *et al.*: Intermittent claudication: an office-based assessment. *J Am Coll Cardiol* 2001, 37:1381–1385.

4. Weyand CM, Goronzy JJ: Giant-cell arteritis and polymyalgia rheumatica. *Ann Intern Med* 2003, 139:505–515.

5. McDaniel MD, Cronenwett JL: Basic data related to natural history of intermittent claudication. *Ann Vasc Surg* 1989, 3:273–277.

6. Reiber GE, Pecoraro RE, Koepsell TD: Risk factors for amputation in patients with diabetes. *Ann Intern Med* 1992, 117:97–105.

7. Gardner AW, Poehlman ET: A longterm walking program is the optimal exercise for increasing endurance in claudication pain. A meta-analysis. *JAMA* 1995, 274:975–980.

8. Lindgarde F, Jehres R, Bjorkman H, *et al.*: Conservative drug treatments in patients with moderately severe chronic occlusive peripheral arterial disease. *Circulation* 1989, 80:1549–1556.

9. Dawson DL, Cutler BS, Meissner MH, Stranduess DE: Cilastazol has beneficial effects in treatment of intermittent claudication. Results from a multicenter, randomized, prospective, double-blind trial. *Circulation* 1998, 98:678–686.

10. Spittell PC, Spittell JA Jr: Occlusive arterial disease of the hand due to repetitive blunt trauma. *Int J Cardiol* 1993, 38:281–292.

11. Gersh BJ, Rihal CS, Rooke TW, Ballard DJ: Evaluation and management of patients with both peripheral vascular and coronary artery disease. *J Am Coll Cardiol* 1991, 18:203–214.

12. ACC/AHA Task Force Report: Guidelines for perioperative cardiovascular evaluation for noncardiac surgery. *Circulation* 1996, 93:1278–1317.

13. Kronzon I, Tuvick PA: Atheromatous disease of the thoracic aorta: Pathologic and clinical implication. *Ann Intern Med* 1997, 126:629–637.

14. Fukumoto Y, Tsutsui H, Tsuchihashi M, *et al.*: The incidence and risk factors of cholesterol embolization syndrome, a complication of cardiac catheterization: a prospective study. *J Am Coll Cardiol* 2003, 42:211–216.

15. Lipoff O, Hoover EL, Diaz C, *et al.*: Initial report of a mycotic aneurysm of the common iliac artery with compression of the ipsilateral ureter and femoral vein. *Texas Heart Inst J* 1986, 13:321–324.

16. Heliboer H, Bueller HR, Lansing AWA, *et al.*: A comparison of real-time compression ultrasonography with impedance plethysmography for the diagnosis of deep-vein thrombosis in symptomatic outpatients. *N Engl J Med* 1993, 329:1365–1369.

17. Verstraete M: The diagnosis and treatment of deep-vein thrombosis. *N Engl J Med* 1993; 329:1418–1419.

18. Levine M, Gent M, Hirsh J, *et al.*: A comparison of low molecular weight heparin administered primarily at home with unfractionated heparin administered in the hospital for proximal deep vein thrombosis. *N Engl J Med* 1996, 334:677–681.

19. Litin SC, Heit JA, Mees KA: Use of low-molecular weight heparin in the treatment of venous thromboembolic disease: answers to frequently asked questions. *Mayo Clin Proc* 1998, 73:545–550.

20. Bauer KA: The thrombophilias: well-defined risk factors with uncertain therapeutic implications. *Ann Intern Med* 2001, 135:367–373.

21. Spittell JA Jr: Occlusive peripheral arterial disease: guidelines for office management. *Postgrad Med* 1982, 71:137–151.

22. Fairbairn JF II: Clinical manifestations of peripheral vascular disease. In *Peripheral Vascular Diseases*, edn 5. Edited by Juergens JL, Spittell JA Jr, Fairbairn JF II. Philadelphia: WB Saunders; 1972:4–25.

23. Nichols WL, Heit JA: Activated protein C resistance and thrombosis. *Mayo Clin Proc* 1996, 71:897–898.

24. Poort SR, Rosendaal FR, Reitsma PH, Bertma RM: A common genetic variation in the 3-untranslated region of the prothrombin gene is associated with elevated plasma prothrombin levels and an increase in venous thrombosis. *Blood* 1996, 88:3698–3703.

25. Juergens JL, Lofgren KA: Chronic venous insufficiency. In *Peripheral Vascular Disease*, edn 5. Edited by Juergens JL, Spittell JA Jr, Fairbairn JF II. Philadelphia: WB Saunders; 1980:820.

SELECT BIBLIOGRAPHY

Bergan JJ, Yao JST: *Venous Disorders.* Philadelphia: WB Saunders; 1991.

Klugherz B, Mobler ER: Current and emerging therapies for lower extremity peripheral arterial disease. *ACC Curr J Rev* 2000, 9:37–39.

Spittell JA Jr: *Contemporary Issues in Peripheral Vascular Disease. Cardiovascular Clinics.* Philadelphia: FA Davis; 1992.

Spittell JA: *Peripheral Vascular Disease for Cardiologists: A Clinical Approach.* Elmsford, NY: Blackwell Publishing, Inc./Futura Division; 2003.

Anticoagulation, Acute and Chronic: Indications and Methods

39

Jack E. Ansell

Key Points

- Failure to rapidly achieve a therapeutic level of heparin therapy is remedied by the use of heparin-dosing nomograms.
- The activated partial thromboplastin time is highly inaccurate unless ex vivo heparin titration curves are used to establish a reagent-specific therapeutic range.
- The advantages of low molecular weight heparin (LMWH) over unfractionated heparin relate to its subcutaneous use, the ability to perform daily dosing once or twice, and the absence of the need for monitoring.
- Studies now document the equivalency or even superiority of LMWH over unfractionated heparin for the treatment of acute deep venous thrombosis. Home therapy is becoming a standard means of treating venous thromboembolism.
- Warfarin therapy is associated with the fewest complications when management is performed by a coordinated system of oversight referred to as an anticoagulation management service.
- Future models of warfarin management include patient self-testing and patient self-management.
- Studies of new oral and parenteral anticoagulants are promising and may substantially change how we treat patients with thrombotic disorders.

Three major classes of antithrombotic drugs are currently in use: anticoagulants, antiplatelet agents, and thrombolytic or fibrinolytic agents. Thrombolytic agents have a direct effect on thrombi by hastening their dissolution, whereas anticoagulants and antiplatelet agents are always prophylactic in that they prevent de novo initiation of thrombosis (primary prophylaxis) or that they prevent extension of established thrombi (secondary prophylaxis). This chapter focuses on those anticoagulant agents of greatest current value: unfractionated heparin, low molecular weight heparin (LMWH), and warfarin, but will also briefly discuss new agents recently approved and others on the horizon.

Anticoagulation entered the therapeutic arena in the mid-1930s with the first clinical use of unfractionated heparin, a drug discovered more than 15 years earlier [1]. Shortly thereafter, the first coumarin-derived oral anticoagulant, dicoumarol, was isolated, and in 1941, it was first put to clinical use [2]. Some 35 years later, further refinements of unfractionated heparin resulted in the identification of LMWH as a suitable anticoagulant with properties more favorable than standard heparin [3•]. Most recently, a further refinement of the heparin molecule came about with the development and approval of fondaparinux [4••]. Unfractionated heparin and LMWH have an immediate onset of action and are indicated for the treatment of acute thromboembolic disorders. Fondaparinux has similar qualities but is currently only approved for prophylaxis in orthopedic surgery. The coumarins have a delayed onset of action of several days and are indicated primarily for the long-term treatment of chronic thromboembolic disorders. All agents are also used for primary prophylaxis in patients at risk.

As we enter the 21st century, we are on the verge of even more dramatic changes in how thromboembolic disorders are treated. There are a number of new antithrombotics or modifications of older agents that have direct inhibitory effects on coagulation factors, can be given orally, and may not require monitoring. These agents have the potential to make our current modalities obsolete. The next few years will be an exciting chapter in the long history of antithrombotic therapy.

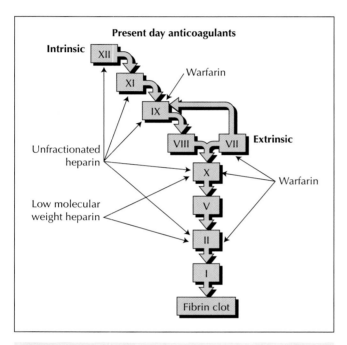

Present day anticoagulants

FIGURE 1 A simplified scheme of the coagulation cascade indicating the factors sensitive to heparin–antithrombin neutralization and the vitamin K–dependent factors reduced by warfarin therapy.

HEPARIN

Unfractionated heparin, also referred to simply as heparin, is a glycosaminoglycan made up of repeating disaccharide units of D-glucosamine and uronic acid with a wide range in molecular weights from 5000 to 30,000 daltons [5]. It is commercially derived primarily from bovine lung or porcine intestinal mucosa. Heparin mediates its effect by binding to a plasma protein, antithrombin (AT, formerly called antithrombin III), altering its conformation and thus enabling AT to bind more rapidly and neutralize the serine protease coagulation factors (IIa, IXa, Xa, XIa, and XIIa) (Fig. 1). Its predominant activity is directed toward factors Xa and IIa. Heparin also binds to another inhibitor, heparin cofactor II, whose principal substrate is thrombin. Heparin contains a unique pentasaccharide essential for binding to AT. To neutralize thrombin, the serine protease must bind to both AT and heparin, forming a ternary complex (Fig. 2). This dual binding requires a minimal chain length of 18 monosaccharides. Factor Xa does not require simultaneous binding to heparin when bound to AT, and thus smaller heparin chain lengths (containing the critical pentasaccharide) can serve to neutralize Xa. Heparin has a half-life of approximately 1 hour after an intravenous bolus. The half-life increases with increasing doses. Heparin is metabolized in part by the liver and is partially excreted by the kidneys [5].

Indications

Heparin is generally indicated as secondary prophylaxis in the treatment of acute thromboembolic disorders (*eg*, deep venous thrombosis [DVT] or pulmonary embolism [PE]), or as primary prophylaxis when an increased risk of thromboembolism exists (*eg*, in surgical patients at risk for postoperative thromboembolism) [6]. Heparin is also used extensively for patients undergoing cardiovascular procedures, percutaneous coronary interventions, and during acute coronary syndromes. The dose and method of

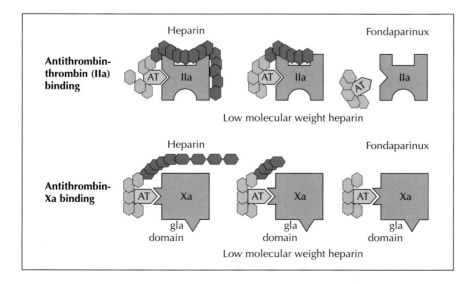

FIGURE 2 Schematic representation of the differential mechanism of heparin-antithrombin's neutralizing effect on thrombin (IIa) and factor Xa compared with the action of low molecular weight heparin and the action of fondaparinux. AT—antithrombin.

administration are determined by the underlying condition and whether it is for primary or secondary prophylaxis. The principal indications for heparin therapy are outlined in Table 1.

Dosing

Although heparin has been an important anticoagulant for over 60 years, it has significant drawbacks as identified in Table 2. Many of these drawbacks are eliminated or reduced

TABLE 1 RECOMMENDED ANTITHROMBOTIC TREATMENT FOR VARIOUS INDICATIONS	
Venous thromboembolic disease	
Prevention of venous thromboembolism	
Low-risk surgery patients	Early ambulation
Moderate-risk general surgery patients	Elastic stockings or intermittent pneumatic compression or low-dose UFH (5000 U SC q12h)
High-risk general surgery patients	Low-dose UFH (q8h) or LMWH
Very high-risk general surgery patients	Low-dose UFH or LMWH combined with intermittent pneumatic compression
Hip and knee joint replacement	LMWH, warfarin (INR 2.0–3.0), adjusted dose SQ UFH, or fondaparinux
Treatment of venous thromboembolism	
Deep venous thrombosis or pulmonary embolism	Acute: UFH IV or adjusted dose SQ sufficient to prolong the activated partial thromboplastin time to a plasma heparin level of 0.2–0.7 U/mL (depending on heparin assay)
	LMWH may be used in place of UFH (dosage varies with product)
	Long-term: Warfarin to maintain an INR 2.0–3.0 for at least 3 months
Arterial thromboembolic disease	
Atrial fibrillation	Warfarin to maintain an INR 2.0–3.0 in high-risk patients (age > 65, previous TIA or stroke, hypertension, heart failure, clinical coronary artery disease, mitral stenosis or prosthetic heart valve, diabetes, or thyrotoxicosis)
Valvular heart disease	
Rheumatic mitral valve disease	Aspirin can be used in low-risk patients
Aortic valve disease	History of systemic embolism or AF: warfarin (INR 2.0–3.0)
Mitral valve prolapse	History of TIA: ASA (160–325 mg/d)
	History of TIA on ASA, systemic embolism, or AF: Oral anticoagulation (INR 2.0–3.0)
	Ticlopidine (or clopidogrel) if warfarin contraindicated
Mitral annular calcification	History of systemic embolism or AF: Oral anticoagulation (INR 2.0–3.0)
Prosthetic heart valves	
Mechanical	Oral anticoagulation (INR 2.5–3.5); consider addition of ASA (80 mg/d) in high-risk patients; consider higher INR in patients with caged ball or disc valve prostheses
	History of systemic embolism: Oral anticoagulation and ASA
Bioprosthetic heart valves	
Mitral position	Oral anticoagulation (INR 2.0–3.0) for 3 months
Aortic position	Oral anticoagulation optional for first 3 months; if not used, consider ASA (325 mg/d)
With AF, systemic embolism or atrial thrombus	Oral anticoagulation (INR 2.0–3.0)
Coronary artery disease	
Myocardial infarction (acute)	
Post-MI (long-term)	ASA (160–325 mg/d) indefinitely unless oral anticoagulation used (warfarin with INR 2.5–3.5)
	Oral anticoagulation (INR 2.5–3.5) in high-risk patients (anterior Q-wave MI, severe left ventricular dysfunction, CHF, mural thrombosis/systemic embolism) for up to 3 months

AF—atrial fibrillation; ASA—aspirin; CHF—congestive heart failure; INR—international normalized ratio; IV—intravenously; LMWH—low molecular weight heparin; MI—myocardial infarction; SQ—subcutaneously; TIA—transient ischemic attack; UFH—unfractionated heparin.

by LMWH as discussed later in this chapter. A major problem with the administration of heparin is the failure to achieve a therapeutic level of anticoagulation early in the course of treatment [7,8,9•,10]. This is principally the result of inadequate dosing to counter the effect of nonspecific heparin binding to plasma proteins and endothelial cells [5]. To remedy this situation, a number of investigators have developed heparin dosing nomograms to standardize therapy across patients and dose adjustments within individual patients [8,9•,10]. These nomograms, some of which are weight based whereas others call for fixed dosing, achieve more rapid therapeutic levels of heparin by requiring higher loading and maintenance doses of the drug. Table 3 outlines a popular dosing nomogram developed by Raschke *et al.* [9•], but others are also available [6].

Monitoring

Another important aspect of therapy is an understanding of the limitations of the activated partial thromboplastin time (aPTT) as a measure of heparin effect. The aPTT's response to heparin is highly dependent on the reagent used in the test (similar to the variability of the prothrombin time [PT] in response to warfarin anticoagulation with different thromboplastins) [6]. There is no conversion or normalizing formula as exists for the PT. Thus, every laboratory is obligated to perform an in vitro or ex vivo heparin titration curve with the reagent currently in use (even with new lots of reagent from the same manufacturer) and establish the reagent-specific therapeutic range (equivalent to 0.2–0.7 U/mL of heparin depending on the type of titration curve used) [11].

Heparin-induced Thrombocytopenia

Besides the complication of bleeding, the major adverse effect of heparin is heparin-induced thrombocytopenia and thrombosis (HITT) [12••]. This phenomenon is due to heparin binding to an endogenous platelet protein, platelet factor 4 (PF4), and eliciting an immune response to a newly created epitope [13]. The binding of IgG to the heparin-PF4 complex leads to clustering of Fc receptors on the platelet surface, binding to these Fc receptors and activation of platelets. Binding of immunoglobulin leads not only to platelet destruction and thrombocytopenia, which by itself is rarely a problem, but it can lead to platelet clumping, thrombosis, and vascular occlusion in either the venous or arterial circulation, with the potential for catastrophic ischemic events [14•]. Once this problem is recognized, heparin therapy must be stopped immediately and, if necessary, an alternative anticoagulant substituted. Two recommended and approved therapeutic alternatives include lepirudin, a direct inactivator of thrombin that binds tightly to thrombin's enzymatic and fibrin binding sites [15,16•], and argatroban, a small molecule direct inhibitor of thrombin that binds reversibly to thrombin's enzymatic site [17,18]. Both drugs are given intravenously and require monitoring. Lepirudin is excreted by the kidney while argatroban is metabolized by the liver. HITT occurs with a frequency of approximately 3% to 5% in patients treated with intravenous heparin for 5 or more days. It can, however, occur at shorter intervals in patients with recent heparin exposure (3 months) [19•] and can also occur in patients receiving subcutaneous therapy or even heparin flushes used to maintain catheter patency. It appears more frequently with bovine lung–derived heparin. Platelet counts should be monitored at baseline in all patients who receive heparin and repeated approximately every 2 or 3 days thereafter in patients receiving intravenous therapy. The ideal frequency of assessing platelet counts in patients receiving low-dose subcutaneous heparin is unknown, but periodic checks are recommended.

LOW MOLECULAR WEIGHT HEPARIN

Low molecular weight heparin is a fragment of unfractionated heparin and is produced by chemical or enzymatic depolymerization of unfractionated heparin [3•]. Various preparations are available, most with an average molecular

TABLE 2 DRAWBACKS OF THERAPY WITH UNFRACTIONATED HEPARIN

Short half-life when given IV; longer when given SQ, but absorption is variable. Therefore usually given by continuous IV infusion.

Binds to plasma proteins, endothelial cells, leukocytes, and platelets, leading to poor recovery and variable aPTT response.

Requires monitoring to maintain a therapeutic range.

Effects on platelets, leading to thrombocytopenia and thrombosis.

Antithrombotic and hemorrhagic potential may reside in different structural components of heparin molecule.

aPTT—activated partial thromboplastin time; IV—intravenously; SQ—subcutaneously.

TABLE 3 WEIGHT-BASED HEPARIN DOSING NOMOGRAM

Initial dose	80 U/kg bolus, then 18 U/kg/h
Maintenance dose	
aPTT < 1.2 x control	80 U/kg bolus, then 4 U/kg/h
aPTT 1.2–1.5 x control	40 U/kg bolus, then 2 U/kg/h
aPTT 1.5–2.3 x control	No change
aPTT 2.3–3 x control	Decrease infusion rate by 2 U/kg/h
aPTT < 3 x control	Hold infusion 1 hour, then decrease rate by 3 U/kg/h

aPTT—activated partial thromboplastin time.

weight of between 4000 and 6500 daltons. They contain the essential pentasaccharide for AT binding, enabling the AT-LMWH complex to neutralize factor Xa, but they lack a substantial number of the larger chains (18 or more monosaccharides) required for binding to thrombin (*see* Fig. 2). Thus, the ratio of the relative neutralizing potency for Xa:IIa, which for unfractionated heparin is 1:1, is approximately 3:1 for LMWH. LMWHs have qualities that make them a better anticoagulant than unfractionated heparin as set out in Table 4. Most important, they have a significantly reduced ability to bind to plasma proteins, endothelial cells, and blood cells, making them more available for binding to AT, producing an anticoagulant effect. Consequently, they have a much greater bioavailability and predictability of response and do not require monitoring. They are also more uniformly absorbed from subcutaneous depots and have a longer plasma half-life, in the range of 3 to 5 hours. LMWHs are excreted predominantly from the kidney. Alteration of dosing is required in renal failure, where it is recommended that full dose therapy be instituted only with the aid of anti-Xa monitoring capability.

Indications

Low molecular weight heparins are approved for many of the conditions for which heparin is used, both for primary and secondary prophylaxis [6]. Enoxaparin is the most commonly used LMWH in the United States. Based on US Food and Drug Administration recommendations, it is formally approved for the prophylaxis of deep vein thrombosis in patients undergoing abdominal surgery, hip and knee replacement surgery, and in acutely ill medical patients [20–22]. However, it is used in many other conditions where patients are at risk of developing venous thromboembolism (VTE) [22,23]. Enoxaparin is also approved for the initial treatment of acute DVT with or without PE and for the outpatient initial treatment of acute DVT without PE [24••,25•,26•]. Although not formally approved for the use in patients with PE alone, enoxaparin is used substantially in patients with PE with or without DVT and in outpatients with PE [27,28]. Finally, enoxaparin is approved for the prophylaxis of ischemic complications of unstable angina and acute coronary syndromes. Although all LMWHs have similar mechanisms of action, indications differ from brand to brand depending on the results of randomized controlled trials, and dosing recommendations may also differ. Thus, it is important to prescribe LMWH by name (generic or brand). Indications for LMWH are listed in Table 1.

LMWH has played an important role in revolutionizing the treatment of acute VTE disorders by moving treatment from the inpatient to the ambulatory arena. Table 5 highlights the results of the two landmark studies that initiated that shift showing that such therapy was not only safe and effective, but by lowering inpatient stays, was potentially very cost effective [25•,26•].

TABLE 4 ADVANTAGES OF LOW MOLECULAR WEIGHT HEPARIN

Observation	Potential advantage
Lack of protein binding	Good bioavailability, predictable dose response, heparin resistance less often encountered
Predictable dose response	Fixed or weight-based dosing possible, monitoring not required
Longer half-life	Once- or twice-daily dosing possible
Smaller molecule	Better subcutaneous absorption
Less effect on platelets and endothelium	Less thrombocytopenia and bleeding

TABLE 5 OUTPATIENT THERAPY FOR TREATMENT OF DEEP VENOUS THROMBOSIS: LOW MOLECULAR WEIGHT HEPARIN VS UNFRACTIONATED HEPARIN

	Levine *et al.* [25•]		Koopman *et al.* [26•]	
Drug	UFH	LMWH	UFH	LMWH
Patients	253	247	198	202
Recurrent thrombosis	17 (6.7%)	13 (5.3%)	17 (8.6%)	14 (6.9%)
Bleeding	3 (1%)	5 (2%)	4 (2%)	1 (0.5%)
Hospital stay (mean days)	6.5	1.1*	8.1	2.7†

*48% never hospitalized.
†36% never hospitalized.
LMWH—low molecular weight heparin; UFH—unfractionated heparin.

Based on the results of clinical studies and on current trends in other countries and in the United States, LMWH is likely to replace unfractionated heparin as the anticoagulant of choice for acute thromboembolic disorders.

FONDAPARINUX

A further refinement on the mechanism of action of heparin is the development of fondaparinux, a synthetically derived, pentasaccharide that binds to and activates AT [29•]. Because fondaparinux lacks longer saccharide chains than in heparin or even LMWH, it has no effect on thrombin and is a specific, indirect inhibitor of activated factor X via its activation of AT (Fig. 2). Fondaparinux is almost 100% bioavailable with little protein binding. It has a predictable antithrombotic effect and requires no coagulation monitoring. Fondaparinux has good absorption from subcutaneous depots, reaches peak concentrations in 1 to 3 hours, and has an effective half-life of approximately 17 hours. Fondaparinux does not induce heparin/platelet factor 4 antibodies or heparin-induced thrombocytopenia. It is excreted entirely by the kidneys and is not recommended in patients with renal impairment (creatinine clearance of < 30 mL/min).

Indications

Fondaparinux has been studied in a large number of patients undergoing hip and knee replacement or hip fracture surgery [30–33]. Tables 6 and 7 show the results of four major trials resulting in an approximate 50% relative risk reduction in VTE without a significant increase in major bleeding. Some controversy surrounds these studies because of differences in the timing of the fondaparinux dose relative to the comparator arm (enoxaparin), but inspite of these differences, fondaparinux still appears to provide substantial benefit. Although not currently approved for the treatment of acute DVT or PE, recently completed studies [34,35] showed that fondaparinux provides equal benefit compared with enoxaparin for DVT or unfractionated heaprin for PE for the prevention of recurrent VTE when used during the first 7 to 14 days of treatment followed by warfarin. Fondaparinux is currently approved for the prophylaxis of VTE in patients undergoing hip or knee replacement surgery or hip fracture surgery.

ORAL ANTICOAGULANTS

Although dicoumarol was the first coumarin anticoagulant identified and isolated from spoiled sweet clover by Link [36] in 1941, crystalline sodium warfarin has been the major formulation used in the United States for over 30 years. In recent years, intense focus has been directed to identifying the appropriate indications for warfarin based on well-designed prospective randomized clinical trials and to qualifying the appropriate intensity of therapy based on an international normalized ratio (INR). Lately, attention has focused on improving the management of oral anticoagulation through coordinated clinical programs known as anti-

---

TABLE 6 VENOUS THROMBOEMBOLISM PROPHYLAXIS: FONDAPARINUX VS LMWH IN ORTHOPEDIC SURGERY

Trial	Fondaparinux, %	LMWH, %	RR, %
Ephesus (hip/2309)*	4	9	56
Pentathalon (hip/2275)*	6	8	25
Penthifra (hip fx/1711)*	8	19	56
Pentamaks (knee/1049)*	13	28	55
Total	7	14	50

*Text in parentheses indicates type of surgery and number of patients.
LMWH—low molecular weight heparin.

TABLE 7 MAJOR BLEEDING: FONDAPARINUX VS LMWH IN ORTHOPEDIC SURGERY

Trial	Fondaparinux, %	LMWH, %
Ephesus (hip)	3.7	2.6
Pentathalon (hip)	1.6	0.7
Penthifra (hip fx)	1.8	1.9
Pentamaks (knee)	1.7	0
Total	2.7	1.6

LMWH—low molecular weight heparin.

coagulation management services or anticoagulation clinics. The latest paradigm of oral anticoagulation management, however, is the model of patient self-management of therapy. This is a direct result of the development of portable, hand-held capillary–whole blood PT monitors that can yield results from a fingerstick sample of blood.

Mechanism of Action

Warfarin exerts its effect by interfering with the reduction and recycling of vitamin K that is oxidized in the process of carboxylating glutamic acid moieties in the precursors of vitamin K–dependent coagulation factors (see Fig. 1) [37]. As a result, poorly functional coagulation precursors are secreted, leading to a defective coagulation cascade. Factor VII has the shortest half-life (~6 hours) and its concentration falls most rapidly. Factor II has a half-life of approximately 60 hours; thus, several days of therapy are required for its concentration to fall, accounting for the reason heparin and warfarin therapy must overlap for a minimum of 3 to 5 days, so that all vitamin K–dependent factors are reduced.

Indications

The effectiveness of warfarin has been established by well-designed clinical trials for primary and secondary prevention of VTE, for prevention of systemic embolism in patients with prosthetic heart valves or atrial fibrillation, for the primary prevention of acute myocardial infarction in high-risk men, and for the prevention of stroke, recurrent infarction, or death in patients with acute myocardial infarction. Achieving and maintaining an optimal target range is essential in all of these indications [37]. Table 1 summarizes these indications. In the past 10 years, the scientific community has thoroughly documented the benefit of warfarin therapy for atrial fibrillation in patients 65 years or older [38]. The question of aspirin therapy in such individuals is no longer debated, since the high incidence of warfarin-associated intracranial hemorrhage found in the Stroke Prevention in Atrial Fibrillation (SPAF) II study [39] has not been confirmed by others.

Although warfarin is not routinely used following an acute myocardial infarction, two recent studies have confirmed its effectiveness with or without concomitant aspirin. In both the ASPECT-2 and WARIS 2 trials [40,41], patients randomized to low-dose aspirin with moderate-intensity warfarin (INR 2.0–2.5) or high-intensity warfarin alone (INR ~3.0–4.0) experienced a significantly lower rate of death, recurrent nonfatal infarction, or stroke compared with those treated with low-dose aspirin alone. How these studies will ultimately influence treatment patterns remains unkown.

Although the combination of aspirin (at low dosage) and warfarin (INR 2.5–3.5) has been shown to reduce the incidence of thromboembolism in patients with prosthetic cardiac valves [42] over warfarin alone, such combined therapy is not routinely used because of the higher risk of hemorrhage.

Management

Oral anticoagulants are challenging to use in clinical practice because they 1) have a narrow therapeutic window, 2) exhibit considerable variability in dose response among subjects, 3) are subject to interactions with drugs and diet, 4) have laboratory control that can be difficult to standardize, and 5) have problems in dosing as a result of patient noncompliance and miscommunication between the patient and physician [37]. Numerous studies have identified the risk of hemorrhage with excessive anticoagulation or thrombosis with inadequate anticoagulation [43,44•]. Based on a study by Cannegeiter et al. [45] of patients with prosthetic valves, a wide range of safety and efficacy exists between an INR of 2.0 and 4.5, although most investigators seek to identify a more narrow range of effectiveness. Besides intensity, patient-specific characteristics also influence the risk of adverse events. Landefeld and Goldman [43] identified heart, liver and kidney disorders, cancer, and anemia as risk factors, as well as a history of stroke, myocardial infarction, or gastrointestinal bleeding. Beyth et al. [44•] developed a bleeding risk index based on age (> 65 or < 65), history of gastrointestinal bleeding or stroke, recent myocardial infarction, hematocrit < 30%, or diabetes mellitus. Finally, because oral anticoagulation management is labor intensive and requires frequent patient contact and communication, a coordinated system of care has been suggested as the ideal system to produce good clinical and more cost-effective outcomes [46]. In a routine setting in which patients are managed by their personal physician along with all other patients, several studies have indicated a high incidence of major hemorrhage in the range of 8% per treatment year. In a coordinated program, an anticoagulation clinic, the rate of major bleeding is closer to 2% to 4%, as is the rate of recurrent thromboembolism. Based on individual studies comparing usual medical care with coordinated care, it is not surprising that a strong impetus exists for the creation of anticoagulation clinics throughout the country.

Dosing

The use of a loading dose of warfarin to initiate therapy induces a rapid, but excessive reduction in factor VII activity, while it fails to achieve a more rapid decline of the other vitamin K–dependent coagulation factors (II, IX, and X). For inpatient therapy, treatment is properly initiated using an average maintenance dose (5 mg) for the first 2 or 3 days [47]. Warfarin should overlap with heparin therapy for a period of 3 to 5 days, since it takes that long to lower the vitamin K–dependent coagulation factors with a longer half-life. If treatment is not urgent (eg, chronic stable atrial fibrillation), warfarin can be commenced out-of-hospital with an anticipated maintenance dose of 4 to 5 mg/d, which usually achieves a therapeutic anticoagulant effect in about 5 days, although a stable INR may take longer to achieve. It has recently been shown that starting outpatients with a 10-mg dose more rapidly achieves therapeutic anticoagulation [48], thus there is room for flexibility in selecting a starting dose of warfarin. Additionally, lower than 5-mg starting doses might be appropriate in the elderly, in patients with impaired nutrition or liver disease, and in patients at high risk of bleeding.

Estimation of the maintenance dose is often based on observations of the INR response following a fixed dose of warfarin over a few days' interval. An individual who rapidly achieves a high therapeutic PT (INR > 2.0) after two doses of warfarin is likely to require a low maintenance dose. The opposite holds for those who show little elevation of the PT (INR < 1.5) after two doses. PT monitoring is usually performed frequently until the therapeutic range has been achieved and maintained for at least two consecutive days, then two or three times weekly for 1 to 2 weeks, then less often, depending on the stability of PT results. If the PT response remains stable, the frequency of testing can be reduced to intervals as long as every 4 weeks. If adjustments to the dose are required, then the cycle of more frequent monitoring is repeated until a stable dose response is again achieved.

Outpatient management of warfarin therapy should aim for simplicity and clarity to avoid patient confusion, poor compliance, and dosing errors that may result in complications. It is recommended that a limited number of warfarin tablet strengths be used in clinical practice and that patients clearly understand the various dosing patterns that are used, such as alternate-day doses or dosing levels based on days of the week.

Management of Nontherapeutic INRs

Patients receiving long-term warfarin therapy often have unexpected fluctuations in dose response that require careful management. These may be due to inaccuracy in PT testing; changes in vitamin K_1 intake (increased or decreased vitamin K_1 in the diet); changes in vitamin K_1 or warfarin absorption (gastrointestinal factors or drug effects); changes in warfarin metabolism (liver disease or drug effects); changes in vitamin K_1–dependent coagulation factor synthesis or metabolism (liver disease, drug effects, other medical conditions); other effects of undisclosed concomitant drug use; or patient compliance issues.

A nontherapeutic (eg, elevated) INR can be managed by discontinuing warfarin, administering vitamin K_1, or infusing fresh frozen plasma, prothrombin concentrate, or recombinant factor VIIa [49]. The choice is based largely on the severity of the clinical situation (eg, the degree of elevation of the INR or the presence of severe bleeding). When warfarin is interrupted, it takes 4 to 5 days for the INR to return to the normal range in patients whose INR is between 2.0 and 3.0. After treatment with oral vitamin K_1 the INR declines substantially within 24 hours. Since the absolute daily risk of bleeding is low even when the INR is excessively prolonged, many physicians manage patients with INR values of 4.0 to 10.0 by stopping warfarin and monitoring more frequently [50], unless the patient is at a higher risk of bleeding or bleeding has already developed.

Vitamin K_1 can be administered by the intravenous, subcutaneous, or oral routes, but intravenous injection may be associated with anaphylactic reactions, and the response to subcutaneous vitamin K_1 may be unpredictable and sometimes delayed [51]. Recent studies show that oral administration is predictably effective, and has the advantages of safety and convenience over parenteral routes. Ideally, vitamin K_1 should be administered in a dose that will quickly lower the INR into a safe but not subtherapeutic range without causing resistance once warfarin is reinstated. High doses of vitamin K_1, though effective, may lower the INR more than is necessary and lead to warfarin resistance for up to a week. Table 8 outlines the 2004 American College of Chest Physicians (ACCP) recommendations for managing patients on coumarin anticoagulants who need their INR lowered because of actual or potential bleeding.

Management of Oral Anticoagulation During Invasive Procedures

Physicians must assess the risk of bleeding from a procedure if anticoagulation is continued versus the risk of thrombosis if anticoagulation is discontinued, as well as the cost of alternative anticoagulation options [52]. Traditionally, full dose, intravenous unfractionated heparin has been the standard for patients who need full anticoagulant protection that is readily reversible before a procedure. Its major drawback is the complexity and cost associated with intravenous heparin therapy and hospitalization. LMHW offers a less complex alternative in that it requires no monitoring and can be given at home. Warfarin is usually discontinued 4 days before the procedure and the INR allowed to decline. Two days before the procedure, LMWH is started, usually at a full treatment dose (100 to 150 antiXa units/kg subcutaneously) once or twice daily depending on the risk of thrombosis, with the last dose given the night before the procedure (~12 hours). It is then restarted about 12 hours after the procedure along with warfarin. When the INR is therapeutic, LMWH is stopped. Several prospective cohort analyses have reported that LMWH is a suitable and less costly alternative and provides therapeutic levels more rapidly and consistently than unfractionated heparin [53–56]. LMWH appears to be at least as effective, if not more effective, and less costly than unfractionated heparin [57–59]. A recent review on the subject summarizes the options and outcomes for a range of surgical procedures including cataract surgery, cutaneous surgery, pacemaker and defibrillator procedures, cardiac catheterization, genitourinary surgery, gastrointestinal endoscopy, and others [60]. Recently, questions have been raised about LMWH's effectiveness in patients with mechanical heart values. Although there are reports of valve thrombosis or systemic embolism with the use of LMWH in this situation, the outcomes may be no different than those achieved with unfractionated heparin, and potentially may be better [57,61–64]. Table 9 summarizes the 2004 ACCP Chest Consensus Conference recommendations for management.

Patient Self-Testing and Self-Management

In 1987, a point-of-care PT instrument was introduced that was able to measure PT from a fingerstick sample of capillary whole blood [65]. This instrument and subsequent models have been shown to be accurate and precise and are suitable for patient self-testing [66]. A number of studies have demonstrated the ability of patients to perform their own PT, communicate the results to their physician, and achieve good outcomes [67–69].

Of greater importance, however, is the potential impact of a self-management model of therapy in which patients adjust their own warfarin dose in response to their own INR testing. Several studies have now shown that such a model of warfarin management results in patients being in therapeutic range a higher percentage of time and experiencing fewer adverse events [70–77]. The differences are greatest when patient self-monitoring is compared with routine medical care as compared with the outcomes achieved by anticoagulation clinics [78]. Such therapy is extremely popular in certain European countries but is just beginning to be introduced in the United States.

Interest in improving the management of oral anticoagulation is timely given the rapid expansion in use of oral anticoagulants. If the benefits of instituting therapy, such as in atrial fibrillation, are outweighed by the occurrence of fatal or serious complications, little has been gained in the effort to combat and prevent thromboembolic disease.

Anticoagulant Therapy in the Future

As identified earlier in this chapter, heparin has many drawbacks as an anticoagulant. LMHW overcomes some of these deficiencies because of its ability to be given once or twice daily by the subcutaneous route and the lack of the need for monitoring. Fondaparinux may further improve upon outcomes, although it is still a parenteral agent and questions about easy reversibility arise in a drug that has a 17-hour half-life should major bleeding occur. Warfarin also has many drawbacks, including the need for monitoring, its slow onset of action, and its narrow therapeutic index. On the horizon are a number of new anticoagulants that may dramatically change how we manage patients with thromboembolic disease. These agents are direct inhibitors of specific coagulation factors (*ie,* no need for antithrombin) such as factors IIa and Xa. Hirudin is a prototype of this type of agent, but hirudin has drawbacks, such as the need for parenteral use and the increased risk of bleeding. Currently in phase I to III clinical trials are a number of agents that can be given orally once or twice daily, have rapid onset of action, may not need laboratory monitoring, and may even have a better risk profile [79••]. Ximelagatran is an example of an oral direct thrombin inhibitor that requires no coagulation monitoring and has been shown in phase III trials to be effective and safe for the acute and chronic treatment of DVT and for the prevention of stroke and systemic embolism in atrial fibrillation compared with standard therapy. Oral direct Xa inhibitors have also already shown effectiveness for the prevention of DVT in

TABLE 8 RECOMMENDATIONS FOR MANAGING ELEVATED INRs OR BLEEDING IN PATIENTS RECEIVING VITAMIN K ANTAGONISTS* [37]	
INR above therapeutic but less than 5.0; no significant bleeding	Lower dose or omit dose, monitor more frequently and resume at lower dose when INR therapeutic; if only minimally above therapeutic range, no dose reduction may be required (grade 2C).
INR > 5.0 but < 9.0; no significant bleeding	Omit next one or two doses, monitor more frequently and resume at lower doses when INR therapeutic. Alternatively, omit dose and give vitamin K1 ($\leq$ 5 mg) orally, particularly if at increased risk of bleeding. If more rapid reversal is required because the patient requires urgent surgery, vitamin K1 (2–4 mg) orally can be given with the expectation that a reduction of the INR will occur in 24 hours. If the INR is still high, additional vitamin K1 (1–2 mg) orally can be given (grade 2C).
INR > 9.0; no significant bleeding	Hold warfarin and give higher dose of vitamin K_1 (5–10 mg) orally with the expectation that the INR will be reduced substantially in 24 to 48 hours. Monitor more frequently and use additional vitamin K_1 if necessary. Resume therapy at lower dose when INR therapeutic (grade 2C).
Serious bleeding at any elevation of INR	Hold warfarin and give vitamin K_1 (10 mg) by slow IV infusion and supplemented with fresh plasma or prothrombin complex concentrate depending on the urgency of the situation; recombinant factor VIIa may be considered as an alternative to prothrombin complex concentrate. Vitamin K_1 can be repeated every 12 hours (grade 1C).
Life-threatening bleeding	Hold warfarin and give prothrombin complex concentrate supplemented with vitamin K_1, 10 mg slow IV infusion; recombinant factor VIIa may be considered as an alternative to prothrombin complex concentrate; repeat if necessary depending on INR (grade 1C).

*Note: If continuing warfarin therapy is indicated after high doses of vitamin K_1, then heparin or LMWH can be given until the effects of vitamin K_1 have been reversed and the patient becomes responsive to warfarin therapy. It should be noted that INR values above 4.5 are less reliable than values in or near the therapeutic range. Thus, these guidelines represent an approximate guide for high INRs.

INR—International Normalized Ratio; IV—intravenous; LMWH—low molecular weight heparin.

TABLE 9 RECOMMENDATIONS FOR MANAGING ANTICOAGULATION IN PATIENTS REQUIRING INVASIVE PROCEDURES (ALL GRADE 2C) [37]

Low risk of thromboembolism*	Stop warfarin approximately 4 days before surgery, allow the INR to return to near normal, briefly use postoperative prophylaxis (if the intervention itself creates a higher risk of thrombosis) with low-dose UFH, 5000 U SC, or prophylactic dose of LMWH, and simultaneously begin warfarin therapy. Alternatively, low-dose UFH or prophylactic dose LMWH can also be used preoperatively.
Intermedicate risk of thromboembolism	Stop warfarin approximately 4 days before surgery, allow the INR to fall, cover the patient beginning 2 days preoperatively with low-dose UFH, 5000 U SC, or a prophylactic dose of LMWH and then commence low-dose UFH (or LMWH) and warfarin postoperatively. Some individuals would recommend a higher dose of UFH or full-dose LMWH in this setting.
High risk of thromboembolism*	Stop warfarin approximately 4 days before surgery, allow the INR to return to normal; begin therapy with full-dose UFH or full-dose LMWH as the INR falls (approximately 2 days preoperatively). UFH can be given as a SC injection as an outpatient; it can then be given as a continuous IV infusion after admission in preparation for surgery and discontinued approximately 5 hours before surgery with the expectation that the anticoagulant effect will have worn off at the time of surgery. It is also possible to continue with SC UFH or LMWH and to stop therapy 12 to 24 hours before surgery with the expectation that the anticoagulant effect will be very low or have worn off at the time of surgery.
With low risk of bleeding	Continue warfarin at a lower dose and operate at an INR of 1.3 to 1.5, an intensity that has been shown to be safe in randomized trials of gynecologic and orthopedic surgical patients. The dose of warfarin can be lowered 4 or 5 days before surgery. Warfarin therapy can then be restarted postoperatively, supplemented with low-dose UFH (5000 U SC), or prophylactic dose LMWH if necessary.

*Low risk of thromboembolism: examples include no recent (> 3 months) venous thromboembolism; atrial fibrillation without a history of stroke or other risk factors; bileaflet mechanical cardiac valve in aortic position. High risk of thromboembolism: examples include recent (< 3 months) history of venous thromboembolism; mechanical cardiac valve in mitral position; old model of cardiac valve (ball/cage).

INR—Internataional Normalized Ratio; IV—intravenous; LMWH—low molecular weight heparin; SC—subcutaneous; UFH—unfractionated heparin.

orthopedic surgery, and phase III trials are under way. In the future, heparin or even LMWH may not be the agent of choice for acute anticoagulation, hospitalization may be a thing of the past, and the problematic PT and aPPT will no longer be necessary as monitoring tools.

KEY REFERENCES

Recently published papers of outstanding interest, as indentified in *References and Recommended Reading*, have been annotated.

•• Turpie AGG, Gallus AS, Hoek JA, *et al.*: A synthetic pentasaccharide for the prevention of deep-vein thrombosis after total hip replacement. *N Engl J Med* 2001, 344:619–625.

The first major report on the effectivenss of fondaparinux in orthopedic surgery.

•• Warkentin TE, Chong BH, Greinacher A: Heparin-induced thrombocytopenia: towards consensus. *Thromb Hemostas* 1998, 79:1–7.

A consensus discussion reviewing the syndrome of heparin-induced thrombocytopenia, its pathophysiology, and treatment.

•• Dolovich LR, Ginsberg JS, Douketis JD, *et al.*: A meta-analysis comparing low-molecular-weight heparins with unfractionated heparin in the treatment of venous thromboembolism. *Arch Intern Med* 2000, 60:181–188.

An excellent review and meta-analysis of the various low molecular weight heparins and their effectiveness, safety, and comparability in venous thromboembolism.

•• Bates SM, Weitz JI: Emerging anticoagulant drugs. *Arterioscler Thromb Vasc Biol* 2003, 23:1491–1500.

A brief, but excellent review of the new anticoagulant drugs on the verge of approval or in the pipeline.

REFERENCES AND RECOMENDED READING

Recently published papers of particular interest have been highlighted as:
• Of interest
•• Of outstanding interest

1. Jacques LB: The new understanding of the drug heparin. Chest 1985, 88:751–754.

2. Butt HR, Allen EV, Bollman JL: A preparation from spoiled sweet clover which prolongs coagulation and prothrombin time of the blood: preliminary reports of experimental and clinical studies. *Mayo Clin Proc* 1941, 16:388–395.

3.• Weitz JI: Low molecular weight heparin. *N Engl Med* 1997, 37:688–698.

4.•• Turpie AGG, Gallus AS, Hoek JA, *et al.* A synthetic pentasaccharide for the prevention of deep-vein thrombosis after total hip replacement. *N Engl J Med* 2001, 344:619–625.

5. Hirsh J: Heparin. *N Engl J Med* 1991, 324:1565–1574.

6. Hirsh J, Warkentin TE, Shaughnessy SG, *et al.*: Heparin and low-molecular-weight heparin: Mechanism of action, pharmacokinetics, dosing monitoring, efficacy, and safety. *Chest* 2001, 119(Suppl):64S–94S.

7. Fennerty A, Thomas P, Blackhouse G, *et al.*: Audit of control of heparin treatment. *BMJ* 1985, 290:27–28.

8. Cruickshank MK, Levine MN, Hirsh J, *et al.*: A standard heparin nomogram for the management of heparin therapy. *Arch Intern Med* 1991, 151:333–337.

9.• Raschke RA, Reilly BM, Guidry JR, *et al.*: The weight-based heparin dosing nomogram compared with a standard care nomogram. *Ann Intern Med* 1993, 119:874–881.

10. Flaker GC, Bartolozzi J, Davis V, *et al.*: and the TIMI 4 Investigators: Use of a standardized heparin nomogram to achieve therapeutic anticoagulation after thrombolytic therapy in myocardial infarction. *Arch Intern Med* 1994, 154:1492–1496.

11. Brill-Edwards P, Ginsberg JS, Johnston M, Hirsh J: Establishing a therapeutic range for heparin therapy. *Ann Intern Med* 1993, 119:104–109.

12.•• Warkentin TE, Chong BH, Greinacher A: Heparin-induced thrombocytopenia: towards consensus. *Hemost Thromb* 1998, 79:1–7.

13. Greinacher A: Antigen generation in heparin-associated thrombcytopenia: The non-immunologic type and the immunologic type are closely linked in their pathogenesis. *Semin Thromb Hemost* 1995;21:108–116.

14.• Warkentin TE, Kelton JG: A 14 year study of heparin-induced thrombocytopenia. *Am J Med* 1996, 101:502–507.

15. Lipirudin for heparin-induced thrombocytopenia. *Med Lett Drugs Ther* 1998, 40:94–95.

16.• Lubenow N, Greinacher A: Hirudin in heparin-induced thrombocytopenia. Semin Thromb Hemost 2002, 28:431–438.

17. Kathirsean S, Argatroban J: *Thrombo Thrombolys* 2002, 13:41–47.

18. Lewis BE: Argatroban anticooagulant therapy in patients with heparin-induced thrombocytopenia. *Circulation* 2001, 103:1838–1843.

19.• Rice L: Delayed-onset heparin-induced thrombocytopenia. *Ann Intern Med* 2002, 136:210–215.

20. Green D, Hirsh J, Heit J, *et al.*: Low molecular weight heparin: a critical analysis of clinical trials. *Pharmacol Rev* 1994, 46:89–109.

21. Samama MM, Cohen AT, Darmon JY, *et al.*: A comparison of enoxaparin with placebo for the prevention of venous thromboembolism in acutely ill medical patients. *N Engl J Med* 1999, 341:793–800.

22. Geerts WH, Heit JA, Clagett GP, *et al.*: Prevention of venous thrombembolism. *Chest* 2001, 119:132S–175S.

23. Ginsberg JS: Thromboembolism and pregnancy. *Thromb Hemostas* 1999, 82:620–625.

24.•• Dolovich LR, Ginsberg JS, Douketis JD, *et al.*: A meta-analysis comparing low-molecular-weight heparins with unfractionated heparin in the treatment of venous thromboembolism. *Arch Intern Med* 2000, 60:181–188.

25.• Levine M, Gent M, Hirsh J, *et al.*: A comparison of low molecular weight heparin administered primarily at home with unfractionated heparin administered in the hospital for proximal deep-vein thrombosis. *N Engl J Med* 1996, 334:677–681.

26.• Koopman MMW, Prandoni P, Piovella F, *et al.*: Treatment of venous thrombosis with intravenous unfractionated heparin administered in the hospital as compared with subcutaneous low molecular weight heparin administered at home. *N Engl J Med* 1996, 334:682–687.

27. Simonneau G, Sors H, Charbonner B, *et al.*: A comparison of low-molecular-weight heparin with unfractionated heparin for acute pulmonary embolism. *N Eng J Med* 1997, 337:663–669.

28. Hull RD Raskob GE, Brant RF, *et al.*: Low-molecular-weight heparin vs heparin in the treatment of patients with pulmonary embolism. Arch Intern Med 2000, 160:229–236.

29.• Bauer KA, Hawkins DW, Peters PC, *et al.*: Fondaparinux, a synthetic pentasaccharide: the first in a new class of antithrombotic agents—the selective factor Xa inhibitors. *Cardiovasc Drug Rev* 2002, 20:37–52.

30. Lassen MR, Bauer KA, *et al.*: Postoperative fondaparinux versus preoperative enoxaparin for prevention of venous thrombembolism in elective hip-replacement surgery: a randomised double-blind comparison. *Lancet* 2002, 359:1715–1720.

31. Turpie AGG, Bauer A, Eriksson BI, *et al.*: Postoperative fondaparinux versus postoperative enoxaparin for prevention of venous thromboembolism after elective hip-replacement surgery: a randomised double-blind trial. *Lancet* 200, 359:1721–1726.

32. Eriksson BI, Bauer KA, Lassen MR, *et al.*: Fondaparinux compared with enoxaparin for the prevention of venous thromboembolism after hip-fracture surgery. *N Engl J Med* 2001, 345:1298–1304.

33. Bauer KA, Eriksson BI, Lassen MR, *et al.*: Fondaparinux compared with enoxaparin for the prevention of venous thromboembolism after elective major knee surgery. *N Engl J Med* 2001, 345:1305–1310.

34. Matisse Investigators: Fondaparinux in comparison to low molecular weight heparin for the initial treatment of symptomatic deep venous thrombosis or pulmonary embolism—The Matisse Clinical Outcome Studies. *Blood* 2002, 100(suppl):83a.

35. Matisse Investigators. Subcutaneous fondaparinux versus intravenous unfractionated heparin in the initial treatment of pulmonary embolism. *N Engl J Med* 2003, 349:1695–1702.

36. Link KP: The discovery of dicumarol and its sequels. *Circulation* 1959, 19:97–107.

37. Ansell J, Hirsh J, Poller L, et al.: The pharmacology and management of the vitamin K antagonists. *Chest* 2004, in press.

38. Atrial Fibrillation Investigators: Risk factors for stroke and efficacy of antithrombotic therapy in atrial fibrillation. *Arch Intern Med* 1994, 154:1449–1457.

39. Stroke Prevention in Atrial Fibrillation Investigators: Warfarin versus aspirin for prevention of thromboembolism in atrial fibrillation: stroke prevention in atrial fibrillation II study. *Lancet* 1994, 343:687–691.

40. Hurlen M, Abdelnoor M, Smith P, *et al.*: Warfarin, aspirin, or both after myocardial infarction. *N Engl J Med* 2002, 347:969–974.

41. van Es RF, Jonker JJC, Verheugt FWA, *et al.*: Aspririn and Coumadin after acute coronary syndromes (the ASPECT-2 study): a randomised controlled trial. *Lancet* 2002, 360:109–113.

42. Turpie AGG, Gent M, Laupacis A, *et al.*: A comparison of aspirin with placebo in patients treated with warfarin after heart-valve replacement. *N Engl J Med* 1993, 329:524–529.

43. Landefeld GS, Goldman L: Major bleeding in outpatients treated with warfarin: incidence and prediction by factors known at the start of outpatient therapy. *Am J Med* 1989, 87:144–152.

44.• Beyth RJ, Quinn LM, Landefeld S: Prospective evaluation of an index for predicting the risk of major bleeding in outpatients treated with warfarin. *Am J Med* 1998, 105:91–99.

45. Cannegieter SC, Rosendaal FR, Wintzen AR, *et al.*: The optimal intensity of oral anticoagulant therapy in patients with mechanical heart valve prostheses: the Leiden artificial valve and anticoagulation study. *N Engl J Med* 1995, 333:11–17.

46. Ansell JE, Hughes R: Evolving models of warfarin management: anticoagulation clinics, patient self-monitoring, and patient self-management. *Am Heart J* 1996, 132:1095–1100.

47. Harrison L, Johnston M, Massicotte MP, *et al.*: Comparison of 5 mg and 10 mg loading doses in initiation of warfarin therapy. *Ann Intern Med* 1997, 126:133–136.

48. Kovacs MJ, Rodger M, Anderson DR, *et al.*: Comparison of 10 mg and 5 mg warfarin initiation nomograms together with low molecular weight heparin for outpatient treatment of acute venous thromboembolism. *Ann Intern Med* 2003, 138:714–719.

49. Deveras RAE, Kessler GM: Reversal of warfarin-induced excessive anticoagulation with recombinant human factor VIIa concentrate. *Ann Intern Med* 2002, 137:884–888.

50. Lousberg TR, Witt DM, Beall DG, *et al.*: Evaluation of excessive anticoagulation in a group model health maintenance organization. *Arch Intern Med* 1998, 158:528–534.

51. Raj G, Kumar R, McKinney P: Time course of reversal of anticoagulant effect of warfarin by intravenous and subcutaneous phytonadione. *Arch Intern Med* 1999, 159:2721–2724.

52. Kearon C, Hirsh J: Management of anticoagulation before and after elective surgery. *N Engl J Med* 1997, 336:1506–1511.

53. Johnson J, Turpie AGG: Temporary discontinuation of oral anticoagulants: role of low molecular weight heparin. *Thromb Hemost* 1999, Aug(suppl):62–63.

54. Tinmouth AH, Morrow BH, Cruickshank M, *et al.*: Dalteparin as periprocedure anticoagulation for patients on warfarin and at high risk of thrombosis. *Ann Pharmacother* 2001, 35:669–674.

55. Spandorfer JM, Lynch S, Weitz HH, *et al.*: Use of enoxaparin for the chronically anticoagulated patient before and after procedures. *Am J Cardiol* 1999, 84:478–480.

56. Amorosi SL, Fanikos J, Tsilimingras K, *et al.*: Bridging therapy during temporary interruption of chronic anticoagulation is less costly with low molecular weigtth heparin than unfractionated heparin. *Circulation* 2002, 106:II-758.

57. Berdague Ph, Boneu B, Soula Ph, *et al.*: Usefulness of low molecular weight heparins during post-operative period in mitral mechanical valve replacement: clinical ischaemic and haemorrhagic complications in 110 cases. *Eur Heart J* 1998, 19(Suppl):534.

58. Smith LK, McKee BD, Schroeder DP: Cost effectiveness and safety of outpatient enoxaparin bridge therapy. *Chest* 1999, 116(Suppl 2):360S.

59. Tsilimingras KV, Grasso-Correnti N, Fanikos J, Goldhaber SZ: Initiation of anticoagulation after cardiac surgery: A prospective cohort study of efficacy, safety, and cost with low molecular weight heparin bridging in lieu of continuous intravenous unfractionated heparin. *J Am Coll Cardiol* 2002, 39:428A.

60. Dunn A, Turpie AGG: Perioperative management of patients on oral anticoagulants: a systematic review. *Arch Intern Med* 2003, 163:901–908.

61. Montalescot G, Polle V, Collet JP, *et al.*: Low molecular weight heparin after mechanical heart valve replacement. *Circulation* 2000, 101:1083–1086.

62. Ferreira IJ, Dos L, Tornos MP, *et al.*: Is low molecular weight heparin a safe alternative to unfractionated heparin in patients with prosthetic mechanical heart valves who must interrupt antithrombotic therapy? *Eur Heart J* 2000, 21(Suppl):301.

63. UPMC Health System: Home LMWH bridge therapy in cardiac valve replacement: safe, effective, and cost saving. *Formulary* 2000, 35:990–991.

64. Tsilimingras K, Grasso-Correnti N, Fanikos J, *et al.*: Initiation of anticoagulation after cardiac surgery: a prospective cohort study of efficacy, safety and cost with low molecular weight heparin bridging in lieu of continuous intravenous unfractionated heparin. *J Am Coll Cardiol* 2002, 39(Suppl A):837–846.

65. Lucas FV, Duncan A, Jay R, *et al.*: A novel whole blood capillary technic for measuring the prothrombin time. *Am J Clin Pathol* 1987, 88:442–446.

66. Leaning KE, Ansell JE: Advanced in the monitoring of oral anticoagulation: point-of-care testing, patient self-monitoring, and patient self-management. *J Thromb Thrombolysis* 1996, 3:377–383.

67. White RH, McCurdy SA, von Marensdorff H, *et al.*: Home prothrombin time monitoring after initiation of warfarin therapy. *Ann Intern Med* 1989, 111:730–737.

68. Anderson D, Harrison L, Hirsh J: Evaluation of a portable prothrombin time monitor for home use by patients who require long-term oral anticoagulant therapy. *Arch Intern Med* 1993, 153:1441–1447.

69. Beyth RJ, Quinn L, Landefeld CS: A multicomponent intervention to prevent major bleeding complications in older patients receiving warfarin. A randomized, controlled trial. *Ann Intern Med* 2000, 133:687–695.

70. Ansell J, Patel N, Ostrovsky D, *et al.*: Long-term patient self-management of oral anticoagulation. *Arch Intern Med* 1995, 155:2185–2189.

71. Sawicki PT: A structured teaching and self-management program for patients receiving oral anticoagulation: a randomized controlled trial. *JAMA* 1999, 281:145–150.

72. Ansell JE: Empowering patients to monitor and manage oral anticoagulation therapy. *JAMA* 1999, 281:181–183.

73. Horstkotte D, Piper C, Wiemer M, *et al.*: Improvement of prognosis by home prothrombin estimation in patients with life-long anticoagulant therapy [abstract]. *Eur Heart J* 1996, 17(Suppl):230.

74. Kortke H, Korfer R: International normalized ratio self-management after mechanical heart valve replacement: Is an early start advantageous? *Ann Thorac Surg* 2001, 72:44–48.

75. Preiss M, Bernet F, Zerkowski HR: Additional information from the GELIA database: analysis of benefit from self-management of oral anticoagulation (GELIA 6). *Euro Heart J* 2001, 3(Suppl Q):Q50–Q53.

76. Watzke HH, Forberg E, Svolba G, *et al.*: A prospective controlled trial comparing weekly self-testing and self-dosing with the standard management of patients on stable oral anticoagulation. *Thromb Haemost* 2000, 83:661–665.

77. Cromheecke ME, Levi M, Colly LP, *et al.*: Oral anticoagulation self-management and management by a specialist anticoagulation clinic: a randomized cross-over comparison. *Lancet* 2000, 556:97–101.

78. Ansell JE: Patient self-testing and patient self-management of oral anticoagulation: is it too late? *Israeli Med J* 2002, 4:1035–1036.

79. ••Bates SM, Weitz JI: Emerging anticoagulant drugs. *Arterioscler Thromb Vasc Biol* 2003, 23:1491–1500.

Cerebrovascular Complications of Cardiac Disorders

Muhammad Ramzan
Marc Fisher

40

> ### Key Points
> - Several cardiac conditions are commonly associated with cerebral embolism.
> - Cardioembolic strokes account for approximately one fourth of all ischemic strokes, and they are potentially more preventable than other causes of stroke.
> - Although potentially preventable, cardioembolic strokes are typically severe, prone to recurrence, and have a poor prognosis.
> - Patent foramen ovale (PFO) with atrial septal aneurysm (ASA), and aortic arch plaques are now recognized embolic sources.
> - Transesophageal echocardiography has proven to increase the yield of embolism source detection, especially aortic atherosclerosis, ASA/PFO, and vegetations.
> - Warfarin is effective in both primary and secondary prevention in nonvalvular atrial fibrillation, but despite the strong evidence and available guidelines, it is still underutilized.
> - New direct thrombin inhibitors are being investigated as alternatives to warfarin therapy.

The relationship between cardiac disorders and stroke has become increasingly evident. A wide variety of cardiac abnormalities are associated with an enhanced potential for stroke occurrence. Significant progress has been made in recent years to better understand the pathophysiologic mechanisms, and to minimize the risk of stroke from well-known cardiac sources. Similarly, with new cardiac imaging techniques it is possible to define the role of potential causes of emboli, such as aortic arch plaques, atrial septal aneurysm, patent foramen ovale, and ventricular strands in cryptogenic stroke. In addition, diagnostic and therapeutic modalities used in cardiology can contribute to cerebral ischemia or hemorrhage. Further adding to the cardiac-cerebrovascular link is the possibility that many of the therapeutic approaches used to treat acute myocardial ischemia are relevant for acute ischemic stroke.

CARDIAC SOURCES OF STROKE

Cardioembolic stroke has assumed increasing importance as diagnostic advances for detecting cardiac sources for emboli have improved [1••,2–4]. Currently, a cardioembolic source for stroke is recognized in 20% to 30% of the approximately 700,000 new or recurrent strokes per year that occur in the United States (*see* the *Heart Disease and Stroke Statistics: 2004 update* from the American Stroke Association [www.strokeassociation.org]). This percentage is even higher in younger stroke patients (*ie*, those younger than 50 years). Potential cardiac sources of emboli are shown in Figure 1, and the frequency of emboli attributed to various sources is shown in Figure 2.

Formation of intracardiac thrombi related to stasis, endothelial disruption, valvular abnormalities, and right-to-left shunts is a common mechanism for embolization in these disparate conditions. These cardiac emboli typically lodge in an intracranial vessel equal to their diameter at right angles to a larger parent artery, causing a clinical stroke syndrome related to the region of ischemic injury (Fig. 3). Cardioembolic stroke is the most likely diagnosis in a stroke patient who has a recognized cardiac disorder, documented cardiac source of embolism, abrupt and maximal neurologic deficits at onset, higher incidence of hemorrhagic transformation, large infarct with involvement of multiple vascular territories (anterior as well as posterior circulation), absence of atherosclerotic disease, or rapid regression of symptoms and initial diminished level of consciousness with likelihood for seizure or syncope [1••,2]. Supportive evidence for the diagnosis of cardioembolic stroke includes the presence of prior or concurrent emboli in other organs or cerebral vascular territories and angiographic demonstration of vascular branch occlusion. The presence of atherosclerotic disease, single vessel territory with either anterior or posterior circulation involvement, single or multiple lacunar infarcts with pure hemiparesis (absence of aphasia, neglect, visual field defects), watershed infarcts, preceding transient ischemic attacks (TIAs), and slow progression are not suggestive of cardioembolic stroke [1••,2]. The presence of a potential cardiac source for emboli does not conclusively establish the diagnosis of cardioembolic stroke because other potential stroke sources, such as large artery atherosclerosis or small intracranial vessel disease, are also present in approximately 33% of such patients. Therefore, the clinical diagnosis of cardioembolic source remains an educated guess. In reviewing the various etiologies for cardioembolic stroke, it is helpful to stratify the causes as high-risk and medium-risk sources (Table 1).

High-Risk Sources

Nonvalvular atrial fibrillation (NVAF) is the most common cardiac disorder that predisposes to stroke occurrence. It is common in the elderly, and the annual stroke risk in untreated patients is approximately 5% (range, 3% to 8%). Stroke risk increases with advancing age, history of hypertension, prior TIA, stroke, and diabetes [5•]. Echocardiographically, left ventricular dysfunction and a dilated left atrium constitute the main predictive factors. Younger patients (< 60 years) without concomitant risk factors have a low risk for stroke.

Congestive heart failure is the second most common cardiac cause of stroke, with a relative risk of two to three times the normal population. It is estimated that 5 million Americans have cardiac failure, and it is associated with a substantial mortality rate (data from the American Heart

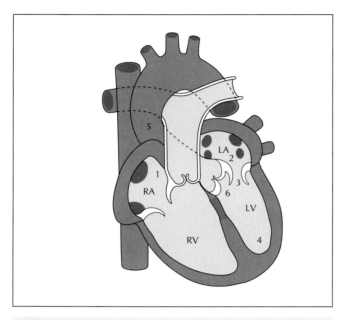

FIGURE 1 Sources of cardiogenic emboli: 1, paradoxical emboli (patent foramen ovale); 2, left atrium (LA) (atrial fibrillation, myxoma); 3, mitral valve (endocarditis, mitral valve prolapse, annulus calcification, prosthetic valve, other vegetations); 4, left ventricle (LV) (dyskinesia or akinesia, cardiomyopathy); 5, aorta (plaques); 6, aortic valve (endocarditis, prosthetic valve). RA—right atrium; RV—right ventricle.

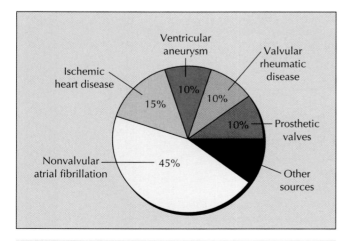

FIGURE 2 Sources of cardioembolism.

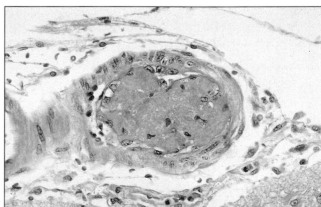

FIGURE 3 Embolus obstructing a cortical vessel.

Association [www.americanheart.org]). Pullicino *et al.* [6••] reported a relative risk of 4.1 in the 50 to 59 age group and 1.5 in the 80 to 89 age group. The risk of recurrent stroke is even higher. In dilated cardiomyopathy, globally impaired ventricular performance promotes stasis and thrombus formation. The annual rate of embolization has been estimated at 3.5% [7]. Warfarin is used for cardiomyopathy and in patients with a left ventricular ejection fraction of less than 30%; however, no randomized trial data are available. Currently two major trials—WATCH (Warfarin and Antiplatelet Therapy in Chronic Heart Failure) and WARCEF (Warfarin Versus Aspirin in Reduced Ejection Fraction) are under way to address this issue.

Acute myocardial infarction (MI) is associated with stroke development in approximately 1% of cases. Patients with transmural anterior wall MI have the greatest risk for thrombus formation and stroke occurrence as compared with the inferior wall MI. Most emboli occur within 4 weeks after the MI, with an incidence of 0.7% to 4.7% in the first 2 weeks [8•]. The risk lessens 4 weeks to 6 months after MI, although at later dates akinetic ventricular segments and left ventricular aneurysms assume greater importance. Randomized trials have shown that warfarin is more effective than placebo in reducing the risk of stroke by 55% [9] and 40% [10] over a period of 37 months. Loh *et al.* [8•] concluded that warfarin had a protective effect against stroke in patients with low ejection fraction after myocardial infarction.

Rheumatic valvular disease has decreased in developed countries but remains an important source for stroke in developing countries. Rheumatic mitral valve disease has the highest incidence of systemic embolism among common forms of heart disease, and it is generally accepted that long-term anticoagulation is effective in lowering the frequency of systemic emboli.

Prosthetic cardiac valves remain an important source of cardiac stroke development, despite advances in valve design. Mechanical valves pose a greater embolic threat than do biologic valves.

Infective endocarditis is a significant source of cardioembolic stroke in both young patients and the elderly. The incidence of native valve endocarditis is reported as 1.5 to six cases per 100,000 per year. In one series of 203 patients, brain ischemia occurred in 19% of patients [11]. Another recent study estimated the stroke incidence of 17% in mitral valve and 9% in aortic valve endocarditis [12]. Echocardiographically documented vegetations did not always correlate with stroke risk. Most strokes occurred at the time of presentation, and recurrent strokes were uncommon if the primary infection was controlled. Many patients develop complication of heart failure with an urgent need of valve replacement surgery, increasing the risk of converting an ischemic stroke into a hemorrhagic one. In general it is recommended to delay the surgery for at least 2 weeks [13]. Mycotic aneurysms leading to rupture or leak is another complication affecting the distal middle cerebral artery branches in 75% of the cases. Mycotic aneurysms can be multiple and may present with subarachnoid hemorrhage. Most of them respond to medical therapy; however, surgery may be required in some cases. MRI with angiography is very helpful in the localization and evaluation of these aneurysms.

Patients with sick sinus syndrome also have a substantial risk for stroke, and it is unclear whether cardiac pacing reduces this risk. Predictors of stroke risk in patients with sick sinus syndrome are a history of cerebrovascular disease, ventricular pacing, and paroxysmal atrial fibrillation [14]. In patients who do require pacemaker insertion for symptomatic bradycardia, a Canadian study found no difference in the stroke risk between physiologic pacing and ventricular pacing [15].

Cardiac myxomas are the most common primary benign cardiac tumors, and they are often quite friable (Fig. 4). They usually develop in atria and 75% of them affect the left atrium [16]. Embolic stroke occurs in nearly 30% to 40% of cases and most often in persons ranging from 30 to 60 years of age. Recurrent emboli before surgery are common (Fig. 5) and surgery is the treatment of choice, with excellent prognosis [17]. Anticoagulation is not always successful in preventing reembolization.

Medium-Risk Sources

The relationship of patent foramen ovale (PFO) and stroke/TIA has been described for decades. Paradoxical emboli were once thought to be a rare cause of stroke; however, several studies in younger stroke patients using contrast echocardiography have demonstrated that a PFO

TABLE 1 SOURCES OF CARDIOEMBOLIC STROKE

High-risk sources
Mechanical prosthetic valves
Mitral stenosis with atrial fibrillation
Atrial fibrillation
Left atrial thrombus
Sick sinus syndrome
Recent myocardial infarction (< 4 wk)
Left ventricular thrombus
Dilated cardiomyopathy
Akinetic segment
Myxoma
Infective endocarditis
Aortic arch plaque

Medium-risk sources
Mitral annulus calcification
Mitral stenosis without atrial fibrillation
Patent foramen ovale
Nonbacterial thrombotic endocarditis
Hypokinetic segment
Myocardial infarction (> 4 wk, < 6 mo)

is four to five times more common in stroke patients than in age-matched controls. The prevalence of PFO is highest in those stroke patients who have no other obvious source for their stroke (cryptogenic stroke). Cryptogenic stroke accounts for 40% of all ischemic stroke. The prevalence of PFO in the general population is estimated to be 25%, whereas in the cryptogenic stroke patients it can be seen in more than 50% of cases. One study compared the echocardiograms of patients with stroke of determined origin with those of patients with cryptogenic stroke [18]. In both the younger (<55 years) and older age groups, a PFO was significantly more common in patients with cryptogenic stroke (48% vs 4% and 38% vs 8%, respectively). In a meta-analysis of several case control studies, Overell et al. [19] showed that PFO was five times more prevalent in young people with cryptogenic stroke and three times more common in the cryptogenic stroke population of all age groups, compared with the healthy controls. The postulated pathogenic mechanisms for paradoxical emboli include peripheral venous thrombosis, stagnation and altered flow pattern in right atrium leading to in situ thrombus formation, and atrial arrhythmias [19,20,21•]. PFO has also been implicated as a cause in patients suffering from migraine with aura, and the effect is stronger when PFO is associated with atrial septal aneurysm (ASA), raising the possibility of an underlying genetic, vascular, or neurochemical mechanism [22–24]. The presence of a PFO in a patient with an otherwise unexplained stroke certainly suggests a relationship, but conclusively establishing that paradoxical embolization has occurred remains difficult. The presence of venous or cardiac thrombus would be supportive; however, it is estimated that only 10% of the patients with PFO have documented venous thrombosis [25]. Elevation of the right heart pressure is another related factor to paradoxical embolization with PFO, and the patient should be carefully questioned for any Valsalva-like episode before stroke onset, although some studies have shown no such relationship. Several studies have tried to define risk stratification for PFO and postulated that the risk is increased

with larger size, increased degree/severity of shunting, presence of atrial septal aneurysm (hypermobile or floppy septum), tunnel-like shunt configuration, and spontaneous echocardiographic shunting [23,26,27•]. The natural history of recurrent stroke in patients with PFO is variable. In one study, the risk of recurrent stroke with PFO was shown to be low (2% per year), but the patients are typically young, complicating decisions about management [28•]. Nedeltchev et al. [29] showed that the annual risk of recurrent stroke is 1.8%, whereas that of recurrent stroke and TIA is 5.5%. This risk was doubled in patients who had multiple cerebrovascular events before the diagnosis of PFO was established. Mas et al. [30•] reported increased risk of recurrent stroke only in those patients who had PFO as well as ASA (hazard ratio, 4.17; 95% CI, 1.47–11.84) at 4-year follow-up. Their study included patients 18 to 55 years age. They reported no increase in risk with isolated PFO (irrespective of the size) or ASA alone. In the PICSS (Patent Foramen Ovale in Cryptogenic Stroke Study) which used the subset of WARSS (Warfarin Aspirin Recurrent Stroke Study) population, there was no evidence of increased adverse events (recurrent stroke or death) in patients with PFO regardless of PFO size, presence of atrial septal aneurysm, or being treated with aspirin or warfarin [21•]. This may be due to their inclusion of patients with noncryptogenic stroke, older age population, and death as one of the endpoints. However this prospective study did confirm the association of PFO with cryptogenic stroke and showed that larger PFOs are associated with cryptogenic stroke.

There are no consensus data on the secondary prevention of stroke in PFO, due to lack of controlled trials. Medical treatment choices include antiplatelet agents or anticoagulation, whereas closure options are open heart surgery or percutaneous PFO closure. The PICSS showed no superiority of warfarin over aspirin. Mas et al. [30•] suggested that aspirin may be sufficient for young patients who have only PFO and a single cerebrovascular event, but patients with both PFO and ASA pose higher risk and alternative thera-

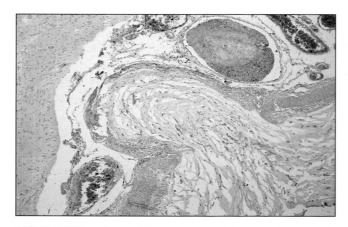

FIGURE 4 Myxomatous tissue within a cerebral vessel.

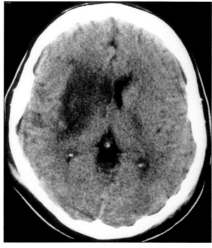

FIGURE 5 Computed tomography scan of a young woman with myxoma-related stroke.

pies should be considered. The meta-analysis of Orgera et al. [31] concluded that warfarin is superior to antiplatelet therapy in reducing the risk of recurrent cerebral ischemic events. Warfarin therapy was reported as equivalent to surgical closure; however, percutaneous closure was not addressed in this study. Recently there has been an increase in reports of the use of percutaneous devices for closure. Khairy et al. [32], in their systematic review of medical therapy and transcatheter closure studies, concluded that the 1-year rate of recurrent thromboembolic events was 3.8% to 12% in medical therapy and 0% to 4.9% in transcatheter closure patients. They reported a 1.5% and 7.9% incidence of major and minor complications associated with transcatheter closure and emphasized the need for randomized clinical trials. Currently, two randomized clinical trials, CLOSURE-1 and RESPECT (Randomized Evaluation of recurrent Stroke comparing PFO closure to Established Current standard of care Treatment), are investigating the efficacy of transcatheter closure versus medical management. It is suggested that antiplatelet agents be used as initial therapy unless there is documented venous or cardiac thrombosis. Endovascular closure may be considered in patients in whom medical therapy fails (recurrent cerebrovascular events despite adequate medical therapy and compliance), patients with contraindication to medical therapy, or high-risk PFO patients [21,24,32]. Although transthoracic contrast echocardiography and transcranial Doppler are used to detect PFO, it is recommended that transesophageal echocardiography (TEE) be used in patients with cryptogenic stroke and suspected PFO [19,30•]. These patients should also have venous Doppler studies to rule out deep venous thrombosis and blood tests to determine whether hypercoagulable status exists.

Ulcerated plaques in the aortic arch (AA) are the other recently recognized source of cerebral emboli that can be classified as a pericardiac source for stroke. Previously, isolated case reports suggested the potential relationship between ulcerated plaques in the AA and embolic stroke. A more comprehensive study evaluated the autopsies of 500 patients with neurologic disease [33•]. It was found that 26% of cerebrovascular disease patients had AA plaques, whereas they were present only in 5% of control subjects with other neurologic disorders. In stroke patients with no other recognized cause, 61% had an ulcerated AA, as compared with 22% of stroke patients with another potential source. Aortic atheromas are also an important cause of strokes associated with cardiac catheterization, cardiopulmonary bypass, or intra-aortic balloon placement, and account for approximately 12% of such occurrences with cardiac surgery [34••]. The two mechanisms that account for the embolic process are either atheroemboli or thromboemboli, the latter being more common. Plaques protruding more than 4 mm and having associated mobile thrombi predict a higher stroke risk [35], with 12% of such patients having a risk of recurrent stroke within 1 year [34••]. One study found that aortic stiffness as calculated by TEE is an independent risk factor irrespective of plaque thickness [36]. TEE can evaluate AA and detect ulcerated plaques, providing a relatively simple (but invasive) method to detect this potential source for embolic stroke. New techniques in the form of CT angiography (CTA), magnetic resonance angiography (MRA), and intraoperative epiaortic ultrasound are emerging to noninvasively detect and characterize the atheromatous disease process. CT and MRI potentially have an advantage in evaluating for the presence of penetrating atherosclerotic ulcers and the associated complications such as intramural hematoma, pseudoaneurysm formation, and aortic rupture, compared with TEE [34••,37]. Still, TEE remains the diagnostic method of choice at present.

A mainstay of therapy are 3-hydoxy-3-methylglutaryl coenzyme-A reductase inhibitors (HMG-CoA inhibitors), commonly known as statins, which have shown to reduce the risk of myocardial infarction or stroke by stabilizing the plaque and preventing the plaque ulceration, hemorrhage, and thrombus formation. In a recent retrospective study of 519 patients with severe thoracic aorta plaque, statins showed an absolute embolic risk reduction of 17%, whereas warfarin and antiplatelet drugs had no significant protective effect [38••]. Anticoagulation with warfarin and antiplatelet therapies is also used, but currently no randomized clinical trials are available to recommend one as compared with the other. Warfarin therapy may be particularly useful when superimposed mobile thrombi are seen on TEE. Aortic endarterectomy is associated with a high risk of emboli and is not performed routinely.

Nonbacterial thrombotic endocarditis, or marantic endocarditis, is believed to be the most common cause of stroke in the cancer patient, at least based on autopsy studies [39]. This condition is characterized by the deposition of small, sterile thrombi on valves and may be responsible for multiple focal deficits in patients with neoplasms.

Mitral valve prolapse (MVP) is a common, although heterogeneous, condition. It is estimated to have a prevalence of 5% in the general population [40]. Studies of stroke in young adults have had widely differing figures, ranging from 2% to more than 30% of strokes attributable to MVP. Certain subgroups of patients are believed to be at increased risk for developing infective endocarditis or peripheral embolization, or both (eg, men older than 45 years with systolic murmurs and patients with myxomatous degeneration of the valve leaflets and chordae). It is unclear if patients with MVP are at an increased risk for stroke [41]. However, recent studies have failed to show any association between MVP and stroke and also reported a markedly decreased prevalence of 2.4% [42].

EVALUATION
Evaluation of patients with cardioembolic stroke includes a history, physical examination, electrocardiogram (including Holter monitor, event monitor, or telemetry), echocardio-

graphy (transthoracic or transesophageal), electrophysiologic studies, transcranial Doppler, and MRI.

The capability to noninvasively detect cardiac sources for embolic stroke has been the main reason for enhanced recognition of the relationship between the two disorders. Echocardiography not only helps in decision making for anticoagulation but also provides guidance regarding medical or surgical treatment. For example, patients with atrial myxoma, infective endocarditis, mitral or aortic stenosis and aortic aneurysm may benefit from surgery, whereas those with left ventricular dysfunction or infective endocarditis will be treated medically with either β- blockers/ACE inhibitors or antibiotics, respectively. Transthoracic echocardiography (TTE) is widely used as an initial screening procedure to detect valvular heart disease, dyskinetic segments, intracardiac thrombi and masses, and cardiomyopathies. The addition of contrast agents, such as agitated saline, is helpful for detecting right-to-left shunts. However, TTE is relatively insensitive, especially for detecting thrombi and left atrial appendage abnormalities and for evaluating the atrial septum. Several studies have compared the diagnostic acumen of TTE with TEE, which provides better visualization of interatrial septum (thus PFO and ASA), left atrium and its appendage, and thoracic aorta. TEE detects potential cardiac sources for emboli significantly better than TTE [43•]. TEE findings, such as spontaneous left atrial contrast and mitral valve strands, are associated with increased stroke risk. The best way to employ TEE in the evaluation of patients with ischemic stroke is continuing to evolve, but it should be the first line of investigation in all patients without an obvious stroke source. TEE is also recommended in patients with endocarditis, valvular heart disease, and in cardiac arrhythmias.

STROKE PREVENTION AND TREATMENT
The substantial stroke risk associated with untreated NVAF prompted five large treatment trials, and the results are now available [44•]. In both the SPAF (Stroke Prevention in Atrial Fibrillation) study and the Danish Atrial Fibrillation, Aspirin, Anticoagulation (AFASAK) study, patients were randomly assigned to receive warfarin, aspirin, or placebo; however, because the trial designs were different, a direct comparison of warfarin with aspirin is not possible. Both studies did demonstrate a significant reduction of ischemic stroke and systemic emboli by warfarin as compared with placebo (Table 2). In SPAF, 325 mg/d of aspirin also significantly reduced end-point occurrence, but in AFASAK, 75 mg/d of aspirin had no effect. A third open-label study, the Boston Area Anticoagulation Trial for Atrial Fibrillation (BAATAF), compared warfarin with placebo. The incidence of ischemic stroke was very low in the warfarin group, 0.4% per year, significantly less than the 3.0% per year rate in the placebo group.

Taken together, these studies and two others strongly support the beneficial effects of warfarin in low doses (international normalized ratio [INR] of 2.0 to 3.0, prothrombin time ratio of 1.2 to 1.5) to reduce primary stroke risk in NVAF patients. A lower INR is associated with less effective stroke prevention, whereas an INR higher than 4.0 has an increased risk for hemorrhage [45•]. The role of aspirin in primary stroke prevention in NVAF has not been established. In the SPAF II trial, a direct comparison of aspirin and warfarin demonstrated no overall difference. Although ischemic stroke incidence was lower in the warfarin group, the risk of hemorrhage was greater [46•]. In SPAF III, a combination of very low-intensity warfarin (INR <1.5) and aspirin (325 mg/d) was less effective than standard-intensity warfarin (INR 2–4) [47•]. Secondary stroke prevention in NVAF patients who have already suffered an initial stroke is another important consideration. The European Atrial Fibrillation Trial demonstrated the efficacy of warfarin in this setting as well, with a decrease in the annual stroke incidence from 12% in the placebo group to 4% in the warfarin group [48].

Therapy with a low to moderate dose of warfarin is indicated in patients with atrial fibrillation who can tolerate this therapy. Patients who are not good candidates for anticoagulation or who do not wish to be placed on warfarin should

				Outcome events per year		
Study	Patients, n	Men, %	Mean age, y	Warfarin vs control, %/%	Aspirin vs control, %/%	Major bleeds per year, %
AFASAK	1007	64	74	2.2/5.5	4.7/5.5	0.8
SPAF	1330	71	67	2.3/7.4	3.6/6.3	1.5
BAATAF	420	72	68	0.4/3.0	—	0.8
CAFA	378	75	68	3.0/4.6	—	2.5
VA	525	100	67	0.9/4.3	—	1.3

TABLE 2 COMPARISON OF STUDIES OF WARFARIN FOR ISCHEMIC STROKE AND SYSTEMIC EMBOLI

AFASAK—The Danish Atrial Fibrillation, Aspirin, Anticoagulation Study; BAATAF—The Boston Area Anticoagulation Trial for Atrial Fibrillation Study; CAFA—The Canadian Atrial Fibrillation Study; SPAF—The Stroke Prevention in Atrial Fibrillation Study; VA—Veterans Administration.

consider aspirin (325 mg/d), clopidogrel, or extended-release dipyridamole/aspirin. A possible alternative being tried for these patients is a procedure in which a device is placed in the left atrial appendage to obliterate it (because the left atrial appendage is the site of 90% to 100% of the thrombus formation in nonvalvular atrial fibrillation). The procedure is called percutaneous left atrial appendage transcatheter occlusion (PLAATO) [49]. Patients are kept on aspirin after the device implantation, and no major adverse events have been reported in more than 50 patients after 1 year of follow-up. However, further clinical trials are needed to establish the long-term safety and efficacy of this procedure before it can be recommended routinely.

Patients younger than 60 years with lone or paroxysmal atrial fibrillation should also consider aspirin at a dose of 325 mg/d. It is unclear whether aspirin or warfarin is better in patients older than 75 years. Risk stratification is recommended to identify those patients with atrial fibrillation who are likely to derive the greatest benefit from anticoagulation treatment [50]. Main contraindications to warfarin are hypersensitivity to warfarin, bleeding dyscrasias, alcohol abuse, renal or hepatic insufficiency, pregnancy, malignant hypertension, and dementia.

The role of warfarin and aspirin for primary stroke prevention in other cardiac disorders has not been as well studied. Warfarin is widely used in patients with rheumatic valvular disease and prosthetic cardiac valves [51]. Currently, only patients with prosthetic valves are recommended to have warfarin-plus-aspirin if they continue to have embolic events while on warfarin only [52–53].

Patients with acute anterior MI and documented ventricular thrombi are also at high risk, and anticoagulants are frequently used. There have been reports of up to a 55% reduction in the cerebral infarction rate in MI patients treated with long-term warfarin after the acute phase, but this area remains somewhat controversial [8•,9,10].

Anticoagulants are frequently used in dilated cardiomyopathy (especially when the ejection fraction is less than 15%), and in other cardiac failure patients with severe left ventricular dysfunction. The ongoing WATCH and WARCEF trials will, hopefully, resolve this issue. The role of anticoagulation in paradoxical embolization, marantic endocarditis, ventricular aneurysms, and other less-common disorders remains uncertain.

Recently, focus has been shifted to alternative therapies other than warfarin, which are easy to administer and monitor. One such class of drugs includes direct thrombin inhibitors. In the SPORTIF III (Stroke Prevention using an ORal Thrombin Inhibitor in atrial Fibrillation) trial, ximelagatran (a direct thrombin inhibitor) was as effective as warfarin in the high-risk group to prevent cardioembolism [54]. Ximelagatran does not require coagulation monitoring and has decreased incidence of bleeding, but a transient increase in liver enzymes was reported in 6% of the patients. The SPORTIF V trial provided additional data about the safety and efficacy of ximelagatran [55]. Argatroban, another

direct thrombin inhibitor, is being used in Japan with some promising results [56]. In past trials, another thrombin inhibitor, hirudin, failed to show positive results. Similarly, idraparinux, a factor Xa–specific pentasaccharide, is being compared with warfarin in the AMADEUS trial. Clopidogrel, a platelet ADP receptor antagonist, in combination with aspirin is being tested against warfarin in the ACTIVE trial.

CONCLUSION

Every patient with cerebral ischemia (either transient or with a completed stroke) should be evaluated by a neurologist, because many neurologic conditions can produce the same symptom complex. In addition, diagnostic and therapeutic advances are occurring at a rapid rate in cerebrovascular disease, and a neurologist would likely be cognizant of the most recent developments.

Regarding cardiogenic embolism, technologic advances have contributed to the increasing recognition of the interconnection between cardiac disorders and stroke. Perhaps many of the currently cryptogenic stroke cases will eventually be assigned to the category of cardioembolic stroke. The similarity between ischemic injury in the heart and the brain implies that therapeutic advances in one area may be helpful and relevant to the other. The exchange of information between cardiologists and neurologists should remain of vital importance to both disciplines.

REFERENCES AND RECOMMENDED READING

Recently published papers of particular interest have been highlighted as:
• Of interest
•• Of outstanding interest

1.•• Ferro JM: Brain embolism: answers to practical questions. *J Neurol* 2003, 250:139–114.

2. Kelley RE, Minagar A: Cardioembolic stroke: an update. *South Med J* 2003, 96:343–399.

3. Brickner ME: Cardioembolic stroke. *Am J Med* 1995, 100:465–474.

4. Wein TH, Bornstein NM: Stroke prevention: cardiac and carotid-related stroke. *Neurol Clin* 2000, 18:321–341.

5.• Atrial Fibrillation Investigators: Risk factors for and efficacy of antithrombotic therapy in atrial fibrillation. *Arch Intern Med* 1994, 154:1449–1457.

6.•• Pullicino PM, Halperin JL, Thompson JL: Stroke in patients with heart failure and reduced left ventricular ejection fraction. *Neurology* 2000, 25:288–294.

7. Falk R:A plea for a clinical trial of anticoagulation in dilated cardiomyopathy. *Am J Cardiol* 1990, 65:914–915.

8.• Loh E, Sutton MSJ, Wun CCC, *et al.*: Ventricular dysfunction and the risk of stroke after myocardial infarction. *N Engl J Med* 1997, 336:251–257.

9. Smith P, Arnesen H, Holme I: The effect of warfarin on mortality and reinfarction after myocardial infarction. *N Engl J Med* 1990, 19:147–152.

10. Anticoagulants in the Secondary Prevention of Events in Coronary Thrombosis (ASPECT) Research Group: Effect of long-term oral anticoagulant treatment on mortality and cardiovascular morbidity after myocardial infarction. *Lancet* 1994, 343:499–503.

11. Hart R, Foster J, Luther M, Kanter M: Stroke in infective endocarditis. *Stroke* 1990, 21:695–700.

12. Anderson DJ, Goldstein LB, Wilkinson WE, *et al.*: Stroke location, characterization, severity, and outcome in mitral vs aortic valve endocarditis. *Neurology* 2003, 25:1341–1346.

13. Sexton DJ, Spelman D: Current best practices and guidelines: assessment and management of complications in infective endocarditis. *Cardiol Clin* 2003, 21:273–282.

14. Sgarbossa EB, Pinski SL, Maloney JD, *et al.*: Chronic atrial fibrillation and stroke in paced patients with sick sinus syndrome. *Circulation* 1993, 88:1045–1053.

15. Connolly SJ, Kerr CR, Gent M, *et al.*: Effects of physiologic pacing versus ventricular pacing on the risk of stroke and death due to cardiovascular causes. *N Engl J Med* 2000, 342:1385–1391.

16. Reynen K: Cardiac myxomas. *N Engl J Med* 1995, 333:1610–1617.

17. Knepper L, Biller J, Adams H, Bruno A: Neurologic manifestations of atrial myxoma. *Stroke* 1988, 19:1435–1440.

18. DiTullio M, Sacco R, Gopal A, *et al.*: Patent foramen ovale as a risk factor of cryptogenic stroke. *Ann Intern Med* 1992, 117:461–465.

19. Overell JR, Bone I, Lees KR: Interatrial septal abnormalities and stroke: a meta-analysis of case-control studies. *Neurology* 2000, 55:1172–1179.

20. Berthet K, Lavergne T, Cohen A, *et al.*: Significant association of atrial vulnerability with atrial septal abnormalities in young patients with ischemic stroke of unknown cause. *Stroke* 2000, 31:398–403.

21.• Homma S, Sacco RL, DiTullio MR, *et al.*: Effect of medical treatment in stroke patients with patent foramen ovale: patent foramen ovale in cryptogenic stroke study. *Circulation* 2002, 105:2625–2631.

22. Lamy C, Giannesini C, Zuber M, *et al.*: Clinical and imaging findings in cryptogenic stroke patients with and without patent foramen ovale: the PFO-ASA Study. Atrial Septal Aneurysm. *Stroke* 2002, 33:706–711.

23. De Castro S, Cartoni D, Fiorelli M, *et al.*: Morphological and functional characteristics of patent foramen ovale and their embolic implications. *Stroke* 2000, 31:2407–2413.

24. Meier B, Lock JE: Contemporary management of patent foramen ovale. *Circulation* 2003, 7:5–9.

25. Lethen H, Flachskampf FA, Schneider R, *et al.*: Frequency of deep vein thrombosis in patients with patent foramen ovale and ischemic stroke or transient ischemic attack. *Am J Cardiol* 1997, 80:1066–1069.

26. Schuchlenz HW, Weihs W, Horner S, Quehenberger F: The association between the diameter of a patent foramen ovale and the risk of embolic cerebrovascular events. *Am J Med* 2000, 15:456–462.

27.• Landzberg M, Khairy P: Indications for the closure of patent foramen ovale. *Heart* 2004, 90:219–224.

28.• Devuyst G, Bogousslavsky J, Ruchat P, *et al.*: Prognosis after stroke followed by surgical closure of patent foramen ovale: a prospective follow-up study with brain MRI and simultaneous transesophageal and transcranial Doppler ultrasound. *Neurology* 1996, 47:1162–1166.

29. Nedeltchev K, Arnold M, Wahl A, *et al.*: Outcome of patients with cryptogenic stroke and patent foramen ovale. *J Neurol Neurosurg Psychiatry* 2002, 72:347–350.

30.• Mas JL, Arquizan C, Lamy C, *et al.*: Patent foramen ovale and atrial septal aneurysm study group: recurrent cerebrovascular events associated with patent foramen ovale, atrial septal aneurysm, or both. *N Engl J Med* 2001, 13:1740–1746.

31. Orgera MA, O'Malley PG, Taylor AJ: Secondary prevention of cerebral ischemia in patent foramen ovale: systematic review and meta-analysis. *South Med J* 2001, 94:699–703.

32.• Khairy P, O'Donnell CP, Landzberg M J: Transcatheter closure versus medical therapy of patent foramen ovale and presumed paradoxical thromboemboli: a systematic review. *Ann Intern Med* 2003, 139:753–760.

33.• Amarenco P, Duyckaerts C, Tzourio C, *et al.*: The prevalence of ulcerated plaques in the aortic arch in patients with stroke. *N Engl J Med* 1992, 326:221–225.

34.•• Tunick PA, Kronzon I: Atheromas of the thoracic aorta: clinical and therapeutic update. *J Am Coll Cardiol* 2000, 35:545–554.

35. Amerenco P, Cohen A, Tzourio C, *et al.*: Atherosclerotic disease of the aortic arch and the risk of ischemic stroke. *N Engl J Med* 1994, 331:1474–1479.

36. Sugioka K, Hozumi T, Sciacca RR, *et al.*: Impact of aortic stiffness on ischemic stroke in elderly patients. *Stroke* 2002, 33:2077–2081.

37. Krinsky GA: Diagnostic imaging of aortic atherosclerosis and its complications. *Neuroimaging Clin N Am* 2002, 12:437–443.

38.•• Tunick PA, Nayar AC, Goodkin GM, *et al.*: NYU Atheroma Group: effect of treatment on the incidence of stroke and other emboli in 519 patients with severe thoracic aortic plaque. *Am J Cardiol* 2002, 15:1320–1325.

39. Rogers L, Cho E, Kempin S, Posner J: Cerebral infarction from non-bacterial thrombotic endocarditis. *Am J Med* 1987, 83:746–756.

40. Cerebral Embolism Task Force: Cardiogenic brain embolism. *Arch Neurol* 1989, 46:727–743.

41. Orencia AJ, Petty GW, Khandheria BK, *et al.*: Risk of stroke with mitral valve prolapse in population-based cohort study. *Stroke* 1995, 26:7–13.

42. Gilon D, Buonanno FS, Joffe MM, *et al.*: Lack of evidence of an association between mitral-valve prolapse and stroke in young patients. *N Engl J Med* 1999, 1:8–13.

43.• Daniel WG, Mugge A: Transesophageal echocardiography. *N Engl J Med* 1995, 332:1268–1279.

44.• Albers GW: Atrial fibrillation and stroke. *Arch Intern Med* 1994, 154:1443–1448.

45.• Hylek EM, Skates SJ, Sheehan MA, Singer DE: An analysis of the lowest effective intensity of prophylactic anticoagulation for patients with nonrheumatic atrial fibrillation. *N Engl J Med* 1996, 335:540–546.

46.• Stroke Prevention in Atrial Fibrillation Investigators: Warfarin versus aspirin for the prevention of thromboembolism in atrial fibrillation. *Lancet* 1994, 343:687–691.

47.• Stroke Prevention in Atrial Fibrillation Investigators: Adjusted-dose warfarin versus low intensity, fixed dose warfarin plus aspirin for high-risk patients with atrial fibrillation. *Lancet* 1996, 348:633–638.

48. European Atrial Fibrillation Trial Study Group: Secondary prevention in non-rheumatic atrial fibrillation after transient ischemic attack or minor stroke. *Lancet* 1993, 342:1255–1262.

49. Sievert H, Lesh MD, Trepels T, *et al.*: Percutaneous left atrial appendage transcatheter occlusion to prevent stroke in high-risk patients with atrial fibrillation: early clinical experience. *Circulation* 2002, 105:1887–1889.

50. Hart RG, Halperin JL: Atrial fibrillation and thromboembolism: a decade of progress in stroke prevention. *Ann Intern Med* 1999, 131:688–695.

51. Stein P, Alpert J, Dalen J, *et al.*: Antithrombotic therapy in patients with mechanical and biological prosthetic heart valves. *Chest* 1998, 114:602S–610S.

52. Turpie AG, Gent M, Laupacis A, *et al.*: A comparison of aspirin with placebo in patients treated with warfarin after heart-valve replacement. *N Engl J Med* 1993, 329:524–529.

53. Hayashi J, Nakazawa S, Oguma F, *et al.*: Combined warfarin and antiplatelet therapy after St. Jude medical valve replacement for mitral valve disease. *J Am Coll Cardiol* 1994, 23:672–677.

54. Olsson SB, and Executive Steering Committee on behalf of the SPORTIF III Investigators: Stroke prevention with the oral direct thrombin inhibitor ximelagatran compared with warfarin in patients with non-valvular atrial fibrillation (SPORTIF III): randomised controlled trial, *Lancet* 2003, 362:1691–1698.

55. Verheugt FW: Can we pull the plug on warfarin in atrial fibrillation? *Lancet* 2003, 362:1686–1687.

56. Urabe T, Tanaka R, Noda K, Mizuno Y: Anticoagulant therapy with a selective thrombin inhibitor for acute cerebral infarction: usefulness of coagulation markers for evaluation of efficacy. *J Thromb Thrombolysis* 2002, 13:155–160.

SELECT BIBLIOGRAPHY

Hinchey JA, Furlan AJ, Barnett HJM: Cardiogenic brain embolism: incidence, varieties, and treatment. In *Stroke*, edn 3. Edited by Barnett H, Mohr J, Stein B, Yatsu F. New York: Churchill Livingstone; 1998:1089–1119.

Kanter M, Sherman D: Embolic stroke of cardiac origin. In *Current Therapy in Neurologic Disease*, edn 3. Edited by Johnson R. Philadelphia: BC Decker; 1990:181–186.

Koudstaal P: Cardioembolic stroke. In *Current Review of Cerebrovascular Disease*. Edited by Fisher M, Bogousslavsky J. Philadelphia: Current Medicine; 1993:41–47.

Sherman D: Prevention of cardioembolic stroke. In *Prevention of Stroke*. Edited by Norris J, Hachinski V. New York: Springer-Verlag; 1991:149–160.

The Heart and Endocrine Diseases

Clifford J. Rosen

41

> ## Key Points
> - Diabetes mellitus profoundly accelerates atherosclerotic disease by micro- and macroangiopathic changes in coronary vessels.
> - Coexistent hypertension and small vessel disease contribute to diabetic cardiomyopathy and congestive heart failure.
> - Cardiac function can be altered by chronic thyrotoxicosis through direct hormonal stimulation or indirectly via sympathetic overactivity.
> - Reduction in cardiac output and asymptomatic pericardial effusions are classic signs of hypothyroidism.
> - Atherosclerotic coronary disease is one of the major manifestations of Cushing's disease.
> - Carcinoid heart disease is caused by endothelial fibrosis as a result of metastatic deposition on surfaces of the right heart and overproduction of vasoactive products such as serotonin.

Hormones are circulating peptides and sterols that regulate tissue activity at sites remote from their points of synthesis. The biologic activity of these endocrine effectors is dependent to a major degree on transport through the circulation. At the same time, the high metabolic requirements of the myocardium demand a fixed proportion of total cardiac output. Thus, as a circulatory pump and as a metabolic factory, the heart plays a central role in targeting hormonal action. A challenge for clinicians is to recognize that organic heart disease can be related to perturbations in hormonal factors or metabolic substrates. This chapter examines how hormonal excess or deficiency states can affect cardiac structure and function.

DIABETES MELLITUS AND THE HEART

The most common endocrine disorder associated with cardiac dysfunction is diabetes mellitus. Coronary artery disease (CAD) is the principle cause of premature death in both insulin-dependent diabetes mellitus (IDDM) and non–insulin-dependent diabetes mellitus (NIDDM) [1]. By the age of 55, one third of diabetics die of CAD compared with a mortality rate of 4% to 8% in the Framingham cohort of men and women without diabetes mellitus [2]. In particular, the incidence of CAD in females with diabetes is five times higher than in nondiabetics, and affected women have a much greater likelihood of dying from the disease than do women without diabetes [3]. Several studies have now confirmed that chronic hyperglycemia in men and women, whether symptomatic or asymptomatic, is a major risk factor for mortality from CAD, independent of all other factors [1–4]. Indeed, type II diabetics have more extensive atherosclerosis compared with euglycemic patients with the same symptoms, as well as greater rates of silent ischemia and poorer outcomes [5]. Moreover, very recent work has suggested that the prediabetic state, which is associated with euglycemia but high insulin levels and obesity, contributes to accelerated atherogenesis [6•,7••]. This is a function of insulin resistance, which increases blood pressure and triglyceride levels as well as reducing high-density lipoprotein (HDL) cholesterol. Moreover, hyperinsulinemia also predisposes to reduced fibrinolysis, increased C-reactive protein, and higher plasminogen activator inhibitor-1 (PAI-1), all of which accelerate the atherosclerotic process [7••].

Although diabetes mellitus ravages the heart by affecting large and small coronary vessels and autonomic nerves, the mechanisms that produce such injury are poorly understood. Several metabolic and structural perturbations seem likely to contribute to the high incidence of CAD in this disease (Table 1). Clearly the most consistent pathologic finding in diabetic heart disease is diffuse atherosclerosis. This *macroangiopathic* process is grossly, radiologically, and microscopically identical to atherosclerosis in coronary vessels of nondiabetic individuals. However, the develop-

ment of atherosclerosis in diabetics is markedly accelerated in part because of deleterious changes in lipids (triglycerides, HDL cholesterol, low-density lipoprotein [LDL] cholesterol) as well as markers of inflammation such as C-reactive protein and PAI-1 [3–5,6•,7••,8]. Indeed, diabetic coronary macroangiopathy, irrespective of phenotype (IDDM vs NIDDM), is more severe and more diffuse than angiopathic disease in nondiabetic patients [5]. Although classical anginal symptoms are frequently reported by diabetics with underlying disease and are more frequent during activities of daily life than in nondiabetics, there is often a mismatch between classic symptomatology and the extent of CAD. Moreover, many diabetic patients have silent myocardial ischemia even though this rate is not statistically different from that in nondiabetic subjects [9]. Unrecognized myocardial infarction (MI) is more common in persons with diabetes and accounts for 39% of diabetic infarctions compared with 22% in patients without diabetes [10]. Therefore, a high index of suspicion is necessary when evaluating diabetic patients for atypical chest pain, nausea, vomiting, or diaphoresis.

Objective tests (angiography, radionuclide studies, exercise examinations) to assess the severity of ischemia are indicated in patients suspected of having occult heart disease, even though exercise-induced angina during treadmill testing is considerably less common in diabetics than in nondiabetics [11]. However, there is ample evidence to suggest that there is impaired exercise tolerance due to left ventricular dysfunction in type II diabetic patients even when their metabolic control is excellent [12••]. There is no evidence, however, to suggest that insulin resistance per se results in impaired left ventricular dysfunction.

The risk of coronary angiography in diabetic patients (compared with nondiabetics of similar age and severity) is *not* increased unless there is superimposed renal disease, in which case pretreatment with intravenous fluids and mannitol can avert serious renal damage [13].

Treatment of myocardial ischemia and silent CAD in diabetics does not differ greatly from therapy for nondiabetics. Therapeutic options include coronary artery angioplasty, arterial stenting, or coronary artery bypass graft (CABG) surgery. A recent multicenter study suggested that diabetics had a higher 5-year survival rate after CABG than after coronary angioplasty [14••]. This is in sharp contrast with nondiabetic patients, whose survival rates are similar for CABG and angioplasty. In respect to heart transplant for those with the most severe forms of cardiomyopathy, there is also no difference in long-term survival, (*ie*, 5 years) between diabetics and nondiabetics, although the former have a much greater risk of infections complicating their postoperative course [15••].

If untreated, the macroangiopathic atherosclerotic process in diabetics can progress rapidly. Both early and later studies confirm significantly higher initial and 1-year mortality rates in diabetics who suffer from myocardial damage compared with patients with heart disease but with-

TABLE 1 POSSIBLE PATHOGENETIC FACTORS CONTRIBUTING TO ACCELERATED ATHEROSCLEROTIC CORONARY ARTERY DISEASE IN DIABETES MELLITUS

Hyperglycemia
Direct toxic effects
Indirect via other risk factors (*eg*, insulin, IGF, LDL)

Hyperinsulinemia

Increased production of endothelial and smooth muscle growth factors
PDGF
IGF-I
EGF
FGF
TGF

Lipoprotein abnormalities including:
Increased LDL and VLDL
Decreased HDL

Altered hormonal milieu
Enhanced growth hormone secretion

Qualitative and quantitative changes in clotting factors

EGF—epidermal growth factor; FGF—fibroblast growth factor; HDL—high-density lipoprotein; IGF-I—insulin-like growth factor-I; LDL—low-density lipoprotein; PDGF—platelet-derived growth factor; TGF—transforming growth factor; VLDL—very low-density lipoprotein.

out glucose intolerance [16,17]. At particularly high risk are younger diabetics (who have a mortality rate three times that of nondiabetics) and diabetic women (who have twice the in-hospital mortality of nondiabetics) [17]. Despite this, the reason for the difference in death rates between diabetics and nondiabetics is not readily apparent. The extent of cardiac damage, the incidence of postinfarction arrhythmias, and the degree of left ventricular dysfunction are not significantly greater in patients with diabetes than in age-and sex-matched euglycemic patients. However, the coexistence of microvascular disease and altered diastolic compliance could be contributing factors. In addition, a higher incidence of coronary vasoconstriction related to autonomic neuropathy may jeopardize potentially viable myocardial tissue and enhance the risk of fatal arrythmias.

Although the management of acute myocardial infarctions (AMIs) for diabetics does not differ from that for nondiabetics, control of hyperglycemia and awareness of other diabetic complications are essential. As noted, the first step in treatment is recognition, a particularly relevant issue for diabetics presenting to the emergency room with hyperglycemia or dyspnea but not chest pain. In the end, increased awareness of the risk of CAD in diabetes should prompt early and aggressive intervention prior to a major myocardial event. Microangiopathy, a process characteristic of diabetic retinopathy and nephropathy, also affects myocardial function and can result in congestive cardiomyopathy. In fact, diabetic cardiomyopathy, with or without coronary vascular involvement, is common and may account for nearly 35% of all cases of idiopathic cardiomyopathy [18]. In the cardiac microvessels and capillaries of both type I IDDM and type II NIDDM patients, basement membrane thickening and microaneurysm have been described [19]. One of the earliest signs of diabetic microangiopathy is microalbuminuria. Recent studies suggest that, even in nondiabetic hypertensive patients, increased albumin excretion is associated with a fourfold greater risk of ischemic heart disease [20]. However, macroangiopathic abnormalities often coexist, making it extremely difficult to interpret the full implication of these changes.

In addition to both micro- and macroangiopathic disease, there are also profound metabolic alterations in carbohydrates and lipids that can alter myocardial function at a cellular level. Reduced glucose uptake, increased fatty acid and triglyceride accumulation, and alterations in calcium transport in the myocardium can contribute to acute and diffuse myocardial dysfunction. The hemodynamic abnormalities described in diabetic cardiomyopathy include reduced cardiac output, impaired left ventricular compliance, increased ventricular wall stiffness, and end-diastolic pressure [21]. Whether these changes are reversible with control of the blood glucose remains controversial, although in vitro studies suggest there is a return to a normal contractile status when extracellular glucose is normalized [22].

Patients with diabetic cardiomyopathy exhibit classical signs of congestive heart failure (CHF) with reduced left ventricular compliance and recurrent pulmonary edema. Because of the high prevalence of atherosclerotic coronary disease in these patients, the premortem diagnosis of primary cardiomyopathy can be difficult. Further complicating the differential diagnosis are other disorders associated with diabetes that can accelerate the disease process, including hypertension and renal failure. Hemochromatosis can also present as a cardiomyopathy or as diabetes mellitus. The management of diabetic cardiomyopathy includes strict control of blood sugars, aggressive therapy for CHF, and control of hypertension.

The clinical course of diabetic heart disease can be dramatically altered by development of autonomic neuropathy. Sudden death, presumably cardiac, is responsible for the marked increase in mortality noted after development of autonomic neuropathy. Several events, in part related to chronic hyperglycemia, lead to autonomic dysfunction (Table 2). Parasympathetic nerve fibers are affected first. This results in a relative increase in sympathetic tone and a resting tachycardia [23]. Alterations in parasympathetic function can also exaggerate coronary vasoconstriction. Sympathetic dysfunction follows soon after parasympathetic involvement and produces orthostatic hypotension, which further reduces coronary artery perfusion [24]. In addition to the changes in the sympathetic and parasympathetic nervous system, atrial axons are also twice as likely to be damaged in diabetic hearts than in metabolically normal individuals [25].

Impaired neurogenic responsiveness to stressors, such as surgery or trauma, diminish cardiac performance and enhance the risk of major postoperative complications. Eventually, autonomic neuropathy can cause sudden death in diabetics. In part, this can be related to malignant arrhythmias from silent ischemia, although there is also evidence that diabetic autonomic neuropathy and a prolonged QT

TABLE 2 DIABETIC AUTONOMIC NEUROPATHY AND ITS DELETERIOUS EFFECTS ON THE HEART

Parasympathetic dysfunction leading to:
Enhanced sympathetic tone
    Increased heart rate
      Coronary vasoconstriction

Sympathetic dysfunction leading to:
Orthostatic hypotension
    Reduced coronary perfusion
Impaired chronotropic response to stress and exercise

Conduction abnormalities leading to:
Sudden death
    Prolonged QT interval + sympathetic dysfunction
      Sympathetic dysfunction + hypokalemia or hypomagnesemia
Syncope

interval shown on electrocardiogram (ECG) may increase the risk of life-threatening ventricular arrhythmias [26]. Other complications seen frequently in diabetics, such as transient hypokalemia, hypomagnesemia, and digitalis toxicity, may also multiply the relative risk of sudden death due to arrhythmia. Primary goals of therapy are correction of any underlying metabolic disorders and treatment of orthostatic hypotension.

THYROID DISEASES AND THE HEART

Hyperthyroidism

The cardiac manifestations of hyperthyroidism are usually the earliest and most prominent parts of the clinical presentation in this disease. Palpitations, tachycardia, and cardiomegaly were first described in hyperthyroid patients more than 200 years ago. Since then, numerous studies have documented the cardiovascular effects of thyrotoxicosis. In general, cardiac manifestations of thyroid overactivity can be divided into direct and indirect effects.

Excess circulating thyroxine *indirectly* affects the heart via the sympathetic nervous system. Anxiety, tremors, tachycardia, increased pulse pressure, and palpitations all can be attributed to the actions of thyroid hormone on the sympathoadrenal system. With active hyperthyroidism, catecholamine synthesis is enhanced and catecholamine uptake and breakdown are reduced. This results in enhanced pressor and chronotropic responses [27]. There also is increased sensitivity of myocardial tissue to catecholamines, possibly due to upregulation of adrenergic receptors [28]. Irrespective of the mechanism, enhanced sympathetic tone contributes greatly to the cardiovascular symptoms in patients with thyrotoxicosis.

Direct actions of thyroxine on the heart, independent of the sympathetic nervous system, have also been described [28]. Excess thyroid hormone can stimulate myocardial contractility, even during experimental states of catecholamine depletion. Furthermore, the marked increase in ionotropy during thyrotoxicosis is not ameliorated by coexistent administration of beta-blockers. This implies that myocardial activity is directly modulated by thyroxine. Stimulation of myocardial adenylate cyclase, changes in intracellular calcium transport, increases in Na/K pump activity, or induction of several contractile proteins contribute to augmented myocardial contractility [29].

The clinical stigmata and hemodynamic alterations that result from thyrotoxicosis often are very apparent. Increased heart rate, pulse pressure, cardiac output, stroke volume, and mean systolic ejection rate are coupled with diminished peripheral vascular resistance and increased circulating blood volume [30]. These findings correlate closely with oxygen utilization and the metabolic needs of the affected individual. Cardiac symptoms of hyperthyroidism also include dyspnea, palpitations, and angina. Patients can appear hypermetabolic, warm, and tachypneic, especially at rest. Frequently there is a third heart sound, and mitral valve prolapse and atrial fibrillation also are associated with thyrotoxicosis.

The diagnosis of hyperthyroidism in elderly individuals can be very elusive, although presenting symptoms are often cardiac. For example, although "apathetic" thyrotoxicosis is associated with profound weight loss and lethargy, it is atrial fibrillation that often points clinicians toward the diagnosis of occult hyperthyroidism [31]. Atrial fibrillation alone occurs in 15% of all patients with hyperthyroidism and is frequently related to underlying CAD, especially in patients older than 40 years. In most cases, atrial fibrillation due to hyperthyroidism is related to the severity of the thyrotoxicosis. It usually resolves following induction of the euthyroid state unless coexistent heart disease is present. Wolff-Parkinson-White syndrome, mitral valve prolapse with arrhythmias, and other supraventricular tachycardias have also been reported in patients with thyrotoxicosis. Echocardiography is generally not useful, although long-standing hyperthyroidism can lead to cardiac hypertrophy.

Treatment of hyperthyroid heart disease centers on controlling thyrotoxic symptoms through the use of beta-blockers (primarily to slow the heart rate) and antithyroid medications (propylthiouracil or methimazole) to reduce intrathyroidal synthesis of thyroxine. As noted previously, induction of the euthyroid state can lead to spontaneous cardioversion. For acute episodes of supraventricular tachycardia, beta-blockers or calcium channel blockers are frequently successful in slowing the heart rate [32••]. On the other hand, failure to control the ventricular response to atrial tachycardia with conventional doses of digitalis suggests that thyrotoxicosis may be an etiologic factor in the arrhythmia.

Thyroid storm is a clinical syndrome characterized by exaggerated organ responsiveness to high circulating levels of thyroxine. But in this era of widespread beta-blocker utilization, thyroid storm can either be masked or missed totally. Cardiac tissue is particularly susceptible to acute rises in thyroid hormone, which results in very rapid heart rates (with or without atrial fibrillation), impending ischemia or infarction, and CHF. Besides beta-blockers and antithyroid medications, high doses of glucocorticoids (which block T_4 to T_3 peripheral conversion), and iodides (which suppress hormone release from the thyroid gland) are usually employed. Lithium carbonate can also be used to further suppress thyroxine release when given for a relatively short period of time (*ie*, < 14 days). Subtle cardiac manifestations are also noted in long-standing, unrecognized hyperthyroidism or in patients treated with radioactive iodine who have not been adequately prepared with antithyroid medications prior to radioiodine ablation.

Hypothyroidism

Not surprisingly, the cardiac manifestations of hypothyroidism are the opposite of those seen with thyrotoxic heart disease. However, in contrast to the overt cardiovascular symptoms that characterize hyperthyroidism (Table 3), signs of hypothyroid heart disease are often subtle. Cardiac signs and symptoms, which result from long-standing hypothyroidism, reflect a profound decrease in left ventricular performance [32••]. This is manifested by a low cardiac output and prolongation of both pre-ejection time and isovolumic contraction. Reduced ionotropy from hypothyroidism can be attributed to altered calcium uptake and release in the myocyte [33]. However, there are also changes in expression of several myocardial contractile proteins. In addition, the slow heart rate can reduce cardiac output during stressful states. In the periphery, hypothyroidism increases systemic vascular resistance; hence, diastolic blood pressure may be very high. Surprisingly, blood volume is reduced even though hypothyroid patients often have non-pitting edema. The pathogenetic factors responsible for edema in hypothyroidism have not been fully elucidated.

As noted previously, few symptoms of hypothyroidism can be directly attributed to cardiac involvement. However, exertional dyspnea and exercise intolerance can be related to altered skeletal and cardiac muscle function. Angina pectoris may be more common in hypothyroidism, but it is unclear if myxedema alone can lead to CHF. Classically, patients with hypothyroidism have a slow heart rate, narrowed pulse pressure, and diminished heart sounds. In addition, diastolic hypertension is common. Laboratory studies generally show an increase in both cholesterol and triglycerides, which contributes to a greater risk of CAD in these patients. Serum creatine phosphokinase (CPK) activity is increased in approximately 30% of patients with hypothyroidism, although the isoenzyme pattern is skeletal rather than myocardial. This increase in enzyme activity is also related to impaired clearance from the circulation.

Electrocardiograms of patients with hypothyroidism show low voltage and sinus bradycardia. However, in contrast to hyperthyroidism, atrial and ventricular arrhythmias are not common. The low voltage noted on ECGs may be related to asymptomatic pericardial effusions, which occur in 30% to 50% of patients with overt hypothyroidism. The severity of pericardial effusion is directly related to the duration and extent of the hypothyroid state [34]. Pericardial aspirates reveal an exudative fluid with high concentrations of cholesterol and protein. However, the risk of pericardial tamponade is very low, with only a handful of cases reported.

Treatment of hypothyroidism reverses most cardiac manifestations. However, it may take a year or more for pericardial effusions to clear. In part this may be related to clinical practice patterns in which concern for arrhythmias in elderly patients has made practitioners more cautious in their approach to the rate of thyroid replacement. Generally, replacement therapy is initiated with very low doses of L-thyroxine (eg, 0.0125 or 0.025 mg/day) and increased gradually. Still, there is considerable controversy surrounding the rapidity of thyroxine replacement in the elderly. Despite anecdotal reports suggesting that thyroxine replacement in full doses to older individuals can increase the risk of arrhythmia, sudden death, or MI, there is little evidence to support that contention. In one prospective study of 55 patients with known symptomatic coronary disease, 38% improved with treatment of their thyroid disease, 46% had no change, and only 16% had more symptoms of ischemic heart disease [35]. Currently the issue of whether thyroid replacement can exacerbate CAD in patients with hypothyroidism remains unresolved. On the other hand, CABG can be safely performed without urgent thyroid replacement in patients with moderate or severe hypothyroidism [32••]. Furthermore, therapeutic introduction of thyroxine immedi-

TABLE 3 CARDIAC MANIFESTATIONS OF THYROID DYSFUNCTION

Hyperthyroidism
Cardiovascular effects
  Increased sympathetic tone
    Increased heart rate
    Widened pulse pressure
    Tachyarrythmias
    Decreased peripheral vascular resistance
    Increased ejection fraction
    Increased blood volume
  Direct effects from excess thyroxine
    Increased ionotropy
    Increased chronotropy
    Shortened ejection and filling times
    ? Cardiac failure
    Increased oxygen demand and utilization
Symptoms and signs
  Dyspnea
  Angina (electrocardiogram changes of ischemia)
  Palpitations, tachycardia
  Anxiety
  Acute myocardial infarction
  Apathy

Hypothyroidism
Cardiovascular effects
  Bradycardia
  Decreased ejection fraction
  Reduced cardiac output
  Narrow pulse pressure
  Diastolic hypertension
  Decreased blood volume
Symptoms and signs
  Low body temperature
  Decreased heart sounds
  Apathy
  Low voltage on electrocardiogram
  Non-pitting edema

ately following CABG has not been associated with an increase in morbidity or mortality [32••].

CALCIUM DISORDERS AND THE HEART

Hypercalcemia

Changes in serum calcium levels do not directly affect myocardial function but can influence electrical activity in the heart. High serum calcium is associated with a reversible shortening of the QT interval and prolongation of the PR interval [36]. First-degree atrioventricular block has been reported in hyperparathyroidism, but ventricular arrhythmias with acute or chronic hypercalcemia are rare. Ventricular arrhythmias are detected only when hypercalcemia is related to an infiltrative granulomatous disorder (eg, sarcoidosis). In contrast, hypertension is reported in nearly 50% of hyperparathyroid patients, which is at least two times higher than the incidence in other adult populations [37]. However, the pathogenesis of hypertension in primary hyperparathyroidism is not well defined, especially after secondary causes of hypertension are excluded. For example, pheochromocytoma can coexist with primary hyperparathyroidism (multiple endocrine neoplasia type II), and should always be considered in patients who present with hypercalcemia and hypertension. Similarly, chronic hypercalcemia can impair renal function because of nephrolithiasis or nephrocalcinosis. In turn this can lead to sustained hypertension. Still, when secondary causes of hypertension are excluded, the incidence of hypertension in hyperparathyroidism remains higher than in the normal population. Unfortunately, like other endocrine disorders associated with hypertension (aldosteronomas, pheochromocytomas), surgical removal of parathyroid adenomas does not always reverse systolic or diastolic hypertension. Finally, with the introduction of parathyroid hormone (PTH 1-34) as an approved treatment for osteoporosis, transient hypercalcemia can develop 1 to 4 hours after a single injection; this occurrence has not been associated with any cardiac symptoms. However, some caution must be exercised in patients receiving daily PTH injections who are coincidentally being treated with digitalis compounds, since this combination may enhance the risk of digitalis toxicity and could induce life-threatening ventricular arrhythmias.

Hypocalcemia

In contrast to hypercalcemia, low serum calcium can be extremely dangerous to the heart. Besides nonspecific ECG changes including ST-T abnormalities, the corrected QT interval (QTc) can be prolonged, enhancing the likelihood of malignant ventricular arrhythmias [36]. Although this is not specific for hypocalcemia, its presence on ECG should alert the clinician to the possibility of hypocalcemia, especially in the setting of the critical care unit. In addition, reversible CHF has been reported in patients with severe hypocalcemia [38].

Hypocalcemia often coincides with another common electrolyte disorder, severe hypomagnesemia [39]. At least 10% of hospitalized patients are hypomagnesemic, and many of those are also mildly hypocalcemic. This occurs because low serum magnesium impairs PTH action and secretion. In addition, magnesium depletion blocks potassium conservation in the kidney, thereby setting up an ominous triad of hypocalcemia, hypokalemia, and hypomagnesemia. These three electrolyte disorders are a major cause of malignant ventricular arrhythmias and sustained atrial tachycardias. In particular, arrhythmias, which result from low serum magnesium, are notoriously resistant to antiarrhythmic treatment unless the magnesium deficit is completely corrected. Principle causes of low calcium and low magnesium include primary hypoparathyroidism (surgery, radiation, or autoimmune), malabsorption due to gastrointestinal disorders (eg, Crohn's disease), vitamin D deficiency syndromes, alcohol, starvation, renal diseases, and diuretic use.

Therapy for hypocalcemia is often urgent in the intensive care setting and generally requires a rapid infusion of 10 mL of a 10% calcium gluconate solution (4.65 mEq (95 mg)/10 mL) over 10 minutes. This should be followed by a slower continuous infusion of 15 mg/kg over 12 to 24 hours. More importantly, the serum magnesium level must also be measured, and if it is low, it must be followed by immediate magnesium replacement (8 to 16 mEq over the first 2 hours followed by continuous infusion of 48 to 64 mEq of magnesium sulfate in 48 hours). Serum magnesium levels provide only a fair gauge of replacement, since most magnesium is not found in the extracellular space. However, levels of serum magnesium greater than 1.8 mEq/L usually are indicative of adequate replacement.

ADRENAL DISORDERS AND THE HEART

Hyperfunction of the Adrenal Gland

Neoplasms of the adrenal gland secrete vasoactive substances (cortisol, aldosterone, epinephrine) that can alter myocardial function. Adrenocortical production of cortisol (Cushing's syndrome) can affect the cardiovascular system in several ways and is the major cause of death if the disease is not successfully treated [40]. More than 75% of patients with Cushing's disease (ie, adrenal hyperfunction caused by pituitary adenomas) have some degree of hypertension, itself a major risk factor for CAD [41]. Hypertension is caused by an increase in plasma volume and stimulation of the renin-angiotensin system, which can sensitize arterioles to the pressor effects of catecholamines [42]. Besides hypertension, lipid abnormalities and coexistent diabetes mellitus (related to insulin resistance) further increase the risk of atherosclerotic cardiovascular disease. Hypokalemia, which also can result from glucocorticoid excess, contributes to a much higher incidence of cardiac arrhythmias.

Aldosterone-producing adenomas (APAs) are characterized by marked diastolic hypertension and profound hypokalemia [43]. Hypertension is due to expansion of plasma volume and can contribute to concentric left ventricular hypertrophy. Malignant arrhythmias due to hypokalemia (and often hypomagnesemia) can strongly influence preoperative morbidity. Surgical removal of these relatively small APAs can reverse long-standing hypertension in the majority of cases and permanently correct the metabolic alkalosis and hypokalemia so characteristic of this syndrome.

Pheochromocytoma is often considered in the differential diagnosis of secondary hypertension, although establishing that diagnosis can be exceedingly difficult. The secretory products from a pheochromocytoma impact the heart and vasculature in several ways. Tachycardia and palpitations result from high circulating levels of norepinephrine or epinephrine [44]. Sustained or episodic hypertension can lead to a hypertensive crisis with heart failure, arrhythmia, or stroke as potential outcomes. Orthostatic hypotension from profound volume depletion following episodes of intense vasoconstriction is not uncommon.

Chronic catecholamine excess can lead to a congestive cardiomyopathy, in part due to sustained hypertension and in part due to a direct toxic effect from catecholamines on the myocardium [44]. Very recently, at least one group has reported left ventricular outflow obstruction in a patient with pheochromocytoma [45]. Many of these manifestations are cured following surgical removal of solitary tumors, although hypertension persists in approximately 25% of patients after complete surgical resection. Medical treatment of hypertension from a pheochromocytoma is generally unsatisfactory and usually involves alpha-blockade as well as competitive inhibition of tyrosine hydroxylation, a critical step in catecholamine synthesis [46]. Beta-blockers can be used to treat tachyarrythmias, but only after complete alpha-blockade has been accomplished. Phentolamine or nitroprusside can be used in the management of acute hypertensive crises.

Adrenal Insufficiency

The principle cardiovascular manifestation of primary adrenal insufficiency is orthostatic hypotension. It is a benchmark of this disorder and can be severe enough to cause syncope [47]. Although hyperkalemia and hyponatremia are frequently present in primary adrenal insufficiency, life-threatening arrhythmias are exceedingly rare. Peaked T waves and nonspecific ST-T changes have been reported in hyperkalemic patients with acute adrenal insufficiency. Secondary adrenal disorders rarely produce orthostasis or hyperkalemia, in part because aldosterone secretion is principally regulated by the renin-angiotensin system.

GROWTH HORMONE AND THE HEART

Cardiac disease is present in approximately one third of patients with growth hormone excess syndrome (ie,

acromegaly) [48]. Cardiovascular complications are the most frequent cause of death in acromegalic patients and are a result of hypertension(which occurs in about 30% of all cases) and excess growth hormone (which can have a direct and deleterious effect on cardiac function). Concentric left ventricular hypertrophy, asymmetric septal hypertrophy, and a reduced ejection fraction are the most frequent signs of cardiac involvement. Cardiac hypertrophy can be very pronounced compared with enlargement of other organs [49]. ECGs are abnormal in more than 50% of patients with acromegaly and reveal nonspecific ST-T changes as well as left ventricular hypertrophy, conduction defects, and ventricular irritability. CAD is relatively frequent in acromegaly and, combined with myocardial dysfunction due to excess growth hormone, contributes to the high incidence of cardiovascular deaths in this disorder. In addition, the high frequency of the sleep apnea syndrome due to macroglossia enhances the likelihood of nocturnal oxygen desaturation, further aggravating latent ischemic disease. The severity of atherosclerotic disease in this syndrome has led some investigators to speculate that high circulating levels of insulin-like growth factor-I (IGF-I), a characteristic feature of acromegaly, enhance the propensity for atherogenesis by stimulating vascular smooth muscle hypertrophy. However, the pathogenesis of accelerated atherosclerosis in acromegaly remains unclear. Interestingly enough, acute growth hormone excess is also associated with cardiac dysfunction. There is a rapid increase in left ventricular mass, normal diastolic function, but a high output state as vascular resistance falls dramatically [50].

Since CAD and left ventricular hypertrophy frequently accompany this disease and may be advanced at the time of diagnosis, it is not surprising that CHF is relatively common in acromegaly. Whether chronic long-standing growth hormone excess results in an "acromegalic" cardiomyopathy remains debatable. In one longitudinal study of patients treated with surgical adenectomy, a sizable proportion of "cured" patients with acromegaly demonstrated improvement in left ventricular size and cardiac function [51]. However, as noted previously, heart disease in this syndrome is multifactorial and exceedingly difficult to define in a single clinical setting. Adult growth hormone deficiency (GHD) is also associated with an increased risk of cardiovascular events. Lipid profiles are unfavorable and there is atherogenesis, possibly due to increased lipoprotein (a) synthesis, although the exact pathophysiology has not been defined. In addition, there appears to be a neuropathic process involved in GHD, since at least one group has noted significant alterations in sympathetic tone among patients with adult onset of GHD [52].

Recombinant human growth hormone (rhGH) recently was approved by the United States Food and Drug Administration for the treatment of adult patients with acquired growth hormone deficiency syndromes. Coincidental with the introduction of this peptide for replacement therapy, studies have been undertaken to examine the role of growth hormone/IGF-I in the pathophysiology and treatment of ischemic CHF. There is now evidence that growth hormone and IGF-I decline significantly in patients with heart failure [53]. In fact, the more severe the heart failure, the more suppressed is the growth hormone/IGF axis. However, trials with rhGH have met with limited success, in part because of the numerous covariates associated with patients who have very low cardiac output [54••]. Some investigators have suggested the use of recombinant human IGF-I in this syndrome, although only very small trials have been undertaken to date [55]. On the other hand, there is no evidence that growth hormone treatment for GHD syndromes has any adverse effects on the heart, or increases the risk of cardiovascular events in adult patients receiving this therapy.

VASOACTIVE PEPTIDES AND THE HEART

The Carcinoid Syndrome

The carcinoid syndrome is characterized by flushing, diarrhea, and heart disease [56]. Tumors that produce this syndrome are almost always metastatic at the time of clinical presentation and arise from enterochromaffin cells scattered throughout the body. Nonfunctioning carcinoids are frequent findings at autopsy, but true secretion of vasoactive material leading to clinical symptoms is relatively rare. Usually these tumors occur in the ileum, bronchus, stomach, ovary, or duodenum. Their secretory products are 5-hydroxytryptamine (serotonin), histamine, and 5-hydroxyindoleacetic acid. The dramatic manifestations of the carcinoid syndrome occur after hepatic metastases, and heart disease is evident only when metastatic disease is clinically apparent. Cardiac symptoms are detected in approximately one third of patients with the carcinoid syndrome and are characterized by right heart failure, tricuspid regurgitation, and pulmonic stenosis [57]. In patients with metastatic bronchial carcinoid (not to the liver), left ventricular dysfunction can be found.

Carcinoid heart disease is caused by fibrosis of the endocardium, especially along the surfaces of the pulmonic and tricuspid valves. Metastatic tumor deposits, which travel directly from the liver to the right heart, are a major pathogenetic factor. However, high levels of serotonin also stimulate endocardial fibrosis and clearly contribute to the clinical manifestations of the carcinoid syndrome. The presentation of cardiac involvement in the carcinoid syndrome includes classic signs of right heart failure such as pitting edema, jugular venous distention, dyspnea, and ascites. Constrictive pericarditis has also been reported in this syndrome [57]. Occasionally the cardiac symptoms occur well after resection of the primary tumor.

Therapy for cardiac-related carcinoid disease centers on controlling metastases with chemotherapy or octreotide acetate while treating symptomatic heart disease with

diuretics and afterload reduction. If possible, surgical removal of the primary disease can halt further cardiac fibrosis. In rare situations, tricuspid valve replacement has been performed [58]. However, cardiac involvement with the carcinoid syndrome usually implies a poor prognosis with a median survival time after diagnosis of 14 months [59].

Secretion of other vasoactive substances can cause orthostatic hypotension. However, they rarely have direct effects on the heart. Vasoactive intestinal peptide (VIP) is secreted from certain gastrointestinal tumors and can lead to diarrhea, hypokalemia, and hypercalcemia. Hypotension is common with VIPomas, and increased cardiac contractility has also been reported [60]. The kinins and kallikreins are also produced by gastrointestinal tumors and have strong vasodilatory properties. These substances, however, do not directly affect cardiac function.

KEY REFERENCES

Recently published papers of outstanding interest, as identified in *References and Recommended Reading*, have been annotated.

•• Haffner SM: Insulin resistance, inflammation and the prediabetic state. *Am J Cardiol* 2003, 92:18–26.

This is an outstanding paper that reviews the San Antonio Heart Study in respect to patients who start with normal glucose tolerance but later develop type II noninsulin-dependent diabetes mellitus. The insulin resistance that occurs in the prediabetic state contributes to increased C-reactive protein and high plasminogen activator inhibitor-1 levels. These contribute to greater risk of atherosclerosis.

•• Poirer P, Garreau C, Bogaty P, *et al.*: Impact of left ventricular dysfunction on maximal treadmill performance in normotensive subjects with well controlled type II NIDDM. *Am J Cardiol* 2000, 85:473–477.

This study demonstrates the importance of recognizing left ventricular dysfunction, even in the patient with well-controlled diabetes. It also implies that factors other than glucose intolerance must be operative.

•• Bypass Angioplasty Revascularization Investigation (BARI). Comparison of coronary artery bypass surgery with angioplasty in patients with multivessel disease. *N Engl J Med* 1996, 335:217–225.

This very large study (BARI) demonstrates for the first time that in diabetic patients coronary artery bypass grafting may be superior to angioplasty in terms of 5-year survival. This is not surprising considering the inherent potential for restenosis in diabetics due to the overproduction of local growth factors that accelerate atherosclerosis.

•• Marelli D, Laks H, Patel B, *et al.*: Heart transplantation in patients with diabetes mellitus in the current era. *J Heart Lung Transplant* 2003, 22:1091–1097.

In this study from a single institution, 101 type I and type II diabetic patients were studied pre- and post-transplant compared with 244 transplant patients without diabetes mellitus. Diabetes mellitus patients tended to have a higher likelihood of ischemic cardiomyopathy, but long-term survival was not different by group. Body mass index was the greatest risk factor for survival in patients undergoing cardiac transplant. Infections were higher in diabetes mellitus than euglycemic controls.

•• Klein I, Ojama K: Thyroid hormone and the cardiovascular system. *J Clin Endocrinol Metab* 1994, 78:1026–1030.

This is an outstanding review of the many and varied manifestations of cardiac disease in thyroidal conditions. In part, this article argues that thyroid hormone replacement in the elderly is not associated with adverse clinical outcomes despite the many anecdotes of numerous clinicians.

•• Fazio S, Salvatini D, Capaldo B, *et al.*: A preliminary study of growth hormone in the treatment of dilated cardiomyopathy. *N Engl J Med* 1996, 334:809–814.

Longstanding acromegaly is associated with cardiac hypertrophy. Short-term growth hormone treatment can increase cardiac function in part due to stimulation of local insulin-like growth factor-I production. Hence it is not surprising that recombinant human growth hormone has been considered as a potential therapeutic modality in end-stage heart disease. This trial is similar to other studies that have suggested that growth hormone can improve muscle performance in elders or in patients with growth hormone deficiency.

REFERENCES AND RECOMMENDED READING

Recently published papers of particular interest have been highlighted as:
• Of interest
•• Of outstanding interest

1. Dunn JP, Ipsen J, Elson KO, Ohtani M: Risk factors in coronary artery disease, hypertension and diabetes mellitus. *Am J Med Sci* 1970, 259:309–315.

2. Garcia MJ, McNamara PM, Gordon T: Morbidity and mortality in diabetics in the Framingham population. *Diabetes* 1974, 23:105–110.

3. Crall FV, Roberts WC: The extramural and intramural coronary arteries in juvenile diabetes mellitus: analysis of nine necropsy patients aged 19–38 years with onset of diabetes before age 15 years. *Am J Med* 1978, 64:221–230.

4. Fisher M: Diabetes and myocardial infarction. *Clin Endocrinol Metab* 1999, 13:331–343.

5. Otel I, Ledru F, Danchin N: Ischemic heart disease in type 2 diabetes. *Metabolism* 2003, 52:6–12.

6.• Solymoss BC, Bourassa MG, Campeau L, *et al.*: Incidence, coronary risk profile and angiographic characteristics of prediabetic and diabetic patients in a population with ischemic heart disease. *Can J Cardiol* 2003, 19:1155–1160.

7.•• Haffner SM: Insulin resistance, inflammation and the prediabetic state. *Am J Cardiol* 2003, 92:18–26.

8. Martin BC, Warram JH, Manson J, Krolewski AS: The excess risk of coronary artery disease increases with duration of diabetes mellitus. *Diabetologia* 1988, 31:518A.

9. Falcone C, Nespoli L, Geroldi D, *et al.*: Silent myocardial ischemia in diabetic and nondiabetic patients with coronary artery disease. *Int J Cardiol* 2003, 90:219–227.

10. Marolis JR, Kannel WB, Feinlieb M, *et al*: Clinical features of unrecognized myocardial infarction-silent and symptomatic; 18 year follow up: the Framingham Study. *Am J Cardiol* 1977, 32:1–7.

11. Murray DP, O'Brien J, Mulrooney R, O'Sullivan DJ: Autonomic dysfunction and silent myocardial ischemia on exercise testing in diabetes mellitus. *Diabet Med* 1990, 7:580–584.

12.•• Poirer P, Garreau C, Bogaty P, *et al.*: Impact of left ventricular dysfunction on maximal treadmill performance in normotensive subjects with well controlled type II NIDDM. *Am J Cardiol* 2000, 85:473–477.

13. Viberti GC, Walker JD: Diabetic nephropathy: etiology and prevention. *Diabetes Metab Rev* 1988, 4:147–167.

14.•• Bypass Angioplasty Revascularization Investigation (BARI). Comparison of coronary artery bypass surgery with angioplasty in patients with multivessel disease. *N Engl J Med* 1996, 335:217–225.

15. •• Marelli D, Laks H, Patel B, *et al.*: Heart transplantation in patients with diabetes mellitus in the current era. *J Heart Lung Transplant* 2003, 22:1091–1097.

16. Kessler II: Mortality experience of diabetic patients: a twenty six year follow-up study. *Am J Med* 1971, 51:715–720.

17. Kannel WB, McGee DL: Diabetes and cardiovascular disease: the Framingham study. *JAMA* 1979, 241:2035–2039.

18. Fein FS, Sonneblick EH: Diabetic cardiomyopathy. *Prog Cardiovasc Dis* 1985, 27:255–265.

19. Factor SM, Okun EM, Minase T: Capillary microaneurysms in the human diabetic heart. *N Engl J Med* 1980, 302:384–390.

20. Jensen JS, Deldt-Rasmussen B, Starndgaard S: Arterial hypertension, microalbuminuria, and risk of ischemic heart disease. *Hypertension* 2000, 35:898–901.

21. Schaffer SW, Artman MF, Wilson GI: Properties of insulin idependent and noninsulin dependent diabetic cardiomyopathies. In: *Pathogenesis of Myocarditis and Cardiomyopathy*. Edited by Kawai C, Abelmann WH. Tokyo: University of Tokyo Press; 1987:149.

22. Schaffer SW, Tan FH, Wilson GL: Development of a cardiomyopathy in a model of noninsulin dependent diabetic. *Am J Physiol* 1985, 248:179–186.

23. Mackay JD, Page MM, Cambridge J, Watkins PJ: Diabetic autonomic neuropathy. *Diabetologia* 1980, 18:471–475.

24. Zander E, Schulz B, Heinke P: Importance of autonomic dysfunction in IDDM subjects with diabetic nephropathy. *Diabetes Care* 1989, 12:259–263.

25. Schramm C, Wagnner M, Nellessen U, *et al.*: Ultrastructural changes of human cardiac atrial nerve endings in diabetes mellitus. *Eur J Clin Invest* 2000, 30:311–316.

26. Clark BF, Ewing DJ: Cardiovascular denervation in diabetic neuropathy. *Ann Intern Med* 1980, 92:304–310.

27. Levey GS, Klein I: Catecholamine-thyroid hormone interactions and the cardiovascular manifestations of hyperthyroidism. *Ann Intern Med* 1990, 88:642–650.

28. Klein I: Thyroid hormone and the cardiovascular system. *Am J Med* 1990, 88:651–656.

29. Balkman C, Ojamaa K, Klein I: Time course of the effects of thyroid hormone on cardiac gene expression. *Endocrinology* 1992, 130:2001–2004.

30. Morkin E, Flink IL, Goldman S: Biochemical and physiologic effects of thyroid hormone on cardiac performance. *Prog Cardiovasc Dis* 1983, 25:455–460.

31. Thomas FB, Massaferri EL, Killman TG: Apathetic thyrotoxicosis: a distinctive clinical and laboratory entity. *Ann Intern Med* 1970, 72:679–689.

32.•• Klein I, Ojama K: Thyroid hormone and the cardiovascular system. *J Clin Endocrinol Metab* 1994, 78:1026–1030.

33. Dillman WH: Biochemical basis of thyroid hormone action in the heart. *Am J Med* 1990, 88;626–635.

34. Kabadi UM, Kumar SP: Pericardial effusion in primary hypothyroidism. *Am Heart J* 1990, 120:1392–1397.

35. Klein I, Ojamaa K: The cardiovascular system in hypothyroidism. In *The Thyroid*. Edited by Bravrman LE, Utiger RD. Philadelphia: Lippincott-Raven Publishers: 1996:799–814.

36. Fitzpatrick L, Bilezikian JP: Primary hyperparathyroidism. In *Principles and Practice of Endocrinology and Metabolism*. Edited by Becker KL. Philadelphia: JB Lippincott Co.; 1991:430–438.

37. Scholz DA. Hypertension and hyperparathyroidism. *Arch Intern Med* 1977, 131:1123–1127.

38. Levine SN, Rheams CN: Hypocalcemic heart failure. *Am J Med* 1975, 78:1022–1032.

39. Rude RK, Singer FR: Magnesium deficiency and excess. *Ann Rev Med* 1981, 32:245–260.

40. Saruta T, Suzuki H, Handa M, *et al.*: Multiple factors contribute to the pathogenesis of hypertension in Cushing's syndrome. *J Clin Endocrinol Metab* 1986, 62:275–279.

41. Krakoff LR, Nicolis G, Ansel B: Pathogenesis of hypertension in Cushing's syndrome. *Am J Med* 1975, 58:216–220.

42. Krakoff LR, Eisenfel AJ: Hormonal control of plasma renin substrate (angiotensionogen). *Circ Res* 1977, 41(suppl II):43–46.

43. Bravo EL, Tarazi RC, Dunston HP *et al.*: The changing clinical spectrum of primary aldosteronism. *Am J Med* 1983, 74:641–651.

44. Hull CJ: Phaechromocytoma: diagnosis, preoperative preparation and anaethestic management. *Br J Anaesthesiol* 1986, 58:1453–1459.

45. Golbisi Z, Sakall M, Ciceh D, *et al.*: Dynamic left ventricular outflow tract obstruction in a patient with pheochromocytoma. *Jpn Heart J* 1999, 40:831–835.

46. Engleman K: Pheochromocytoma. *Clin Endocrinol Metab* 1977, 6:769–789.

47. Loriaux DL: The polyendocrine deficiency syndromes. *N Engl J Med* 1983, 312:1568–1572.

48. Molitch ME: Clinical manifestations of acromegaly. *J Clin Endocrinol Metab* 1992, 21:597–613.

49. Martin JB, Kerber RE, Sherman BM, *et al.*: Cardiac size and function in acromegaly. *Circulation* 1977, 56:863–870.

50. Fazio S, Cittadivin A, Biondi B, *et al.*: Cardiovascular effects of short term GH hypersecretion. *J Clin Endocrinol Metab* 2000, 86:179–182.

51. McGuffin WL, Sherman BM, Roth J, *et al.*: Acromegaly and cardiovascular disorders. A prospective study. *Ann Intern Med* 1974, 81:11–15.

52. Leung KS, Muin P, Wallynahmed M, *et al.*: Abnormal heart rate variability in adults with growth hormone deficiency. *J Clin Endocrinol Metab* 2000, 85:628–633.

53. Osterzie KJ, Blum WF, Strohm O: Severity of chronic heart failure due to coronary heart disease predicts the endocrine effects of short term rhGH. *J Clin Endocrinol Metab* 2000, 85:1533–1539.

54.•• Fazio S, Salvatini D, Capaldo B, *et al.*: A preliminary study of growth hormone in the treatment of dilated cardiomyopathy. *N Engl J Med* 1996, 334:809–814.

55. Donoth MY, Zapf J: IGF-I an attractive option for CHF. *Drugs Aging* 1999, 15:251–254.

56. Feldman JM: Carcinoid tumors and syndrome. *Semin Oncol* 1987, 14:237–257.

57. Maton PN: The carcinoid tumor and the carcinoid syndrome. In *Principles and Practices of Endocrinology and Metabolism*. Edited by Becker KL. Philadelphia: JB Lippincott Co.; 1991:1641–1643.

58. Codd JE, Proxda J, Merjavy J: Palliation of carcinoid heart disease. *Arch Surg* 1987, 122:1076–1080.

59. Moertel CG: An odyssey in the land of small tumors. *J Clin Oncol* 1987, 5:1503–1507.

60. Said SI: Vasoactive intestinal peptide. *J Endocrinol Invest* 1986, 9:191–201.

SELECT BIBLIOGRAPHY

American Diabetes Association: Consensus statement on the detection and management of lipid disorders in diabetes. *Diabetes Care* 1993, 16:106–112.

Aron DC, Tyrrel JB: Cushing's syndrome. *Endocrinol Metab North Am* 1994, 23:487–509.

Bonow R, Bohoman N, Hazzard W: Stratification in CAD and special populations. *Am J Med* 1996, 101(suppl)17–25.

Krahn AD, Klein GJ, Kerr CR, *et al.*: How useful is thyroid function testing with recent onset atrial fibrillation? *Arch Intern Med* 1996, 2221–2226.

Luscher TF, Creager MA, Beckman JA, Cosentino F: Diabetes and vascular disease: pathophysiology, clinical consequences, and medical therapy. *Circulation* 2003, 108:1655–1661.

Rheumatic Diseases and the Heart

Deborah M. DeMarco
Bonnie J. Bidinger

Key Points
- Physicians must have an awareness of the resurgence of rheumatic fever and the importance of antibiotic prophylaxis.
- Recognition of Lyme disease and spondyloarthropathies as a cause of bradycardia and conduction disturbances is important.
- There is potential involvement of all components of the heart in patients with systemic lupus erythematosus, rheumatoid arthritis, and scleroderma.
- Premature atherosclerosis has been recognized with increasing frequency in lupus and rhematoid arthritis.
- Coronary artery thrombosis can be secondary to either phospholipid antibodies or vasculitis.
- The high frequency of asymptomatic cardiac involvement in scleroderma indicates the need for cardiac evaluation in all newly diagnosed patients.

The heart can suffer involvement in a spectrum of rheumatic diseases (Table 1). Cardiac disease is usually the result of the primary inflammatory, metabolic, or infiltrative process or is secondary to other organ system disease. Although the pathophysiologic mechanisms of these rheumatic diseases are quite diverse, some or all of the components of the heart may be affected by each of these conditions.

ACUTE RHEUMATIC FEVER

Acute rheumatic fever (ARF) is a rare sequela of group A streptococcal infection of the upper respiratory tract. Its manifestations, as outlined in the Jones criteria (Table 2) [1], remain the means of diagnosis for the initial attack. Carditis is its principal cardiac manifestation and has decreased in incidence in adults from 65% to 30% since the 1940s, but it remains at 70% to 90% in children. In chronic rheumatic heart disease, carditis may result in scarring of the heart valves and subsequent valvular heart disease. In a few patients, severe carditis occurs with rapid onset of complications, possibly leading to death.

Often, carditis in ARF is asymptomatic and is diagnosed by detection of a new murmur during the physical examination. Other major criteria for diagnosis include the presence of cardiomegaly, congestive heart failure, and pericardial friction rub or other signs of pericardial effusion. The most common murmur associated with ARF is mitral regurgitation followed by aortic insufficiency. First-degree heart block may be seen on the electrocardiogram, but it is neither specific nor prognostically important. There is no characteristic electrocardiogram pattern for ARF.

TABLE 1 SITES OF INVOLVEMENT OF RHEUMATIC DISEASES AND THE HEART

Disease	Aortic root	Pericardium	Myocardium	Endocardium	Coronary arteries	Conduction abnormality	Arrhythmias
Acute rheumatic fever	—	Pericarditis	Cardiomyopathy	Valvulitis, chronic valvular disease	—	+	—
Lyme disease	—	Pericarditis	Cardiomyopathy	—	—	Atrioventricular block	Atrial and ventricular tachyarrhythmias
Systemic lupus erythematosus	Aortitis (rare)	Pericarditis (tamponade, constriction)	Myocarditis (rare)	Libman-Sacks syndrome, thrombosis (antiphospholipid antibody syndrome)	Vasculitis, accelerated atherosclerotic disease, thrombosis (antiphospholipid antibody syndrome), embolic antiphospholipid antibody syndrome	Atrioventricular block (neonatal)	Ventricular
Rheumatoid arthritis	Granulomatous vasculitis	Pericarditis, constriction	Granulomatous myocarditis, interstitial myocarditis	Valvulitis	Vasculitis, accelerated atherosclerotic disease	+	—
Systemic sclerosis (scleroderma)	—	Pericarditis	Myocardial fibrosis, cor pulmonale	—	Intimal hyperplasia	+	Supra and ventricular
Dermatomyositis and polymyositis	—	—	Myocarditis	—	Vasculitis	+	+
Vasculitis	—	Pericarditis	Myocardial infarction	—	Vasculitis	+	+
Spondyloarthropathies (ankylosing spondylitis, Reiter's syndrome)	Aortitis	—	—	Aortic regurgitation	—	+	—
Polychondritis	Aortitis	Pericarditis (rare)	—	Aortic and mitral valvulitis	Vasculitis	+	+
Marfan syndrome	Dilatation, dissection	—	—	Mitral valve prolapse, aortic insufficiency	—	—	—
Ehlers-Danlos syndrome	Dilatation	—	Ventricular and atrial septal defects	Aortic insufficiency, mitral prolapse, tricuspid prolapse, bicuspid aortic valves, pulmonary regurgitation	—	—	—
Amyloidosis	—	Constrictive pericarditis	Restrictive cardiomyopathy	Valvular disease (tricuspid, mitral)	Intra-arterial deposition	+	+

Diagnosis

Establishing a definitive diagnosis of rheumatic fever is important not only for acute management of disease manifestations, but also because of the potential need for antibiotic prophylaxis. In addition to the Jones criteria (Table 2), the diagnosis depends on establishing an antecedent streptococcal infection by laboratory tests; an elevated titer of at least one antibody on the antistreptolysin-O assay, anti-DNAse B, or antihyaluronidase test can be detected in approximately 95% of patients with ARF [2]. The rapid Streptozyme (Wampole Laboratories, Cranbury, NJ) slide test is not recommended because of its variable results.

Treatment

The current recommended treatment course is outlined in Table 3. All household members should have throat cultures taken, because reinfection may occur if the organism is not eradicated from the environment. Anti-inflammatory medication is usually administered for arthritis, fever, and mild carditis, although it is not protective against the subsequent development of chronic rheumatic heart disease. Patients with severe carditis require prompt administration of corticosteroid therapy as an adjunct to their cardiac medications.

Secondary prophylaxis is recommended for patients who have had ARF (Table 3). Duration of prophylaxis remains controversial, but it can safely be discontinued if 1) the patient is older than 20 years; 2) the most recent attack occurred more than 5 years previously; 3) there was no carditis with the previous attack; and 4) there is no evidence of rheumatic heart disease [3]. The likelihood of the patient's exposure to children and the patient's reliability are considerations.

LYME DISEASE

Lyme disease, a systemic illness caused by the spirochete *Borrelia burgdorferi*, has cardiac manifestations in 4% to 10% of untreated patients. The cardiac complications usually develop 4 to 8 weeks after exposure to an infected tick, but they can occur as early as 4 days after the onset of the initial illness [4•]. Sometimes, they may predate the initial antibody response.

The most common cardiac abnormalities (Table 1) include atrioventricular block, myopericarditis, and left ventricular dysfunction, but atrial and ventricular tachycardias have been reported [4•]. In Europe, dilated cardiomyopathy has been observed as a chronic manifestation of Lyme disease, and *B. burgdorferi* has been isolated from some endomyocardial biopsies of such patients [5••]. Almost all patients with atrioventricular conduction disturbances manifest first-degree block at some time during their course; high-grade block occurs in up to 50% of patients, and symptomatic complete heart block, in approximately 8% [4•]. The block is usually at or above the level of the atrioventricular node, predicting a benign prognosis, but more sinister conduction disturbances may occur. Temporary cardiac pacing is frequently needed by patients who have severe heart block with hemodynamic instability. Permanent pacemaker insertion is rarely indicated. The block generally resolves completely with antibiotic treatment, and the long-term prognosis is excellent (Table 4).

SYSTEMIC LUPUS ERYTHEMATOSUS

Cardiovascular involvement occurs in 29% to 66% of patients with systemic lupus erythematosus (SLE) (Table 1) [6,7]. Autopsy and even echocardiographic studies may

---

TABLE 2 JONES CRITERIA (REVISED) FOR DIAGNOSIS OF INITIAL ATTACK OF RHEUMATIC FEVER

Major manifestations
Carditis
Polyarthritis
Chorea
Erythrema marginatum
Subcutaneous nodules
Minor manifestations
Clinical
    Arthralgia
    Fever
Laboratory
    Elevated erythrocyte sedimentation rate
    C-reactive protein
    Leukocytosis
    Prolonged P-R interval
Supporting evidence of streptococcal infection
Increased titer of antistreptococcal antibodies
    (antistreptolysin-O or others)
Positive throat culture for group A *Streptococcus*

TABLE 3 TREATMENT RECOMMENDATIONS FOR ACUTE RHEUMATIC FEVER	
Drug	**Dosage**
Acute treatment	
Penicillin	250 mg four times daily for 10 days
Erythromycin	250 mg four times daily for 10 days
Prophylaxis	
Penicillin G benzathine	1.2×10^6 U intramuscularly every 4 weeks
Penicillin V	250 mg orally twice daily
Sulfadiazine	0.5 g orally once daily
Erythromycin	250 mg orally twice daily

document significant findings in the heart without clinically apparent disease.

Pericardial disease is the most common cardiac manifestation of SLE, documented at autopsy in approximately 80% of patients but seen as symptomatic disease in 8% to 50% of patients. It usually presents in association with SLE disease activity in other organs.

Patients with symptomatic pericarditis generally present with anterior or substernal chest pain that is characteristically pleuritic and relieved by leaning forward. The pain may be associated with dyspnea or arrhythmias. A pericardial friction rub may be heard on auscultation. A chest roentgenogram may reveal an enlarged cardiac silhouette. Transient electrocardiographic changes (ST-segment elevation and PR-interval depression) may be seen. Echocardiography may reveal pericardial effusions or pericardial thickening. Life-threatening complications of pericarditis include cardiac tamponade and constriction, but both are rare. Pericardial fluid is usually exudative with high protein and normal to low glucose levels compared with serum.

Symptomatic pericarditis can often be successfully treated with nonsteroidal anti-inflammatory drugs such as indomethacin, 50 mg three times daily [8], and, occasionally, oral corticosteroids at low dosages (15 to 30 mg/d). Hemodynamically compromising effusions require pericardial aspiration and high-dose intravenous corticosteroids.

Myocardial involvement in SLE should be categorized as primary or secondary. Primary myocarditis is rare, occurring clinically in 2.1% to 14% of patients with SLE. Patients present with unexplained tachycardia, congestive heart failure (rarely), ventricular arrhythmias, conduction defects, electrocardiogram abnormalities (including ST-T wave changes), and cardiomegaly without evidence of valvular or pericardial disease. Endocardial biopsy specimens may confirm histologically the presence of myocarditis.

Secondary causes of myocardial dysfunction in SLE include systemic hypertension, valvular disease [9], pulmonary disease, coronary artery ischemia, drug toxicity, and amyloidosis. These secondary causes are often clinically more important than true lupus myocarditis.

Treatment of SLE patients with carditis includes distinguishing primary from secondary disorders and appropriately treating any secondary cardiac insult. Anti-inflammatory and immunosuppressive therapy should be reserved for active lupus carditis.

Coronary artery involvement in SLE includes embolic events, thromboses [7], vasculitis, and premature atherosclerosis [10,11,12•]. Women with SLE have a variety of atherosclerotic risk factors, some of which are "nontraditional," including the cumulative prednisone dose. Accelerated atherosclerosis has become recognized as a significant late complication of SLE as the prognosis of the disease in general has improved. The treatment of the SLE patient with acute myocardial ischemia initially should be similar to that of patients with atherosclerotic coronary artery disease. However, the etiology of the ischemia must be determined by arteriography because coronary arteritis must be treated with corticosteroids and immunosuppressant agents.

The most characteristic cardiac manifestation of SLE is nonbacterial verrucous endocarditis, so-called Libman-

TABLE 4 ANTIBIOTIC THERAPY FOR LYME DISEASE		
Stage-symptoms	**Regimen***	**Length, _d_**
Early Lyme disease	Doxycycline, 100 mg b.i.d. or amoxicillin, 500 mg t.i.d. or erythromycin, 250 mg q.i.d.	10–21
Neurologic symptoms		
Bell's palsy only	Doxycycline, 100 mg b.i.d. or amoxicillin, 500 mg t.i.d.	21
Meningitis, encephalitis Radiculoneuropathy	Penicillin G, 20 million U/d IV or ceftriaxone, 2 g/d	14–21
Lyme carditis		
Mild (first-degree AV block, normal left ventricular function)	Doxycycline, 100 mg b.i.d.	30
Moderate to severe (high-degree AV block)	Penicillin G, 20 million U/d IV or ceftriaxone, 2 q/d IV May require temporary pacemaker	14–21
Lyme arthritis	Doxycycline, 100 mg b.i.d. or amoxicillin, 500 mg q.i.d. plus probenecid, 500 mg q.i.d. or penicillin G, 20 million U/d IV or ceftriaxone, 2 g/d IV	30
Pregnancy		
Early-localized	Amoxicillin, 500 mg t.i.d.	21
Late-disseminated	Penicillin G, 20 million U/d IV or ceftriaxone 2 g/d IV	14–21

*Failures occur with all regimens.
AV—atrioventricular; b.i.d.—twice per day; IV—intravenous; q.i.d.—four times per day; t.i.d.—three times per day.
(*Adapted from* Steere [5••].)

Sacks endocarditis, which occurs on the ventricular surface of the mitral valve. A similar lesion involving the aortic valve has also been described, as well as a necrotizing valvulitis secondary to vasculitis of the smaller vessels supplying the valve. Libman-Sacks lesions rarely produce significant valvular dysfunction. However, hemodynamically significant aortic and mitral insufficiency may occur. Valve replacements may be required, but the associated mortality has been as high as 25%. Rarely, lesional material of Libman-Sacks endocarditis may dislodge and embolize.

Conduction abnormalities and arrhythmias owing to SLE are not usually clinically significant and should be managed the same way as in patients without SLE. If acute conduction disease is suspected clinically to be secondary to myocarditis or arteritis, a short trial of corticosteroids should be initiated in the hemodynamically compromised patient [6].

The infants of mothers with SLE also may suffer cardiac disease, most commonly in the form of neonatal heart block. This syndrome in infants is referred to as permanent neonatal lupus and is associated with maternal anti–Ro (SSA) antibodies.

RHEUMATOID ARTHRITIS

Rheumatoid arthritis (RA) may involve all structures of the heart as the result of granulomatous proliferation or vasculitis (Table 1). Echocardiography can detect pericarditis and valvular disease, whereas endocardial biopsies can diagnose myocardial involvement [13].

Pericarditis, the most common of the rheumatoid cardiac manifestations with an incidence of approximately 50% by autopsy studies, rarely causes impairment of left ventricular function. However, constrictive pericarditis or a large pericardial effusion may compromise cardiac output and require pericardial aspiration or pericardiectomy.

Pericardial effusions generally respond to administration of 30 to 40 mg/d of prednisone over a several-week period. Pericardiocentesis should be performed early if tamponade is suspected or if there is a question of septic or suppurative pericarditis. In cases of constrictive pericarditis, pericardiectomy is the only effective therapy.

The myocardium may be affected by granulomatous inflammation, interstitial myocarditis, and coronary artery vasculitis. Cardiac conduction abnormalities, including complete heart block, may develop as a result of rheumatoid nodules. The heart block tends to occur in patients with severe, erosive, nodular-forming disease and is generally permanent. Coronary arteritis and amyloidosis are less common causes of heart block.

Arteritis in the rheumatoid patient may affect the coronary arteries and aorta, resulting in myocardial infarction, dilatation of the aortic root, and aortic valvular insufficiency, respectively.

Endocardial involvement is generally a result of granulomatous inflammation that may affect all four valves.

Aortic valvular insufficiency is well documented [14]. Mitral and tricuspid disease so severe as to cause symptoms is very rare. As in SLE, RA has also been associated with an increased risk of cardiovascular disease. This elevated risk is independent of traditional risk factors such as smoking, diabetes mellitus, and hypercholesterolemia [15], but instead is thought to be related to the systemic inflammation associated with RA. Potential mechanisms contributing to atherosclerosis in RA include upregulation of inflammatory cytokines and adhesion molecules, immune complex–mediated endothelial damage, and production of a hypercoagulable state due to thrombocytosis and elevated levels of fibrinogen and other proteins [16]. This raises the question of whether early and aggressive treatment of RA with disease-modifying antirheumatic drugs could have a positive impact on lowering the risk of cardiovascular disease and events in this patient population.

Newer therapies found useful in the treatment of RA over the past several years include the tumor necrosis factor (TNF)-α inhibitors infliximab, etanercept, and adalimumab. These medications block the effects of TNF-α, a proinflammatory cytokine important in the pathogenesis of RA. Generally well tolerated, these therapies may increase the risk of infection in patients and should not be given to those with pre-existing clinically significant infections [17]. Other potential adverse effects include infusion and injection site reactions and the development of autoantibodies. TNF-α inhibitors may also worsen symptoms of heart failure and should be used with caution in this patient population.

Another relatively new class of drugs used extensively in RA is the cyclo-oxygenase-2 (COX-2) inhibitors. These drugs are marketed as anti-inflammatory drugs with fewer gastrointestinal side effects and may therefore be tolerated by a larger number of individuals. However, their ability to alter the balance of vasoactive eicosanoids and their potential prothrombotic effects have raised concerns about possible harmful cardiovascular effects [18,19]. Currently, there are no prospective, randomized, controlled trials that directly address the cardiovascular risks of COX-2 inhibitors, but caution is advised when prescribing these drugs to at-risk patients. There are retrospective data that suggest concomitant low-dose aspirin should be used in patients with coronary artery disease who are taking COX-2 inhibitors.

SCLERODERMA

Systemic sclerosis (scleroderma) is a generalized disorder of connective tissue characterized by fibrosis and vascular obliteration. Cardiac involvement (Table 1) may be primary or secondary to involvement of other organ systems and, together with renal disease, is the leading cause of early death [20•]. Cardiac disease in systemic sclerosis may also be secondary to other organ system involvement, such as malignant hypertension, uremia, and cor pulmonale as a result of severe pulmonary hypertension or severe interstitial lung disease.

Pericardial disease, although common at autopsy, is not often recognized clinically. Pericardial involvement presents most commonly as an indolent chronic pericardial effusion of variable size in an asymptomatic patient or in one who may have nonspecific findings such as chest pain, dyspnea, and cardiomegaly or symptoms of congestive heart failure. Chronic pericardial effusions may be a premonitory indicator of the development of renal failure within 6 months. Less commonly, pericardial disease may occur as an acute inflammatory process with dyspnea, chest pain, fever, and pericardial friction rub.

Asymptomatic pericardial disease usually does not predict a poor clinical course in contrast to symptomatic involvement. Pericardial tamponade may occur but is thought to be uncommon. Constrictive and restrictive pericarditis have been reported but appear to be extremely rare.

Involvement of the myocardium, specifically focal myocardial fibrosis, has been found in autopsied scleroderma patients, but clinically evident disease occurs much less frequently. Vasospasm of the coronary microvasculature may be the primary etiology [21]. Fibrosis and/or ischemia may also lead to diastolic dysfunction [22]. In patients with the CREST (calcinosis, Raynaud's disease, esophageal dysfunction, sclerodactyly, telangiectasia) variant of scleroderma, resting right ventricular function is abnormal more commonly than in generalized scleroderma (systemic sclerosis) and is usually secondary to pulmonary vascular disease.

Conduction and electrocardiogram abnormalities in systemic sclerosis are common and diverse. The electrocardiogram is normal in approximately 50% of patients. Only 10% of patients had electrocardiogram infarct patterns, most commonly in the septal region. Low-voltage and nonspecific ST segment abnormalities are the most common electrocardiogram disturbances. Ventricular conduction abnormalities occur in approximately 2% to 5% of systemic sclerosis patients. Infarcts and conduction disease also are thought to be caused by diffuse myocardial fibrosis. These abnormalities may lead to complete heart block or asystole. Thus, myocardial fibrosis and thallium perfusion abnormalities are common in patients with systemic sclerosis, but global left ventricular function is usually maintained. Ventricular arrhythmias are the primary cause of sudden death in up to 60% of patients.

Diagnosis

Because of the frequency of subclinical cardiac involvement and the high cardiac mortality in patients with systemic sclerosis, baseline cardiac evaluation should be performed in all newly diagnosed patients, including ambulatory 24-hour electrocardiogram monitoring, electrocardiograms, and radionucleotide imaging (thallium perfusion scans). If patients have symptoms suggestive of coronary artery disease, cardiac catheterization should be considered to evaluate for coexistent atherosclerosis.

Treatment

Treatment of cardiac manifestations of systemic sclerosis and CREST remains somewhat empiric but should be directed at the specific symptoms or problems. Angiotensin-converting enzyme inhibitors or calcium channel blockers should be used to manage hypertension. Angina resulting from coronary vasospasm may respond to calcium channel blockers. Angina secondary to coronary artery disease should be treated as it is for non–systemic sclerosis patients. Symptomatic pericardial effusions usually respond to nonsteroidal anti-inflammatory agents, but corticosteroids are occasionally required. Drugs that can exacerbate underlying conduction disturbances should be avoided. Because of a possible increased mortality associated with use of antiarrhythmic agents, systemic sclerosis patients so treated should be monitored closely with repeated ambulatory electrocardiograms.

There is preliminary evidence that corticosteroids may improve myocardial function in scleroderma patients. In a small uncontrolled study, investigators found that 20 mg prednisolone given over 20 days to patients with systemic sclerosis resulted in an 18% improvement in left ventricular function [23]. This effect was found to be greater in those with diffuse disease and in those with poorer baseline left ventricular function. As this was a small uncontrolled study of short duration, certainly larger controlled studies will be required to further delineate the potential therapeutic effects of steroids on myocardial function in this population, particularly as corticosteroids can increase the risk of scleroderma renal crisis, a potentially fatal condition.

POLYMYOSITIS AND DERMATOMYOSITIS

Cardiac abnormalities in polymyositis and dermatomyositis (Table 1) have been identified in as many as 40% of patients, perhaps more commonly in dermatomyositis. Only approximately 15% of patients have symptomatic cardiac involvement, while up to 70% of all those with polymyositis will have some cardiac involvement diagnosed noninvasively during the course of their illness. Some have suggested that cardiac disease is an important prognostic factor in polymyositis and dermatomyositis [24].

The electrocardiogram is abnormal in 25% to 100% of patients. The most common abnormalities are nonspecific ST-T wave changes, atrioventricular block, and axis deviation. Rarely, complete heart block requiring permanent pacemaker implantation may occur. Abnormal Q waves resembling myocardial infarction may occur without underlying coronary artery disease. Arrhythmias occur less frequently.

Congestive heart failure may occur either as a result of the disease or secondary to hypertension associated with long-term corticosteroid therapy. Myocarditis has been found at autopsy in some patients with histories of congestive heart failure as well as in patients who have not had congestive heart failure prior to death. Myocardial fibrosis has not been a common histologic finding.

Studies of coronary arteries have shown vasculitis, arteritis obliterans, and angiographically normal vessels despite ischemic changes on the electrocardiogram. Coexistent atherosclerotic disease also may be found.

The diagnostic evaluation of patients with polymyositis and dermatomyositis should include a baseline electrocardiogram, creatine phosphokinase with MB fraction, and echocardiogram. It is not clear if 24-hour ambulatory electrocardiogram monitoring should be performed as a screening study in all newly diagnosed patients or only those with symptoms of rhythm disturbances. Persistent elevation of creatine phosphokinase-MB despite normal skeletal muscle strength may indicate ongoing myocarditis and should prompt further noninvasive testing such as thallium perfusion scanning.

There are no controlled trials that specifically evaluate treatment of cardiac disease in polymyositis and dermatomyositis. High-dose prednisone (60 to 80 mg/d) is usually required for at least 6 weeks at diagnosis, with tapering as indicated by clinical examination and muscle enzyme testing. Management of congestive heart failure, in addition to the conventional measures, may also require use of high-dose corticosteroids.

VASCULITIS

The vasculitides are a group of disorders in which inflammation and necrosis of blood vessel walls result in organ system abnormalities caused by thrombosis and hemorrhage. Several forms of necrotizing systemic vasculitis may involve the heart. Kawasaki syndrome, which causes giant coronary artery aneurysms, occurs in children. Polyarteritis nodosa, Wegener's granulomatosis, and the Churg-Strauss syndrome may affect the heart and are discussed herein. Cardiac involvement in these disorders requires no special treatment.

Wegener's Granulomatosis

This relatively rare form of vasculitis shows cardiac involvement (Table 1) in up to 30% of untreated patients but in only 10% to 15% of those treated with cytotoxic agents. Coronary arteritis leading to myocardial infarction and pericarditis are the most common cardiac complications. Pericarditis often is symptomatic and may lead to tamponade. Any portion of the heart may be involved, leading to congestive heart failure, heart block, or arrhythmias, but these complications are much less common [25•].

Polyarteritis

Polyarteritis is a necrotizing vasculitis involving small and medium-sized muscular arteries. Cardiac involvement (Table 1) is observed in nearly 60% of patients in autopsy series but is often clinically silent. Congestive heart failure, pericarditis, myocardial infarction, and conduction abnormalities are the most common manifestations. Congestive heart failure may be caused by hypertension, which is seen in greater than 50% of patients, or by coronary insufficiency.

Churg-Strauss Syndrome

Also called allergic granulomatous angiitis, Churg-Strauss syndrome usually occurs in patients with a history of asthma or allergic rhinitis. The heart is a primary target organ (Table 1). Cardiac granulomas are commonly found at autopsy [26•]. Widespread myocardial damage may result from vasculitis affecting the coronary vessels. Cardiac disease may present as acute pericarditis, constrictive pericarditis, congestive heart failure, or myocardial infarction and accounts for approximately 50% of deaths of patients with Churg-Strauss syndrome. Electrocardiograms are abnormal in at least 50% of patients. Careful cardiovascular evaluation should be done early in patients with suspected Churg-Strauss syndrome because delayed treatment can lead to myocardial infarction and intractable congestive heart failure [26•].

SPONDYLOARTHROPATHIES

The seronegative spondyloarthropathies are a group of disorders that include ankylosing spondylitis, Reiter's syndrome or reactive arthritis, psoriatic arthritis, and the arthritis of inflammatory bowel disease (ulcerative colitis and regional enteritis, or Crohn's disease).

Cardiac involvement (Table 1) occurs in approximately 5% of individuals with ankylosing spondylitis, generally in patients with long-standing disease [27]. Inflammation of the aortic valve and root [28] and of the atrioventricular node may cause aortic regurgitation and conduction abnormalities that may also occur in patients with Reiter's syndrome. Aortic valve fibrosis and thickening may be appreciated by echocardiography. Fibrosis extending to the interventricular system may cause complete heart block or milder forms of atrioventricular conduction abnormalities in 5% to 10% of men with ankylosing spondylitis. HLA-B27 has also been associated with isolated aortic regurgitation and with aortic regurgitation associated with severe conduction abnormalities. Subtle abnormalities of diastolic function have been found frequently in patients with ankylosing spondylitis.

Heart block and aortitis have been reported in up to 10% of individuals with severe, longstanding Reiter's syndrome. Conduction defects, such as P-R interval prolongation, second-degree block with Wenckebach's phenomenon, and complete heart block, may occur early in Reiter's syndrome [29].

RELAPSING POLYCHONDRITIS

Polychondritis is an episodic disorder of cartilage associated with inflammatory arthritis, aortitis, and inflammation of the aortic and mitral valves. It affects predominately middle-aged, white individuals, although cardiac involvement is more common in men.

Cardiac involvement (Table 1) occurs in 20% to 40% of patients and is the second most common cause of death, beyond respiratory tract involvement. Abnormalities include aortic insufficiency and mitral insufficiency and, less commonly, pericarditis, abnormal electrocardiograms, paroxysmal atrial tachycardia, cardiac ischemia, and the conduction abnormalities, including complete heart block [30].

Because cardiac involvement may be asymptomatic, some authors suggest baseline electrocardiograms, chest roentgenograms, and echocardiograms in all patients with relapsing polychondritis. If valvular disease is detected, the echocardiogram can be useful for follow-up.

Corticosteroids have been the mainstay of therapy, but immunosuppressives also have been used for organ-threatening, corticosteroid-resistant disease activity. Successful valvuloplasty and valve replacements have been reported, but valve dehiscence may occur as a result of persistent inflammation [31].

CONNECTIVE TISSUE DISEASE, INCLUDING MARFAN SYNDROME AND EHLERS-DANLOS SYNDROME

Cardiovascular abnormalities associated with Marfan syndrome (Table 1) include aneurysmal dilatation of the ascending aorta, aortic valve insufficiency, coarctation of the aorta, mitral valve prolapse, mitral annulus calcification with mitral regurgitation, atrial and ventricular septal defects, tetralogy of Fallot, patent ductus arteriosus, and pulmonary artery aneurysms. Aneurysmal dilatation of the ascending aorta with rupture and aortic regurgitation are the causes of the shortened lifespan of 32 years in patients with Marfan syndrome. Annual echocardiographic monitoring is recommended until the aorta exceeds 50% of normal for body surface area, at which time echocardiographic monitoring should be done every 6 months. Management of aortic dilatation in Marfan syndrome includes β-blockade, specifically propranolol, and avoidance of vigorous activity. Pregnancy appears to be safe if aortic dilatation is not present. Surgical intervention with aortic grafting repair has proved beneficial when aortic dilatation reaches 6 cm [32,33].

Cardiovascular abnormalities in patients with Ehlers-Danlos syndrome (Table 1) include large artery aneurysms (the most serious manifestation of the syndrome), atrial septal defects, aortic valve insufficiency, ventricular papillary muscle dysfunction, dextrocardia, and conduction abnormalities. In patients with type IV Ehlers-Danlos syndrome, the so-called vascular or ecchymotic type, death generally occurs within the first two decades of life because of rupture of major arteries and gastrointestinal bleeding. Tetralogy of Fallot, peripheral pulmonary stenosis, bifid pulmonary artery, and dextrocardia also have been reported [34].

Mitral valve prolapse is a fairly common cardiac manifestation of both Marfan syndrome and Ehlers-Danlos syndrome. Therefore, patients with mitral valve prolapse should be evaluated clinically for these diseases.

AMYLOIDOSIS

The heart is a common site of amyloid deposition in both systemic and localized forms of amyloidosis (Table 5). Cardiac involvement is universally present in primary and myeloma-associated amyloidosis and is a major cause of death [34]. Amyloid also frequently affects the hearts of individuals with familial-hereditary amyloidosis but rarely occurs in those with secondary amyloidosis.

The primary manifestations of amyloid heart disease are cardiomegaly and low-output congestive heart failure. Cardiac amyloidosis also may present as constrictive pericarditis, restrictive cardiomyopathy, cardiac conduction disorders, and arrhythmias and may simulate ischemic heart disease with typical or atypical angina and "pseudoinfarct" electrocardiogram findings [35]. The diagnosis of amyloid heart disease should be considered in elderly individuals with heart disease of unknown etiology, particularly in those without atherosclerosis and valvular heart disease, and in patients in their fifth and sixth decades of life who have multisystem disease consistent with systemic amyloidosis and have the previously mentioned cardiac presentations.

Intractable heart failure may be the first manifestation and the cause of death in systemic amyloidosis. Amyloid is

TABLE 5 COMPARISONS OF CARDIAC AMYLOIDOSIS IN PRIMARY AMYLOID VERSUS SENILE CARDIAC AMYLOID		
	Heart in primary amyloid (*n* = 21)	**Senile cardiac amyloid (*n* = 26)**
Cardiac amyloid deposits	Higher grade deposits, perifiber and mixed, frequent vascular involvement	Lower grade deposits, predominantly nodular distribution pattern, infrequent vascular involvement
Mean age of patients, *y*	57.6	83
Male-to-female ratio	1.6:1	5.5:1
Congestive heart failure, %	76	35
Pseudoinfarction electrocardiogram findings, %	45	Uncommon
Sudden death, %	33	19

deposited diffusely in the myocardium but also may involve the pericardium, endocardium, and heart valves. The atrioventricular valves are more commonly involved than the pulmonary and aortic valves [35]. Murmurs are present occasionally.

Pericardial effusions are rare, but signs of constrictive pericarditis or restrictive myocardiopathy may develop. Pericardial involvement tends to occur in patients with high-grade amyloid deposits [35]. The demonstration of left ventricular diastolic pressures greater than those on the right helps to distinguish restrictive cardiomyopathy from constrictive pericarditis.

Ischemic heart disease secondary to amyloid deposition in intramyocardial arteries occurs in less than 2% of patients. Electrocardiograms may reveal the pattern of anteroseptal infarction in the absence of evidence of infarction at autopsy.

Amyloid deposits in the sinus node or fibrosis of the conduction system may cause rhythm disturbances in both patients with primary amyloid and senile cardiac amyloid [36]. Amyloid-induced neuropathy resulting in orthostatic hypotension may also cause dizziness, light-headedness, or syncope in the patient with amyloid heart disease.

Various invasive and noninvasive procedures are used to evaluate for cardiac amyloidosis. Echocardiograms may reveal thick-walled ventricles with normal or reduced-sized cavities. Left ventricular diastolic abnormalities are detectable by echocardiography even prior to development of clinically apparent amyloid heart disease. Ejection fractions may be normal despite significant heart failure, reflecting impaired cardiac relaxation (impaired diastolic function). Two-dimensional echocardiograms may reveal "granular sparkling." Diffuse uptake of 99m pyrophosphate may reflect the severity of myocardial Tc2 amyloid infiltration. Endomyocardial biopsy is the only definitive means of detecting amyloid deposits in the heart [35].

The median survival after diagnosis of primary or multiple myeloma–associated amyloid is approximately 12 months, with median survival of only 6 months from the onset of congestive heart failure in those with cardiac involvement. Of patients with primary amyloid, cardiac disease is reported to be the cause of death in 30% to 50% and is probably underreported [35]. The three variables of congestive heart failure, amount of weight loss, and presence of monoclonal light chains in urine predict poor outcome.

Although there is no specific therapy for amyloidosis, treatment of a predisposing disease may be useful. Alkylating agents have been used to treat primary amyloidosis, but they do not reverse the disease. Colchicine prevents acute febrile attacks in familial Mediterranean fever and retards amyloid deposition and further renal function deterioration in these individuals. Colchicine also may prolong survival in patients with primary amyloid.

Congestive heart failure secondary to amyloid heart disease should be treated with salt restriction and judicious use of diuretics. Hypovolemia should be avoided because ventricular filling may be compromised secondary to ventricular wall stiffening. Postural hypotension also may result from volume depletion secondary to decreased fluid intake or protein–osmotic diuresis, adrenal insufficiency, autonomic neuropathy, and low-output cardiac failure. Mineralocorticoids, elastic stockings, treatment of malabsorption, and fluid supplementation are supportive therapies. Great care should be used when treating with digitalis because of the risk of conduction abnormalities and arrhythmias in patients with cardiac amyloid.

References and Recommended Reading

Recently published papers of particular interest have been highlighted as

- Of interest
- •• Of outstanding interest

1. Shulman ST, Kaplan EL, Bisno AL, et al.: Jones criteria (revised) for guidance in the diagnosis of rheumatic fever. *Circulation* 1984, 69:203A–208A.

2. Gaasch WH: Guidelines for the diagnosis of rheumatic fever. *JAMA* 1992, 268:2069–2073.

3. Berrios X, del Campo E, Guzman B, et al.: Discontinuing rheumatic fever prophylaxis in selected adolescents and young adults. *Ann Intern Med* 1993, 118:401–406.

4.• Nagi KS, Joshi R, Thakur, RF: Cardiac manifestations of Lyme disease: a review. *Canadian J Cardiol* 1996, 12:503–506.

5.•• Steere AC: Lyme disease. *N Engl J Med* 2001, 345:115–125.

6. Roberts WC, High ST: The heart in systemic lupus erythematosus. *Curr Probl Cardiol* 1999, 24:1–56.

7. Moder KG, Miller TD, Tazelaar HD: Cardiac involvement in systemic lupus erythematosus. *Mayo Clin Proc* 1999, 74:275–84.

8. Schifferdecker B, Spodick DH: Nonsteroidal anti-inflammatory drugs in the treatment of pericarditis: clinical review. *Cardiol Rev* 2003, 11:211–217.

9. Hojnik M, George J, Ziporen L, Shoenfeld Y: Heart valve involvement (Libman-Sacks endocarditis) in the antiphospholipid syndrome. *Circulation* 1996, 93:1579–1587.

10. Doria A, Shoenfeld Y, Wu R, et al.: Risk factors for subclinical atherosclerosis n a prospective cohort of patients with systemic lupus erythematosus. *Ann Rheum Dis* 2003, 62:1071–1077.

11. Kao AH, Sabatine JM, Manzi S: Update on vascular disease in systemic lupus erythematosus. *Curr Opin Rheumatol* 2003. 15:519–527.

12.• Bruce IN, Urowitz MB, Gladman DD, et al.: Risk factors for coronary heart disease in women with systemic lupus erythematosus. *Arthritis Rheum* 2003, 48:3159–3167.

13. Carrao S, Salli L, Arnone S, et al.: Cardiac involvement in rheumatoid arthritis: evidence of silent heart disease. *Eur Heart J* 1995, 16:253–256.

14. Levine AJ, Dimitri WR, Bonser RS: Aortic regurgitation in rheumatoid arthritis necessitating aortic valve replacement. *Euro J Cardio-Thoracic Surg* 1999, 15:213–214.

15. Del Rincon I, Williams K, Stern MP, et al.: High incidence of cardiovascular events in a rheumatoid arthritis cohort not explained by traditional cardiac risk factors. *Arthritis Rheum* 2001, 44:2737–2745.

16. Van Doornum S, McColl G, Wicks IP: Accelerated atherosclerosis: an extraarticular feature of rheumatoid arthritis? *Arthritis Rheum* 2002, 46:862–873.

17. Keystone EC: Tumor necrosis factor-a blockade in the treatment of rheumatoid arthritis. *Rheum Dis Clin North Am* 2001, 27:427–443.

18. Weir MR, Sperling RS, Reicin A, Gertz BJ: Selective COX-2 inhibition and cardiovascular effects: a review of the rofecoxib development program. *Am Heart J* 2003, 146:591–604.

19. Mandami M: Effect of selective cyclooxygenase-2 inhibitors and naproxen on short-term risk of acute myocardial infarction in the elderly. *Arch Intern Med* 2003, 163:481–486.

20.• Deswal A, Follansbee WP: Cardiac involvement in scleroderma. *Rheum Dis Clin North Am* 1996, 22:841–860.

21. Steen VD, Follansbee WP, Conte CG, *et al.*: Thallium perfusion defects predict subsequent cardiac dysfunction in patients with systemic sclerosis. *Arthritis Rheum* 1996, 39:677–681.

22. Valentini G, Vitale DF, Giunta A, *et al.*: Diastolic abnormalities in systemic sclerosis: evidence for associated defective cardiac functional reserve. *Ann Rheum Dis* 1996, 55:455–460.

23. Antoniades L, Sfikakis PP, Mavrikakis M: Glucocorticoid effects on myocardial performance in patients with systemic sclerosis. *Clin Exp Rheumatol* 2001, 19:431–437.

24. Spiera R, Kagen L: Extramuscular manifestations in idiopathic inflammatory myopathies. *Curr Opin Rheumatol* 1998, 10:556–561.

25.• Goodfield NE, Bhandari S, Plant WD, *et al.*: Cardiac involvement in Wegener's granulomatosis. *Br Heart J* 1995, 73:110–115.

26.• Abril A, Calamia KT, Cohen MD: The Churg Strauss syndrome (allergic granulomatous andiitis): review and update. *Semin Arthritis Rheumatol* 2003, 33:106–114.

27. Arnett FC: Seronegative spondyloarthropathies. *Bull Rheum Dis* 1987, 37:1–12.

28. Roldan CA, Chavez J, Wiest PW, *et al.*: Aortic root disease and valve disease associated with ankylosing spondylitis. *J Am Coll Cardiol* 1998, 32:1397–1404.

29. Dier T, Rosencrance JG, Chillag SA: Cardiac conduction manifestations of Reiter's syndrome. *South Med J* 1991, 84:799–800.

30. Bowness P, Hawley IC, Morris T, *et al.*: Complete heart block and severe aortic incompetence in relapsing polychondritis: clinicopathologic findings. *Arthritis Rheum* 1991, 34:97–100.

31. Lan-Lazdunski L, Hvass U, Paillole C, *et al.*: Cardiac valve replacement in relapsing polychondritis. A review. *J Heart Valve Dis* 1995, 4:277–235.

32. Gott VL, Pyeritz RE, Magovern GJ, *et al.*: Surgical treatment of aneurysms of the ascending aorta in the Marfan syndrome: results of composite-graft repair in 50 patients. *N Engl J Med* 1986, 314:1070–1074.

33. Safi HJ, Vinnerkuist A, Bhama JK, *et al.*: Aortic valve disease in Marfan syndrome. *Curr Opin Cardiol* 1998, 13:91–95.

34. Leier CV, Call TD, Fulkerson PK, *et al.*: The spectrum of cardiac defects in the Ehlers-Danlos syndrome. *Ann Intern Med* 1980, 92:171–178.

35. Kyle RA: Amyloiditis. *Circulation* 1995, 91:1269–1271.

36. Reisinger J, Dubrey SW, Lavalley M, *et al.*: Electrophysiologic abnormalities in AL (primary) amyloidosis with cardiac involvement. *J Am Coll Cardiol* 1997, 30:1046–1051.

SELECT BIBLIOGRAPHY

Askari AD, Huetter TL: Cardiac abnormalities in polymyositis/dermatomyositis. *Semin Arthritis Rheum* 1982, 12:208–219.

Bergfeldt L: HLA-B27 associated rheumatic diseases with severe cardiac bradyarrhythmias. *Am J Med* 1983, 75:210–215.

Buyon JP: Neonatal lupus syndromes. *Curr Opin Rheumatol* 1994, 6:523–529.

Dubrey S, Mendes L, Skinner M, *et al.*: Resolution of heart failure in patients with AL amyloidosis. *Ann Intern Med* 1996, 125:482–484.

Esdaaile JM, Abrahamowicz M, Groddzicky T, Li Y: Traditional Framingham risk factors fail to fully account for accelerated atherosclerosis in systemic lupus erythematosus. *Arthritis Rheum* 2001, 44:2331–2337.

Grant SCD, Levy RD, Venning MC, *et al.*: Wegener's granulomatosis and the heart. *Br Heart J* 1994, 71:82–86.

Hankey GJ, Eikelboom JW: Cyclooxygenase-2 inhibitors: are they really atherothrombotic, and if not, why not? *Stroke* 2003, 34:2736–2740.

Morrison I, McEntegart A, Capell H: Polymyositis with cardiac manifestations and unexpected immmunology. *Ann Rheum Dis* 2002, 61:1110–1111.

Nesher G, Ilany J, Rosenmann D, *et al.*: Vascular dysfunction in antiphospholipid syndrome: prevalence, clinical features, and treatment. *Semin Arthritis Rheum* 1997, 27:27–35.

O'Neill TW, King G, Graham IM, *et al.*: Echocardiographic abnormalities in ankylosing spondylitis. *Ann Rheum Dis* 1992, 51:652–654.

Roldan CA, Crawford M: Reply [letter]. *J Am Coll Cardiol* 1993, 22:1269–1270.

Schattner A, Liang MH: The cardiovascular burden of lupus: a complex challenge. *Arch Intern Med* 2003, 163:1507–1513.

Stollerman GH: Rheumatic fever in the 21st century. *Clin Infect Dis* 33:806–814.

The Aging Heart
J. V. Nixon

> ### *Key Points*
> - Morphologic, physiologic, and cellular changes in the cardiovascular system are associated with the normal aging process.
> - The prevalence of cardiovascular disease processes, including chronic ischemic heart disease, acute myocardial infarction, hypertension, arrhythmias, and valvular heart disease, changes with age.
> - Medical therapy should be focused on cardiovascular risk factor modification as well as preservation of cardiac preload, heart rate, and contractility.
> - The value of surgical or interventional therapy must be assessed for age.
> - Peer recommendations for the management of cardiovascular diseases in the older patient must be considered.

Clinical assessment of the older cardiovascular patient must incorporate a series of unique variables. Aging is accompanied by changes in the cardiovascular system [1]. Furthermore, lifestyle impacts the extent and rate of these cardiovascular functions, and must encompass changes in lifestyle and disease prevalence as well as alterations caused by aging [2•].

CHANGES IN CARDIAC ANATOMY AND PHYSIOLOGY

Aging is associated with a gradual increase in cardiac weight, principally in left ventricular mass and wall thickness [3] (Table 1). Aortic root dilatation and left atrial enlargement have been demonstrated. Importantly, left ventricular volumes remain unchanged. Furthermore, there is an age-related decline in vascular endothelial function [4]. Experimental studies have shown that an increase in collagen-tissue laydown with a diffuse development of fibrous tissue as well as an increase in myocardial cell size are associated with the age-related cardiac hypertrophy [5] (Fig. 1). These data generally agree with morphologic and biopsy studies in older patients [6]. In addition, several experimental studies have documented the myocardial cellular changes associated with aging (Table 2).

Details of functional changes in the aging cardiovasculature of humans are limited by the suitability of the population selected, the lifestyle of such a study population, and the utility of noninvasive diagnostic technologies with specific self-imposed limitations. Nevertheless, systolic function is maintained both at rest and during exercise [7] (Fig. 2). The response of heart rate to exercise is attenuated in the elderly. Thus, during exercise, the older heart compensates for the attenuated heart-rate response by increasing end-diastolic and stroke volumes to preserve cardiac output [7]. The increased left ventricular wall mass serves to maintain a normal wall stress in the presence of increased left ventricular volumes during exercise. When exercise responses of older men are compared with those of women, both sexes show parallel declines in peak exercise performance with age despite an overall higher exercise capacity in men. Only men show an age-related decrease in cardiac volumes at rest and exercise; cardiac index and ejection fraction decline equally with age in both sexes [8]. Also, the attenuated chronotropic and inotropic responses and the cardiac dilatation associated with dynamic exercise in the elderly are due to the age-related blunting of beta-adrenergic responsiveness [9] (Table 3). Furthermore, this increasing stiffness with age does not appear to be slowed or reversed by dynamic training programs or by prolonged endurance training [10–12].

Although the altered diastolic function or compliance clearly shown in experimental studies is difficult to document accurately in humans by noninvasive methods,

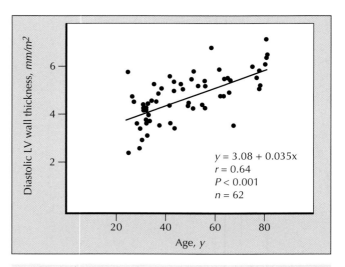

FIGURE 1 Linear regression plot showing the relation between increased age and increased diastolic left ventricular (LV) wall thickness in male participants in the Baltimore Longitudinal Aging Population. (*Adapted from* Gerstenblith *et al.* [3].)

TABLE 1 AGE-RELATED CHANGES IN CARDIAC ANATOMY

Experimental studies
Myocardial hypertrophy
Individual cellular enlargement
Increased collagen
Increased fibrous tissue

Human studies
Increased left ventricular mass
Increased interventricular septal and posterior left
  ventricular wall thickness
Left atrial enlargement
Aortic root dilatation

TABLE 2 AGE-RELATED CHANGES IN CARDIAC PHYSIOLOGY

Experimental studies
Prolonged calcium transit
Prolonged transmembrane potential
Prolonged contraction duration
Prolonged relaxation
Increased resting and dynamic stiffness
Diminished responses to digitalis glycosides,
  norepinephrine, and isoproterenol

Human studies
Increased left ventricular wall mass
Increased left ventricular stroke volume during exercise
Decreased diastolic stiffness
Decreased diastolic filling

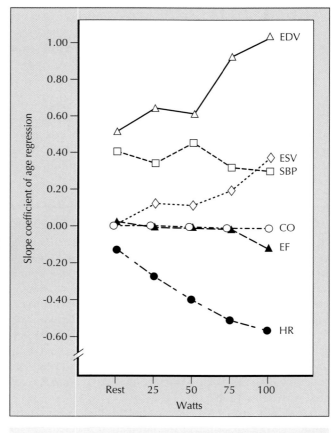

FIGURE 2 The slopes of the regression functions of age for end-diastolic volume (EDV), end-systolic volume (ESV), systolic blood pressure (SBP), cardiac output (CO), ejection fraction (EF), and heart rate (HR) at rest and at increasing incremental workloads from 25 to 100 W during dynamic exercise in the Baltimore Longitudinal Aging Population. (*Adapted from* Rodeheffer *et al.* [7].)

several noninvasive parameters of diastolic filling have consistently been shown to be altered with age [10]. Both Doppler echocardiographic and radionuclide techniques show the reduction in early rapid diastolic filling and the increased dependence on atrial contraction seen with aging (Figs. 3, 4, and 5). These findings reflect the increased stiffness associated with the morphologic changes of the aging heart.

AGING AND CARDIOVASCULAR DISEASE

Table 3 summarizes the changes that occur in the cardiovascular system with aging. Any treatment algorithm in an older cardiovascular patient has many branches. In the older patient, prevalence of the disease process and any unique forms of presentation must be considered. The value of surgical or interventional therapy must be assessed for age. Furthermore, medical therapy is directed at the preservation of cardiac preload, heart rate, and contractility, emphasizing controlled afterload reduction as an option.

CHRONIC ISCHEMIC HEART DISEASE

Prevalence

The prevalence of atherosclerotic heart disease increases significantly with age; more than 50% of people older than 65 years die from the effects of coronary artery disease [2•]. Furthermore, the prevalence of diagnosed coronary disease in this age group is only 30% to 50% of the prevalence of significant disease found at autopsy.

Diagnosis

Because of an age-related, altered lifestyle, including a decline in physical activity, presenting symptoms are often different than with younger patients. As a manifestation of systolic or diastolic dysfunction, dyspnea is a more prominent symptom than pain, which is usually a manifestation of physical exertion. Also, silent myocardial ischemia is more prevalent in older patients [13]. Added heart sounds and mitral regurgitation are normal variants related to age. Exercise stress testing may be of limited value in older patients because of their altered physical capability and the increased incidence of resting ST-segment electrocardiogram abnormalities. Thus, stress-imaging techniques, both stress echocardiography and stress thallium perfusion, and in particular pharmacologic stress-imaging technology, may be more productive in older patients [14].

Therapy

The guidelines for the management of patients with ischemic heart disease have been well established [15]. Unless contraindicated, the principles of management are not altered by the age of the patient. Appropriate management of risk factors, including hypertension, diabetes mellitus, lipid therapy, and smoking cessation applies at all ages including the elderly [15–18]. Recent reviews have outlined the benefits of cholesterol management and the reduction of cardiovascular risk utilizing coenzyme-A reductase inhibitor drugs (statins) [17]. All anti-ischemic agents, nitrates, beta-blockers, and calcium channel blockers, in addition to aspirin therapy, are effective in older patients. Concomitant consideration of the higher prevalence of silent ischemia in these patients suggests the selection of medications with a prolonged intrinsic half-life to maintain constant therapeutic plasma levels. Percutaneous transluminal coronary angioplasty is a therapeutic option in older patients in whom low mortality rates persist regardless of age [19] (Table 7). Data from the Coronary Artery Surgery Study (CASS) show increased intraoperative mortality and morbidity rates in older patients after bypass surgery, yet long-term survival and pain relief are compatible with results in younger patients (Fig. 6) [20].

Cardiovascular risk management is no longer limited by age. Trials of risk factor modification utilizing global risk assessment have shown that morbidity and mortality rates may be improved irrespective of the age population studied [18]. In addition, more information is now available regarding the use of statin drugs for the cardiovascular preventative management of the older individual (Table 7) [17]. Secondary preventive management is now clear irrespective of the age of the patient. All patients irrespective of their age with a diagnosis of coronary artery disease and/or who have suffered an acute cardiac event are now placed on a statin drug irrespective of their cholesterol level for the rest of their lives. Primary preventive care of patients without a history of coronary artery disease in an older population is less clearly defined. In the individual at high cardiovascular risk with an elevated cholesterol level, a statin is indicated. However, in the similar individual at low cardiovascular risk, there appears to be no association between age, cholesterol level, and mortality [17].

TABLE 3 PHYSIOLOGIC IMPLICATIONS OF AGE-RELATED CHANGES IN THE CARDIOVASCULAR SYSTEM

Central effects
Preload: attenuated
Contractility: not attenuated
Heart rate: attenuated at all levels of exercise
Afterload: not attenuated

Peripheral effects
Decreased vascular distensibility
Decreased β-adrenergic responsiveness

ACUTE MYOCARDIAL INFARCTION
Prevalence

The increased prevalence of coronary atherosclerosis was discussed in the previous section.

Diagnosis

The diagnostic methods used in younger patients are equally accurate in older patients. Presenting symptoms may be altered by age. Older patients with acute myocardial infarction may present more often with dyspnea or arrhythmias rather than chest pain (Table 4).

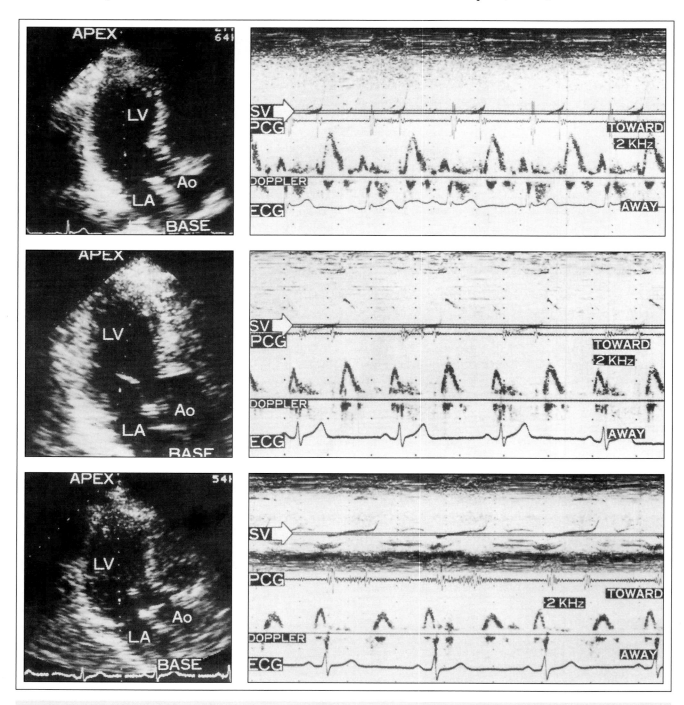

FIGURE 3 Changes in Doppler echocardiographic left ventricular (LV) diastolic filling patterns in normal subjects. **Top**, A 26-year-old man. **Middle**, a 48-year-old man. **Lower**, A 59-year-old man.

Ao—aorta; ECG—electrocardiogram; LA—left atrium; PCG—phonocardiogram; SV—sample volume. (*From* Miyatake *et al.* [45]; with permission.)

Therapy

Mortality and morbidity rates are higher in older patients [2•]. These higher rates may be age-related, caused by the higher prevalence of ischemic heart disease, or they may be caused by the greater frequency of concomitant diseases, particularly hypertension. Results vary among trials of thrombolytic therapies in older patients with acute myocardial infarction, although recent data show lower mortality rates in the treated groups. Contraindications to thrombolytic therapy increase with age. Secondary preventative therapy with aspirin, beta-blockers, angiotensin-converting enzyme (ACE) inhibitors, and lipid-lowering agents are equally effective in older and younger patients who have had myocardial infarction [17,21,22]. Recent published reviews of older patients have shown the comparatively infrequent use of secondary preventative agents and confirmed the validity of these recommendations [23,24].

HYPERTENSION

Prevalence

Hypertension is increasingly more common with increasing age [16,25,26]. In Americans older than 60 years,

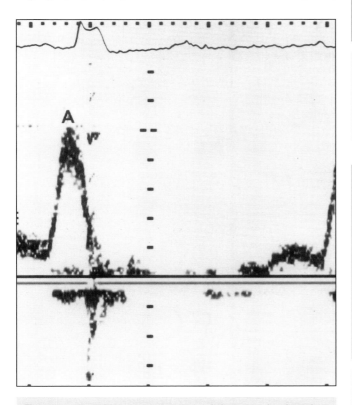

FIGURE 4 Doppler echocardiographic left ventricular diastolic filling pattern in an elderly patient with hypertension showing slow deceleration of the E wave, prolonged deceleration time, prominent A wave, and altered E:A ratio. (*From* Shah and Pai [46]; with permission.)

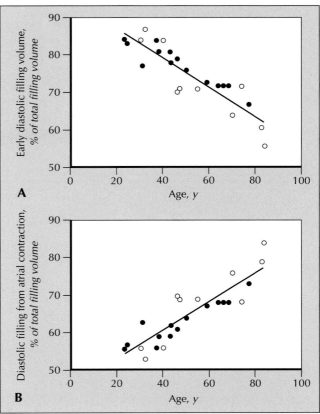

FIGURE 5 The relative contribution of early diastolic filling (**A**) and atrial contraction (**B**) to left ventricular filling as assessed by Doppler echocardiography in healthy men (*closed circles*) and women (*open circles*) ranging from 20 to 80 years of age. (*Adapted from* Lakatta [47].)

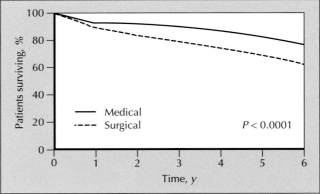

FIGURE 6 Cumulative 6-year survival in surgical and medical groups among 1491 patients 65 years of age or older from the Coronary Artery Surgery Study (CASS) registry. Survival is adjusted for left ventricular wall motion, congestive heart failure, number of diseased vessels, associated medical diseases, and age at angiograpy. (*Adapted from* Gersch *et al.* [20]).

hypertension exists in 60% of whites, 71% of blacks, and 61% of Hispanics [26]. Effective antihypertensive therapy significantly reduces mortality and morbidity in patients older than 65 [27,28]. In this age population, systolic blood pressure (isolated systolic hypertension) is a better predictor of both mortality and cardiovascular events (stroke, coronary heart disease, heart failure, and end-stage renal disease), although diastolic hypertension remains a significant independent cardiovascular risk factor (Fig. 7) [16,29]. Furthermore, the prevalence of associated left ventricular hypertrophy substantially compounds the cardiovascular risk [30].

Diagnosis

The importance of the diagnosis of hypertension in this age population lies in its identification [31]. Other identifiable causes of hypertension (eg, renovascular hypertension, primary aldosteronism) may occur with greater frequency in this age population. Identification of pseudohypertension in this age group also significantly reduces the frequency of the diagnosis of hypertension (Fig. 8) [31].

Therapy

Recent data provide suitable end points above which the mortality and morbidity risk of the disease significantly increases. It appears to be clearly established that blood pressure targets are the same for older individuals as for middle-aged and younger hypertensives (120/80) [16]. The Systolic Hypertension in the Elderly Program (SHEP) showed that morbidity rates are reduced when patients older than 60 years with isolated systolic hypertension above 160 mm Hg are effectively treated with diuretics or diuretics and beta-blockers (Fig. 9) [32]. Subsequently, the Syst-Eur trial has shown similar reductions in fatal and nonfatal stroke rates in patients effectively treated with a long-acting dihydropyridine calcium channel blocker, nitrendipine [33]. These studies appear to be reaffirmed in the results of the Antihypertensive and Lipid-Lowering Treatment to Prevent Heart Attack Trial (ALLHAT) [28]. ALLHAT was an outcomes based prospective trial of more than 42,000 mild to moderate

	Older (> 65 y)*	Younger (< 65 y)†
Total series		
Primary success	98 (81%)	412 (80%)
Mean CSA stenosis	92 → 35	87 → 15
Gradient, mm Hg	41 → 8	57 → 15
Last 200 cases	43	157
Primary success	40 (93%)	142 (90%)
Major complications		
Emergency CABG	5 (4.1%)	24 (4.7%)
MI (Q wave)	3 (2.5%)	15 (2.9%)
Death	1 (0.8%)	0

TABLE 4 RESULTS OF CORONARY ANGIOPLASTY IN THE ELDERLY

*n = 121.
†n = 518.
CABG—coronary artery bypass surgery; CSA—cross-sectional area; MI—myocardial infarction.

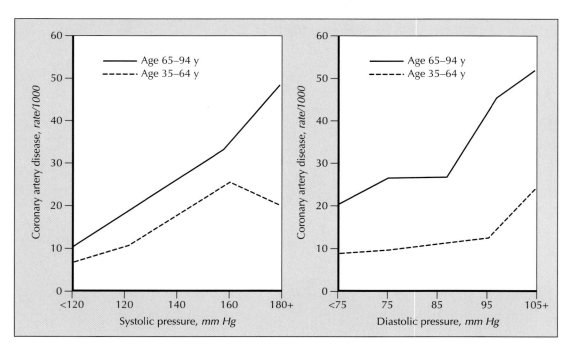

FIGURE 7 Biennial rate of coronary artery disease according to blood pressure and relation to age for men in the Framingham study. (Adapted from Levy et al. [48].)

hypertensives, 33,300 of whom completed the 4.9 year duration of the trial, addressing the outcomes associated with a diuretic, a calcium channel blocker, and an ACE inhibitor utilized to control hypertension. Mortality rates and morbidity rates were the same with all three forms of therapy in the patients in the trial over the age of 65 years, with the exception of a higher incidence of peripheral vascular disease in the group treated with the ACE inhibitor compared with the diuretic group [28].

Recommended nonpharmacologic modalities of management include dietary modifications, weight loss, consistent exercise, sodium restrictions, reduction in alcohol consumption, and smoking restriction [30]. Lifestyle modifications appear to be equally important in hypertension management in older persons as in their younger cohorts [29]. Pharmacologic therapy may be more favorably directed in the older patient by maintaining cardiac preload, heart rate, and contractility, and by emphasizing the suitability of afterload reduction. Also, both contraindications to and the adverse effects of all medications are more frequent in older patients. Furthermore, certain therapies are better suited to the older patient. As stated previously, diuretics effectively reduce mortality and morbidity rates in older patients with systolic hypertension [32]. Their less desirable characteristics include their primary physiologic effect on cardiac preload and their potential for precipitating hypokalemic arrhythmias, particularly in the presence of left ventricular hypertrophy [31].

The negative inotropic and chronotropic effects of beta-blockers may reduce their suitability in older patients, as does their tendency to suppress conduction system activity. Nevertheless, beta-blockers are the optimal form of secondary prophylaxis after myocardial infarction in all age groups [21]. The incidence of postural hypotension after application of primary vasodilators is higher in the elderly [31].

The dose response to an ACE inhibitor may be lower in an older patient, because plasma renin activity levels are attenuated with age [30]. The incidences of adverse effects,

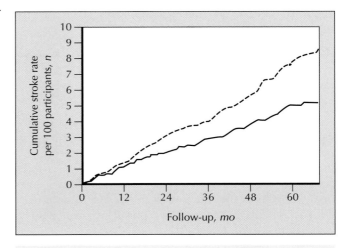

FIGURE 9 Cumulative fatal plus nonfatal stroke rate per 100 participants in the active treatment (*solid line*) and placebo (*broken line*) groups during the Systolic Hypertension in the Elderly Program (SHEP). (*Adapted from* SHEP Cooperative Research Group [32].)

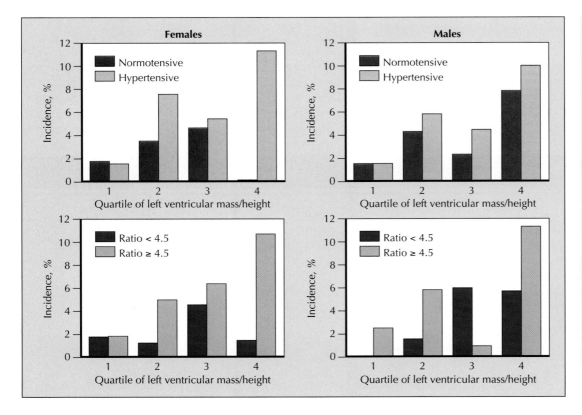

FIGURE 8 Four-year incidence (per 100 subjects) of initial coronary disease events according to gender-specific quartiles of left ventricular mass/height in women (*left panels*) and men (*right panels*). **Top**, Rates stratified by hypertension status. **Bottom**, Rates stratified by ratio of total/high-density lipoprotein cholesterol. (*Adapted from* Levy *et al.* [48].)

such as coughing, and contraindications are higher in older patients. Nevertheless, recent studies show these compounds to be effective agents in older patients with mild hypertension [28,34]. Calcium channel blockers, particularly dihydropyridines, are the vasodilator of choice in patients with low renin activity. These compounds also effectively induce regression of left ventricular hypertrophy. Furthermore, calcium channel blockers may suppress ventricular arrhythmias in patients with left ventricular hypertrophy, improve abnormal diastolic function, and potentially regress atherosclerotic plaques [26,30] (Table 5).

ARRHYTHMIAS
Prevalence

Arrhythmias occur with greater frequency in older cardiovascular patients because of their increased prevalence of coronary artery disease and hypertension; however, this increased prevalence of arrhythmias does not appear to be associated with increased mortality or morbidity [2•]. Also, bradyarrhythmias may occur with greater frequency in older patients because of the increased prevalence of nodal and conduction system disease [2•].

Atrial fibrillation is the most common arrhythmia in patients over the age of 65 years [35]. There are an estimated 2.2 million people in the United States with atrial fibrillation, with a projected increase to more than 5.6 million by 2050 [36]. It may precipitate or worsen congestive heart failure or ischemia and is a specific marker for both an increased incidence of stroke and increased mortality [2•,18].

Diagnosis

Arrhythmias, particularly tachyarrhythmias, may have more profound hemodynamic manifestations in older patients because of age-related diastolic dysfunction, requiring a sustained diastolic filling period and a significant atrial contraction. Furthermore, arrhythmias, particularly atrial

fibrillation in this age population, may be clinically silent [37]. The diagnosis may be critical because asymptomatic atrial fibrillation appears to carry the same thromboembolic risk as the symptomatic form of the condition, both requiring anticoagulation. An uncontrolled ventricular rate may lead to progressive ventricular dysfunction if untreated [37].

Therapy

As with other forms of cardiovascular therapy, the frequency of contraindications to and the adverse effects of antiarrhythmic drugs are greater in an older population. Sequential pacing is useful in older patients [2•]. Effective management of atrial fibrillation includes anticoagulation. There is no current evidence that anticoagulants should be withheld in an older age population, even among patients not perceived to have high-risk factors for thromboembolism [36]. Maintenance of normal sinus rhythm, if possible, or the control of the ventricular rate response are other important components of management with consideration of the use of flecainide, sotalol, or amiodarone [2•,38,39].

VALVULAR DISEASE
Prevalence

As previously discussed, added heart sounds and systolic murmurs such as mitral regurgitation are normal variant findings in an elderly population. The cause and prevalence of valvular pathology in the elderly relates primarily to degenerative disease. Senile degeneration and calcification of the aortic valve renders aortic stenosis a disease of the sixth, seventh, and eighth decades [40] (Fig. 10). Although aortic regurgitation may result from a congenitally bicuspid valve, it is mainly a condition of middle rather than old age [41]. Furthermore, aortic stenosis may be asymptomatic in this age population [42]. The diminishing incidence of rheumatic heart disease has resulted in a reducing prevalence of mitral stenosis among the older population. The prevalence of coexisting coronary artery

TABLE 5 PREVENTIVE CARDIOVASCULAR MANAGEMENT IN THE OLDER PATIENT		
Trial/study	**Age**	**Significance**
Association between age, cholesterol, and mortality		
Framingham Study	> 70	Not significant
Epidemiological Study of the Elderly	79±9	Not significant
Honolulu Heart Study	71–93	Not significant
Primary prevention trial		
AFCAPs/TexCAPs	> 65	Not significant
Secondary prevention trials		
4S	> 65	Significant
CARE	> 65	Significant
Heart Protection Study	> 65	Significant

disease is higher in this age population, which may impact both diagnosis and management.

Diagnosis

The clinical characteristics of different valvular diseases may be altered or suppressed by the presence of age-related characteristics that are normal variants. The clinical suspicion of coexistent valvular pathology in an older patient warrants careful assessment by Doppler echocardiography, which is capable of accurately quantifying valvular stenosis and estimating valvular regurgitation [42,43].

Therapy

In general, surgical intervention in the management of valvular heart disease is only affected by an increased intra-operative surgical risk and any concomitant age-related conditions such as coronary artery disease [2•,41]. The outcome after valve replacement for aortic stenosis and mitral stenosis does not appear to be impacted by age [41] (Fig. 11). Balloon aortic valvuloplasty is a therapeutic option in older patients with significant aortic stenosis; however, restenosis rates of up to 80% within 6 months leave questions of therapeutic efficacy [42,44]. Thus aortic balloon valvuloplasty tends to be utilized as a bridge procedure prior to other surgical treatment [42]. Balloon mitral valvuloplasty appears to be a therapeutic option for a younger mitral stenosis patient as confirmed by experience and limitations imposed by a preoperative echocardiographic scoring system [41,43]. Clinical indications for valvular replacement in aortic regurgitation and mitral regurgitation also do not appear to be affected by age [41]; however, the same reservations regarding age-related concomitant diseases do apply.

CONGESTIVE HEART FAILURE

Prevalence

The prevalence of congestive heart failure as a manifestation of end-stage ischemic, hypertensive, or valvular heart disease is as high as 2 million patients in the United States, with an additional 400,000 being diagnosed each year [2•,41]. Mortality is 50% within 5 years of the diagnosis [41]. Furthermore, the prevalence is expected to double over the next 30 years. Although the mortality associated with coronary disease and stroke has diminished in the last 20 years, it has continued to increase with congestive heart failure.

Diagnosis

When a patient is evaluated for congestive heart failure, it is necessary to determine whether the predominant component is systolic or diastolic dysfunction [2•,10]. This differential diagnosis is optimally made by echocardiography. Predominant diastolic dysfunction with a normal ejection fraction is usually associated with hypertension and often occurs in conjunction with left ventricular hypertrophy.

Systolic dysfunction with a depressed ejection fraction is often associated with ischemic heart disease or hypertension.

Management

A critical part of the management of congestive heart failure is management of the principal etiology. In addition, diastolic dysfunction and regression of increased left ventricular mass is optimally treated with long-acting calcium channel blocking agents or ACE inhibitors [42]. Comprehensive management of congestive heart failure incorporates multiple modalities, especially in this age population. These include diet, physical therapy, and psychosocial issues in addition to medical therapies. High rates of hospitalization

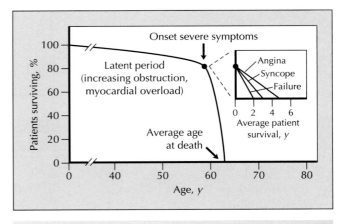

FIGURE 10 The natural history of aortic stenosis. (*Adapted from* Ross and Braunwald [49].)

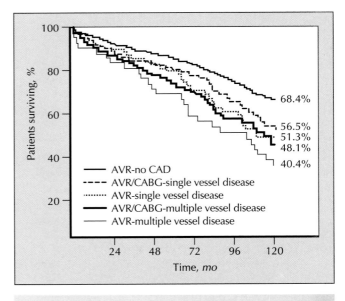

FIGURE 11 Late survival for patients undergoing isolated aortic valve replacement (AVR) and AVR plus coronary artery bypass grafting (CABG), grouped according to no coronary artery disease (CAD), single-vessel CAD, and multiple-vessel CAD. (*Adapted from* Lytle *et al.* [50].)

and rehospitalization with congestive heart failure in elderly patients are due to several factors, including underutilization of effective therapies, noncompliance of diet and medications, in addition to other environmental, psychosocial, and economic considerations. Systolic dysfunction usually necessitates the use of several modalities, *eg*, the decreased neurohormonal activation and ventricular remodeling produced by an ACE inhibitor, a diuretic, and digoxin. Furthermore, it is well established that prognosis in congestive heart failure is significantly improved by the use of ACE inhibitor therapy, aldosterone antagonists, and beta-blockers [22].

TABLE 6 PRESENTING SYMPTOMS OF ACUTE MYOCARDIAL INFARCTION IN ELDERLY PATIENTS

	Patients, %	
Symptoms	65–74 y	75–84 y
Chest pain	78	60
Dyspnea	41	44
Sweating	34	23
Syncope	3	18
Confusion	3	8
Stroke	2	7

DRUG USE IN THE OLDER PATIENT

Aging may influence the cardiovascular response to any drug, including any cardiovascular drug. The aging process also affects other organ systems, including the kidney and the liver, both of which are significantly involved in the metabolism and excretion of drugs. Because cardiovascular disease and the administration of cardiovascular agents is more prevalent in the elderly, drug heterogeneity of response, absorption rates, drug interactions, and associated system morbidity become important considerations in the appropriate therapeutic management of these older patients.

TABLE 7 ADVANTAGES AND DISADVANTAGES OF VARIOUS CLASSES OF ANTIHYPERTENSIVE AGENTS IN ELDERLY PATIENTS

Clinical variables	Diuretic	α-Blocker	ACE inhibitor	β-Blocker	Calcium antagonist
Volume depletion	+	–	–	–	–
Suppression of heart rate	–	–	–	+	±
Suppression of cardiac output	–	–	–	+	±
Regression of LVH	–	+	+	±	+
Suppression of VEA	–	–	–	+	+
Preservation of renal function	+	–	+	–	+
Regression of atherosclerosis	–	±	–	±	+
Improved lipid profile	–	±	±	±	±
Effective with low PRA	+	+	–	–	+

+—variable associated with this class of drug; – —variable not associated with this class of drug; ±—variable associated with this class of drug in some cases, but not others; ACE—angiotensin-converting enzyme; LVH—left ventricular hypertrophy; PRA—plasma renin activity; VEA—ventricular ectopic activity.

REFERENCES AND RECOMMENDED READING

Recently published papers of particular interest have been highlighted as:
• Of interest

1. Nixon JV: Effects of aging on the heart. *Choices Cardiol* 1993, 7:119–120.

2.• Lakatta EG, Gerstenblith G, Weisfeldt ML: The aging heart: structure, function and disease. In *Heart Disease*, edn 5. Edited by Braunwald E. Philadelphia: WB Saunders; 1997:1687–1703.

3. Gerstenblith G, Fredrickson J, Yin FCP, *et al.*: Echocardiographic assessment of a normal adult aging population. *Circulation* 1977, 56:273.

4. Celemajer DS, Sorensen KE, Spiegelhalter DJ, *et al.*: Aging is associated with endothelial function in healthy men years before the age-related decline in women. *J Am Coll Cardiol* 1994, 24:471–476.

5. Lakatta EG: Alterations in the cardiovascular system that occur with advancing age. *Fed Proc* 1979, 38:163.

6. Unverforth DV, Fetter JK, Unverforth BJ, *et al.*: Human myocardial histologic characteristics in congestive heart failure. *Circulation* 1983, 68:1194.

7. Rodeheffer RJ, Gerstenblith G, Becker LC, *et al.*: Exercise cardiac output is maintained with advancing age in healthy human subjects: cardiac dilatation and increased stroke volumes compensate for diminished heart rate. *Circulation* 1984, 69:203.

8. Fleg JL, O'Connor F, Gerstenblith G, *et al.*: Impact of age on the cadiovascular response to upright exercise in healthy men and women. *J Appl Physiol* 1995, 78:890–900.

9. Fleg JL, Schulman S, O'Connor F, *et al.*: Effects of acute beta-adrenergic receptor blockage on age-associated changes in cardiovascular performance during dynamic exercise. *Circulation* 1994, 90:2333–2341.

10. Nixon JV, Burns CA: Cardiac effects of aging and diastolic dysfunction in the elderly. In *Heart Failure and Left Ventricular Diastolic Dysfunction*, edn 1. Edited by Gaasch WH, LeWinter M. Philadelphia: Lea & Febiger; 1994:427–435.

11. Fleg JL, Shapiro EP, O'Connor F, *et al.*: Left ventricular filling performance in older male athletes. *JAMA* 1995, 273:1371–1375.

12. Tran UL, Arrowood JA, Nixon JV: Effects of long-term dynamic conditioning on cardiac function in the older human heart. *J Invest Med* 1995, 43:299.

13. Miller PF, Sheps DS, Bragdon EE, *et al.*: Aging and pain perception in ischemic heart disease. *Am Heart J* 1990, 120:22.

14. Lam JYT, Chaitman BR, Glaenzer M: Safety and diagnostic accuracy of dipyridamole-thallium imaging in the elderly. *J Am Coll Cardiol* 1988, 11:585.

15. Gibbons RJ, Chatterjee K, Daley J, *et al.*: ACC/AHA/ACP-ASIM guidelines for the management of patients with chronic stable angina: a report of the American College of Cardiology/American Heart Association Task Force on Practice Guidelines. *J Am Coll Cardiol* 1999, 33:2092–2197.

16. The Seventh Report of the Joint National Committee on the Detection, Evaluation, and Treatment of High Blood Pressure (The JNC 7 Report). *JAMA* 2003, 289:2560–2572.

17. Nixon JV: Cholesterol management and the reduction of cardiovascular risk. *Preventive Cardiol* 2004, 7:34–41.

18. Kannel WB: Coronary heart disease risk factors in the elderly. *Am J Geriatr Cardiol* 2002, 11:101–107.

19. Raisner AE, Hust RG, Lewis JM, *et al.*: Transluminal coronary angioplasty in the elderly. *Am J Cardiol* 1986, 57:29.

20. Gersch BJ, Krenmal RA, Schaff HV, *et al.*: Comparison of coronary artery bypass surgery and medical therapy in patients 65 years of age or older. *N Engl J Med* 1985, 313:217.

21. Norwegian Multicenter Study Group: Timolol-induced reduction in mortality and reinfarction in patients surviving acute myocardial infarction. *N Engl J Med* 1981, 304:801.

22. Pfeffer MA, Braunwald E, Moye LA, *et al.*: Effect of captopril on mortality and morbidity in patients with left ventricular dysfunction after myocardial infarction. *N Engl J Med* 1992, 327:669.

23. Krumholz HM, Radford MJ, Ellerbeck EF, *et al.*: Aspirin for secondary prevention after acute myocardial infarction in the elderly: prescribed use and outcomes. *Ann Intern Med* 1996, 124:292–298.

24. Krumholz HM, Radford MJ, Wang Y, *et al.*: National use and effectiveness of beta blockers for the treatment of elderly patients after acute myocardial infarction: National Cooperative Cardiovascular Project. *JAMA* 1998, 280:623–629.

25. Hypertension Detection and Follow-up Program Cooperative Group: Five year findings of the Hypertension Detection and Follow-Up Program. Mortality by race, sex, and age. *JAMA* 1979, 242:2572.

26. Burt VL, Whelton P, Rocella EJ, *et al.*: Prevalence of hypertension in the US adult population: results from the third National Health and Nutrition Examination Survey, 1988–1991. *Hypertension* 1995, 25:305–313.

27. Insura JT, Sacks HS, Lau TS, *et al.*: Drug treatment of hypertension in the elderly. *Ann Intern Med* 1994, 121:355.

28. ALLHAT Cooperative Research Group: Major outcomes in high-risk hypertensive patients randomized to angiotensin-converting enzyme inhibitor or calcium channel blocker vs. diuretic: the Antihypertensive and Lipid-Lowering Treatment to Prevent Heart Attack Trial (ALLHAT). *JAMA* 2002, 288, 2981–2997.

29. National High Blood Pressure Education Program Working Group. National High Blood Pressure Education Program working group report on hypertension in the elderly. *Hypertension* 1994, 23:275–285.

30. Levy D, Garrison RJ, Savage DD, *et al.*: Left ventricular mass and incidence of coronary heart disease in an elderly cohort. *Ann Intern Med* 1989, 110:101.

31. Nixon JV: Treating hypertension in the elderly: a physiological basis for selections of therapy. *Cardiol Elderly* 1993, 1:441–446.

32. SHEP Cooperative Research Group: Prevention of stroke by antihypertensive drug treatment in older persons with isolated systolic hypertension: final results in the systolic hypertension in the elderly program (SHEP). *JAMA* 1991, 265:3255.

33. Staessen JA, Fagard R, Thijs L, *et al.*: Randomized double blind comparison of placebo and active treatment for older patients with isolated systolic hypertension. *Lancet* 1997, 350:757–764.

34. Applegate WB: Hypertension in elderly patients. *Ann Intern Med* 1989, 110:901.

35. Furberg CD, Psaty BM, Manolio TA, *et al.*: Prevalence of atrial fibrillation in elderly subjects (the Cardiovascular health Study). *Am J Cardiol* 1994, 74:236.

36. Dhond AJ, Michelena HI, Ezekowitz MD: Anticoagulation in the Elderly. *Am J Geriatr Cardiol* 2003, 12:243–250.

37. Camm AJ: Atrial fibrillation—a near epidemic. *Am J Geriatr Cardiol* 2003, 11:352.

38. Stevenson WG, Stevenson LW, Middlekoff HR, *et al.*: Improving survival for patients with atrial fibrillation and advanced heart failure. *J Am Coll Cardiol* 1996, 28:1458–1463.

39. Stevenson WG, Stevenson LW: Atrial fibrillation in heart failure. *N Engl J Med* 1999, 341:910–921.

40. Carabello BA: Timing of surgery in mitral and aortic stenosis. *Cardiovasc Clin* 1991, 9:229.

41. Braunwald E: Valvular heart disease. In *Heart Disease*, edn 4. Edited by Braunwald E. Philadelphia: WB Saunders; 1992:1007.

42. Alipour MS, Shah PM: Diagnosis of aortic stenosis in the elderly: role of echocardiography. *Am J Geriatr Cardiol* 2003, 12:201–206.

43. Feigenbaum H: Echocardiography. In *Heart Disease*, edn 4. Edited by Braunwald E. Philadelphia: WB Saunders; 1992:81.

44. Safian RD, Kentz RE, Berman AD: Aortic valvuloplasty. *Cardiovasc Clin* 1991, 9:289.

45. Miyatake K, Okamoto M, Kinoshiter N, *et al.*: Augmentation of atrial contribution to left ventricular inflow with aging as assessed by intracardiac Doppler flowmetry. *Am J Cardiol* 1984, 53:586.

46. Shah PM, Pai RG: Diastolic heart failure. *Curr Probl Cardiol* 1992, 12:821.

47. Lakatta EG: The aging heart. *Ann Intern Med* 1990, 113:456.

48. Levy D, Wilson PWF, Anderson KM, *et al.*: Stratifying the patient at risk from coronary disease: new insights from the Framingham Study. *Am Heart J* 1990, 119:712.

49. Ross J Jr, Braunwald E: Aortic stenosis. *Circulation* 1968, 38(suppl 5):61.

50. Lytle BW, Cosgrove DM, Gill CC, *et al.*: Aortic valve replacement combined with myocardial revascularization: late results and determinants of risk for 471 in-hospital survivors. *J Thorac Cardiovasc Surg* 1988, 95:402.

SELECT BIBLIOGRAPHY

Wenger NK: Cardiovascular disease in the elderly. In *Current Problems in Cardiology*. Edited by O'Rourke RA. St. Louis: Mosby–Year Book; 1992:10.

Pregnancy and the Heart

Brad S. Burlew
Howard R. Horn

Key Points

- Pregnancy imposes a hemodynamic burden on the cardiovascular system.
- Severe valvular stenotic lesions are poorly tolerated; regurgitant lesions have better outcomes.
- Mitral valve prolapse is rarely a problem.
- Anticoagulation worsens the outcome during pregnancy.
- Pulmonary hypertension is associated with a very poor outcome.
- With careful medical care and appropriate hemodynamic monitoring, most patients with cardiac disease can be safely carried through pregnancy and delivery.

Pregnancy is a condition that places temporary but significant hemodynamic stresses on the woman with underlying cardiac disease. The risk of complications from these stresses depends on the nature of the maternal cardiac abnormality, ranging from negligible risk with mitral valve prolapse to a very high likelihood of maternal and fetal death in patients with advanced pulmonary hypertension. Skillful management of the gravid patient with cardiac disease depends on an understanding of the normal clinical findings associated with the gravid state, the recognition of cardiac disease in the pregnant woman, and an understanding of the likely response of a specific disorder to the hemodynamic changes.

Fortunately, the prevalence of heart disease in the reproductive female population is fairly low (between 0.4% and 4.1%) [1,2]. Worldwide, rheumatic heart disease accounts for up to 90% of the cardiac disorders seen in pregnant women. Mitral stenosis is the most common lesion, occurring in approximately 90% of women with rheumatic heart disease. In the United States, Canada, and Western Europe, rheumatic heart disease now accounts for a diminishing portion (approximately 45% to 75%) of all cases of heart disease [2–4]. Congenital heart disease accounts for much of the remainder, with patients with surgically corrected congenital heart disease and those with prosthetic valves forming a relatively new category of pregnant women with heart disorders.

SIGNS AND SYMPTOMS ASSOCIATED WITH PREGNANCY

The signs and symptoms of pregnancy are a consequence of the normal physiologic changes that occur. These changes include an increase in maternal total blood volume, which reaches maximal values of 50% above baseline (nongravid) values. Plasma volume increases more than the red blood cell mass, which increases by only approximately 10%, resulting in a relative hemodilution [1]. This accounts for the physiologic anemia of pregnancy (Fig. 1).

Resting cardiac output also increases during pregnancy approximately 40% to 50% above that of the nongravid state (Fig. 2) [5]. Increased cardiac output is initially mediated through an increased stroke volume; the stroke volume then returns toward the normal range while the heart rate progressively increases. The gravid uterus occasionally compresses the inferior vena cava in the recumbent and standing positions, reducing venous return and cardiac output (Fig. 3) [6,7].

As pregnancy progresses, variations occur in cardiac output, stroke volume, and regional perfusion patterns. As the uterus enlarges, alterations occur in venous return to the central circulation as well. These changes are associated with the development of symptoms and signs that may mimic heart disease. For example, exertional dyspnea normally occurs in over 50% of pregnant women. Orthopnea, paroxysmal nocturnal dyspnea, dizziness, and easy fatigability are quite common. Syncope and presyncope may occur in the normal gravid woman, presumably caused by compression of the inferior vena cava by the uterus. Patients also may experience chest discomfort, mimicking angina pectoris.

On physical examination, normal patients may have prominent neck veins, inspiratory rales, ventricular (S_3) gallops, cardiomegaly, and peripheral edema. Murmurs, particularly systolic flow murmurs with an intensity of up to grade 2 (out of 6), are often heard (Fig. 4). Although diastolic murmurs are unusual in pregnancy, a diastolic murmur over the pulmonic area similar to the Graham Steell murmur is sometimes heard. This murmur, which is believed to be related to a physiologic dilatation of the pulmonary artery, vanishes soon after delivery [1]. A diastolic flow murmur arising from the tricuspid valve is occasionally heard; it likewise disappears after delivery. Venous sounds such as venous hums and mammary souffles also can be heard [8].

ACQUIRED VALVULAR HEART DISEASE
Worldwide, mitral stenosis is the most frequently observed acquired valvular lesion in reproductive women. It also poses one of the most substantial risks to the survival of the mother and the fetus. Depending on the degree of stenosis, a pressure gradient develops across the valve, resulting in elevated pressures in the left atrium and the pulmonary veins. Factors that increase the left atrial pressure are those that increase the diastolic mitral valvular flow rate through an increase in cardiac output or heart rate (which diminishes the duration of diastole, increasing the diastolic transvalvular gradient).

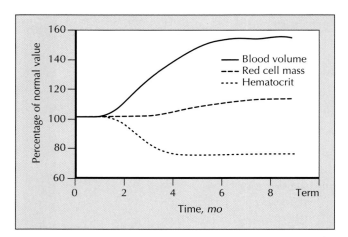

FIGURE 1 Hematologic effects of pregnancy.

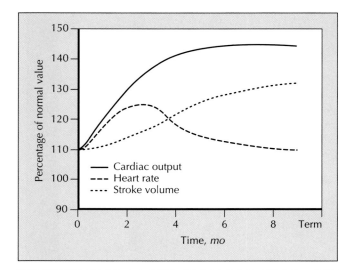

FIGURE 2 Hemodynamic effects of pregnancy.

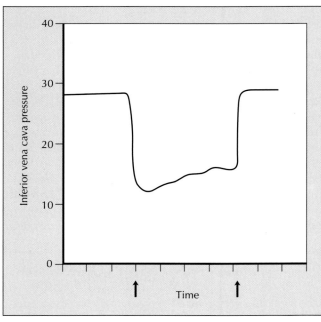

FIGURE 3 Hemodynamic effect of the gravid uterus. The uterus is lifted between the *arrows*. (*Adapted from* Kerr [6].)

Because of the normal physiologic increases in cardiac output during pregnancy and delivery, left atrial pressures tend to be more severely elevated in the gravid state as the diastolic flow across the stenotic mitral valve increases. The elevation in left atrial pressure can result in pulmonary edema and hypoxemia. Clinically, patients develop dyspnea, tachypnea, orthopnea, and paroxysmal nocturnal dyspnea, which are also symptoms often experienced by the normal gravid woman. Frank pulmonary edema and hemoptysis can occur in the third trimester and in the immediate postpartum period. Even patients who appear to be doing well can decompensate suddenly with the onset of rapid atrial tachycardia. Symptomatic tachycardias therefore must be treated promptly and effectively with digoxin and perhaps beta-blockade, because pulmonary edema frequently ensues. Patients with refractory symptomatic atrial fibrillation should have cardioversion. Infection and even mild hyperthyroidism also need to be treated promptly in this setting, because these disorders can similarly trigger tachycardia and subsequent pulmonary edema. At parturition, monitoring of the patient's volume status with a pulmonary artery catheter is recommended [1,9,10].

Aortic stenosis appears to affect pregnancy adversely, with a 17% overall maternal mortality rate [11]. Patients with severe aortic stenosis are preload dependent with a fixed stroke volume. Any increase in cardiac output is mediated through an increase in heart rate. Medications that decrease heart rate or preload should be avoided if possible. Vasodilators should also be avoided. If critical stenosis is diagnosed before pregnancy, surgical correction should be recommended.

Mitral and aortic valvular insufficiency are typically well tolerated in the gravid patient. The severity of valvular regurgitation may actually decrease during pregnancy because of the physiologic decrease in peripheral vascular resistance. Patients generally respond well to conservative therapy if they become symptomatic.

Mitral valve prolapse unassociated with other cardiovascular abnormalities does not increase maternal or fetal risk [12]. The use of prophylactic antibiotics in this setting remains controversial.

PROSTHETIC VALVES

Hemodynamically, patients with prosthetic valves tend to fare quite well throughout pregnancy. However, the combined fetal wastage and spontaneous abortion rates in patients receiving anticoagulant therapy approaches 60% [13]. An additional concern in these patients is the teratogenesis associated with warfarin therapy. Warfarin exposure at 6 to 9 weeks of gestation carries an 8% incidence of warfarin embryopathy [14]. Although heparin does not cross the placenta, prolonged intravenous therapy is associated with maternal complications, including development of heparin-induced osteopenia. In view of these issues, widely followed recommendations for anticoagulation during pregnancy include the administration of intravenous heparin during the first trimester, usually from weeks 6 through 12, and use of oral warfarin therapy during the second and third trimesters [15]. During the last weeks of pregnancy, intravenous heparin is again administered, because late exposure to warfarin is clearly associated with increased peripartum hemorrhage.

Although this protocol was designed to minimize risk to the fetus and the mother, the use of intravenous heparin does not appear to result in a significantly better outcome [16]. Indeed, on substitution or oral anticoagulation with unfractionated heparin as just described, there is an increase in maternal thromboembolic complications and death [13].

The development of low molecular weight heparins has provided an opportunity for alternatives to intravenous heparin in this setting. Review of the limited information currently available suggests the incidence of valve thrombosis and maternal death when these agents are used in the first trimester is unfortunately significantly increased as compared with heparin [17]. Low molecular weight heparin therefore cannot be recommended in this setting.

Pregnancy in patients requiring systemic anticoagulation continues to present significant risks to the fetus and the mother, and should perhaps be avoided. Management of the anticoagulated pregnant patient with a mechanical prosthetic valve is probably best accomplished in consulta-

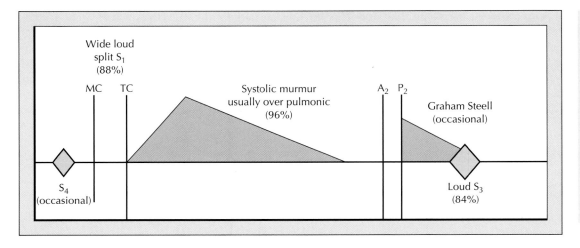

FIGURE 4
Auscultatory findings during pregnancy. A$_2$—aortic second sound; P$_2$—pulmonic second sound; S$_1$—first heart sound; S$_3$—third heart sound; S$_4$—fourth heart sound. (*Adapted from* Cutforth and MacDonald [26].)

tion with a cardiologist or another physician familiar with this problem.

PERIPARTUM CARDIOMYOPATHY

Peripartum cardiomyopathy is a disease of unknown etiology associated with development of congestive heart failure during the final month of pregnancy or during the 5 months after delivery. This disorder occurs initially in people who have not previously had heart disease and in whom other explanations for congestive heart failure are not apparent. It is more common among blacks, is more likely to occur in a woman 30 years of age or older who is pregnant with twins or who has toxemia, and is more likely to occur during a third or subsequent pregnancy. If the patient has ever acquired peripartum cardiomyopathy, it is likely to return in subsequent pregnancies, particularly if the patient had persistent postpartum cardiomegaly. Hypertension, myocarditis, and dietary factors may play roles in the development of peripartum cardiomyopathy [18•,19].

Standard therapy with digoxin and diuretics is usually sufficient. If needed, hydralazine and nitrates also can be used, because no studies have demonstrated the induction of teratogenesis in humans with the use of these agents. Prepartum use of angiotensin-converting enzyme inhibitors is strictly contraindicated during pregnancy because of their association with neonatal craniofacial deformities, renal failure, and death. However, postpartum use of angiotensin-converting enzyme inhibitors is appropriate, although breast-feeding should be strongly discouraged.

MYOCARDIAL INFARCTION

Fortunately, ischemic heart disease during pregnancy is quite uncommon, undoubtedly because women of reproductive age are at extremely low risk for its development. In view of the current US trend toward bearing children later in life, myocardial infarction among pregnant women will probably be seen more frequently in the future. The present frequency of myocardial infarction in pregnancy is very low, with an incidence of only approximately 10,000 pregnancies [20••]; the overall maternal mortality rate in this population is approximately 21%.

Current management recommendations include bed rest, aspirin, heparin, intravenous nitroglycerin, and beta-blockade. There are anecdotal reports of successful preterm percutaneous transluminal coronary angioplasty (PTCA) and stent deployment, although routine use of interventional techniques has not yet been extensively studied. Similarly, there are a number of reports of thrombolytic therapy in the gravid female, usually for pulmonary embolism. There does not appear to be any teratogenic effect of thrombolytic agents, although experience with their use in acute myocardial infarction is limited. It was previously recommended that oxytocin not be used in patients with ischemic heart disease. Currently, however, synthetic oxytocin, which does

not contain arginine vasopressin, is available; in appropriate doses, it is unlikely to increase coronary vasoconstriction. With the intravenous bolus administration of 5 to 12 U, oxytocin does produce a 30% decrease in mean arterial pressure and a 50% increase in cardiac output among healthy patients undergoing tocolysis. These hemodynamic effects can be avoided by the administration of oxytocin as a dilute solution [21]. Synthetic oxytocin has been used successfully in pregnant patients after myocardial infarction.

SELECTED DEVELOPMENTAL ABNORMALITIES

Primary pulmonary hypertension is associated with high fetal and maternal mortality rates. Generally, cardiac abnormalities associated with pulmonary hypertension (with or without right-to-left communication) are associated with a maternal mortality rate of approximately 50% [8]. Avoidance or interruption of pregnancy is indicated. Congenital heart disease in the pregnant woman usually poses some hazard to the mother. These patients are best treated in conjunction with a specialist familiar with these abnormalities. Genetic counseling also may be appropriate.

Other developmental abnormalities include Marfan syndrome and hypertrophic cardiomyopathy. With its connective tissue abnormality, Marfan syndrome is associated with a high incidence of aneurysmal dilatation of the aortic root. In one study [22], dissection or rupture of the aortic root occurred in 50% of affected pregnant women, although in our experience the frequency of these events is much lower. Serial echocardiography has been recommended to monitor the progression of dilatation or the development of dissection of the aortic root. The risk of sudden death is believed to be proportional to the diameter of the aortic root [22]. Nonetheless, undetected dissections have occurred despite close echocardiographic monitoring; the availability of endoscopic echocardiography may improve sensitivity in this regard. Meticulous control of blood pressure with beta-blockade is an approach we have used for this condition.

Hypertrophic obstructive cardiomyopathy is usually associated with uneventful pregnancies. The outflow obstruction is dynamic and dependent on factors such as blood pressure and ventricular preload, both of which should be maintained if possible. During pregnancy, patients should be encouraged to lie preferentially in the lateral decubitus positions. This maneuver relieves inferior vena caval obstruction, preserving ventricular preload. Because of the likelihood of marked worsening of the dynamic outflow obstruction, beta-sympathomimetic tocolytic agents are strictly contraindicated in this disorder. Regional anesthesia, with its risk of hypotension, should also be avoided [23].

CONCLUSIONS

With careful medical care and appropriate hemodynamic monitoring, most patients with cardiac disease can be safely carried through pregnancy and delivery [24]. Unfortunately, termination of the pregnancy is still sometimes indicated. In patients with severe congestive heart failure, termination should be considered during early pregnancy, because continuation of the pregnancy is likely to result in an unacceptable outcome for both the mother and fetus. Similarly, therapeutic abortion should be considered in patients with primary or secondary pulmonary hypertension (with or without right-to-left communications) and in those with cyanotic congenital heart disease. These clinical conditions can be associated with maternal mortality rates in excess of 50%. Termination of the pregnancy during the first or second trimester presents a more favorable risk to the patient [25].

KEY REFERENCE

A recently published paper of outstanding interest, as identified in *References and Recommended Reading*, has been annotated.

•• Roth A, Elkayam U: Acute myocardial infarction associated with pregnancy. *Ann Intern Med* 1996, 125:751–762.

Excellent, comprehensive review of the epidemiology, course, diagnosis, prognosis, and treatment of acute myocardial infarction during pregnancy.

REFERENCES AND RECOMMENDED READING

Recently published papers of particular interest have been highlighted as:
• Of interest
•• Of outstanding interest

1. Conradsson T, Werkö L: Management of heart disease in pregnancy. *Prog Cardiovasc Dis* 1974, 16:407–419.

2. McFaul PB, Dornan JC, Lamki H, Boyle D: Pregnancy complicated by maternal heart disease: a review of 519 women. *Br J Obstet Gynaecol* 1988, 95:861–867.

3. Szekely P, Snaith L: *Heart Disease and Pregnancy*. London: Churchill Livingstone; 1974:53.

4. Shime J, Mocarski EJM, Hastings D, *et al.*: Congenital heart disease in pregnancy: short and long term implications. *Am J Obstet Gynecol* 1987, 156:313–322.

5. Robson SC, Hunter S, Boys RJ, Dunlop W: Serial study of factors influencing changes in cardiac output during pregnancy. *Am J Physiol* 1989, 256:H1060–H1065.

6. Kerr MG: The mechanical effects of the gravid uterus in late pregnancy. *J Obstet Gynaecol Br Comm* 1965, 72:513–529.

7. Metcalf J, Ueland K: Maternal cardiovascular adjustment to pregnancy. *Prog Cardiovasc Dis* 1974, 16:363–374.

8. McAnulty JH, Metcalfe J, Ueland K: General guidelines in the management of cardiac disease. *Clin Obstet Gynecol* 1981, 24:773–789.

9. Lang RM, Borow KM: Pregnancy and heart disease. *Clin Perinatol* 1985, 12:551–569.

10. Ueland K, Hansen JM: Maternal cardiovascular dynamics II: posture and uterine contractions. *Am J Obstet Gynecol* 1969, 103:1–7.

11. Arias F, Pineda J: Aortic stenosis and pregnancy. *J Reprod Med* 1978, 20:229–232.

12. Tang LCH, Chan SYW, Wong VCW, Ma H: Pregnancy in patients with mitral valve prolapse. *Int J Gynaecol Obstet* 1985, 23:217–221.

13. Chan WS, Anand S, Ginsberg JS: Anticoagulation of pregnant women with mechanical valves: a systematic review of the literature. *Arch Intern Med* 2000, 160:191–196.

14. Pauli RM, Hall JG, Wilson KM: Risks of anticoagulation during pregnancy. *Am Heart J* 1980, 100:761–762.

15. Hirsch J, Cade JF, O'Sullivan EF: Clinical experience with anticoagulation therapy during pregnancy. *BMJ* 1970, 1:270–275.

16. Hall JG, Pauli RM, Wilson KM: Maternal and fetal sequelae of anticoagulation during pregnancy. *Am J Med* 1980, 68:122–140.

17. Leyh RG, Fischer S, Ruhparwar A, Haverich A: Anticoagulation therapy in pregnant women with mechanical heart valves. *Arch Gynecol Obstet* 2003, 268:1–4.

18.• Lampert MB, Lang RM: Peripartum cardiomyopathy. *Am J Heart J* 1995, 130:960–970.

19. O'Connell JB, Costanzo-Nordin MR, Subramanian R, *et al.*: Peripartum cardiomyopathy: clinical, hemodynamic, histologic and prognostic characteristics. *J Am Coll Cardiol* 1986, 8:52–56.

20.•• Roth A, Elkayam U: Acute myocardial infarction associated with pregnancy. *Ann Intern Med* 1996, 125:751–762.

21. Weis FR, Markello R, Mo B, Bochiecho P: Cardiovascular effects of oxytocin. *Obstet Gynecol* 1975, 46:211–214.

22. Pyeritz RE: Maternal and fetal complications of pregnancy in the Marfan syndrome. *Am J Med* 1981, 71:784–790.

23. Shah DM, Sunderji SG: Hypertrophic cardiomyopathy and pregnancy: report of a maternal mortality and review of literature. *Obstet Gynecol Surv* 1985, 40:444–448.

24. Whittemore R, Hobbins JC, Engle MA: Pregnancy and its outcome on women with and without surgical treatment of congenital heart disease. *Am J Cardiol* 1982, 50:641–651.

25. Elkayam U, Gleicher N: Cardiac problems in pregnancy. *JAMA* 1984, 251:2838–2839.

26. Cutforth R, MacDonald CB: Heart sounds and murmurs during pregnancy. *Am Heart J* 1966, 71:741–747.

Heart Transplantation

Jorge E. Massare
John B. O'Connell

45

Key Points

- Heart transplantation stands as a successful and often the only therapeutic alternative for patients with end-stage heart disease.

- Heart transplantation remains strictly limited by the availability of donor hearts.

- The 5-year survival rate in heart transplant recipients averages 70%. The overall functional status of surviving heart transplant recipients is excellent.

- Any cardiac condition associated with substantial morbidity and mortality not amenable or unresponsive to medical therapy constitutes a potential indication for heart transplantation.

- Exercise testing with measurement of peak oxygen consumption is a useful adjunct in assessing the need for transplantation.

- The most frequent regimen for maintenance immunosuppression following heart transplantation uses cyclosporine, mycophenolate mofetil, and prednisone.

- Although the incidence of infection has decreased with improved immunosuppressive agents, it remains the main cause of death from day 31 to 365 after heart transplantation.

- Cardiac-allograft vasculopathy or "chronic rejection" is a process of accelerated coronary artery disease that represents the leading cause of death after the first year of heart transplantation.

BACKGROUND

Following its highly publicized beginnings in the late 1960s, the relatively poor survival rate of heart transplantation limited the application of this procedure to just a few centers worldwide through the 1970s. With evolving surgical techniques and medical advances such as the development of the transvenous endomyocardial biopsy, and especially the introduction of the immunosuppressant cyclosporine in 1981, the success rate improved dramatically and led to a rapid increase in the use of cardiac transplantation throughout the United States. Today, with the sustained rise in the prevalence of congestive heart failure, heart transplantation stands as a successful, and often the only, therapeutic alternative for patients with end-stage heart disease.

TRANSPLANT VOLUME

After the introduction of cyclosporine in the early 1980s, the number of reported heart transplantations and centers performing this procedure rapidly proliferated both worldwide and in the United States [1]. These numbers, however, have been declining since 1995 [2] (Fig. 1). In contrast, the size of the waiting list for heart transplantation has grown exponentially until 1998 just to level off thereafter at a

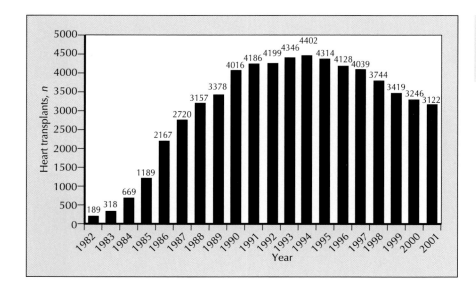

FIGURE 1 Number of heart transplants worldwide reported by year. (*Adapted from* the International Society for Heart and Lung Transplantation Registry [22].)

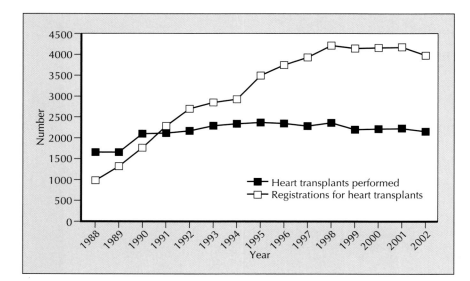

FIGURE 2 Number of heart transplants performed yearly compared to number of new registrations for heart transplant waiting list in the United States between 1988 and 2002. (*Adapted from* the Organ Procurement and Transplantation Network [4].)

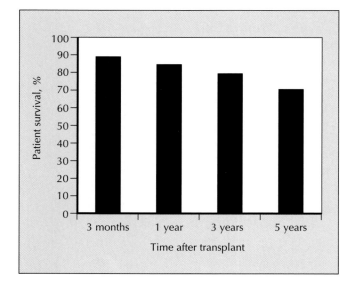

FIGURE 3 Patient survival among heart transplant recipients. (*Adapted from* the Organ Procurement and Transplantation Network [7].)

number close to 4000 patients per year [3] (Fig. 2), representing almost twice the number of patients who can possibly be transplanted, according to the number of transplants per year performed over the last decade [4]. Equally important, the time on the waiting list has dramatically increased. From 1992 to 2001, the percentage of patients waiting less than 1 year decreased by almost 50% from 68% to 35%, and those waiting more than 2 years quadrupled from 11% to 46% of the waiting list population [3].

It is unclear whether the decline in the number of heart transplantations is due to a decrease in the number of transplants; a decrease in the reporting of procedures performed, especially by non-US centers [5,6]; or clinical stabilization of the patients on the waiting lists with medical therapy, surgery, revascularization procedures, defibrillators and/or cardiac pacing, which make deferral or even avoiding transplantation possible in many cases. Nevertheless, heart transplantation still remains strictly limited by the availability of donor hearts.

CURRENT RESULTS

The dramatic improvement in survival after heart transplantation is illustrated in Figure 3 [4]. Many centers achieve 1-year survival rates exceeding 90%. Five-year actuarial survival rate averages 70%, and individual heart transplant recipients have survived more than 20 years. Mortality during the first year of transplantation is 1.4 times that of the next 4 years combined, but after a steep fall during the first 6 months, survival decreases in a linear rate of 4% per year thereafter. Patient half-life (time to 50% survival) and conditional half-life (time to 50% survival for patients who survived beyond 1 year) for patients transplanted between 1982 and 2001 are 9.3 years and 12 years, respectively [5] (Fig. 4).

Equally important, the functional status of surviving heart transplant recipients is excellent, with more than 90%

reported as having no activity limitations at 1, 3, and 5 years after transplantation and close to 40% reported full-time or part-time employment [5].

RECIPIENT SELECTION

The increasing prevalence of congestive heart failure (CHF) added to the improved survival rate after heart transplantation has led to an increase in the number of patients that will likely benefit from transplantation. Although the size of the waiting list has stabilized for the past 5 years, the supply of donor hearts has also been stagnant over the last 10 years; *ie*, the number of patients on the waiting list is almost double the number of transplants performed every year, reflected in a transplant rate of 55% in 2002 [7].

Although the death rate on the waiting list remains high (14% in 2002) [7], it has substantially decreased compared with previous years. Part of this decline could be attributed to successive modifications in the transplant candidate selection process through the revision of the policies for the allocation of candidates over the last 10 years.

INDICATIONS

Any cardiac condition associated with substantial morbidity and mortality not amenable or unresponsive to medical therapy constitutes a potential indication for heart transplantation. The primary underlying cause of heart failure leading to adult heart transplantation has been equally balanced between coronary heart disease and noncoronary cardiomyopathy [5] (Fig. 5). Other possible indications are shown in Table 1. Regardless of the cause of heart failure, severe symptoms despite maximal medical management (New York Heart Association [NYHA] functional class III to IV) and a poor expected 12-month survival related to the heart condition should be present. The determination of prognosis in

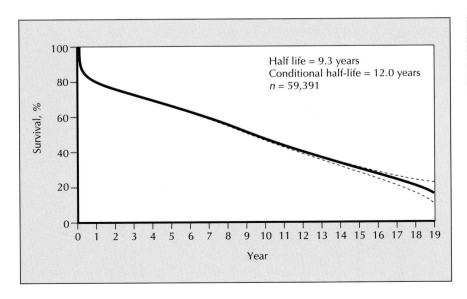

FIGURE 4 Actuarial survival for heart transplantations performed between January 1982 and June 2001. (*Adapted from* Taylor *et al.* [5].)

patients with advanced heart failure is difficult due to the complexity of numerous factors playing a role (Table 2). Low left ventricular ejection fraction alone is not sufficient for transplant candidacy because only those patients with associated advanced symptoms of heart failure or life-threatening arrhythmias carry a 6- to 12-month mortality risk great enough to warrant immediate transplant consideration.

Exercise testing with measurement of oxygen consumption by expired gas analysis is a useful adjunct in assessing the need for transplantation. It not only provides an objective confirmation of the subjective determination of NYHA functional class, but also has been shown to predict 12-month survival in patients with severe left ventricular dysfunction and resultant CHF [8]. Table 3 illustrates generally accepted indications for heart transplantation, independently of the primary cause.

CONTRAINDICATIONS

Although a transplant candidate's present level of symptoms and cardiovascular prognosis are critical to the selection process, expected morbidity and mortality after heart

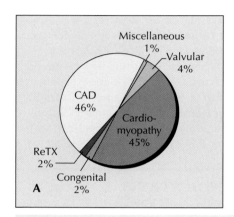
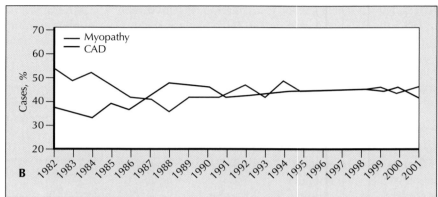

FIGURE 5 Diagnoses leading to heart transplantation. CAD—coronary artery disease; ReTX—retransplantation. (*Adapted from* Taylor *et al.* [5].)

TABLE 1 CONDITIONS THAT MAY LEAD TO HEART TRANSPLANTATION*
Cardiomyopathy
Ischemic cardiomyopathy
Dilated cardiomyopathy: idiopathic, familial
Restrictive cardiomyopathy: idiopathic, amyloidosis, sarcoidosis, endocardial fibrosis, secondary to radiation or chemotherapy
Hypertrophic cardiomyopathy
Myocarditis: viral, peripartum, toxic (ethanol, adriamycin)
Valvular heart disease
Coronary heart disease
Refractory angina
Ischemia not amenable to revascularization
Inoperable primary cardiac tumors
Refractory life-threatening arrhythmias not controllable with implantable cardioverter-defibrillator
Uncorrectable congenital heart disease
Retransplant/graft failure
Cardiac-allograft vasculopathy
Rejection
*Adapted from the Organ Procurement and Transplantation Network (www.optn.org).

TABLE 2 ADVERSE PROGNOSTIC FACTORS IN HEART FAILURE
Ischemic origin
Advanced NYHA functional class
Presence of ventricular S_3 gallop
Left bundle branch block
Intraventricular conduction delay
Ventricular tachycardia
Decreased heart rate variability
Antiarrhythmic drug use
Low left ventricular ejection fraction
Left atrial enlargement
Deceleration time of E wave on Doppler echocardiography
Reduced cardiac index
Increased pulmonary capillary wedge pressure
Low peak exercise oxygen consumption
Reduced serum sodium
Increased plasma levels of vasoactive neurohormones (catecholamines, BNP, endothelin-1, aldosterone, angiotensin)
Accelerated myocardial adrenergic activity
BNP—B-type natriuretic peptide; NYHA—New York Heart Association.

transplantation must also be addressed. Patients with end-stage heart disease and irreversible, uncontrollable, or untreatable comorbid conditions are not suitable candidates for transplantation. Coexisting medical problems may independently affect posttransplantation outcomes adversely, or they may do so in combination with the toxicity of the immunosuppressive drugs.

As experience with heart transplantation has grown, the list of the traditional absolute contraindications has changed to the extent that most transplant physicians would now agree that these are relative contraindications that require discussion and individual patient exemptions [9] (Table 4). For example, some patients with diabetes mellitus now routinely undergo transplantation and appear to have similar outcomes to patients without diabetes at 1 year [10] and 5 years after transplantation [11]. Heart transplantation has been successfully performed in the setting of well-controlled HIV infection [12]. Active systemic infection is a strong reason to delay transplantation; paradoxically, candidates with implanted ventricular assist devices complicated with infection of the device are now treated with heart transplantation. The upper age limit has steadily increased to the degree that 12% of patients on the waiting list in 2001 were over 65 years old and the percentage of heart transplant recipients older than 65 increased from 4% in 1992 to 10% in 2001 [3].

THE SELECTION PROCESS

Patients with CHF and NYHA class III or IV symptoms not amenable to other treatment modalities and without clear contraindications should be referred to a heart transplant center for consideration. Such patients will undergo an extensive evaluation directed at identifying and assessing all the factors noted previously. A committee of physicians and other health care personnel generally makes a decision on each candidate. Some patients will be judged unacceptable because of one or more contraindications, whereas others may have transplantation deferred due to symptoms of insufficient severity or a relatively favorable prognosis. Those patients deemed acceptable and in imminent need of transplantation will be actively "listed" on a computerized, nationwide waiting list. Each patient awaiting heart transplantation is assigned a status code that corresponds to the urgency for that patient to receive a transplant (Table 5). Organs are allocated based on age group, body size, blood group, urgency status and time on the waiting list. The distribution of organs follows a geographic sequence centered at the organ donor hospital location. The waiting time for a suitable candidate ranges from as little as 1 day to more than 2 years, with a median time to transplantation of approximately 100 days for patients in status 1A or 1B in 2000 and 2001 [3].

MANAGEMENT

At the time of transplantation, the recipient trades terminal heart disease for other significant problems: medication toxicities and complications of the immunosuppression. Despite introduction of more specific immunosuppressive agents, optimal posttransplantation care requires constant vigilance for potential complications.

TABLE 3 INDICATIONS FOR HEART TRANSPLANTATION*
Generally accepted
Refractory NYHA functional class III or IV heart failure
Sustained dependence on inotropic or mechanical circulatory support
Refractory life-threatening ventricular arrhythmias
Severe myocardial ischemia not amenable to revascularization
Peak oxygen consumption (VO_2 max) < 10 mL/kg/min
High-risk heart failure survival score (HFSS)†
Probable
Refractory fluid status and/or renal function instability
Peak oxygen consumption (VO_2 max) < 14 mL/kg/min
Medium-risk HFSS†
*Adapted from Deng [38].
†HFSS is calculated based on heart rate, mean blood pressure, etiology, QRS duration, serum sodium, left ventricular ejection fraction, and peak oxygen uptake [39].
NYHA—New York Heart Association.

TABLE 4 TRADITIONAL CONTRAINDICATIONS FOR HEART TRANSPLANTATION*
Age
Coexistent systemic illness with a poor prognosis
Myocardial infiltrative or inflammatory disease
Irreversible major organ dysfunction (pulmonary, hepatic, renal)
Irreversible pulmonary arterial hypertension
Acute or irreversible pulmonary parenchymal disease
Severe peripheral or cerebrovascular disease
Active peptic ulcer disease
Active diverticular disease
Insulin-dependent diabetes with end-organ damage
Active infection
Coexisting neoplasm
Psychosocial instability and/or substance abuse
Severe obesity
Severe osteoporosis
*Adapted from Cimato and Jessup [9].

Normal Allograft Physiology

The surgical technique of a traditional orthotopic heart transplantation is simplified by anastomosing a residual cuff of the recipient's left and right atria tissue to the donor atria rather than separately anastomosing the two venae cava and four pulmonary veins (Fig. 6). As a result, two sinus nodes are present postoperatively. After this operation, atrial activity from the recipient's sinus node can often be seen on the electrocardiogram dissociated from the sinus rhythm of the donor heart. This recipient's atrial activity is electrically isolated from the donor heart by the suture line. Most operations now apply a modification of this technique in which the donor right atrium is left intact and is anastomosed to the recipient inferior and superior vena cava.

Another unique feature of the donor heart is denervation. All transplanted hearts remain denervated for at least 1 year and partially denervated thereafter. Without the dominant inhibitory parasympathetic influence, the resting heart rate in the transplant recipient is usually between 90 and 110 bpm. Loss of afferent neural signaling blunts the perception of angina in response to myocardial ischemia. Likewise, denervation impairs normal vasoregulatory responses to elevated cardiac filling pressures. Response to hemodynamic stressors and exercise is also altered; without direct sympathetic innervation, reflex tachycardia is lost and the transplanted heart responds to circulating catecholamines, an inherently delayed mechanism, taking at least twice as long for a transplanted heart to achieve the same heart rate as that of a normal subject during exercise. Despite these differences in physiology, heart transplant recipients are generally capable of achieving normal exercise tolerance; some even participate in competitive athletics.

Importantly, as a consequence of denervation, the transplanted heart responds differently than the native heart to many pharmacologic agents (Table 6).

Immunosuppression

Immunosuppressive agents are applied for induction of immunosuppression at the time of transplantation, prevention of acute rejection (maintenance therapy), and treatment of acute rejection episodes.

TABLE 5 ADULT PATIENT STATUS*†

Each patient awaiting heart transplantation is assigned a status code that corresponds to the urgency for that patient to receive a transplant.

Status 1A

At least one of the following:

1. Patients requiring mechanical circulatory support for acute hemodynamic decompensation, including:
   Left and/or right ventricular assist device
   Total artificial heart
   Intra-aortic balloon pump
   Extracorporeal membrane oxygenator
2. Patients requiring mechanical circulatory support with objective evidence of device-related complications such as:
   Thromboembolism
   Device infection
   Mechanical failure
   Life-threatening ventricular arrhythmias
3. Patients requiring mechanical ventilation
4. Patients requiring continuous infusion of single high-dose or multiple intravenous inotropes and continuous hemodynamic monitoring

Status 1B

At least one of the following:

1. Left and/or right ventricular assist device implanted
2. Continuous infusion of intravenous inotropes

Status 2

Patients who do not meet criteria for status 1A or 1B

Status 7

Patients considered temporarily unsuitable to receive a transplant

*Adapted from the Organ Procurement and Transplantation Network Policies for Organ Distribution: Allocation of Thoracic Organs, as of 7/27/03 (www.optn.org).

†A pediatric patient status has been created and is available online at www.optn.org/policiesAndBylaws/policies.asp.

The goal of induction immunosuppression is to prevent acute rejection during the first weeks after transplantation and "induce" a state of relative tolerance. Commonly used agents are polyclonal antibody preparations such as antithymocyte globulin (ATG) and antilymphocyte globulin (ALG), as well as the monoclonal antibody OKT3 (muromonab CD3) and the interleukin-2 receptor blockers basiliximab and daclizumab. These preparations are effective at extending the time to first rejection, but they do not affect the overall survival [13,14] and are associated with higher rates of infection and posttransplant lymphoproliferative disorders [15,16]. Therefore, the use of induction therapy has been in decline [5].

Maintenance immunosuppression is based on multidrug regimens. A standard regimen includes a calcineurin inhibitor, an antiproliferative agent, and corticosteroids. Two calcineurin inhibitors are widely used: cyclosporine and tacrolimus (formerly called FK506). Although molecularly different, they inhibit lymphocyte activation and block B- and T-cell proliferation. They were equally efficacious when compared in randomized controlled trials [17,18]. Their side effect profiles are also similar, although the incidence of hypertension and dyslipidemia are lower with tacrolimus, and it does not cause hirsutism or gingival hyperplasia [19,20]. The antiproliferative agents inhibit nucleotide biosynthesis. Mycophenolate mofetil is replacing azathioprine as a first-line agent within this group due to its superior efficacy and less bone marrow suppression. Corticosteroids are used at high doses perioperatively and then tapered down to a low maintenance dose and even discon-

tinued. Currently, the most frequent regimen for maintenance immunosuppression is cyclosporine, mycophenolate mofetil, and prednisone [5].

In addition to the intrinsic toxicity of the immunosuppressive drugs (Table 7), significant interactions with other commonly prescribed medications pose a real threat to the heart transplant recipient. Calcineurin antagonists are metabolized by the cytochrome P-450 3A, interacting with many other drugs that utilize this metabolic pathway, leading to either elevated serum levels and toxicity (eg, renal

TABLE 6 EFFECT OF CARDIOVASCULAR DRUGS ON TRANSPLANTED HEARTS

Drug	Effect on the Transplanted Heart
Digoxin	Normal increase of contractility; minimal effect on atrioventricular node
Atropine	No activity
Epinephrine	Increased contractility
	Increased heart rate
Norepinephrine	Increased contractility
	Increased heart rate
Isoproterenol	Increased contractility
	Increased heart rate
Adenosine	Increased depression of sinus rate
β-Blockers	Increased antagonist effect

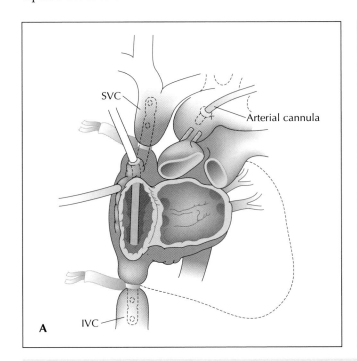

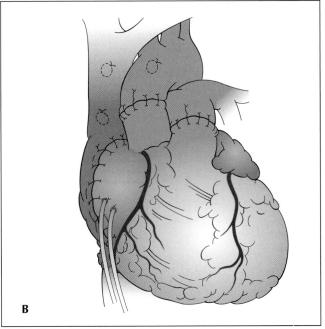

FIGURE 6 Heart transplantation. **A,** Diagram of recipient's mediastinum with heart resected and cannulas in place. **B,** Diagram of donor heart anastomosed in the orthotopic position. IVC—inferior vena cava; SVC—superior vena cava. (*Adapted from* Hunt *et al.* [40].)

failure) or decreased serum levels and transplant rejection (Table 8). Nonsteroidal anti-inflammatory drugs (NSAIDs), amphotericin, aminoglycosides, and radiocontrast agents potentiate the nephrotoxicity of calcineurin inhibitors. These agents also inhibit metabolism of 3-hydroxy-3-methylglutaryl coenzyme A (HMG-CoA) reductase inhibitors (statins) making them potentially more

toxic, particularly with rhabdomyolysis, at lower doses. Allopurinol dramatically impairs the metabolism of azathioprine and can lead to suppression of the bone marrow [21]. Mycophenolate mofetil mainly interacts with drugs that impair its absorption, such as aluminum-containing antacids, cholestyramine, and antibiotics, and drugs that inhibit its renal excretion, such as probenecid.

In view of these important drug interactions, recipients are routinely advised to contact the heart transplant center before starting therapy with any new drugs.

COMPLICATIONS

Rejection

Posttransplant management is focused on the prevention and treatment of allograft rejection. Periodic assessment of allograft function by echocardiography and hemodynamic measurements and screening with transvenous right ventricular endomyocardial biopsies allow detection of most episodes of acute rejection before symptoms develop. Acute rejection is diagnosed by histologic examination of endomyocardial biopsy specimens. Signs and symptoms that may suggest acute rejection are shown in Table 9. Suspicion of acute rejection is a medical emergency and warrants immediate consultation with the transplant center. When allograft function is not compromised and the histologic grade of rejection is low, it often resolves without treatment or with optimization of maintenance immunosuppression. For more severe cases, treatment options are numerous, but pulse therapy with intravenous methylprednisolone and high-dose oral prednisone are the most common. When there is allograft failure (decreased left ventricular ejection fraction or overt congestive heart failure), or rejection episodes are resistant to corticosteroids, potent polyclonal or monoclonal antilymphocyte antibody

TABLE 7 SIDE EFFECTS OF IMMUNOSUPPRESSIVE AGENTS

Calcineurin inhibitors
  Cyclosporine
    Nephrotoxicity
    Neurotoxicity
    Diabetes mellitus
    Hypertension
    Hyperlipidemia
    Hirsutism
    Gingival hyperplasia
  Tacrolimus
    Nephrotoxicity
    Neurotoxicity
    Diabetes mellitus
    Hypertension
    Dyslipidemia
Antiproliferative agents
  Azathioprine
    Leukopenia
    Anemia
    Thrombocytopenia
    Pancreatitis
    Hepatitis
    Peptic ulcer disease
    Lymphoproliferative disorders
  Mycophenolate mofetil
    Nausea, vomiting, diarrhea
    Gastritis, peptic ulcer disease
    Urinary urgency, dysuria
    Leukopenia
Corticosteroids
  Cushing's syndrome
  Osteoporosis
  Osteonecrosis
  Myopathy
  Acne
  Cataracts
  Peptic ulcer disease
  Impaired wound healing
  Dyslipidemia
  Glucose intolerance/diabetes mellitus
  Emotional lability/psychosis

TABLE 8 COMMON DRUG INTERACTIONS OF CYCLOSPORINE AND TACROLIMUS

Increase cyclosporine and tacrolimus blood levels
  Erythromycin, clarithromycin
  Ketoconazole, fluconazole, itraconazole, voriconazole
  Diltiazem, nifedipine, nicardipine, verapamil
  Metoclopramide
  Bromocriptine
Decrease cyclosporine and tacrolimus blood levels
  Carbamazepine
  Phenobarbital
  Phenytoin
  Rifampin
  Nafcillin

preparations are available (*eg*, antithymocyte globulin and muromonab-CD3).

Infections

Suppression of the immune system to prevent rejection also increases the susceptibility of the transplant recipient to typical and atypical infections. Although the overall incidence of infection has decreased with improved immunosuppressive agents, it continues to be a major cause of morbidity and mortality. From day 31 to 365 after transplant, infections are the most frequent cause of death, accounting for almost 35% of all the deaths. This decreases to about 13% between years 3 and 5, and to less than 10% thereafter [5]. Infections are also responsible for half of the re-hospitalizations during the first year after transplantation [22].

Bacterial pathogens account for the majority of severe infections, but viral, fungal, and protozoal agents each play a role. The most common sites of bacterial infections are the lungs, urinary tract, surgical wound, and bloodstream, and the most common responsible agents are *Pseudomonas aeruginosa*, *Escherichia coli*, *Streptococcus aureus*, and coagulase-negative *Staphylococci*. The viral agents most frequently implicated in posttransplant infections are cytomegalovirus (CMV), in the form of disseminated infection, pneumonia, hepatitis or gastroenteritis; herpes simplex virus (HSV), mainly causing stomatitis; and herpes zoster virus (HZV). Fungal infections are mostly caused by *Aspergillus* and *Candida*, mainly as pulmonary and disseminated infections. *Pneumocystis carinii* pneumonia (PCP) remains an important complication, although most programs administer oral trimethoprim-sulfamethoxazole prophylaxis. Protozoal infections are mostly caused by *Toxoplasma gondii*, *Giardia*, and *Trichomonas* [23].

The time of occurrence of an infectious episode can help identify the likely responsible organism, because many of these infections typically manifest during a specific time after transplantation. Most of the infections occurring during the first month are the same bacterial or candidal infections of surgical wounds, lungs, urinary tract, or catheter-related that occur in any surgical patient. Between the first and sixth months, opportunistic infections produced by viruses (*eg*, CMV, HSV, and HZV), fungi (especially *Aspergillus*), and PCP are particularly common. After the sixth month, infectious complications are usually similar to those of the general population. However, these patterns of infection are not fixed and are influenced by duration and intensity of immunosuppression, environmental exposure, and epidemiologic patterns [24].

Antimicrobial prophylaxis has been successful in reducing the incidence of infection. Perioperative cephalosporins have reduced early staphylococcal infections [25]. Pyrimethamine and trimethoprim-sulfamethoxazole have been shown to be efficacious in decreasing the incidence of posttranplant toxoplasmosis and PCP, respectively [26,27]. For CMV prophylaxis, high-dose ganciclovir decreases the incidence of reactivation of CMV infections. CMV-seronegative recipients of CMV-seropositive donors constitute the highest risk group for CMV infections. For these patients, most programs prolong the duration of ganciclovir administration and add intravenous hyperimmune globulin to the prophylactic regimen.

Cardiac-Allograft Vasculopathy

The donor heart is susceptible to a process of accelerated intimal hyperplasia and vascular smooth-muscle cell proliferation that leads to diffuse and concentric narrowing and occlusion of the coronary arteries, in contrast to the more focal and eccentric lesions of atherosclerosis. This process has been termed cardiac-allograft vasculopathy (CAV), or chronic rejection. The incidence of CAV depends on the method used for its detection. By angiography, it is estimated to be 10% at 1 year and nearly 50% at 5 years posttransplant [28]; these numbers are even higher when coronary intravascular ultrasound is used [29]. It is clear that the incidence of CAV increases with each successive year following heart transplantation, and it represents the leading cause of death after the first year of heart transplantation [5,30]. Current pathophysiologic hypotheses propose that the vasculature of the donor heart stimulates an immune response that culminates in cell proliferation and myointimal thickening. Non-immunologic factors seem to be implicated as well, with older donor age, donor history of hypertension, and pretransplant coronary artery disease, among others, identified as risk factors for the development of CAV [5]. An increasing body of evidence suggests that viral infections, particularly CMV, may also contribute to CAV. Clinically, because of denervation of the heart, most patients with advanced CAV do not experience angina. It rather manifests as new-onset heart failure, tachy- or bradyarrhythmias, syncope, or sudden cardiac death. Most transplant programs perform yearly coronary examination with angiography to screen for this process. The addition of intravascular ultrasound to conventional angiography greatly increases the sensitivity for the

TABLE 9 SIGNS AND SYMPTOMS OF ACUTE CARDIAC ALLOGRAFT REJECTION
Signs
Relative hypotension
Elevated jugular venous pressure
S$_3$ gallop
Pulmonary rales
Peripheral edema
Low-grade fever
Arrhythmias
Symptoms
Dyspnea
Orthopnea
Fatigue

diagnosis. Treatment options for CAV are limited, because the diffuse coronary lesions are rarely amenable to percutaneous transluminal coronary angioplasty or coronary artery bypass surgery. Current therapeutic strategies mainly focus on its prevention. Some agents have proven to be beneficial in this setting, such as calcium channel blockers, particularly diltiazem [31], and HMG-CoA reductase inhibitors, such as pravastatin [32] and simvastatin [33]. In addition to preventing CMV infection, administration of ganciclovir early after transplant reduces the incidence of CAV [34]. Aspirin is routinely prescribed to transplant recipients, despite the lack of evidence that it prevents CAV. Ultimately, in severely symptomatic patients due to this condition, cardiac retransplantation may be advised.

Malignancies

An increased incidence of malignancy is a well-recognized complication of chronic immunosuppression in heart transplant recipients. The latest data from the International Society for Heart and Lung Transplantation Registry showed a cumulative prevalence of malignancy of 3.3% and 18% at 1 and 5 years after transplantation, respectively. Skin cancers, primarily squamous cell carcinoma, and a particular type of B-cell lymphoma called posttransplant lymphoproliferative disorder (PTLD), account for the majority of cancers [22]. Therefore, regular assessment of transplant recipients should include careful examination of the skin and lymph nodes. As in the general population, skin cancers are more frequent in patients who have had excessive exposure to the sun. PTLD has been associated with intense immunosuppression, particularly potent antilymphocyte antibody preparations, and Epstein-Barr virus infection. The mainstay of treatment for these malignancies is reduction of immunosuppressive therapy. Patients who do not respond to this approach may benefit from surgical debulking of the tumor and adjuvant chemotherapy or radiotherapy. The prognosis in those cases is poor.

Other Complications

Hypertension is a very predictable complication of heart transplant, with over 90% of patients receiving immunosuppressive maintenance therapy that includes cyclosporine and corticosteroids requiring antihypertensive therapy by 6 months [35]. The incidence of hypertension is lower with tacrolimus. Treatment of hypertension in transplant recipients may be complicated, considering the interactions of many traditional antihypertensives with the immunosuppressive agents. Dyslipidemia is also increased after heart transplantation and should be treated early. HMG-CoA reductase inhibitors are often routinely prescribed in all cardiac transplant recipients irrespective of the lipid levels in view of the favorable effects of these drugs on CAV [36]. Severe renal dysfunction, defined by creatinine greater than 2.5 mg/dL, need for dialysis or need for renal transplant, occurs in over 25% of heart recipients 5 years after transplant [22]. Myriad other complications may strike the heart transplant recipient, as illustrated in Table 10.

ROLE OF THE PRIMARY CARE PHYSICIAN

Despite a relatively favorable survival and quality of life after heart transplantation, regular and thorough general medical care is critical in minimizing complications. Most transplant programs encourage continued participation by the patient's primary care provider, especially when frequency of visits to the transplant center for biopsies diminishes. The patient is best cared for during the first 3 to 6 months by the transplantation center. Afterward, if there are no significant complications, patients may return to the primary care provider for all general medical care. Safe management of posttransplant patients by primary care physicians requires, however, in-depth knowledge of drug interactions with

TABLE 10 COMPLICATIONS FOLLOWING HEART TRANSPLANTATION
Acute rejection
Infection
Cardiac-allograft vasculopathy
Malignancies
Systemic hypertension
Dyslipidemia
Chronic kidney disease
Osteoporosis
Osteonecrosis
Gout
Obesity
Glucose intolerance

TABLE 11 INDICATIONS FOR THE PRIMARY CARE PHYSICIAN TO CONTACT OR REFER A HEART TRANSPLANT RECIPIENT TO THE TRANSPLANT CENTER*
Suspected allograft rejection (unexplained fever, relative hypotension, new signs or symptoms of congestive heart failure)
New-onset renal failure
Fever without an obvious source
Complicated infections
Cardiovascular events (myocardial infarction, syncope, complicated arrhythmias, sudden death)
Suspected major abdominal disease
Malignancies
Medication changes or intolerance
Possible noncompliance
*Adapted from Wagoner [37].

immunosuppressive agents as well as clear understanding of the differences in the physiology of the transplanted heart [37]. Close communication between primary care physicians and the transplant team allows most problems to be appropriately handled close to the patient's home, obviating travel to the sometimes distant transplant center. Table 11 outlines indications for the primary care physician to contact or refer to the transplant center.

REFERENCES AND RECOMMENDED READING

1. O'Connell JB, Gunnar R, Evans R, *et al.*: Task Force 1: Organization of Heart Transplantation in the US. *J Am Coll Cardiol* 1993, 22:8–14.

2. Hertz MI, Mohacsi PJ, Taylor DO, *et al.*: The Registry of the International Society for Heart and Lung Transplantation: Introduction to the Twentieth Official Report. *J Heart Lung Transplant* 2003, 22:610–615.

3. Grover FL, Barr ML, Edwards LB, *et al.*: Thoracic transplantation. *Am J Transplant* 2003, 3 (Suppl 4):91–102.

4. The Organ Procurement and Transplantation Network Data 2002 Report: Data as of September 19, 2003. Available at *www.optn.org*.

5. Taylor DO, Edwards LB, Mohacsi PJ, *et al.*: The Registry of the International Society for Heart and Lung Transplantation: Twentieth Official Adult Heart Transplant Report—2003. *J Heart Lung Transplant* 2003, 22:616–624.

6. Hertz MI, Taylor DO, Trulock EP, *et al.*: The Registry of the International Society for Heart and Lung Transplantation: Nineteenth Official Report. *J Heart Lung Transplant* 2002, 21:950–970.

7. University Renal Research and Education Association: 2002 Annual Report of the US Organ Procurement and Transplantation Network and the Scientific Registry of Transplant Recipients: Transplant Data 1992–2001. Rockville, MD: HHS/HRSA/OSP/DOT; 2003. Accessible at *http://www.optn.org/data/annualreport.asp*.

8. Mancini D, Eisen H, Kussmaul W, *et al.*: Value of peak exercise oxygen consumption for optimal timing of cardiac transplantation in ambulatory patients with heart failure. *Circulation* 1991, 83:778–786.

9. Cimato TR, Jessup M: Recipient selection in cardiac transplantation: contraindications and risk factors for mortality. *J Heart Lung Transplant* 2002, 21:1161–1173.

10. Ladowski JS, Kormos RL, Uretsky BF, *et al.*: Heart transplantation in diabetic recipients. *Transplantation* 1990, 49:303–305.

11. Mancini D, Beniaminovitz A, Edwards N, *et al.*: Survival of diabetic patients following cardiac transplant. *J Heart Lung Transplant* 2001, 20:168.

12. Calabrese LH, Albrecht M, Young J, *et al.*: Successful cardiac transplantation in an HIV-1-infected patient with advanced disease. *N Engl J Med* 2003, 348:2323–2328.

13. Barr ML, Sanchez JA, Seche LA, *et al.*: Anti-CD3 monoclonal antibody induction therapy: immunological equivalency with triple-drug therapy in heart transplantation. *Circulation* 1990, 82(Suppl 5):IV291–IV294.

14. Beniaminovitz A, Itescu S, Lietz K, *et al.*: Prevention of rejection in cardiac transplantation by blockade of the interleukin-2 receptor with a monoclonal antibody. *N Engl J Med* 2000, 342:613–619.

15. Smart FW, Naftel DC, Costanzo MR, *et al.*: Risk factors for early, cumulative, and fatal infections after heart transplantation: a multiinstitutional study. *J Heart Lung Transplant* 1996, 15:329–341.

16. Swinnen LJ, Costanzo-Nordin MR, Fisher SG, *et al.*: Increased incidence of lymphoproliferative disorder after immunosuppression with the monoclonal antibody OKT3 in cardiac transplant recipients. *N Engl J Med* 1990, 323:1723–1728.

17. Trompeter R, Filler G, Webb NJ, *et al.*: Randomized trial of tacrolimus versus cyclosporin microemulsion in renal transplantation. *Pediatr Nephrol* 2002, 17:141–149.

18. Rinaldi M, Pellegrini C, Martinelli L, *et al.*: FK506 effectiveness in reducing acute rejection after heart transplantation: a prospective randomized study. *J Heart Lung Transplant* 1997, 16:1001–1010.

19. Taylor D, Barr M, Radovancevic B, *et al.*: A randomized, multicenter comparison of tacrolimus and cyclosporine immunosuppressive regimens in cardiac transplantation: decreased hyperlipidemia and hypertension with tacrolimus. *J Heart Lung Transplant* 1999, 18:336–345.

20. Reichart B, Meiser B, Vigano M, *et al.*: European multicenter tacrolimus heart pilot study: three year follow-up [abstract]. *J Heart Lung Transplant* 2001, 20:249–250.

21. Kirklin JK, Young JB, McGiffin DC, George JF: Immunosuppressive modalities. In *Heart Transplantation*. Edited by Kirklin JK, Young JB, McGiffin DC. New York: Churchill Livingstone; 2002:390–463.

22. International Society for Heart and Lung Transplantation Registry 2003: www.ishlt.org/registries/.

23. Montoya JG, Giraldo LF, Efron B, *et al.*: Infectious complications among 620 consecutive heart transplant patients at Stanford University Medical Center. *Clin Infect Dis* 2001, 33:629–640.

24. Fishman JA, Rubin RH: Infection in organ-transplant recipients. *N Engl J Med* 1998, 338:1741–1751.

25. Petri WA Jr.: Infections in heart transplant recipients. *Clin Infect Dis* 1994, 18:141–146.

26. Holliman RE, Johnson JD, Adams S, Pepper JR: Toxoplasmosis and heart transplantation. *J Heart Transplant* 1991, 10:608–610.

27. Olsen SL, Renlund DG, O'Connell JB, *et al.*: Prevention of *Pneumocystis carinii* pneumonia in cardiac recipients by trimethoprim-sulfamethoxazole. *Transplantation* 1993, 56:359–362.

28. Constanzo MR, Naftel DC, Pritzker MR, *et al.*: The Cardiac Transplant Research Database: heart transplant coronary artery disease detected by coronary angiography: a multiinstitutional study of preoperative donor and recipient risk factors. *J Heart Lung Transplant* 1998, 17:744–753.

29. Kapadia SR, Ziada KM, L'Allier PM, *et al.*: Intravascular ultrasound imaging after cardiac transplantation: advantage of multivessel imaging. *J Heart Lung Transplant* 2000, 19:167–172.

30. Miller L: Long-term complications of cardiac transplantation. *Prog Cardiovasc Dis* 1991, 33:229–282.

31. Schroeder JS, Gao SZ, Alderman EL, *et al.*: A preliminary study of diltiazem in the prevention of coronary artery disease in heart-transplant recipients. *N Engl J Med* 1993, 328:164–170.

32. Kobashigawa JA, Katznelson S, Laks H, *et al.*: Effects of pravastatin on outcomes after cardiac transplantation. *N Engl J Med* 1995, 333:621–627.

33. Wenke K, Meiser B, Thiery J, Nagel D, *et al.*: Simvastatin reduces graft vessel disease and mortality after heart transplantation: a four-year randomized trial. *Circulation* 1997, 96:1398–1402.

34. Valantine HA, Gao SZ, Menon SG, *et al.*: Impact of prophy-lactic immediate posttransplant gancyclovir on development of transplant atherosclerosis: a post hoc analysis of a randomized, placebo-controlled study. *Circulation* 1999, 100:61–66.

35. Olivari M, Antolick A, Ring W: Arterial hypertension in heart transplant recipients treated with triple-drug immunosuppressive therapy. *J Heart Lung Transplant* 1989, 8:34–39.

36. Kirklin JK, Young JB, McGiffin DC, Rayburn BK: Other long-term complications of heart transplantation. In *Heart Transplan-tation*. Edited by Kirklin JK, Young JB, McGiffin DC. New York: Churchill Livingstone; 2002:666–702.

37. Wagoner LE: Management of the cardiac transplant recipient: roles of the transplant cardiologist and primary care provider. *Am J Med Sci* 1997, 314:173–184.

38. Deng MC: Cardiac transplantation. *Heart* 2002, 87:177–184.

39. Aaronson KD, Schwartz JS, Chen TMC, *et al.*: Development and prospective validation of a clinical index to predict survival in ambulatory patients referred for cardiac transplant evaluation. *Circulation* 1997, 95:2660–2667.

40. Hunt SA, Schroeder JS, Berry GJ: Cardiac transplantation, mechanical ventricular support, and endomyocardial biopsy. In *Hurst's The Heart*. Edited by Fuster V, Wayne Alexander R, O'Rourke RA, eds. New York: McGraw-Hill; 2001:725–747.

Atrial Fibrillation: Practical Approaches

Hongsheng M. Guo
Brian Olshansky

46

Key Points

- Atrial fibrillation is common and is associated with hypertensive, ischemic, and valvular heart disease and cardiomyopathies, but can also occur without any obvious cause. Aging, pericarditis, endocarditis, alcohol intoxication, hyperthyroidism, and cardiac surgery are also associated with atrial fibrillation.

- Atrial fibrillation can be classified as acute onset, persistent, permanent, paroxysmal or postoperative. Each clinical presentation requires a specific, individualized therapeutic approach.

- The treatment goal is to eliminate symptoms; improve exercise tolerance; and prevent hemodynamic collapse, stroke, and ventricular dysfunction caused by impaired atrial mechanical function, atrioventricular dysynchrony, and presence of an irregular, inappropriate (often rapid) rate.

- Prevention of thromboembolic complications with chronic anticoagulation is of crucial significance. A newly developed direct thrombin inhibitor, ximelagatran, is expected to replace warfarin with a much superior safety and efficacy profile.

- The fact that atrial fibrillation, especially the paroxysmal form, is often triggered from the pulmonary veins advances our understanding about mechanisms and new forms of treatment including catheter ablation. Nonpharmacologic treatments are diverse and evolving. A cure of atrial fibrillation is now achievable in many patients, particularly those with paroxysmal atrial fibrillation who remain severely symptomatic despite medical therapy. However, dramatic changes in management are likely.

Atrial fibrillation, an irregular, rapid, atrial arrhythmia, prevents effective atrial contraction and causes an irregular, often rapid, ventricular response. Although not immediately life threatening, atrial fibrillation can impair hemodynamics; cause troublesome, even intolerable, symptoms; and increase the risk for stroke and heart failure. It has been associated with a twofold-increased risk of death in the elderly, but it is unclear whether atrial fibrillation is the direct cause [1,2]. Complexities in atrial fibrillation presentations and a plethora of treatment options make atrial fibrillation management difficult. Different guidelines developed by different authors and organizations [3,4] truly have not made the issue any easier. In fact, some of these deal with limited aspects of this complex issue, and may only apply to certain patient populations [4].

PREVALENCE AND INCIDENCE

More than 2.2 million American adults (1.5 million over the age of 70 years) have atrial fibrillation; this number is increasing concomitant with an increase in the elderly [5–10]. Atrial fibrillation is present in 0.4% of the population, but more than 10% of the very elderly have atrial fibrillation [11]. By 2020, a 46% increase in atrial fibrillation prevalence is expected.

SOCIOECONOMIC IMPACT

Atrial fibrillation, the most common arrhythmia diagnosis leading to hospitalization, causes 33% of all hospitalizations for arrhythmia therapy and more than 1,000,000 hospital days per year. The average length of stay, 4.2 days, costs $6333 ± $7368 per patient [12]. (These statistics underestimate management costs and time commitment because atrial fibrillation is mainly treated outside the hospital.) A trend toward outpatient management is apparent even though, because of Food and Drug Administration (FDA) mandate, some antiarrhythmic drugs for atrial fibrillation must be started in the hospital. Loss of work, stroke, heart failure, and the need for repeated physician contacts further compound the problem.

CAUSES

Various conditions have been associated with and suspected to cause atrial fibrillation, although atrial fibrillation also occurs without apparent cause or heart disease. This is known as "lone" atrial fibrillation and occurs in about 30% of patients. ALFA (Etude en Activite Liberale de la Fibrillation Auriculaire), a study of 756 atrial fibrillation patients, indicated that hypertensive, ischemic, and valvular heart disease and dilated cardiomyopathy are major conditions associated with atrial fibrillation [13] (Table 1). Toxin exposure (eg, alcohol), hypoxia, enhanced vagal or sympathetic tone, elevated diastolic pressures, pulmonary embolus, hyperthyroidism, pericarditis, endocarditis, and cardiac surgery are associated with atrial fibrillation; however, hypertension and congestive heart failure remain the major predisposing factors [14,15] (Table 2). Hereditary forms of atrial fibrillation exist [16]. Myocardial infarction is a suspected but rare cause for atrial fibrillation. The relationship between atrial fibrillation and other medical conditions may be unclear, but knowledge of these conditions is crucial to determine the management approach because hemodynamic consequences of atrial fibrillation, the need for long-term treatment, proarrhythmic risk, and thromboembolic risk are disease dependent.

MECHANISMS

Atrial fibrillation is manifest as rapid, random (or "chaotic") electrical atrial activation. The two important aspects regarding the mechanisms responsible for atrial fibrillation are 1) initiating focal triggers, and 2) a substrate for perpetuation and sustenance of atrial fibrillation. Focal triggers have been reported from the atrial, the vena cava, and most often pulmonary veins [17–20]. Reentry, particularly micro-reentrant with multiple wavelets, rotators, and spiral waves, has been suggested to be responsible for atrial fibrillation maintenance [21–25]. Also, fibrillatory conduction can occur from a rapidly firing focus. Atrial fibrillation initiated from focal discharge can be eliminated by ablation [18,19,26,27], but cure might be more difficult when atrial fibrillation involves large portions of the atria. Atrial fibrillation can perpetuate (and perhaps change the mechanism of) atrial fibrillation by "electrical remodeling" [28]. The longer atrial fibrillation occurs, the more difficult it is to prevent and treat and the more likely there will be atrial dilatation and mechanical dysfunction ("mechanical remodeling"). The larger the atria, the more likely atrial fibrillation will persist. There is a poorly defined relationship between atrial fibrillation and other atrial tachyarrhythmias, such as atrial flutter.

CLASSIFICATION

Despite its heterogeneous clinical presentation, atrial fibrillation classification has significant clinical importance. Atrial fibrillation can be classified by etiology, mechanism, or electrocardiographic (ECG) appearance, but the most practical classification is based on clinical presentation [13]. Distinctive characteristics include length of episodes, patient age, symptoms, need for treatment, and chronicity. The American College of Cardiology/American Heart Association/European Society of Cardiology (ACC/AHA/ESC) Practice Guidelines for the Management of Patients With Atrial Fibrillation recommends a classification scheme of first-detected and recurrent atrial fibrillation, in addition to lone atrial fibrillation [3]. A first-detected episode of atrial

TABLE 1 SYMPTOMS BY ATRIAL FIBRILLATION (AF) PRESENTATION

Symptoms (%)	Total population, (n = 756)	Paroxysmal AF, (n = 167)	Chronic AF, (n = 389)	Recent onset AF, (n = 200)
Palpitations	409 (54.1)	132 (79.0)	174 (44.7)	103 (51.5)
Chest pain	76 (10.1)	22 (13.2)	32 (8.2)	22 (11.0)
Dyspnea	336 (44.4)	38 (22.8)	182 (46.8)	116 (58.0)
Syncope, dizzy spells	79 (10.4)	29 (17.4)	31 (8.0)	19 (9.5)
Fatigue	108 (14.3)	21 (12.6)	51 (13.1)	36 (18.00)
Other	7 (0.9)	0	7 (1.8)	0
None	86 (11.4)	9 (5.4)	63 (16.2)	14 (7.0)

fibrillation can be either or not symptomatic, or self-limited. It recognizes there can be uncertainty about the duration and about previously undetected episodes. When a patient has had two or more episodes, atrial fibrillation is considered recurrent. It then can be further classified into paroxysmal (generally last less than or equal to 7 days), persistent (usually more than 7 days), and permanent (cardioversion failed or not attempted) [3].

First-detected Atrial Fibrillation

Initial presentation can result in hemodynamic compromise and often requires urgent intervention (Fig. 1). This may be caused by transient, reversible triggers, such as alcohol, hypoxia, pericarditis, etc. as mentioned above, and does not necessarily implicate need for chronic treatment.

Paroxysmal Atrial Fibrillation

Paroxysmal atrial fibrillation (Fig. 2) is characterized by short, repetitive, self-limited episodes lasting seconds to minutes or up to several days. Treatment depends on episode length and frequency and associated symptoms. Paroxysmal atrial fibrillation is more common in younger individuals. Because it is frequently associated with severe symptoms, there is generally a need to maintain sinus rhythm. Untreated, atrial fibrillation paroxysms tend to become more severe and prolonged.

Persistent or Permanent Atrial Fibrillation

Persistent atrial fibrillation (Fig. 3) is characterized by intermittent episodes that last more than several days, and requires pharmacological or electrical cardioversion for termination. It tends to become a repetitive, recurrent problem. Drug therapies can convert more permanent forms of

atrial fibrillation to persistent atrial fibrillation. Ultimately, attempts to maintain sinus rhythm may become futile as the patient shows resistance to drugs. Some patients benefit from frequent cardioversions.

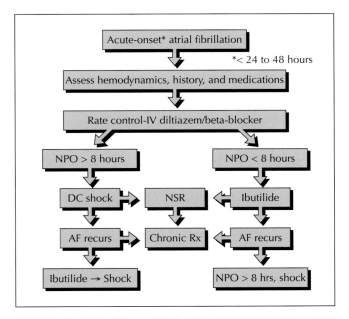

FIGURE 1 Approach to the patient with acute-onset atrial fibrillation (< 24 to 48 hours). AF—atrial fibrillation; IV—intravenous; NPO—nothing by mouth; NSR—normal sinus rhythm.

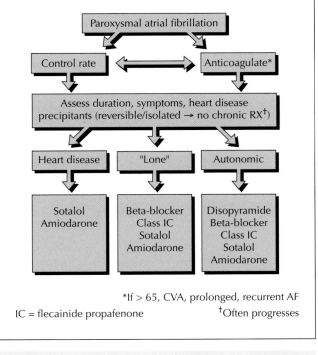

FIGURE 2 Approach to the patient with paroxysmal atrial fibrillation (AF). CVA–cerebrovascular accident.

TABLE 2 ASSOCIATED CLINICAL CONDITIONS IN 756 PATIENTS WITH ATRIAL FIBRILLATION (ALFA TRIAL)	
Condition	Patients, %
Heart disease	
None	29.2
Hypertensive heart disease	21.4
Ischemic heart disease	16.6
Valvular heart disease	18.5
Dilated cardiomyopathy	15.2
Miscellaneous	4.9
Other predisposing or associated factors	
Hypertension	39.4
Hyperthyroidism	3.1
Bronchopulmonary disease	11.2
Diabetes	10.7
Congestive heart failure	29.8
Prior thromboembolic events	8.4

Permanent atrial fibrillation (Fig. 3) is present for prolonged periods (> 1 month). Attempts at cardioversion, perhaps initially successful, fail, and the patient ultimately remains in atrial fibrillation. Restoration of sinus rhythm is unlikely or impossible, particularly if atrial fibrillation is present over 1 year and when there are very large atria (> 5 cm).

Chronic atrial fibrillation is not necessarily the same as permanent atrial fibrillation. It could be a chronic condition that has responded at least intermittently to therapies. This should be distinguished from permanent atrial fibrillation as management options differ.

Postoperative Atrial Fibrillation

Postoperative atrial fibrillation is a common, generally self-limited, persistent, or paroxysmal form of atrial fibrillation that occurs after cardiac surgery. Paroxysmal atrial fibrillation and permanent atrial fibrillation are associated with different clinical conditions. Valvular heart disease and other structural abnormalities, including hypertrophy and ischemia, are more closely associated with chronic atrial fibrillation [13].

"Gray zones" between these forms of atrial fibrillation exist; one can transition into, or be associated with, another. This classification does not pertain to all clinical situations. Consider an asymptomatic patient who presents with unknown duration atrial fibrillation (Fig. 4). Atrial fibrillation may also be surreptitious (ie, not documented) but can be a cause for stroke in a young patient.

CONSEQUENCES OF ATRIAL FIBRILLATION

No effective atrial contraction is present with atrial fibrillation. Loss of "atrial kick" can decrease cardiac output by more than 30%, especially when diastolic function is impaired (aortic stenosis, hypertrophic cardiomyopathy, cardiac surgery, myocardial infarction, hypertensive heart disease, and heart failure). Restoring sinus rhythm may

greatly improve hemodynamics. Atrial fibrillation can create an inappropriate rate at rest, during exercise, or both. "Uncontrolled" atrial fibrillation is generally rapid and physiologically inappropriate. Heart rate control with a drug may not correct the physiologically inappropriate chronotropic response under all conditions.

Persistent rapid rates may result in electrical remodeling of the atria, lead to changes in atrial refractoriness, and cause persistent or permanent atrial fibrillation [29]. Mechanical remodeling also occurs in the atria and ventricles. Tachycardia-mediated (or induced) cardiomyopathy caused by persistent, rapid ventricular rates is an underrec-

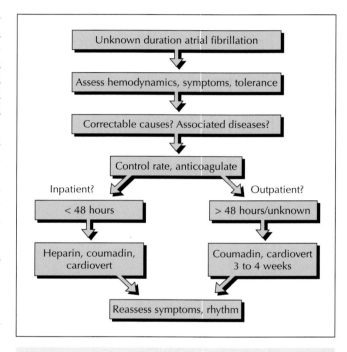

FIGURE 4 Approach to the patient with unknown duration atrial fibrillation.

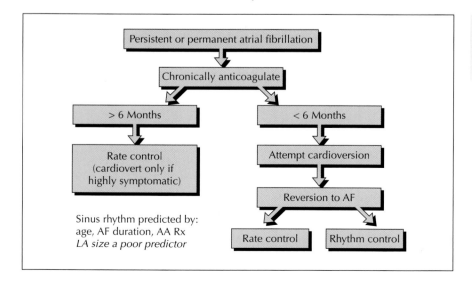

FIGURE 3 Approach to the patient with persistent or permanent atrial fibrillation (AF) AA—antiarrhythmia; LA—left atrium.

ognized condition that can progress to end-stage cardiomyopathy similar to dilated cardiomyopathy. Chronic rapid rates in atrial fibrillation should never be allowed to occur, even if a patient is asymptomatic. Rate control can normalize ejection fraction [30] but, even so, the myocardium of a chronically fibrillated heart does not return to normal histologically despite normalization in ejection fraction. The risk of sudden death might not be reduced. Heart rate control as a part of early and chronic atrial fibrillation management is required.

Atrial fibrillation can cause "tachycardia-mediated" atrial cardiomyopathy as well as ventricular cardiomyopathy. Ineffective rapid atrial contraction can cause atrial dilatation and create the milieu for atrial thrombi leading to stroke.

Rapid, irregular heart rates can initiate ischemia and malignant ventricular arrhythmias. An irregular rate (even if the rate is controlled) may impair cardiac output [30], cause symptoms, and alter autonomic function. Atrial fibrillation can inspire need for treatment that may be worse than the disease.

Perhaps one of the most disturbing issues regarding atrial fibrillation is the risk of stroke. A higher risk is associated with advanced age, hypertension, diabetes mellitus, coexistent cardiovascular disease and heart failure, prior history of stroke, or transient ischemic attack [31–36]. Conversion from atrial fibrillation to sinus rhythm, no matter by what means, is also associated with an increased risk for stroke [37]. Female sex, blood pressure greater than 160 mm Hg,

and left ventricular dysfunction have been associated with increased risk for stroke [33,38]. A similar annual stroke rate has been reported in patients with either recurrent or permanent atrial fibrillation in the SPAF (Stroke Prevention in Atrial Fibrillation) study [39]. It does not appear related to treatment approach (rate vs rhythm control). Proper use of anticoagulation can significantly reduce, if not completely abolish, the risk of stroke (detailed discussion later in the Management section).

SYMPTOMS

The reason to treat a patient with atrial fibrillation is not to prevent death, because no treatment, except radiofrequency ablation in a single-centered nonrandomized report [26], has been shown to help in this regard. Rather, the goal is to prevent symptoms and other premorbid consequences. No "symptom scale" for patients with atrial fibrillation has been devised, but atrial fibrillation is associated with subtle (an identifiable change in heart rhythm) or blatant (cardiogenic shock) symptoms and impaired quality of life. Symptoms are related to the clinical presentation, underlying condition, and age and activities of the patient. A young athlete with exercise-induced atrial fibrillation is likely to be symptomatic and in need of aggressive therapy in contrast to an octogenarian unaware that atrial fibrillation is even present.

Common symptoms from atrial fibrillation include fatigue (chronic atrial fibrillation) and palpitations (paroxysmal atrial fibrillation) [13] (Table 1). Chronic atrial fibrillation may be less symptomatic than frequent, annoying, paroxysms. All symptoms are not of equal importance and do not require the same treatment [13] (Table 3). The patient's interpretation of the intensity of the symptoms and importance of atrial fibrillation must be considered. The end point to measure successful therapy is difficult but includes the number of episodes of recurrent atrial fibrillation, the improvement in symptoms, and the length of episodes. There has been an interest in measuring the "burden" of atrial fibrillation (ie, total number and length of episodes and number of symptomatic episodes) as a marker of success.

A rare paroxysm of atrial fibrillation may incur little health risk but can be perceived as a serious issue to a patient who demands aggressive treatment. This issue becomes important regarding referral for potentially risky therapies, such as ablation. Alternatively, a patient with poorly controlled, asymptomatic, chronic atrial fibrillation may develop heart failure and yet request no treatment at all. A total of 21.8% of males and 28.9% of females with atrial fibrillation have heart failure.

Symptoms of atrial fibrillation depend on patient activities, the chronicity of atrial fibrillation, the ventricular rate in atrial fibrillation, and underlying conditions. Many patients are completely asymptomatic, although the percentage of patients who are truly asymptomatic is

TABLE 3 PAROXYSMAL ATRIAL FIBRILLATION		
Characteristics	Pts	%
Frequency		
≥ 1 per d	22	13.2
≥1 per wk	20	12.0
≥1 per mo	34	20.4
≥1 per y	66	39.5
Undetermined	25	14.9
Duration		
2–59 min	27	16.2
1–23 h	73	43.7
≥ 24 h	32	19.2
Undetermined	35	21.0
Precipitating factors		
Exercise, emotion	31	18.6
Postprandial	13	7.8
Caffeine	4	2.4
Fever	5	3.0
Hypoxia	3	1.8
Miscellaneous	10	6.0
Total	66	39.5

unknown because they may not present for evaluation. Symptoms of atrial fibrillation may abate over time. The reason for this is not clear; chronic atrial fibrillation may lead to physiologic compensatory mechanisms. Alternatively, patients with chronic atrial fibrillation may limit their physical activity.

CLINICAL EVALUATION

Evaluation starts with a complete history and physical examination. If atrial fibrillation is identified, it should be classified. The severity of the symptoms, the potential consequences of atrial fibrillation, and the risks to the patient must be determined. An effort to identify an underlying cause or associated condition is mandatory. Hemodynamic impairment and patient tolerance of the rhythm must be considered.

Evaluation of a patient with atrial fibrillation varies with the clinical presentation. An elderly, hypertensive individual with atrial fibrillation has a higher likelihood of heart disease than does a young athlete. But a young athlete has a greater chance of having an associated accessory pathway (Wolff-Parkinson-White syndrome). The evaluation must be comprehensive yet reasonable. Not all patients need an extensive evaluation. This would require expensive testing and would be unwise, potentially dangerous, and unnecessary. Alternatively, missing a serious treatable cause for atrial fibrillation (such as an accessory pathway) is tragic.

Atrial fibrillation can contribute to or be the primary cause for symptoms and hemodynamic impairment or simply be an epiphenomenon. The distinction is critical. Consider a patient admitted to an emergency room with pulmonary edema and atrial fibrillation. Cardioversion must be considered but may be inappropriate (and dangerous) if atrial fibrillation has been present for years. An arrhythmia consultant may be needed to formulate the best treatment plans.

An ECG is the next step. It is inexpensive, can confirm the presence of atrial fibrillation, and may reveal its etiology. Patients with atrial fibrillation may have a normal ECG if atrial fibrillation has resolved. If symptoms suggest atrial fibrillation, further diagnostic evaluation will be required to rule out atrial fibrillation.

Ambulatory ECG (ie, Holter monitoring) can be diagnostic. It can assess efficacy of therapy, but this approach may miss atrial fibrillation if it is infrequent. The ambulatory ECG can also be used to correlate symptoms with atrial fibrillation. It has a role in the assessment of the adequacy of rate control.

Event monitoring is emerging as a method for diagnosing atrial fibrillation and correlating symptoms to atrial fibrillation. This approach uses an external or implanted monitor with automatic or manual triggering to detect atrial fibrillation. A good strategy to treat a patient with atrial fibrillation is to confirm that the symptoms are caused by atrial fibrillation; otherwise, treatment may be futile. Alternatively, symptomatic atrial fibrillation patients may have asymptomatic episodes; treatment of atrial fibrillation may prevent symptoms but may mislead the patient and the physician into believing that atrial fibrillation is controlled. Surreptitious episodes of atrial fibrillation may persist and lead to stroke, heart failure, and electrical remodeling, with the consequence of chronic atrial fibrillation.

All patients should have at least one measurement of thyroid hormone levels because hyperthyroidism is a potential treatable cause of atrial fibrillation. Hyperthyroidism can usually be easily diagnosed without even measuring the thyroid hormone level; however, in the elderly, in particular, it may be difficult to diagnose "apathetic" hyperthyroidism. Thyroid hormone level should also be measured in patients who are being treated with amiodarone and have recurrent atrial fibrillation because amiodarone, especially in low doses, may cause hyperthyroidism. More amiodarone, in this instance, would make the patient with atrial fibrillation more resistant to treatment [40].

Transthoracic echocardiography can provide evidence of an underlying heart condition (eg, ventricular dysfunction, valvular disease, ventricular hypertrophy) and information about atrial size. The transthoracic echocardiogram should be performed at least once in any patient who does not have an explainable cause for atrial fibrillation.

MANAGEMENT

Four strategies are used to manage patients with atrial fibrillation: 1) restoration and maintenance of sinus rhythm (rhythm control), 2) ventricular rate control (rate control), 3) anticoagulation, and 4) treatment of the underlying disorder [41]. A patient may require all four strategies.

Data from several large, multicenter, prospective, randomized, controlled clinical trials indicate that rate control of atrial fibrillation and anticoagulation has a substantial, if not preferred, role in the management of patients with atrial fibrillation [42–46] and studies are ongoing [47,48]. However, the patient populations in these trials are typically elderly (65 years or older) with persistent or permanent atrial fibrillation, many with structural heart diseases. Pharmacological approaches are used to achieve either rate control or rhythm control. Younger patients with paroxysmal atrial fibrillation, with no structural heart disease, and nonpharmacologic approaches, are underrepresented in these trials (Table 4).

Rate Control

Rate control is an effective approach for many patients, especially those with permanent and persistent atrial fibrillation as suggested by recent clinical trials as discussed above. It is a reasonable strategy for those with paroxysmal atrial fibrillation, especially for the elderly who are not highly symptomatic, who have structural heart disease, or who have failed antiarrhythmic drugs. Rate control is not associated with greater risk of stoke than rhythm control in the elderly. Anticoagulation should be considered for all at risk for stroke, unless contraindicated.

Rate control is more favored by internists and family practitioners but is less favored by cardiologists and electrophysiologists as a sole approach [49]. Ventricular rate control can be extremely difficult; although rate control may appear to be achieved at rest, it may not be really controlled, and the physiologic response to exercise can be inadequate. The term "rate control" has never been defined satisfactorily. A resting heart rate of 60 to 90 beats per minute may not be appropriate or even achievable. In the AFFIRM (Atrial Fibrillation Follow-up Investigation of Rhythm Management) study, a heart rate ≤ 80 beats per minute at rest and ≤ 110 beats per minute during 6-minute walk is considered adequately controlled. Adequate rate control really implies adequate rate response and a normal physiologic and autonomic response to stresses.

Rate control has some advantages over maintaining sinus rhythm: 1) patients can improve symptomatically, 2) management is straightforward, and 3) life-threatening proarrhythmia is not an issue. Ventricular rate control can be achieved pharmacologically and nonpharmacologically. Drug therapy includes calcium channel blockers, beta-blockers, or digitalis. Nonpharmacologic therapy (selected for drug-resistant patients) includes atrioventricular (AV) nodal ablation with a rate-responsive permanent ventricular pacer (or dual chamber pacing with "mode-switching" for patients with intermittent atrial fibrillation).

For first-detected atrial fibrillation, rate control is favored as the initial approach if the patient is not hemodynamically compromised. Depending on the urgency to treat, rate control can be accomplished with an intravenous (IV) calcium blocker (verapamil or diltiazem), beta-blocker (metoprolol or esmolol), or digoxin. The safest, most effective approach uses a short-acting beta-blocker (*eg*, esmolol) or diltiazem.

Digitalis has been widely used, but it takes time to work and is much less effective, particularly in patients who are physically active. Stafford *et al.* [49] and McAlister *et al.* [50] in retrospective studies of 493 and 2490 patients, respectively, found digoxin was used in 53% and 79%, calcium blockers were used in 15% and 29%, and beta-blockers were used in 13% and 24% of patients. Digoxin must never be given to patients with atrial fibrillation who have the Wolff-Parkinson-White syndrome because it is associated with cardiac arrest.

Calcium channel blockers (verapamil and diltiazem) or beta-blockers are first-line therapies [51]. Digoxin,

TABLE 4 RHYTHM CONTROL VERSUS RATE CONTROL: SUMMARY OF PUBLISHED CLINICAL TRIALS

Clinical trial	Patients, *n*	Patient population	Follow-up	End points and results
AFFIRM [42]	4060	Age ≥65 (mean 69.7) or with ≥1 stroke or death risk factor	3.5 years	*Primary*: Mortality: no difference *Secondary*: More hospitalization and drug adverse effects in rhythm control group; more strokes associated with discontinued or inadequate anticoagulation in both groups.
RACE [46]	522	All had persistent (≥1 year) atrial fibrillation and had 1–2 cardioversions. Median atrial fibrillation duration 309 days for rhythm control and 337 days for rate control group. Mean age 68.	2.3 years	*Primary*: Cardiovascular mortality + CHF + thromboembolism + bleeding + pacemaker implantation + severe drug adverse effects: no difference
PIAF [48]	252	New-onset or permanent symptomatic atrial fibrillation (mean atrial fibrillation duration ≈4 months). Diltiazem was used for rate control and cardioversion + amiodarone for rhythm control. Mean age 61.	1 year	*Primary*: Improvement in atrial fibrillation related symptoms: no difference *Secondary*: Better 6-min walking distance, but more hospital admission and drug adverse effects with rhythm control.
STAF [45]	200	Persistent atrial fibrillation (>4 weeks), left atrium >45 mm, CHF and NYHA ≥2, EF <45%, ≥1 prior cardioversion. Permanent (>2 years) and paroxysmal atrial fibrillation was excluded. Mean age 67.	19.6 months	*Primary*: Death + stroke/TIA + CPR+ thromboembolism: no difference *Secondary*: More cardiovascular admission with rhythm control; no difference in quality of life, bleeding, and syncope. All but one end point events occurred during atrial fibrillation.

CHF—congestive heart failure; CPR—cardiopulmonary resuscitation; EF—ejection fraction; NYHA—New York Heart Association; TIA—transient ischemic attack.

combined with a calcium blocker or a beta-blocker, may provide synergistic benefit. Few data support one drug over another, but digoxin is more likely to lead to an irregular ventricular response and is less likely to work with exercise. If a regular response rate is seen with digoxin, consider digoxin toxicity. Digoxin is best suited for an elderly, inactive patient with left ventricular dysfunction. A beta-blocker is best for controlling heart rate in patients with atrial fibrillation during exercise, but it may slow the rate too much, causing fatigue, and this symptom is one reason to treat atrial fibrillation.

According to a recently published analysis of National Ambulatory Medical Care Survey data from 1355 visits among patients with atrial fibrillation [52], the overall use of agents for ventricular rate control decreased significantly in the last decade, from 71.6% in 1991–1992 to 56.2% in 1999–2000. This was primarily due to a significant decrease in digoxin use, from 64.4% to 36.7%. There was no significant change in either beta-blocker use (from 16.3% to 22.2%, $P = 0.09$), or calcium channel blocker use (from 15.8% to 13.5%, $P = 0.13$) [52].

If rate control cannot be achieved pharmacologically, AV nodal ablation with implantation of a pacemaker is a reasonable option. This approach has been shown to improve symptoms, exercise tolerance, New York Heart Association (NYHA) function class, quality of life, and health care use, but has no long-term survival benefits [53–55]. The patient becomes pacemaker dependant, which leads to potential long-term risks and increased risk of sudden death early after ablation of the AV node. To offset this risk, the pacemaker must be programmed to a faster rate (around 90 beats per minute) for the first several weeks. In addition, possible adverse effects from the resultant right ventricular pacing and ventricular activation dysynchrony need to be considered. We learned from a recently published study that right ventricular pacing in patients without indications for cardiac pacing might be detrimental by increasing death and hospitalization for heart failure [56].

It is best to consider ventricular rate control as primary, long-term therapy for 1) asymptomatic atrial fibrillation with no compelling reason to restore sinus rhythm, 2) documented permanent atrial fibrillation, and 3) conditions in which the risk of antiarrhythmic drugs exceeds the extent of symptoms. Adequate rate control can be difficult to determine; there are no gold standards. There is little evidence that rate control attempts have improved; the use of rate control drugs for atrial fibrillation has decreased from 79% to 62% from 1980 to 1996 [57].

One must remember that no matter what means used, pharmacologic or nonpharmacologic, rate control does not cure atrial fibrillation, and will not eliminate thromboembolic risk.

Rhythm Control

Rhythm control includes cardioversion (electrical or chemical) and maintenance of sinus rhythm. Sinus rhythm can be maintained pharmacologically or nonpharmacologically. General principles are outlined in the following. A comprehensive review of cardioversion of atrial fibrillation along with other atrial tachycardias, and prevention of cardioversion-associated thromboembolic complications is available elsewhere [37].

Cardioversion

Direct-current (DC) cardioversion remains a standard, common, accepted outpatient procedure used to treat a growing number of patients with symptomatic atrial fibrillation. Antiarrhythmic drugs are another but less successful method to convert atrial fibrillation and maintain sinus rhythm. Despite renewed interest in the rate control of atrial fibrillation, based on controlled multicenter randomized trials [42,43,45,46], clinically necessary cardioversion of atrial fibrillation to return the patient to sinus rhythm is a time-honored approach [58] that will likely continue despite the well-known potential for complications [59,60].

Several populations of patients with atrial fibrillation can benefit from cardioversion and/or maintenance of normal sinus rhythm. Those who may benefit the most include patients who 1) have hemodynamic intolerance or development of congestive heart failure directly due to atrial fibrillation; 2) may remain in sinus rhythm after cardioversion relatively long term without requiring extended antiarrhythmic drug use; 3) have only one episode of persistent, possibly symptomatic atrial fibrillation; 4) have developed tachycardia-induced cardiomyopathy; 5) develop severe symptoms directly from atrial fibrillation despite rate control (*ie*, not due to rapid rate alone); and 6) have paroxysmal or chronic atrial fibrillation during and immediately after ablative therapy. Other select populations may benefit as well.

It is unlikely that recent randomized controlled clinical trials will have a substantial impact on the use of cardioversion for atrial fibrillation. Cardioversion indications may become even more complex as increasing use of nonpharmacologic therapies become integrated into clinical practice. The management of anticoagulation before and after ablative therapy for atrial fibrillation poses new problems regarding management to prevent stroke.

Outpatient DC cardioversion can be performed safely and effectively with properly trained personnel, even without use of an antiarrhythmic agent [61,62]. The success rate of about 80% to 90% to return patients to sinus rhythm depends on the length of the atrial fibrillation episode. Sinus rhythm is less likely to be maintained if it has existed chronically for more than 1 year, even with addition of an antiarrhythmic agent. In one report [63], 81% of those with atrial fibrillation lasting for less than 1 year versus 42% of those with atrial fibrillation lasting for more than 1 year maintained sinus rhythm 100 days after cardioversion. Similar data were found at 1 year [64]. In addition, although DC cardioversion is generally safe and effective, it has a small associated risk.

The efficacy of DC cardioversion may be enhanced with new technologies (ie, biphasic or multiphasic external shock [37,65–67], internal DC shocks) or preloading with IV ibutilide, a class III antiarrhythmic drug [68]. The authors favor at least one attempt to maintain sinus rhythm, even if the patient is without symptoms, because return to sinus rhythm may surprisingly improve exercise tolerance, even in an asymptomatic patient. However, opinions vary on this point [69]. DC cardioversion should not be considered for elderly patients with asymptomatic, permanent atrial fibrillation.

Direct-current cardioversion should always be performed with anticoagulation if the episodes last more than 24 hours, unless transesophageal echocardiography (TEE) shows no left atrial clots. The risk for thromboembolism is greatest in the first 3 to 5 days after cardioversion without proper anticoagulation. DC cardioversion can be repeated if atrial fibrillation recurs.

There are no prospective, randomized, placebo-controlled studies regarding anticoagulation for cardioversion-related thromboembolic risk. However, several retrospective case-control series [61,62,70–76] have repeatedly shown that adequate periprocedure anticoagulation effectively minimizes, if not completely abolishes, this risk related to reversion of atrial tachyarrhythmias to normal sinus rhythm (Table 1). Based on these observational data, the ACC/AHA/ESC Guidelines for the Management of Patients with Atrial Fibrillation recommend that anticoagulation be used for 3 to 4 weeks before and after cardioversion for patients with atrial fibrillation of unknown duration or with atrial fibrillation for more than 48 hours (class I, level of evidence B) [3].

Transesophageal echocardiography–guided cardioversion

Transesophageal echocardiography can determine accurately presence of a left atrial thrombus provided that the entire left atrium, including left atrial appendage, is visualized and that it is interpreted properly. The issue of left atrial clot is complicated by presence of "smoke," spontaneous ultrasound contrast, which is common in atrial fibrillation. While smoke does not necessarily indicate clot, it indicates slow atrial flow, a potential predisposing factor for atrial thrombus. Slow atrial flow is seen frequently in atrial flutter and fibrillation [77,78].

Experience and controlled trials support the use of TEE-guided cardioversion [79]. It appears safe to cardiovert a patient with atrial fibrillation who has no left atrial thrombi on TEE as long as acute anticoagulation with heparin for 24 to 48 hours is undertaken at the time of cardioversion and maintained therapeutic with warfarin thereafter or if the patient has been adequately anticoagulated with warfarin at the time of cardioversion. Left atrial appendage thrombi can form rapidly early after cardioversion even if not present on a TEE immediately before cardioversion [80].

The Assessment of Cardioversion Using Transesophageal Echocardiography (ACUTE) trial was a randomized prospective multicenter trial that evaluated two cardioversion strategies for atrial fibrillation of more than 2 days' duration: TEE-guided cardioversion (with proper anticoagulation at time of cardioversion) versus a conventional approach (3 weeks of adequate warfarin anticoagulation followed by electrical cardioversion) [81]. The composite primary end point was cerebrovascular accident, transient ischemic attack, and peripheral embolism within 8 weeks. Secondary end points were functional status, successful restoration and maintenance of sinus rhythm, hemorrhage, and death.

Normal sinus rhythm restoration was greater initially with TEE guidance than with conventional therapy, but this immediate advantage faded at 8 weeks. Interestingly, although embolic events in both groups were similar (< 5/619 in the TEE group and 3/603 in the conventional arm, < 1% in each), hemorrhagic events in the conventional group significantly exceeded those of TEE-guided therapy (18 events [2.9%] vs 33 events [5.5%], $P = 0.03$). This was due presumably to the longer duration of warfarin therapy in the conventional group. Patients in the TEE group also had a shorter time to cardioversion (mean [±SD], 3.0±5.6 vs 30.6±10.6 days, $P < 0.001$) and a greater rate of successful restoration of sinus rhythm (440 patients [71.1%] vs 393 patients [65.2%], $P = 0.03$). At 8 weeks, there were no significant differences between the two groups in the rates of death or maintenance of sinus rhythm or in functional status [81]. Ultimately, risks, benefits, and costs were similar for both groups.

In a substudy of the ACUTE trial, patients in the conventional group did convert to sinus rhythm of an antiarrhythmic drug at a higher rate due to the 3 to 4 week waiting period compared with the TEE group, so that some did not require electrical cardioversion. One hundred sixty-seven of 1041 patients were identified in the TEE-guided and conventional groups who converted spontaneously, with twice as many in the conventional compared with the TEE-guided group (110/523 [21%] vs 57/518 [11%]; $P < 0.001$). Those who had converted spontaneously had a higher rate of maintaining sinus rhythm at 8 weeks (87.2% vs 48.9%, $P < 0.001$). The conventional treatment strategy allowed greater opportunity for spontaneous conversion. In the absence of favorable predictors of spontaneous cardioversion (short duration of atrial fibrillation, lower NYHA class, and smaller left atrial size), the TEE-guided approach should be considered first [82].

The reasons to use TEE are actually more complex. TEE guidance should be considered for patients who are unlikely to tolerate atrial fibrillation well for a protracted period, for patients in whom effective anticoagulation cannot be maintained easily with large fluctuations in international normalized ratio (INR) values for the 3- to 6-week periods, and patient preference. Otherwise, it is not unreasonable to anticoagulate for 3 to 4 weeks and then cardiovert as long as the INR values are consistently greater than 2.0.

Retrospective data are also persuasive [62]. Such data do not exclude patients undergoing cardioversion who do not fit into a prospective trial and do conform to present clinical management strategies of patients with atrial fibrillation.

The absence of a left atrial appendage thrombus on TEE does not guarantee absence of thromboembolism after cardioversion. There are multiple reports of thromboembolism in patients who had a negative TEE followed by cardioversion when anticoagulation was not performed [83–86]. If a left atrial appendage thrombus is seen on TEE, cardioversion should not be performed. Therapeutic anticoagulation for at least 3 weeks should be achieved and then the TEE should be repeated. If a thrombus is still present, the risk of cardioversion resulting in thromboembolism may be excessive. The risk of cardioverting an anticoagulated patient with a long-standing atrial clot seen on TEE, however, is not completely clear. There may be specific TEE markers that may help stratify which patient is at higher and which is at lower risk.

Maintenance of Sinus Rhythm and Antiarrhythmic Drugs

Maintenance of sinus rhythm after cardioversion can be very difficult, often impossible, even with help of antiarrhythmic drug use. In the AFFIRM study, the prevalence of sinus rhythm in the rhythm-control group at was 82.4%, 73.3%, and 62.6% at 1-, 3-, and 5-year follow-up, respectively [42].

However, recurrence of atrial fibrillation with usual clinical follow-up (ECG and symptoms) might be significantly underestimated. In a recent prospective study [87] of 110 patients with a history of paroxysmal or persistent atrial fibrillation and a class I indication for physiological pacing, a pacemaker with dedicated functions for atrial fibrillation detection and electrogram storage was implanted, and antiarrhythmic drug treatment was optimized. Patients were regularly followed up with evaluation of atrial fibrillation–related symptoms, a resting ECG, and interrogation of device memory. During 19 months and 678 follow-up visits, atrial fibrillation was documented in 51 patients (46%) by ECG recording and in 97 patients (88%) by a review of stored electrograms ($P < 0.0001$). Device interrogation revealed atrial fibrillation recurrences lasting more than 48 hours in 50 patients, 19 of whom (38%) were completely asymptomatic and in sinus rhythm at subsequent follow-up. In 11 (16%) of 67 patients with device-confirmed freedom from atrial fibrillation for 3 months or more, atrial fibrillation lasting more than 48 hours recurred subsequently [87].

Antiarrhythmic drug selection must be individualized and depends on the patient, underlying disease, and atrial fibrillation characteristics. The most effective drugs are sotalol and amiodarone [88]. A substudy of the AFFIRM trial suggests amiodarone was more effective at 1 year than either sotalol or class I agents for the strategy of maintenance of sinus rhythm without cardioversion [89]. Amiodarone is effective in controlling ventricular rate, maintaining sinus rhythm, and preventing postoperative atrial fibrillation. Guidelines have been developed regarding amiodarone use [40].

Antiarrhythmic drug use is changing: 2.9 million antiarrhythmic drug prescriptions were given in 1986 compared with 2.04 million prescriptions in 1992 [57]; 22% of cardiologists, 11% of general practitioners, and 9% of internists use antiarrhythmic drugs for patients with atrial fibrillation. There has been a trend to reduce class IA drug use because of their inherent risks and side effects.

An analysis of National Ambulatory Medical Care Survey data from 1355 visits among patients with atrial fibrillation showed although there was no change in overall use of antiarrhythmic agents for sinus rhythm maintenance from 1991–1992 to 1999–2000, class IA drug use decreased from 9.2% to 2.2% while class IC drug use increased from 0.5% to 2.9%; quinidine use decreased from 5.0% to 0.0%, while amiodarone use increased from 0.2% to 6.4%. There was, however, no significant change in sotalol use [52].

Class IC drugs are reserved for patients without structural heart disease who have paroxysmal atrial fibrillation. Class III drug use has increased recently. Amiodarone tends to be used as a drug of last resort when other drugs fail or for patients with congestive heart failure. Sotalol tends to be used for patients with intact left ventricular function who have no renal or pulmonary disease. Dofetilide is a new antiarrhythmic with no negative inotropic or beta-blocking properties (in contrast to sotalol). The Food and Drug Administration (FDA) mandates a physician-training course for using this drug.

It is difficult to predict which antiarrhythmic drug will most effectively maintain sinus rhythm. The efficacy at 1 year is about 50% for all drugs except amiodarone. An end point of complete control of atrial fibrillation may be unachievable for some patients, but the burden of prolonged, frequent occurrences may be reduced. A recurrence can be managed, but it may be expensive and have a devastating psychological effect on the patient. Also, if atrial fibrillation recurs when a patient is taking an antiarrhythmic agent, atrial fibrillation may be slower, shorter, or better tolerated. A drug such as sotalol is associated with slower rates in atrial fibrillation. In addition, sotalol is associated with slower rates in sinus rhythm, which may cause symptoms. Quinidine may accelerate the ventricular rate in atrial fibrillation and must be used with an AV nodal blocking drug. Flecainide can cause atrial fibrillation to become a slow flutter with rapid AV conduction.

Antiarrhythmic drugs are selected on a safety-first basis and tailored to the underlying clinical situation. Significant variations in antiarrhythmic agent use have been observed among subspecialties of treating physicians [90]. Failure of one antiarrhythmic drug, even in the same class, does not imply that a similar drug would not work. A patient may fail sotalol but achieve complete control with amiodarone.

A recurrence does not necessarily imply that another drug is needed. Also, antiarrhythmic drugs are often not titrated appropriately. Sotalol, for example, has only beta-blocking properties at low doses. Higher doses are required to achieve a class III effect. A recent multicenter trial of sotalol indicated that the most efficacious dose for most patients is 120 mg twice a day [91]. Regarding amiodarone, patients require a long "load." What appears a failure may be, in reality, lack of effective loading.

The Canadian Trial of Atrial Fibrillation (CTAF) has shown that amiodarone is superior to sotalol and propafenone in maintaining sinus rhythm and with low incidence of side effects [92]. Studies have compared amiodarone with quinidine (79% vs 46% and 33% vs 13% efficacy, respectively) [93], amiodarone with flecainide (60% vs 34% efficacy, respectively) [94], amiodarone with sotalol (71% vs 40% efficacy, respectively) [95,96], and amiodarone with propafenone [97]. In addition, amiodarone has been 87%, 80%, and 57% effective at 1, 2, and 5 years, respectively, in patients refractory to an average of 2.5 antiarrhythmic drugs [98].

A randomized, double-blind, placebo-controlled study (Sotalol-Amiodarone Fibrillation Efficacy Trial [SAFE-T]) [88] is ongoing at 20 Veterans Affairs medical centers to test the superiority of the two most frequently used antiarrhythmic agents, sotalol and amiodarone, against each other and a placebo in patients with persistent atrial fibrillation. The authors expect the results to help guide physicians in choosing drugs(s) to maintain normal sinus rhythm.

Nevertheless, these data do not imply that all patients should be started first on amiodarone. Amiodarone has long-term risks; other drugs should be considered as appropriate before amiodarone is given.

Anticoagulation

Atrial fibrillation is responsible for 15% of all strokes. Patients with rheumatic mitral valve disease have a 17-fold increased risk for stroke compared with the general population [7]. Patients with nonvalvular atrial fibrillation have a 5.6 times greater risk of stoke compared with the general population. In the Framingham Study, the "attributable" risk of stroke from atrial fibrillation varied from 1.5% for those age 50 to 59 years to 9.9% for those age 70 to 79 years and 23.5% for those age 80 to 89 years [6,7,99–101]. Stroke risk in patients with nonvalvular atrial fibrillation is highest for those older than 65 years (annual risk increases from 4.9% for those age < 65 to 8.1% for those age > 75 years) and those with diabetes, hypertension, heart failure, and previous stroke. The annual risk of stroke in an elderly atrial fibrillation patient with one risk factor (excluding hypertension) is 7.9% (0.022% daily risk) without anticoagulation, 3.6% with hypertension, and 1.1% with no risk factors. For those with several risk factors, the annual risk for stroke can approach 20%.

Anticoagulation in patients with atrial fibrillation can reduce stroke risk two- to 18-fold. Five randomized, placebo-controlled trials of high-risk patients with atrial fibrillation have been performed [6,99–101] (Fig. 5). All showed marked benefit of warfarin, except CAFA (Canadian Atrial Fibrillation Anticoagulation Study), which was stopped when other studies showed clear benefit of anticoagulation (it was not ethical to continue). The annual stroke risk for those in the warfarin group was 0.4% to 3.4% compared with 4.3% to 6.2% in the placebo group. The overall reported risk reduction of 67% is likely an underestimate of benefits of anticoagulation because the studies used an intention-to-treat analysis. The risk for bleeding and

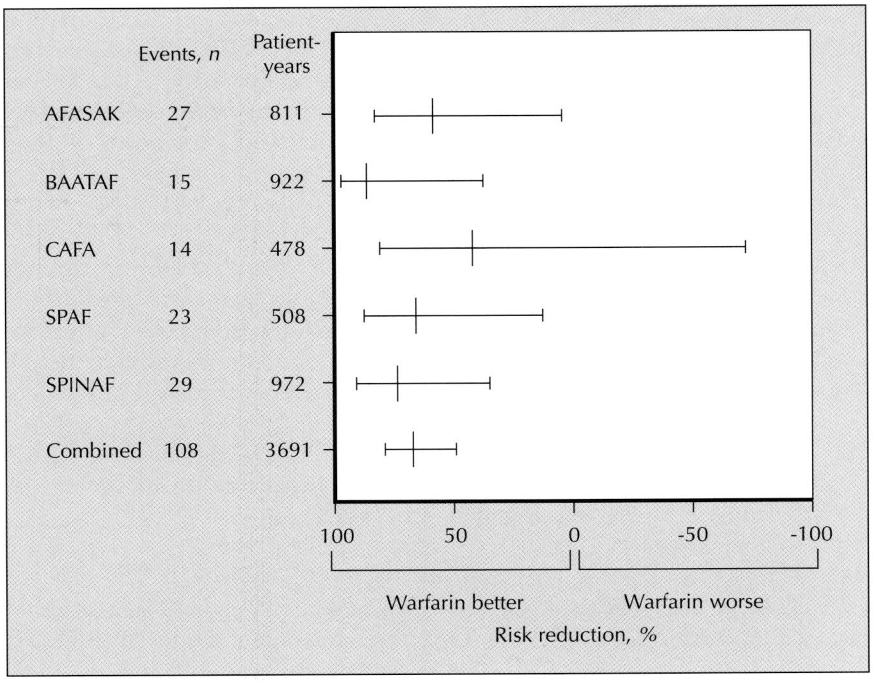

FIGURE 5 Multicenter, randomized use of warfarin to prevent stroke.

stroke was nearly absent for those who actually had an INR of 2.0 to 3.0 (not the selected values for all studies and not present for all patients). Aspirin was associated with small and inconsistent benefit. It is doubtful that aspirin has any role in low-risk or younger patients, and it cannot be recommended with certainty.

A compilation of data from six major multicenter trials shows a 45% relative risk reduction for any stroke, 52% for ischemia stroke, and 29% for cardiovascular events with warfarin given chronically based on an intention-to-treat analysis [102], but the benefits may really be greater than that.

A recently published large retrospective study of 13,559 patients with nonvalvular atrial fibrillation reported that anticoagulation with warfarin with an INR of 2.0 or greater reduces not only the frequency of ischemic stroke but also its severity and the risk of death from stroke when compared with aspirin or warfarin with an INR less than 2.0 [103].

Anticoagulation for atrial fibrillation is now more common because of results of randomized trials that show consistent benefit [52,104]. Still, only 32% to 58% of practicing clinicians are anticoagulating atrial fibrillation patients appropriately [104–108]. The older the atrial fibrillation patient, the greater the risk of a stroke but also the greater the risk of falls and bleeding. The risk-to-benefit ratio of anticoagulation for high-risk patients appears to favor anticoagulation, but patients at highest risk for bleeding were not tested in clinical trials. American College of Chest Physicians (ACCP) guidelines mandate anticoagulation for atrial fibrillation patients older than 75 years and those age 65 to 75 years with risk factors. We also advocate anticoagulation for patients younger than 65 when there are persistent and recurrent episodes of atrial fibrillation requiring cardioversion and when there are risk factors. Anticoagulation must be considered for any patient undergoing cardioversion.

Paroxysmal atrial fibrillation is as risky because persistent or permanent atrial fibrillation and the type of atrial fibrillation should not be a factor to consider in whether a patient should be anticoagulated. If a patient has one episode of atrial fibrillation and it is clear that he or she is not having more episodes (this can be difficult because asymptomatic episodes of atrial fibrillation occur even in symptomatic patients), anticoagulation may not be necessary. There is no evidence, however, that anticoagulation can be stopped in a patient who is taking an antiarrhythmic drug and is having no recurrences of atrial fibrillation. Despite this, many physicians stop anticoagulation in a patient who maintains sinus rhythm for long periods while taking an antiarrhythmic drug.

Anticoagulation can be performed acutely with heparin intravenously and warfarin given orally. The goal is to maintain, with warfarin, an INR of 2.0 to 3.0. A higher INR increases the risk of bleeding but provides no additional benefit, and a lower INR is inadequate. The risk for stroke increases rapidly below an INR of 2.0. There is no proven benefit of ticlopidine or combinations of aspirin with warfarin.

Proper warfarin anticoagulation can be difficult. Changes in diet, medications, and dietary supplements can cause the INR to fluctuate substantially. It is recommended that the INR be determined at least weekly during initiation and monthly after stabilization. Home INR monitoring is now being used for individual patients but is expensive. For a patient undergoing cardioversion, consistent weekly INR values of greater than 2.0 are required for 3 to 4 weeks. Afterward, warfarin should be given for at least 4 weeks and the patient should be heparinized acutely if the patient is not fully anticoagulated.

Warfarin is presently the drug of choice for anticoagulation patients with atrial fibrillation. Due to its inherent pharmacokinetic and pharmacodynamic disadvantages, there are problems using this drug. Several caveats apply: 1) INR values fluctuate. 2) The INR value, even if elevated at the time of initial anticoagulation, may not reflect full anticoagulant. Efficacy is not always assured despite an INR > 2.0. It can take time to achieve therapeutic anticoagulation. 3) Termination of warfarin can induce a prothrombotic state (although this is not completely clear and is disputed) [109]. 4) Proper management requires frequent INR measurements. It can take time to reverse its effect, when necessary.

Anticoagulants for nonvalvular atrial fibrillation cause about 17,000 major hemorrhagic complications in the United States per year, of which about 4000 are fatal [110]. In five randomized trials with follow-up periods of 1.3 to 2.3 years, 10% to 38% of patients permanently discontinued anticoagulants. Perhaps this is one of the reasons that many physicians turn away from the use of warfarin in atrial fibrillation patients, particularly the elderly, who are at highest risk for stroke due to atrial fibrillation. Scrupulous attention to detail may be required for safe warfarin use long term [111]. In contrast to the concept that warfarin is inappropriately underutilized in atrial fibrillation patients, perhaps it is underutilized for good reason [112], and better alternatives are needed. Other means of anticoagulation are often considered for patients at risk of thromboembolism in atrial fibrillation.

Unfractionated heparin

Historically, heparin has been considered a surrogate for warfarin for atrial fibrillation. In fact, anticoagulants are often used in an inconsistent pattern from patient to patient [113]. This appears to be similar worldwide [114]. However, heparin and warfarin have marked differences and the risk/benefit ratio of heparin has not been explored carefully. Despite recent guidelines that advocate its use [3], the efficacy and safety of heparin anticoagulation is not well established for atrial fibrillation.

Fractionated heparin

Interest in the use of low molecular weight heparin is growing [115–117]. A multicenter, randomized trial (ACUTE II) is enrolling 200 patients with atrial fibrillation for more than 48 hours requiring cardioversion. TEE-guided IV unfractionated heparin bridge therapy to warfarin is being compared with TEE-guided subcutaneous enoxaparin bridge therapy to warfarin [117].

While awaiting the results from the ongoing ACUTE II trial [117], findings from several observational clinical series are encouraging. De Luca *et al.* [118] studied the use of enoxaparin in TEE-guided cardioversion of 48 patients with atrial fibrillation lasting more than 48 hours. Enoxaparin was started and cardioversion was performed after a TEE showing no intracardiac thrombi or spontaneous echo contrast. TEE was then repeated 7 days after cardioversion. Enoxaparin was discontinued in 24 patients after a repeated TEE showing no intracardiac thrombi. There was no thromboembolic event during 2-month follow-up [118].

Dalteparin, another low molecular weight heparin, has been tested in 125 patients with TEE-guided cardioversion [119]. The authors suggest that simple, well-tolerated and effective anticoagulation was possible [119]. In another study of 172 patients [120], the feasibility and safety of TEE-guided early cardioversion with short-term dalteparin (2 × 5,000 U) (90 patients) was compared with 82 patients receiving heparin (5000 U bolus and infusion). All received warfarin for 1 month after cardioversion. No patient had a thromboembolic event noted in 4 weeks [120].

While low molecular weight heparin may be as effective as warfarin, more information is needed before it can be recommended without restraint. Two ongoing prospective randomized multicenter trials [117,121] will provide more insights into this issue.

Ximelagatran

An ideal anticoagulant would fulfill these criteria: easy administration (oral or topical), predictable absorption, rapid onset and offset of action, no or rare interaction of other drugs, favorable side effect profile, and no monitoring or frequent dose adjustment required. While warfarin effectively reduces stroke risk in patients with atrial fibrillation, it causes bleeding and is difficult to manage, requiring regular blood monitoring and frequent dose adjustments. Furthermore, warfarin interacts with a host of foods and other medications. As a result, warfarin is underutilized. There have been continuous efforts searching for a replacement [122].

Ximelagatran, the first oral compound from a novel class of anticoagulants, direct thrombin inhibitors, might solve many of these current difficulties [122–125].

Several parenteral direct thrombin inhibitors, *ie*, argatroban, hirudin, and bivalirudin, have been successfully developed and commercially available. However, these agents are less suitable for long-term anticoagulation. Ximelagatran, one of the two oral direct thrombin inhibitors (BIBR 1048, the other) currently in clinical development, is a prodrug that, after absorption, is biotransformed into melagatran, a potent competitive inhibitor of human alphathrombin. Melagatran inhibits both free and clot-bound

thrombin. It effectively reduces thrombin generation and thrombin activity [126,127]. Figure 6 shows the mechanisms of how ximelagatran works on the coagulation cascade in relationship to heparin and warfarin. In addition, melagatran potently inhibits thrombin-induced platelet activation and aggregation [128–130].

The results of the second Oral Thrombin Inhibitor in Atrial Fibrillation (SPORTIF-II) trial suggested an acceptable safety profile of the drug [131]. In this 12-week randomized and double-blind study (ximelagatran vs warfarin) of 254 patients with at least one risk factor for stroke in addition to atrial fibrillation, ximelagatran given in fixed doses up to 60 mg twice daily was well tolerated without the need for coagulation monitoring or dose adjustment. In the ximelagatran-treated group, there were only two thromboembolic events: one patient with hypertension, left ventricular dysfunction, and diabetes and a previous history of transient ischemic attacks experienced a nonfatal ischemic stroke; another patient had a transient ischemic attack. Two transient ischemic attacks occurred in the warfarin group. No major hemorrhages were observed in the ximelagatran group, while one occurred in the warfarin group. Elevated liver enzymes while taking ximelagatran were observed in eight patients, but normalized with continuous treatment in five patients and after cessation of the drug in three patients [131].]

The preliminary results from the SPORTIF-III trial, recently presented at the American College of Cardiology 52nd Annual Scientific Session, are very promising. This open-label trial enrolled 3407 patients with atrial fibrillation in 23 nations. The design has been reported [132]. All patients had nonvalvular atrial fibrillation and some additional risk factor for stroke, such as hypertension, congestive

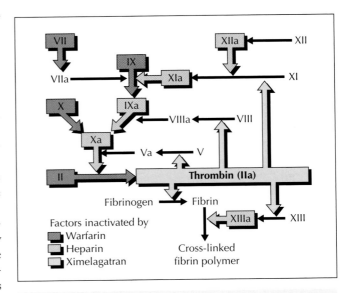

FIGURE 6 The mechanisms of how the direct thrombin inhibitor ximelagatran works on the coagulation cascade in relationship to heparin and warfarin.

heart failure, previous stroke, thromboembolism, or various combinations involving diabetes or coronary artery disease. The trial compares adjusted-dose warfarin regulated by monthly measurements of the prothrombin time (INR: 2–3) against ximelagatran of a fixed oral dose (36 mg twice daily) without coagulation monitoring or dose adjustment. Ximelagatran did prove as effective as well-controlled warfarin in preventing both ischemic and hemorrhagic strokes and systemic embolic events. In addition, ximelagatran caused less bleeding than warfarin.

This trial is complemented by the results from the double-blind North American SPORTIF V trial, the largest-ever clinical trial conducted to date to address the issue. The efficacy of ximelagatran is equivalent to warfarin but it has not been tested for efficacy in light of cardioversion. These data, however, address the long-term use of anticoagulation of atrial fibrillation but do not directly focus on the short-term benefits in those patients who have acute-onset atrial fibrillation or require cardioversion. There is also some concern about liver toxicity. This issue has not been completely resolved at this time.

Nonpharmacologic approaches

Nonpharmacologic approaches are being tested to reduce the risk of thrombus formation in the left atrium. One, percutaneous left atrial appendage occlusion, involves placement of an occlusive device in the left atrial appendage to eliminate it from the circulation [133]. These approaches are not well tested nor are they widely available. While they may reduce the risk of thromboembolism long-term, there is no indication that they would be effective for short-term management of the patient requiring cardioversion. During acute episodes of atrial fibrillation requiring cardioversion, even if these devices are used, anticoagulation should be considered as it is for other patients with similar conditions and episode lengths of atrial fibrillation [133–135].

There is a growing role for TEE. Several studies have shown this approach is safe and cost-effective. The ACUTE trial has demonstrated that this approach is safe as long as the patient is anticoagulated at time of cardioversion, even with a negative TEE [19]. An advantage of this approach is that the time to cardioversion is shortened. The 3- to 4-week wait for adequate anticoagulation before cardioversion can drag on for months. A survey of seven regions in the United States showed that the TEE-guided approach is used in only 12% of cardioversions; 75% of practices indicated they use TEE only occasionally. The highest use of the TEE-guided approach was found at academic institutions and tertiary referral centers. There was little consensus on the most appropriate clinical indications for this approach.

For lone atrial fibrillation in young patients with short and rare episodes, anticoagulant therapy is not recommended. For older patients with frequent episodes, warfarin is probably best. Intermittent or paroxysmal atrial fibrillation should inspire the possibility of using warfarin with an

INR of between 2 to 3 if atrial fibrillation is not controlled. If the rhythm does not stay in sinus rhythm, these patients should be chronically anticoagulated.

Atrial Fibrillation Ablation and Other Curative Approaches

Lack of a favorable outcome from a rhythm control approach compared to a rate control approach [42,48] may be due to adverse effects from and inefficacy of antiarrhythmic drugs as a means to restore and maintain sinus rhythm [26]. The efficacy and certainty of antiarrhythmic drugs to maintain sinus rhythm are also questioned [87].

The search for curative therapies remains vibrant with promising initial results [18,19,26,27,136–138]. The pioneering work by Haissaguerre et al. [19] highlighted the importance of the pulmonary veins as a frequent source of focal triggers for initiation of atrial fibrillation. In their original study of 45 patients with paroxysmal atrial fibrillation, frequent isolated atrial ectopic beats, the sites of origin of these beats initiating atrial fibrillation were localized in the pulmonary veins, with 48% in the left superior, 26% in the right superior, 17% in the left inferior, and 9% in the right inferior pulmonary veins. After radiofrequency ablation of these foci and a mean follow-up of 8 months, atrial fibrillation was completely eliminated in 62% of the patients [19]. Since then, triggers have been reported from many nonpulmonary vein foci, including left atrium (frequently posterior left atrium), right atrium (including crista terminalis), interatrial septum, coronary sinus, superior vena cava (occasionally left-sided), and ligament of Marshall [17,20,139–141].

Different approaches with a variety of ablative techniques (Figs. 7 and 8) have been reported with success rates ranging from 21% to 75% for persistent or permanent atrial fibrillation, and from 60% to 88% for paroxysmal atrial fibrillation [18–20,26,27,136,138,139,142–145]. All of these studies are exclusively single-center studies, and all but two [26,27] are case series. There is no prospective, multicenter, randomized, controlled study available to date.

Catheter ablation for atrial fibrillation has evolved from targeting ectopic foci within the pulmonary veins with an initially relatively high complication rate of pulmonary vein stenosis to various and still-evolving techniques that offer a fairly safe, moderately effective option for patients with atrial fibrillation. However, several issues must be considered before the procedure is recommended. First, the procedure is highly invasive and highly technically challenging. An experienced tertiary center with a reasonable procedure volume is highly recommended. Second, as previously stated, the techniques are relatively new and still evolving. Time is needed for them to mature, and their efficacy needs to be confirmed by prospective multicenter randomized, controlled studies.

Based on these, we currently consider the following patients better candidates for catheter ablation: paroxysmal atrial fibrillation patients who remain symptomatic despite medical therapy and younger patients without severe structural heart disease.

WHEN TO HOSPITALIZE

Patients with atrial fibrillation are generally managed on an outpatient basis. Hospital admission is reserved for those with impaired hemodynamics, especially with intolerable symptoms (*eg*, heart failure, pulmonary edema, hypotension, and syncope); a thromboembolic event; treatment of associated conditions; initiation of urgent anticoagulation; initiation of a class IA or class III antiarrhythmic drug; and urgent cardioversion.

For a nonanticoagulated patient with atrial fibrillation lasting more than 24 hours, urgent cardioversion should be planned. TEE may need to be performed, but anticoagulation should be initiated in any case. Hospitalization may be required to acutely anticoagulate such patients and then to switch them to heparin. Recent interest in use of low molecular weight heparin started as an outpatient, followed by warfarin, may be valid (although it is untested). For a patient with chronic atrial fibrillation, warfarin can be initiated as an outpatient in most instances, although there is a small risk of a prothrombotic state that can occur with warfarin before full anticoagulation is anticipated. This is balanced against the risk of admitting such a patient and starting heparin in the hospital.

The reason to admit a patient for select antiarrhythmic drug initiation is to monitor the patient for a potential life-threatening arrhythmia that may occur because of the drug. Patients with structural heart disease are at highest risk for

drug proarrhythmia and should be considered for admission. Amiodarone can be started on an outpatient basis in "stable" patients.

All antiarrhythmic drugs have potential risk. No data indicate that hospital admission improves safety or efficacy of an antiarrhythmic drug. Many problems with antiarrhythmic drugs occur after discharge. In one meta-analysis of all proarrhythmic occurrences on quinidine, flecainide, and propafenone for hospitalized patients, 50%, 62%, and 100% occurred for quinidine, flecainide, and propafenone, respectively, after discharge [146].

Class IA drugs should be started in a hospitalized setting because of the risk of torsades de pointes and other proarrhythmic risks. However, a patient with vagally mediated atrial fibrillation who has no heart disease could have disopyramide started carefully as an outpatient if he or she is not at high risk for torsades de pointes. When structural heart disease is present, the incidence of proarrhythmia is higher. In one report, 93% of the proarrhythmic events occurred in patients with structural heart disease as opposed to 7% without structural heart disease [147].

In a patient who has paroxysmal atrial fibrillation and no structural heart disease, the class IC antiarrhythmic drugs can be started out of the hospital. Sotalol (a new class III agent), dofetilide, and any other class II agent need to be started and titrated in a hospitalized setting because of the risk of death and torsades de pointes. The FDA now

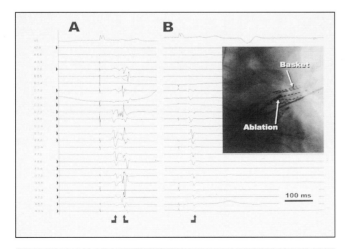

FIGURE 7 Catheter ablation of atrial fibrillation: approach targeting at pulmonary vein (PV) potentials and atriopulmonary vein disconnection. PV potentials are recorded in the left superior PV during distal coronary sinus pacing (**A**) using a basket mapping catheter (Constellation; Boston Scientific, Boston, MA). These PV potentials, but not atrial (A) signals, disappear after segmental radiofrequency applications to the atrial side outside of the PV ostium (**B**). All PVs are targeted and electrically disconnected from the left atrium.

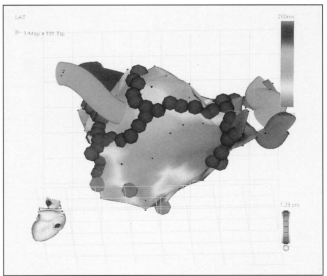

FIGURE 8 Catheter ablation of atrial fibrillation: approach with ablation lesion lines created in the left atrium encircling all pulmonary veins. A three-dimensional representation of left atrium and pulmonary veins (caudal posteroanterior projection) is constructed with an electroanatomic mapping system (CARTO; Biosense-Webster, Diamond Bar, CA). Red tags represent sites at which radiofrequency energy is delivered. Left- and right-sided pulmonary veins are encircled. Also shown are ablation lines in mitral isthmus and posterior left atrium. (*See* Color Plate.)

mandates that sotalol and dofetilide be started in the hospital because of the potential risks. When an antiarrhythmic drug is initiated in the hospital, the patient should remain in the hospital during the loading phase, which is approximately 5 half-lives for the antiarrhythmic drugs. For sotalol, it is 5 doses or 3 days. There may be ways to safely shorten the period of hospitalization.

Any patient with structural heart disease undergoing drug ("chemical conversion") of atrial fibrillation should have this performed in the hospital. The only exception to this is the "pill-in-the-pocket" approach, whereby a class IC antiarrhythmic drug (flecainide, 300 mg, or propafenone, 600 mg) is given as a large oral dose outside the hospital [148]. This approach appears to be safe and effective based on small series in the United States and Italy, but more information is needed. This approach should not be used without additional AV nodal blocking drug use.

MANAGEMENT OF ATRIAL FIBRILLATION
First-detected Atrial Fibrillation

The initial step is to stabilize the patient hemodynamically with rate control or cardioversion (admit if unstable). Achieve rate control with an IV calcium blocker (*eg*, diltiazem) or a beta-blocker (*eg*, esmolol) if the patient is not hypotensive (Fig. 1).

Cardiovert (under anesthesia) if there is an acute infarct (rare), hypotension, pulmonary edema, or unstable angina. If there are severe uncontrollable symptoms, or hemodynamic collapse, urgent cardioversion may need to be considered. If there is a question about the need for cardioversion and there is a high risk of thromboembolism, cardioversion (electrical or chemical) should be avoided until after adequate anticoagulation. An alternate approach is to perform TEE before cardioversion. If TEE does not detect intracardiac thrombi, early cardioversion could be performed in lieu of 4 weeks of anticoagulation. If intracardiac thrombi are detected, cardioversion should be deferred. A follow-up TEE is recommended to ensure resolution of intracardiac thrombi before cardioversion can be anticipated.

Direct-current shock is preferable, but IV ibutilide may chemically cardiovert the patient or facilitate cardioversion. Ibutilide is more effective than procainamide; both can cause torsades de pointes. The patient will need to be observed for at least 4 hours after a dose of ibutilide. Magnesium sulfate given before ibutilide may decrease the risk of torsades de pointes. If atrial fibrillation recurs after immediate DC cardioversion or if the patient has an ineffective shock, ibutilide could be given followed by another shock. Some patients treated with diltiazem also cardiovert, but adenosine is ineffective. Ibutilide and calcium blockers can also prevent an early recurrence of atrial fibrillation after DC cardioversion.

After resolution of a first episode of atrial fibrillation, it is possible that no more therapy would be needed; it is safe to use a beta-blocker or calcium channel blocker.

Undetermined Duration

As mentioned previously, atrial fibrillation is frequently asymptomatic. For many patients, initial and recurrent atrial fibrillation events are silent. In a recent study [149,150], a total of 848 patients with chronic atrial fibrillation were randomized to receive sotalol, quinidine, and verapamil, or placebo after cardioversion. The patients were followed with daily transtelephonic ECG recording. Within 1 year, about two thirds of the patients had recurrence. Of these patients, 70% had at least one asymptomatic event, and the incidence of stroke was the same with or without symptoms. Therefore, it is often difficult, impossible sometimes, to determine how long the patient has been in atrial fibrillation.

If a patient has atrial fibrillation of unknown duration with mild symptoms or an absence of symptoms, hospitalization is unnecessary (Fig. 4). Rate control and anticoagulation are cornerstones to therapy. Elective cardioversion after 3 to 4 weeks of anticoagulation could be considered but, if there are clearly no symptoms and the rate is well controlled, cardioversion is not preferable, especially in the elderly.

Paroxysmal

The duration, frequency, and severity of episodes are assessed. Heart disease is ruled out (Fig. 2). Precipitants (*eg*, changes in autonomic tone, alcohol use, acute illnesses, vagal surges from vomiting, hypokalemia, and hyperthyroidism) should be evaluated. If atrial fibrillation paroxysms recur, long-term therapy or curative catheter ablation should be considered. Anticoagulation is unnecessary for younger patients unless episodes are frequent (more than one to two times per week), prolonged (more than 6 hours), repetitive, or associated with structural heart disease.

Initially, rate control is recommended. Beta-blockade is the best initial approach. If heart disease is present and symptoms are severe, antiarrhythmic therapy should be started in the hospital. Sotalol is recommended for those with structural heart disease who have good ventricular function and is generally started in the hospital. Amiodarone therapy can be initiated on an outpatient basis if the systolic function is impaired. Dofetilide can also be used for those with paroxysmal atrial fibrillation (although it is generally recommended for persistent atrial fibrillation). Sotalol and dofetilide are FDA approved for treating patients with atrial fibrillation.

In patients with "lone" atrial fibrillation (*ie*, no obvious heart disease, no left ventricular hypertrophy), especially in younger patients (age less than 65 years), flecainide and propafenone are effective, safe, FDA-approved choices. Sotalol is a second-line agent because it can cause bradycardia and torsades de pointes (in a dose-dependent manner). The risk of torsades de pointes increases when there is left ventricular hypertrophy. Amiodarone is also effective and may have a low proarrhythmic risk, but it can cause troublesome bradyarrhythmias and other forms of toxicity. It is reserved as the last choice, especially for younger patients. In addition, serious consideration must be given whether it is worth using amiodarone or if ablation should be attempted instead.

For vagally mediated atrial fibrillation, disopyramide or propantheline can be effective. Beta-blockers may be effective if episodes are sympathetically mediated. Paroxysmal atrial fibrillation can progress to more chronic forms of atrial fibrillation.

For patients with recurrent episodes, particularly if drugs are ineffectice or associated with symptoms, pulmonary vein ablation is a reasonable choice.

Persistent or Permanent, Drug Refractory

Assessing hemodynamics, symptoms, and atrial fibrillation tolerance helps formulate a plan (Fig. 3). Repeated attempts at cardioversion may be necessary to alleviate symptoms. Drug therapy must be titrated and used appropriately, and risks and underlying conditions must be considered. Amiodarone appears to be more effective than other drugs for this form of atrial fibrillation [151]. There may be a role for the implanted atrial defibrillators for persistent atrial fibrillation.

Figure 3 also summarizes an approach to managing patients with permanent atrial fibrillation. Anticoagulation is required. If the patient has atrial fibrillation for less than 1 year, an attempt at cardioversion may be warranted. Aggressive attempts at cardioversion (including internal cardioversion and use of devices capable of external biphasic shock) might be useful but futile. If atrial fibrillation is present for more than 1 year, rate control is only recommended for asymptomatic or mildly symptomatic patients. This recommendation may change with newer therapies. Cardioversion for permanent atrial fibrillation is recommended only if the patient is highly symptomatic. Rate control should be documented. If not achieved with drugs, AV nodal ablation with pacemaker implantation is the next step. Pulmonary vein ablation or linear ablation lesion delivery in the left atrium may be effective to maintain sinus rhythm.

Postoperative

Atrial fibrillation after cardiac surgery is common and has a frequency of 5% to 40% [152]. Atrial fibrillation usually occurs 2 to 4 days after cardiac surgery; it can cause symptoms, thromboembolism, heart failure, and prolonged hospital stays, and can increase costs. It rarely causes death. Postoperative atrial fibrillation is frequently self-limited, transient, and paroxysmal. It tends to respond to beta-blockers. Leave this rhythm untreated when the episodes are transient, the patient is asymptomatic, and the hemodynamics are not impaired. Otherwise, management is complex and outside the scope of this review.

THE ARRHYTHMIA CONSULTANT

Patients with atrial fibrillation are often managed by physicians with no specific expertise in managing patients with arrhythmias. Problems arise with 1) the selection and knowledge of the safety and efficacy of antiarrhythmic agents, 2) anticoagulation, 3) cardioversion, 4) proper rate control, and 5) failing to recognize consequences of atrial fibrillation [153]. An arrhythmia consultant should be called if a patient is not responding adequately to the prescribed medication, if atrial fibrillation rates cannot be controlled, if the patient has a stroke, if there are questions about anticoagulation, or if an antiarrhythmic drug is needed. The consultant may be aware of newer, potentially effective therapies. Always consider which patient needs referral for specialized treatment.

NEW DEVELOPMENTS

Treatment options are expanding for atrial fibrillation and are complex. These new treatments have new dangers but also hold promise to markedly improve the quality of life of patients with atrial fibrillation and possibly improve survival [26,154].

Dofetilide and other new antiarrhythmic drugs may be more effective and safer for patients with atrial fibrillation and may serve a role, especially for those with heart failure [155,156]. It is not yet known if these drugs represent simply another drug selection or if there are real additional benefits over other drugs. Drugs are being developed, including azimilide [157], trecetilide [158], dronederone, and others.

There are also promising nonpharmacologic therapies [154,159–161]. Atrial pacing may effectively prevent atrial fibrillation in patients with sinus bradycardia. Dual chamber pacing is associated with a lower risk of recurrent atrial fibrillation and stroke [162,163]. Perhaps one reason for this is that it is known whether the patient has atrial fibrillation and is treated appropriately for this. A patient with a VVI pacemaker may have their atrial fibrillation and the need of anticoagulation ignored. Recent controversial evidence suggests that dual site atrial pacing can be effective. Multicenter trials are under way.

As mentioned previously, techniques for atrial fibrillation catheter ablation are still evolving [164]. While initial results are very promising, particularly for those patients with paroxysmal atrial fibrillation, the efficacy needs to be approved by prospective multicenter randomized, controlled studies. Their long-term effects have not been tested.

A pacing algorithm that detects and overdrive suppresses native rhythm merges (atrial premature beats and atrial tachycardia) has been tested in patients with sinus node dysfunction and atrial fibrillation [165]. After 6-month follow-up, the symptomatic atrial fibrillation burden was decreased by 25%. However, there was no significant difference in quality of life, mean number of atrial fibrillation episodes, total hospitalizations, incidence of complications, adverse events, and deaths between treatment group and control group [165]. Therefore, its clinical significance is not clear.

The implantable atrial defibrillator is another emerging technology [166–170]. The therapy is effective, but a limitation is that shocks at a level needed to cardiovert are extremely painful. This technique may become refined to the point that it will ultimately become useful for select patients.

The role of the varied array of device therapeutic approaches (including "hybrid therapy") is evolving and not presently clear.

A surgical "maze" procedure has been developed. This appears a successful procedure and may be indicated for those refractory patients who require sinus rhythm [171].

CONCLUSIONS

Based on the complexities of management, atrial fibrillation treatment must be individualized. Symptom reduction and prevention of serious consequences, including stroke and heart failure, are the primary goals for the majority of patients. Several valid approaches exist, and treatment algorithms are evolving. For some patients, a cure is now achievable. The management of patients with atrial fibrillation is likely to change dramatically.

REFERENCES AND RECOMMENDED READING

1. Kannel WB, Wolf PA, Benjamin EJ et al.: Prevalence, incidence, prognosis, and predisposing conditions for atrial fibrillation: population-based estimates. Am J Cardiol 1998, 82:2N–9N.

2. Iacovino JR: Mortality of atrial fibrillation in a population selected to be free of major cardiovascular impairments. J Insur Med 1999, 31:8–12.

3. Fuster V, Ryden LE, Asinger RW et al.: ACC/AHA/ESC guidelines for the management of patients with atrial fibrillation: executive summary. A report of the American College of Cardiology/American Heart Association Task Force on Practice Guidelines and the European Society of Cardiology Committee for Practice Guidelines and Policy Conferences (Committee to Develop Guidelines for the Management of Patients With Atrial Fibrillation) developed in collaboration with the North American Society of Pacing and Electrophysiology. Circulation 2001, 104:2118–2150.

4. Snow V, Weiss KB, LeFevre M, et al.: Management of newly detected atrial fibrillation: a clinical practice guideline from the American Academy of Family Physicians and the American College of Physicians. Ann Intern Med 2003, 139:1009–1017.

5. Furberg CD, Psaty BM, Manolio TA, et al.: Prevalence of atrial fibrillation in elderly subjects (the Cardiovascular Health Study). Am J Cardiol 1994, 74:236–241.

6. Wolf PA, Abbott RD, Kannel WB: Atrial fibrillation: a major contributor to stroke in the elderly. The Framingham Study. Arch Intern Med 1987, 147:1561–1564.

7. Wolf PA, Abbot RD, Kannel WB: Atrial fibrillation as an independent risk factor for stroke: the Framingham Study. Stroke 1991, 22:983–988.

8. Ryder KM, Benjamin EJ: Epidemiology and significance of atrial fibrillation. Am J Cardiol 1999, 84:131R–138R.

9. Feinberg WM, Blackshear JL, Laupacis A, et al.: Prevalence, age distribution, and gender of patients with atrial fibrillation. Analysis and implications. Arch Intern Med 1995, 155:469–473.

10. Levy S: Epidemiology and classification of atrial fibrillation. J Cardiovasc Electrophysiol 1998, 9(Suppl):S78–S82.

11. Go AS, Hylek EM, Phillips KA, et al.: Prevalence of diagnosed atrial fibrillation in adults: national implications for rhythm management and stroke prevention: the AnTicoagulation and Risk Factors in Atrial Fibrillation (ATRIA) Study. JAMA 2001, 285:2370–2375.

12. Benjamin EJ, Wolf PA, D'Agostino B, et al.: Impact of atrial fibrillation on the risk of death: the Framingham Heart Study. Circulation 1998, 98:946–952.

13. Levy S, Maarek M, Coumel P, et al.: Characterization of different subsets of atrial fibrillation in general practice in France: the ALFA study. The College of French Cardiologists. Circulation 1999, 99:3028–3035.

14. Lowenstein SR, Gabow PA, Cramer J et al.: The role of alcohol in new-onset atrial fibrillation. Arch Intern Med 1983, 143:1882–1885.

15. Levy S: Factors predisposing to the development of atrial fibrillation. Pacing Clin Electrophysiol 1997, 20:2670–2674.16. Allessie MA: Is atrial fibrillation sometimes a genetic disease? N Engl J Med 1997, 336:950–952.

17. Chen SA, Lee SH, Tai CT, Yu WC: High incidence of focal atrial fibrillation (AF) from the right atrium (RA). J Cardiovasc Electrophysiol 2001, 12:120.

18. Chen SA, Hsieh MH, Tai CT, et al.: Initiation of atrial fibrillation by ectopic beats originating from the pulmonary veins: electrophysiological characteristics, pharmacological responses, and effects of radiofrequency ablation. Circulation 1999, 100:1879–1886.

19. Haissaguerre M, Jais P, Shah DC, et al.: Spontaneous initiation of atrial fibrillation by ectopic beats originating in the pulmonary veins. N Engl J Med 1998, 339:659–666.

20. Lin WS, Tai CT, Hsieh MH, et al.: Catheter ablation of paroxysmal atrial fibrillation initiated by non-pulmonary vein ectopy. Circulation 2003, 107:3176–3183.

21. Moe GK, Abildskov JA: Atrial fibrillation as a self-sustaining arrhythmia independent of focal discharge. Am Heart J 1959, 58:59–70.

22. Jalife JO, Berenfeld J, Mansour M: Mother rotors and fibrillatory conduction: a mechanism of atrial fibrillation. Cardiovasc Res 2002, 54:204–216.

23. Jalife J: Rotors and spiral waves in atrial fibrillation. J Cardiovasc Electrophysiol 2003, 14:776–780.

24. Jalife J, Berenfeld O, Skanes A, Mandapati R: Mechanisms of atrial fibrillation: mother rotors or multiple daughter wavelets, or both? J Cardiovasc Electrophysiol 1998, 9:S2–S12.

25. Gray RA, Pertsov AM, Jalife J: Spatial and temporal organization during cardiac fibrillation. Nature 1998, 392:75–78.

26. Pappone C, Rosanio S, Augello G, et al.: Mortality, morbidity, and quality of life after circumferential pulmonary vein ablation for atrial fibrillation: outcomes from a controlled nonrandomized long-term study. J Am Coll Cardiol 2003, 42:185–197.

27. Oral H, Scharf C, Chugh A, et al.: Catheter ablation for paroxysmal atrial fibrillation: segmental pulmonary vein ostial ablation versus left atrial ablation. Circulation 2003, 108:2355–2360.

28. Wijffels MC, Kirchhof CS, Dorland R, et al.: Atrial fibrillation begets atrial fibrillation. A study in awake chronically instrumented goats. Circulation 1995, 92:1954–1968.

29. Wijffels MC: The natural history of atrial fibrillation: what is the role of atrial remodeling and what can we learn from the atrial defibrillator? *J Cardiovasc Electrophysiol* 1999, 10:1210–1213.

30. Van Gelder IC, Crijns HJ, ValGilst WH, *et al.*: Decrease of right and left atrial sizes after direct-current electrical cardioversion in chronic atrial fibrillation. *Am J Cardiol* 1991, 67:93–95.

31. Adjusted-dose warfarin versus low-intensity, fixed-dose warfarin plus aspirin for high-risk patients with atrial fibrillation: Stroke Prevention in Atrial Fibrillation III randomised clinical trial. *Lancet* 1996, 348:633–638.

32. Secondary prevention in non-rheumatic atrial fibrillation after transient ischaemic attack or minor stroke. EAFT (European Atrial Fibrillation Trial) Study Group. *Lancet* 1993, 342:1255–1262.

33. Hart RG, Pearce LA, McBride R, *et al.*: Factors associated with ischemic stroke during aspirin therapy in atrial fibrillation: analysis of 2012 participants in the SPAF I-III clinical trials. The Stroke Prevention in Atrial Fibrillation (SPAF) Investigators. *Stroke* 1999, 30:1223–1239.

34. Predictors of thromboembolism in atrial fibrillation: I. Clinical features of patients at risk. The Stroke Prevention in Atrial Fibrillation Investigators. *Ann Intern Med* 1992, 116:1–5.

35. Predictors of thromboembolism in atrial fibrillation: II. Echocardiographic features of patients at risk. The Stroke Prevention in Atrial Fibrillation Investigators. *Ann Intern Med* 1992, 116:6–12.

36. Moulton AW, Singer DE, Haas JS: Risk factors for stroke in patients with nonrheumatic atrial fibrillation: a case-control study. *Am J Med* 1991, 91:156–161.

37. Guo HM, *et al.*: Cardioversion of atrial tachyarrhythmias: anticoagulation to reduce thromboembolic complications. *Prog Cardiovasc Dis* 2004, in Press.

38. Boysen G, Nyboe J, Appleyard M, *et al.*: Stroke incidence and risk factors for stroke in Copenhagen, Denmark. *Stroke* 1988, 19:1345–1353.

39. Hart RG, Pearce LA, Rothbart RM, *et al.*: Stroke with intermittent atrial fibrillation: incidence and predictors during aspirin therapy. Stroke Prevention in Atrial Fibrillation Investigators. *J Am Coll Cardiol* 2000, 35:183–187.

40. Goldschlager N, Epstein AE, Naccarelli G, *et al.*: Practical guidelines for clinicians who treat patients with amiodarone. Practice Guidelines Subcommittee, North American Society of Pacing and Electrophysiology. *Arch Intern Med* 2000, 160:1741–1748.

41. Prystowsky EN: Management of atrial fibrillation: therapeutic options and clinical decisions. *Am J Cardiol* 2000, 85(10A):3D–11D.

42. Wyse DG, Waldo AL, DiMarco JP, *et al.*: A comparison of rate control and rhythm control in patients with atrial fibrillation. *N Engl J Med* 2002, 347:1825–1833.

43. Hohnloser SH, Kuck KH: Atrial fibrillation—maintaining sinus rhythm versus ventricular rate control: the PIAF trial. Pharmacological Intervention in Atrial Fibrillation. *J Cardiovasc Electrophysiol* 1998, 9(8 Suppl):S121–126.

44. Saxonhouse SJ, Curtis AB: Risks and benefits of rate control versus maintenance of sinus rhythm. *Am J Cardiol* 2003, 91:27D–32D.

45. Carlsson J, Miketic S, Windeler J, *et al.*: Randomized trial of rate-control versus rhythm-control in persistent atrial fibrillation: the Strategies of Treatment of Atrial Fibrillation (STAF) study. *J Am Coll Cardiol* 2003, 41:1690–1696.

46. Van Gelder IC, Hagens VE, Bosker HA, *et al.*: A comparison of rate control and rhythm control in patients with recurrent persistent atrial fibrillation. *N Engl J Med* 2002, 347:1834–1840.

47. Yamashita T, Ogawa S, Aizawa Y, *et al.*: Investigation of the optimal treatment strategy for atrial fibrillation in Japan. *Circ J* 2003, 67:738–741.

48. Hohnloser SH, Kuck KH, Lilienthal J: Rhythm or rate control in atrial fibrillation—Pharmacological Intervention in Atrial Fibrillation (PIAF): a randomised trial. *Lancet* 2000, 356:1789–1794.

49. Stafford RS, Robson DC, Misra B, *et al.*: Rate control and sinus rhythm maintenance in atrial fibrillation: national trends in medication use, 1980-1996. *Arch Intern Med* 1998, 158:2144–2148.

50. McAlister FA, Ackman ML, Tsuyuki RT, *et al.*: Contemporary utilization of digoxin in patients with atrial fibrillation. Clinical Quality Improvement Network Investigators. *Ann Pharmacother* 1999, 33:289–293.

51. Falk RH: Pharmacologic control of heart rate in atrial fibrillation. *Cardiol Clin* 1996, 14:521–536.

52. Fang MC, Stafford RS, Ruskin JN, Singer DE: National trends in antiarrhythmic and antithrombotic medication use in atrial fibrillation. *Arch Intern Med* 2004, 164:55–60.

53. Ozcan C, Jahangir A, Friedman PA, *et al.*: Long-term survival after ablation of the atrioventricular node and implantation of a permanent pacemaker in patients with atrial fibrillation. *N Engl J Med* 2001, 344:1043–1051.

54. Wood MA, Brown-Mahoney C, Kay GN, Ellenbogen KA: Clinical outcomes after ablation and pacing therapy for atrial fibrillation : a meta-analysis. *Circulation* 2000, 101:1138–1144.

55. Kay GN, Ellenbogen KA, Guidici M, *et al.*: The Ablate and Pace Trial: a prospective study of catheter ablation of the AV conduction system and permanent pacemaker implantation for treatment of atrial fibrillation. APT Investigators. *J Interv Card Electrophysiol* 1998, 2:121–135.

56. Wilkoff BL, Cook JR, Epstein AE, *et al.*: Dual-chamber pacing or ventricular backup pacing in patients with an implantable defibrillator: the Dual Chamber and VVI Implantable Defibrillator (DAVID) Trial. *JAMA* 2002, 288:3115–3123.

57. Phillips BG, Bauman JL: Prescribing trends and pharmacoeconomic considerations in the treatment of arrhythmias. Focus on atrial fibrillation and flutter. *Pharmacoeconomics* 1995, 7:21–33.

58. Lown B, Perlroth MG, Kaidbey S, *et al.*: Cardioversion of atrial fibrillation. *N Engl J Med* 1963, 269:325–331.

59. Resnekov L, McDonald L: Complications in 220 patients with cardiac dysrhythmias treated by phased direct current shock, and indications for electroconversion. *Br Heart J* 1967, 29:926–936.

60. Aberg H, Cullhed I: Direct current countershock complications. *Acta Med Scand* 1968, 183:415–421.

61. Botkin SB, Dhanekula LS, Olshansky B: Outpatient cardioversion of atrial arrhythmias: efficacy, safety, and costs. *Am Heart J* 2003, 145:233–238.

62. Gallagher MM, Hennessey BJ, Edvardsson N, *et al.*: Embolic complications of direct current cardioversion of atrial arrhythmias: association with low intensity of anticoagulation at the time of cardioversion. *J Am Coll Cardiol* 2002, 40:926–933.

63. Duytschaever M, Haerynck F, Tavernier R, Jordaens L: Factors influencing long term persistence of sinus rhythm after a first electrical cardioversion for atrial fibrillation. *Pacing Clin Electrophysiol* 1998, 21:284–287.

64. Verhorst PM, Kamp O, Welling RC, *et al.*: Transesophageal echocardiographic predictors for maintenance of sinus rhythm after electrical cardioversion of atrial fibrillation. *Am J Cardiol* 1997, 79:1355–1359.

65. Page RL, Kerber RE, Russell JK, *et al.*: Biphasic versus monophasic shock waveform for conversion of atrial fibrillation: the results of an international randomized, double-blind multicenter trial. *J Am Coll Cardiol* 2002, 39:1956–1963.

66. Zhang Y, Ramabadren RS, Boddicker KA, *et al.*: Triphasic waveforms are superior to biphasic waveforms for transthoracic defibrillation: experimental studies. *J Am Coll Cardiol* 2003, 42:568–575.

67. Zhang Y, *et al.*: Quadraphasic shocks for transthoracic defibrillation: experimental studies. *Circulation* 2003, 108:IV–319.

68. Kerber RE: Transthoracic cardioversion of atrial fibrillation and flutter: standard techniques and new advances. *Am J Cardiol* 1996, 78:22–26.

69. Levy S: Cardioversion of chronic atrial fibrillation—towards a more aggressive approach. *Eur Heart J* 2000, 21:263.

70. Arnold AZ, Mick MJ, Mazurek RP, *et al.*: Role of prophylactic anticoagulation for direct current cardioversion in patients with atrial fibrillation or atrial flutter. *J Am Coll Cardiol* 1992, 19:851–855.

71. Elhendy A, Gentile F, Khandheria BK, *et al.*: Safety of electrical cardioversion in patients with previous embolic events. *Mayo Clin Proc* 2001, 76:364–368.

72. Elhendy A, Gentile F, Khandheria BK, *et al.*: Thromboembolic complications after electrical cardioversion in patients with atrial flutter. *Am J Med* 2001, 111:433–438.

73. Gentile F, Elhendy A, Khandheria BK, *et al.*: Safety of electrical cardioversion in patients with atrial fibrillation. *Mayo Clin Proc* 2002, 77:897–904.

74. Lanzarotti CJ, Olshansky B: Thromboembolism in chronic atrial flutter: is the risk underestimated? *J Am Coll Cardiol* 1997, 30:1506–1511.

75. Mehta D, Baruch L: Thromboembolism following cardioversion of "common" atrial flutter. Risk factors and limitations of transesophageal echocardiography. *Chest* 1996, 110:1001–1003.

76. Seidl K, Hauer B, Schwick NG, *et al.*: Risk of thromboembolic events in patients with atrial flutter. *Am J Cardiol* 1998, 82:580–583.

77. Kamp O, Verhorst PM, Welling RC, Visser CA: Importance of left atrial appendage flow as a predictor of thromboembolic events in patients with atrial fibrillation. *Eur Heart J* 1999, 20:979–985.

78. Irani WN, Grayburn PA, Afridi I: Prevalence of thrombus, spontaneous echo contrast, and atrial stunning in patients undergoing cardioversion of atrial flutter. A prospective study using transesophageal echocardiography. *Circulation* 1997, 95:962–966.

79. Klein AL, Grimm RA, Murray RD, *et al.*: Use of transesophageal echocardiography to guide cardioversion in patients with atrial fibrillation. *N Engl J Med* 2001, 344:1411–1420.

80. Kamalesh M, Subbiah S, Sharan L, *et al.*: Rapid formation of left atrial appendage thrombus after unsuccessful cardioversion of atrial fibrillation. *Echocardiography* 2001, 18:157–158.

81. Klein AL, Murray RD, Grimm RA: Role of transesophageal echocardiography-guided cardioversion of patients with atrial fibrillation. *J Am Coll Cardiol* 2001, 37:691–704.

82. Stollberger C, Schneider B, Finsterer J: Is percutaneous left atrial appendage transcatheter occlusion an alternative to oral anticoagulation in patients with atrial fibrillation? *Circulation* 2003, 107:e11–e12.

83. Manning WJ, Silverman DI, Douglas PS: Thromboembolism after negative TEE. *Circulation* 1994, 90:3121–3122.

84. Missault L, Jordaens L, Gheeraert P, *et al.*: Embolic stroke after unanticoagulated cardioversion despite prior exclusion of atrial thrombi by transoesophageal echocardiography. *Eur Heart J* 1994, 15:1279–1280.

85. Seidl K, Rameken M, Drgemuller A, *et al.*: Embolic events in patients with atrial fibrillation and effective anticoagulation: value of transesophageal echocardiography to guide direct-current cardioversion. Final results of the Ludwigshafen Observational Cardioversion Study. *J Am Coll Cardiol* 2002, 39:1436–1442.

86. Black IW, Fatkin D, Sagar KB, *et al.*: Exclusion of atrial thrombus by transesophageal echocardiography does not preclude embolism after cardioversion of atrial fibrillation. A multicenter study. *Circulation* 1994, 89:2509–2513.

87. Israel CW, Gronefeld G, Ehrlich JR, *et al.*: Long-term risk of recurrent atrial fibrillation as documented by an implantable monitoring device: implications for optimal patient care. *J Am Coll Cardiol* 2004, 43:47–52.

88. Singh SN, Singh BN, Reda DJ, *et al.*: Comparison of sotalol versus amiodarone in maintaining stability of sinus rhythm in patients with atrial fibrillation (Sotalol-Amiodarone Fibrillation Efficacy Trial [Safe-T]). *Am J Cardiol* 2003, 92:468–472.

89. Maintenance of sinus rhythm in patients with atrial fibrillation: an AFFIRM substudy of the first antiarrhythmic drug. *J Am Coll Cardiol* 2003, 42:20–29.

90. Zimetbaum P, Ho KK, Olshansky B, *et al.*: Variation in the utilization of antiarrhythmic drugs in patients with new-onset atrial fibrillation. *Am J Cardiol* 2003, 91:81–83.

91. Benditt DG, Williams JH, Jin J, *et al.*: Maintenance of sinus rhythm with oral d,l-sotalol therapy in patients with symptomatic atrial fibrillation and/or atrial flutter. d,l-Sotalol Atrial Fibrillation/Flutter Study Group. *Am J Cardiol* 1999, 84:270–277.

92. Roy D, Talajic M, Dorian P, *et al.*: Amiodarone to prevent recurrence of atrial fibrillation. Canadian Trial of Atrial Fibrillation Investigators. *N Engl J Med* 2000, 342:913–920.

93. Vitolo E, Tronci M, Larovere MT, *et al.*: Amiodarone versus quinidine in the prophylaxis of atrial fibrillation. *Acta Cardiol* 1981, 36:431–444.

94. Zarembski DG, Nolan PE Jr, Slack MK, *et al.*: Treatment of resistant atrial fibrillation. A meta-analysis comparing amiodarone and flecainide. *Arch Intern Med* 1995, 155:1885–1891.

95. Kochiadakis GE, Marketou ME, Igoumenidis NE, *et al.*, Amiodarone, sotalol, or propafenone in atrial fibrillation: which is preferred to maintain normal sinus rhythm? *Pacing Clin Electrophysiol* 2000, 23:1883–1887.

96. Kochiadakis GE, Igoumenidis NE, Marketou ME, *et al.*: Low dose amiodarone and sotalol in the treatment of recurrent, symptomatic atrial fibrillation: a comparative, placebo controlled study. *Heart* 2000, 84:251–257.

97. Kochiadakis GE, Igoumenidis NE, Marketou ME, *et al.*: Amiodarone versus propafenone for conversion of chronic atrial fibrillation: results of a randomized, controlled study. *J Am Coll Cardiol* 1999, 33:966–971.

98. Chun SH, Sager PT, Stevenson WG, *et al.*: Long-term efficacy of amiodarone for the maintenance of normal sinus rhythm in patients with refractory atrial fibrillation or flutter. *Am J Cardiol* 1995, 76:47–50.

99. Wolf PA, Singer DE: Preventing stroke in atrial fibrillation. *Am Fam Physician* 1997, 56:2242–2250.

100. Wolf PA, D'Agostino RB, Belanger AG, *et al.*: Secular trends in the prevalence of atrial fibrillation: The Framingham Study. *Am Heart J* 1996, 131:790–795.

101. Wolf PA: Prevention of stroke. *Lancet* 1998, 352(Suppl 3):SIII15–SIII18.

102. van Walraven C, Hart RG, Singer DE, *et al.*: Oral anticoagulants vs aspirin in nonvalvular atrial fibrillation: an individual patient meta-analysis. *JAMA* 2002, 288:2441–2448.

103. Hylek EM, Go AS, Chang Y, *et al.*: Effect of intensity of oral anticoagulation on stroke severity and mortality in atrial fibrillation. *N Engl J Med* 2003, 349:1019–1026.

104. Osseby GV, Benatru I, Sochurkova D, *et al.*: Trends in utilization of antithrombotic therapy in patients with atrial fibrillation before stroke onset in a community-based study, from 1985 through 1997. From scientific evidence to practice. *Prev Med* 2004, 38:121–128.

105. Mendelson G, Aronow WS: Underutilization of warfarin in older persons with chronic nonvalvular atrial fibrillation at high risk for developing stroke. *J Am Geriatr Soc* 1998, 46:1423–1424.

106. Stafford RS, Singer DE: Recent national patterns of warfarin use in atrial fibrillation. *Circulation* 1998, 97:1231–1233.

107. Flaker GC, McGowen DJ, Bocchler M, *et al.*: Underutilization of antithrombotic therapy in elderly rural patients with atrial fibrillation. *Am Heart J* 1999, 137:307–312.

108. Smith NL, Psaty BM, Furberg CD, *et al.*: Temporal trends in the use of anticoagulants among older adults with atrial fibrillation. *Arch Intern Med* 1999, 159:1574–1578.

109. Zeuthen EL, Lassen JF, Husted SE: Is there a hypercoagulable phase during initiation of antithrombotic therapy with oral anticoagulants in patients with atrial fibrillation? *Thromb Res* 2003, 109:241–246.

110. Cundiff DK: Anticoagulants for nonvalvular atrial fibrillation (NVAF)—drug review. *Gen Med* 2003, 5:4.

111. Schulman S: Clinical practice. Care of patients receiving long-term anticoagulant therapy. *N Engl J Med* 2003, 349:675–683.

112. Weisbord SD, Whittle J, Brooks RC: Is warfarin really underused in patients with atrial fibrillation? *J Gen Intern Med* 2001, 16:743–749.

113. Mayet J, Wasan B, Sutton GC: Cardioversion of atrial arrhythmias: audit of anticoagulation management. *J R Coll Physicians Lond* 1997, 31:313–316.

114. Leung CS,. Tam KM: Antithrombotic treatment of atrial fibrillation in a regional hospital in Hong Kong. *Hong Kong Med J* 2003, 9:179–185.

115. Camm AJ: Atrial fibrillation: is there a role for low-molecular-weight heparin? *Clin Cardiol* 2001, 24(3 Suppl):I15–I19.

116. Wodlinger AM, Pieper JA: Low-molecular-weight heparin in transesophageal echocardiography-guided cardioversion of atrial fibrillation. *Pharmacotherapy* 2003, 23:57–63.

117. Murray RD, Shah A, Jasper SE, *et al.*: Transesophageal echocardiography guided enoxaparin antithrombotic strategy for cardioversion of atrial fibrillation: the ACUTE II pilot study. *Am Heart J* 2000, 139:1–7.

118. de Luca I, Sorino M, Del Salvatore B, de Luca L: A new therapeutic strategy for electrical cardioversion of atrial fibrillation. *Ital Heart J* 2001 2:831–840.

119. Bechtold H, Gunzenhauser D, Sawitzki H, *et al.*: Anticoagulation with the low-molecular-weight heparin dalteparin (Fragmin) in atrial fibrillation and TEE-guided cardioversion. *Z Kardiol* 2003, 92:532–539.

120. Yigit Z, Kucukoglu MS, Okcun B, *et al.*: The safety of low-molecular weight heparins for the prevention of thromboembolic events after cardioversion of atrial fibrillation. *Jpn Heart J* 2003, 44:369–377.

121. Stellbrink C, Hanrath P, Nixdorff U, *et al.*: Low molecular weight heparin for prevention of thromboembolic complications in cardioversion—rationale and design of the ACE study (Anticoagulation in Cardioversion using Enoxaparin). *Z Kardiol* 2002, 91:249–254.

122. Sarich TC, Wolzt M, Eriksson UG, *et al.*: Effects of ximelagatran, an oral direct thrombin inhibitor, r-hirudin and enoxaparin on thrombin generation and platelet activation in healthy male subjects. *J Am Coll Cardiol* 2003, 41:557–564.

123. Eriksson UG, Bredberg U, Hoffmann KJ, *et al.*: Absorption, distribution, metabolism, and excretion of ximelagatran, an oral direct thrombin inhibitor, in rats, dogs, and humans. *Drug Metab Dispos* 2003, 31:294–305.

124. Kaplan KL, Francis CW: Direct thrombin inhibitors. *Semin Hematol* 2002, 39:187–196.

125. Hopfner R: Ximelagatran (AstraZeneca). *Curr Opin Investig Drugs* 2002, 3:246–251.

126. Gustafsson D: Oral direct thrombin inhibitors in clinical development. *J Intern Med* 2003, 254:322–334.

127. Gustafsson D, Elg M: The pharmacodynamics and pharmacokinetics of the oral direct thrombin inhibitor ximelagatran and its active metabolite melagatran: a mini-review. *Thromb Res* 2003, 109(Suppl 1):S9–S15.

128. Gustafsson D, Antonsson T, Bylund R, *et al.*: Effects of melagatran, a new low-molecular-weight thrombin inhibitor, on thrombin and fibrinolytic enzymes. *Thromb Haemost* 1998, 79:110–118.

129. Nylander S, Mattsson C: Thrombin-induced platelet activation and its inhibition by anticoagulants with different modes of action. *Blood Coagul Fibrinolysis* 2003, 14:159–167.

130. Mattsson C, Menschik-Lundin A, Nylander S, *et al.*: Effect of different types of thrombin inhibitors on thrombin/thrombomodulin modulated activation of protein C in vitro. *Thromb Res* 2001, 104:475–486.

131. Petersen P, Grind M, Adler J: Ximelagatran versus warfarin for stroke prevention in patients with nonvalvular atrial fibrillation. SPORTIF II: a dose-guiding, tolerability, and safety study. *J Am Coll Cardiol* 2003, 41:1445–1451.

132. Halperin JL: Ximelagatran compared with warfarin for prevention of thromboembolism in patients with nonvalvular atrial fibrillation: Rationale, objectives, and design of a pair of clinical studies and baseline patient characteristics (SPORTIF III and V). *Am Heart J* 2003, 146:431–438.

133. Sievert H, Lesh MD, Trepels T, *et al.*: Percutaneous left atrial appendage transcatheter occlusion to prevent stroke in high-risk patients with atrial fibrillation: early clinical experience. *Circulation* 2002, 105:1887–1889.

134. Crystal E, Lamy A, Connolly SJ, *et al.*: Left Atrial Appendage Occlusion Study (LAAOS): a randomized clinical trial of left atrial appendage occlusion during routine coronary artery bypass graft surgery for long-term stroke prevention. *Am Heart J* 2003, 145:174–178.

135. Nakai T, Lesh MD, Gerstenfeld EP, *et al.*: Percutaneous left atrial appendage occlusion (PLAATO) for preventing cardioembolism: first experience in canine model. *Circulation* 2002, 105:2217–2222.

136. Haissaguerre M, Jais P, Shah DC, *et al.*: Electrophysiological end point for catheter ablation of atrial fibrillation initiated from multiple pulmonary venous foci. *Circulation* 2000, 101:1409–1417.

137. Haissaguerre M, Jais P, Shah DC, *et al.*: Right and left atrial radiofrequency catheter therapy of paroxysmal atrial fibrillation. *J Cardiovasc Electrophysiol* 1996, 7:1132–1144.

138. Pappone C, Oreto G, Lamberti F, *et al.*: Catheter ablation of paroxysmal atrial fibrillation using a 3D mapping system. *Circulation* 1999, 100:1203–1208.

139. Shah D, Haissaguerre M, Jais P, Hocini M: Nonpulmonary vein foci: do they exist? *Pacing Clin Electrophysiol* 2003, 26:1631–1635.

140. Hwang C, Peter CT, Chen PS: Radiofrequency ablation of accessory pathways guided by the location of the ligament of Marshall. *J Cardiovasc Electrophysiol* 2003, 14:616–620.

141. Tsai CF, Tai CT, Hsieh MH, *et al.*: Initiation of atrial fibrillation by ectopic beats originating from the superior vena cava: electrophysiological characteristics and results of radiofrequency ablation. *Circulation* 2000, 102:67–74.

142. Jais P, Haissaguerre M, Shah DC, *et al.*: A focal source of atrial fibrillation treated by discrete radiofrequency ablation. *Circulation* 1997, 95:572–576.

143. Natale A, Pisano E, Shewchik J, *et al.*: First human experience with pulmonary vein isolation using a through-the-balloon circumferential ultrasound ablation system for recurrent atrial fibrillation. *Circulation* 2000, 102:1879–1882.

144. Kanagaratnam L, Tomassoni G, Schweikert R, *et al.*: Empirical pulmonary vein isolation in patients with chronic atrial fibrillation using a three-dimensional nonfluoroscopic mapping system: long-term follow-up. *Pacing Clin Electrophysiol* 2001, 24:1774–1779.

145. Oral H, Knight BP, Ozaydin M, *et al.*: Clinical significance of early recurrences of atrial fibrillation after pulmonary vein isolation. *J Am Coll Cardiol* 2002, 40:100–104.

146. Thibault B, Nattel S: Optimal management with Class I and Class III antiarrhythmic drugs should be done in the outpatient setting: protagonist. *J Cardiovasc Electrophysiol* 1999, 10:472–481.

147. Simons GR, Eisenstein EL, Shaw LJ, *et al.*: Cost effectiveness of inpatient initiation of antiarrhythmic therapy for supraventricular tachycardias. *Am J Cardiol* 1997, 80:1551–1557.

148. Capucci A, Villani GQ, Piepoli MF, Aschieri D: The role of oral 1C antiarrhythmic drugs in terminating atrial fibrillation. *Curr Opin Cardiol* 1999, 14:4–8.

149. Fetsch T, Burschel G, Breithardt G, *et al.*: Medicamentous prevention after electric cardioversion of chronic atrial fibrillation. Goals and design of the PAFAC Study. *Z Kardiol* 1999, 88:195–207.

150. Ferguson JJ III: Meeting highlights: Highlights of the XXIII Congress of the European Society of Cardiology. *Circulation* 2001, 104:111e–116e.

151. Weinfeld MS, Drazner MH, Stevenson WG, Stevenson LW: Early outcome of initiating amiodarone for atrial fibrillation in advanced heart failure. *J Heart Lung Transplant* 2000, 19:638–643.

152. Olshansky B: Management of atrial fibrillation after coronary artery bypass graft. *Am J Cardiol* 1996, 78:27–34.

153. Mead GE, Elder AT, Faulkner S, Flapan AD: Cardioversion for atrial fibrillation: the views of consultant physicians, geriatricians and cardiologists. *Age Ageing* 1999, 28:73–75.

154. Cannom DS: Atrial fibrillation: nonpharmacologic approaches. *Am J Cardiol* 2000, 85:25D–35D.

155. Hohnloser SH, Li YG, Bender B, *et al.*: Pharmacological management of atrial fibrillation: an update. *J Cardiovasc Pharmacol Ther* 2000, 5:11–16.

156. McClellan KJ, Markham A: Dofetilide: a review of its use in atrial fibrillation and atrial flutter. *Drugs* 1999, 58:1043–1059.

157. Karam R, Marcello S, Brooks RR, *et al.*: Azimilide dihydrochloride, a novel antiarrhythmic agent. *Am J Cardiol* 1998, 81:40D–46D.

158. Sager PT: New advances in class III antiarrhythmic drug therapy. *Curr Opin Cardiol* 2000, 15:41–53.

159. Baerman JM, Olshansky B, Wilber DJ: Advances in the nonpharmacologic treatment of atrial fibrillation. *J Invasive Cardiol* 1992, 4:160–166.

160. Keane D, Zou L, Ruskin J: Nonpharmacologic therapies for atrial fibrillation. *Am J Cardiol* 1998, 81:41C–45C.

161. Murgatroyd FD, Leenhardt A: Non-pharmacological treatments for atrial fibrillation. A critical perspective on the status quo. *Arch Mal Coeur Vaiss* 2000, 93:7–16.

162. Saksena S, Delfaut P, Prakash A, *et al.*: Multisite electrode pacing for prevention of atrial fibrillation. *J Cardiovasc Electrophysiol* 1998, 9(8 Suppl):S155–S162.

163. Connolly SJ, Kerr CR, Gent M, *et al.*: Effects of physiologic pacing versus ventricular pacing on the risk of stroke and death due to cardiovascular causes. Canadian Trial of Physiologic Pacing Investigators. *N Engl J Med* 2000, 342:1385–1391.

164. Pappone C, Santinelli V, Manguso F, *et al.*: Pulmonary vein denervation enhances long-term benefit after circumferential ablation for paroxysmal atrial fibrillation. *Circulation* 2004, 109:327–334.

165. Carlson MD, Ip J, Messenger J, *et al.*: A new pacemaker algorithm for the treatment of atrial fibrillation: results of the Atrial Dynamic Overdrive Pacing Trial (ADOPT). *J Am Coll Cardiol* 2003, 42:627–633.

166. Ayers GM: New concepts in atrial defibrillation. *J Interv Card Electrophysiol* 2000, 4(Suppl 1):155–161.

167. Chen L, Keane AT, Every NR: The Food and Drug Administration and atrial defibrillation devices. *Am J Manag Care* 1999, 5:899–909.

168. Griffin JC: Indications for an atrial defibrillator. *J Cardiovasc Electrophysiol* 1998, 9:S187–S192.

169. Jung J, Hahn SJ, Heisel A, *et al.*: Defibrillation efficacy and pain perception of two biphasic waveforms for internal cardioversion of atrial fibrillation [atrial defibrillators]. *J Cardiovasc Electrophysiol* 2003, 14:837–840.

170. Josephson ME: New approaches to the management of atrial fibrillation. The role of the atrial defibrillator. *Circulation* 1998, 98:1594–1596.

171. Cox JL, Ad N, Palazzo T, *et al.*: Current status of the Maze procedure for the treatment of atrial fibrillation. *Semin Thorac Cardiovasc Surg* 2000, 12:15–19.

D

Dallas criteris
  in endomyocardial biopsy, 299t, 299–300
D-dimer
  in pulmonary embolism, 362, 364
DeBakey classification
  of aortic dissection, 390, 390f–391f, 390t
Deep venous thrombosis
  diagnosis of, 359–360, 360t, 401
  prevention and treatment of, 360t, 360–361,
    401, 402f, 403, 409t, 413
Denervation
  of transplanted hearts, 472–473
Depression
  heart failure and, 278
Dermatomyositis, 444–445
Diabetes mellitus
  atherosclerosis risk and, 116
  cardiac effects of, 429–432, 430t–431t
  heart failure and, 278
  hypertension in, 159
  myocardial infarction in, 213
  noninvasive testing in, 40–41
  palpitations in, 79
Diastolic dysfunction
  in congestive cardiomyopathy, 278
  pulmonary hypertension in, 356
Diastolic murmurs
  in infectious endocarditis, 311–314
  in patient evaluation, 8t, 8–9
Dicoumarol, 407, 412
Diet
  behaviors to improve, 142t, 142–143
  cardiac arrest associated with, 96
  fatty acids in, 134, 135t
Differential diagnosis
  cost-benefit ratio in, 10–11
Difficult patients
  referrals and, 14
Digoxin
  in aortic valve disease, 247, 251
  in atrial fibrillation, 485–486
  in cardiomyopathy
    congestive, 275
    restrictive, 284
  in mitral regurgitation, 230
Dilated cardiomyopathy
  infectious, 297, 300–301, 304
Diphtheria
  myocarditis in, 303
Dipyridamole
  in stress testing, 35
    in chest pain evaluation, 53
    in preoperative assessment, 23, 23f
Direct-current cardioversion
  in atrial fibrillation, 486–488
Disability
  in patient evaluation, 1, 2t
Disopyramide
  in hypertrophic cardiomyopathy, 264
  in syncope, 89
Diuretics
  in cardiomyopathy
    congestive, 273, 275
    restrictive, 284, 287
  in edema management, 107–108, 108t
  in hypertension, 160t, 161
    pulmonary, 357
  in mitral stenosis, 228
Dizziness
  cardiac arrest and, 99
Dobutamine
  in cardiogenic shock, 73
  in congestive cardiomyopathy, 275
  in stress testing, 35, 38
    echocardiographic, 23, 24f, 54
Dofetilide
  in atrial fibrillation, 488, 493–495
Dopamine
  in cardiogenic shock, 73
Doppler echocardiography, 36, 37f
  in aortic stenosis, 246f, 246–247, 337
  in heart failure, 62f
  in mitral valve prolapse, 235, 237
  in restrictive cardiomyopathy, 283
  in valvular heart disease, 42
Doxorubicin
  congestive cardiomyopathy from, 268
Draining
  in pericardial effusion, 324

Drug interactions
  with immunosuppressives, 473–474, 475t
  with statins, 146
Drugs. *See also* Pharmacotherapy
  aging and, 458
  cardiac arrest associated with, 95–96, 97f
  fibrous endocarditis induced by, 290
  interactions with antihypertensives of, 157t
  palpitations associated with, 80, 80t
Dual chamber pacemaker implantation
  in hypertrophic cardiomyopathy, 264
Duke Prognostic Treadmill Score, 53, 53t
Duration of chest pain
  in patient evaluation, 47
Dyslipidemia
  after heart transplantation, 476
Dyspnea
  in congestive cardiomyopathy, 267, 268t
  in patient evaluation, 2
  in pulmonary embolism, 361, 361t

E

Ebstein's anomaly, 341–343, 342f
  adult postoperative, 348
  tricuspid valve in, 255–257, 256f
Echinococcosis
  myocarditis in, 305
Echocardiography, 36–38
  after cardiac arrest, 96
  in amyloidosis, 447
  in aortic dissection, 391
  in aortic regurgitation, 250–251, 251f
  in aortic stenosis, 245–247, 246f, 337
  in atrial fibrillation, 484
  of cardiac tumors, 373, 373t, 374f
  cardioembolic stroke risk and, 424
  in cardiomyopathy
    congestive, 271f, 271t, 271–272
    hypertrophic, 262, 263f
    restrictive, 282–283, 287, 298
  in chest pain, 52
  in coarctation of the aorta, 338
  contrast, 36–37
  dobutamine stress
    in chest pain evaluation, 54
    in preoperative assessment, 23, 24f
  Doppler, 36, 37f
  in Ebstein's anomaly, 256, 342
  in heart failure, 60, 62f
  in infectious endocarditis, 309, 314, 314t
  in infectious myocarditis, 297–298, 298f, 302–304
  in mitral regurgitation, 229f, 229–230
  in mitral stenosis, 226–227, 227f
  in mitral valve prolapse, 235, 236f, 237
  M-mode, 36
  in myocardial contusion, 382
  in patent ductus arteriosus, 334–335, 335f
  in pericardial effusion, 323–324
  in pericarditis
    acute, 320–321
    constrictive, 325–327
  in pulmonary hypertension, 354–355
  in pulmonic valve disease, 259–260
  in septal defects, 331, 331f, 333, 333f
  stress, 23, 24f, 38
  in ST-segment elevation myocardial infarction, 206
  in syncope, 88
  transesophageal, 37f, 37t, 37–38
  in tricuspid stenosis and regurgitation, 257–258
  two-dimensional, 36, 37f
  in valvular heart disease
    adult postoperative congenital, 347–348
    assessment of, 42
Edema
  causes of, 104f
  in congestive cardiomyopathy, 269
  defined, 103
  formation of, 103
  in hypothyroidism, 433
  patient evaluation in, 2, 103–110
    generalized, 104–106, 105t–106t
    localized, 104
  treatment of, 106–110, 109t
    diuretics in, 107–108, 108t
    generalized, 106–110, 107t–109t
    indications for, 107
    localized, 104
  types of, 104
    cardiac, 104–105, 105t–106t
    hepatic, 105, 105t–106t

  idiopathic, 106
  renal, 105–106, 106t
Effort
  chest pain during, 48
Ehlers-Danlos syndrome, 440t, 446
Eisenmenger's syndrome, 339f–340f, 339–340
  as surgical contraindication, 334
Ejection fraction
  in congestive cardiomyopathy, 268–269, 273
Ejection murmurs
  systolic
    in patient evaluation, 7–8, 8t
Electrocardiography, 30–33
  in aortic regurgitation, 250
  in aortic stenosis, 244–245, 245f, 336–337, 337f
  in arrhythmias, 31, 31t
  in atrial fibrillation, 95f, 484
  in Brugada syndrome, 94–95, 96f
  in bundle branch block, 31, 32t, 33
  in calcium disorders, 434
  in cardiomyopathy
    congestive, 270f, 270–271
    hypertrophic, 262
    restrictive, 282, 285, 287–288, 290
  in chest pain, 50–51, 51f
    emergency evaluation of, 46
  in chronic ischemic heart disease, 186–187
  in corrected transposition of the great vessels, 343
  in Ebstein's anomaly, 256, 256f, 342
  in exercise stress testing, 33f, 33–34, 52–53, 53t
  in heart failure, 59, 60f
  in infarction, 30f, 30–31
  in infectious myocarditis, 297, 304–305
  in interventricular septal defect, 333
  in ischemia, 30
  in left ventricular hypertrophy, 31, 32t
  in mitral stenosis, 227
  in myocardial contusion, 379, 379f, 381t, 381–382
  overview of, 30
  in palpitations, 78f, 81, 82t
  in pericardial effusion, 323
  in pericarditis, 30f, 31
    acute, 320f–321f, 320–321
    constrictive, 325
  in polymyositis and dermatomyositis, 444–445
  in preoperative assessment, 22–24
  in pulmonary embolism, 361–362, 362t
  in pulmonic valve disease, 258–260, 259f
  in scleroderma, 444
  signal average, 38
  in ST-segment elevation myocardial infarction, 204f, 204–206, 205t
  in syncope, 88
  in thyroid disorders, 433
  in tricuspid stenosis and regurgitation, 257f, 257–258
  in unstable angina pectoris, 197, 197f–198f
  in ventricular fibrillation, 94f
Electrolyte abnormalities
  palpitations in, 79–80
Electron beam computed tomography, 39–40, 40f
  in chronic ischemic heart disease, 187
Electrophysiologic abnormalities
  sudden cardiac death from, 94f–96f, 94–95
Electrophysiologic studies, 38
  in adult postoperative congenital heart disease, 346
  after cardiac arrest, 97
  in congestive cardiomyopathy, 271
  in heart failure, 59
Embolism. *See also* Pulmonary embolism
  anticoagulants in, 409t
  in cardioembolic stroke, 419–425, 420f–423f, 421f, 424t
  in infectious endocarditis, 314, 316
  in mitral valve disease, 226, 229
  in peripheral arterial disease, 400–401
  pulmonary hypertension in, 356–357
Emergency evaluation
  of chest pain, 46
Emergency treatment
  of unstable angina pectoris, 198–199
Enalapril
  in congestive cardiomyopathy, 275
Endocarditis
  drug-induced, 290
  in hypereosinophilic syndrome, 285
  infectious, 309–316, 310f–313f, 310t, 313t–316t.
    See also Infectious endocarditis
  nonbacterial thrombotic
    stroke risk in, 423
  in systemic lupus erythematosus, 442–443

Color Plates

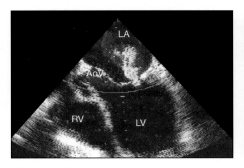

Chapter 4, Figure 6, p. 37

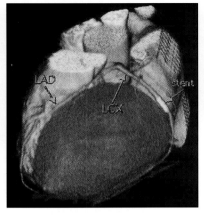

Chapter 4, Figure 8A, p. 39

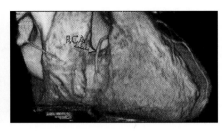

Chapter 4, Figure 8B, p. 39

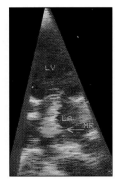

Chapter 6, Figure 3B, p. 62

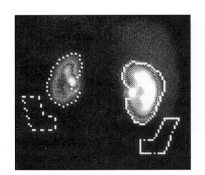

Chapter 16, Figure 5, p. 166

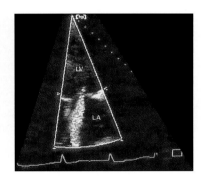

Chapter 21, Figure 3, p. 229

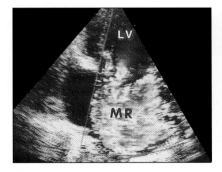

Chapter 22, Figure 11, p. 240

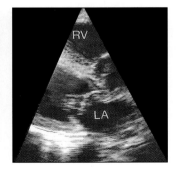

Chapter 23, Figure 8B, p. 251

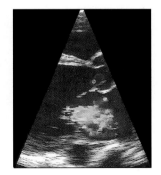

Chapter 26, Figure 5C, p. 271

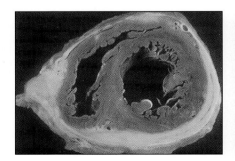

Chapter 30, Figure 4, p. 324

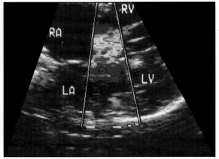

Chapter 31, Figure 2, p. 331

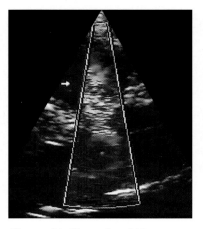

Chapter 31, Figure 3, p. 333

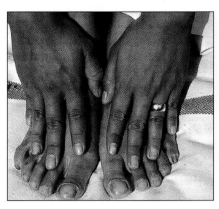

Chapter 31, Figure 4, p. 335

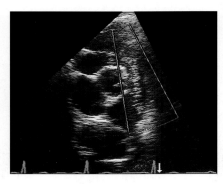

Chapter 31, Figure 5, p. 335

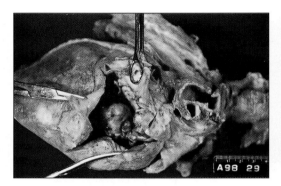

Chapter 35, Figure 2a, p. 372

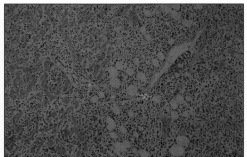

Chapter 35, Figure 2b, p. 372

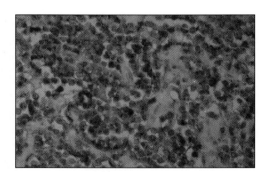

Chapter 35, Figure 2c, p. 372

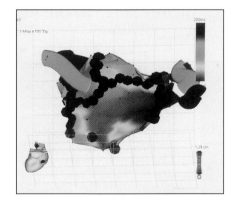

Chapter 46, Figure 8, p. 493